tial Geriatrics

EDITION

HENRY WOODFORD

BSc, FRCP

Consultant Geriatrician

Northumbria Healthcare NHS Foundation Trust

Foreword by

JAMES GEORGE

Consultant Geriatrician, Carlisle

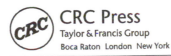

CRC Press

Taylor & Francis Group

Boca Raton London New York

CRC Press is an imprint of the
Taylor & Francis Group, an **informa** business

CRC Press
Taylor & Francis Group
6000 Broken Sound Parkway NW, Suite 300
Boca Raton, FL 33487-2742

Printed on acid-free paper
Version Date: 20150710

International Standard Book Number-13: 978-1-910227-65-7

Visit the Taylor & Francis Web site at
http://www.taylorandfrancis.com

and the CRC Press Web site at
http://www.crcpress.com

Contents

To my wife, Leanne

Foreword to the third edition

Geriatric medicine, with over a thousand consultants, is now the largest medical specialty in the UK. With the ageing population, the development of subspecialties in geriatrics and the increasing acute workload, the specialty is expected to expand rapidly over the next decade. Dr Woodford has highlighted a gap in the market which this book fills. Although there are now numerous large textbooks on geriatric medicine, there is no concise practical evidence-based guide for the beginner in the specialty. Geriatrics is both an 'old' and a 'new' specialty. 'Old' in the sense that it dates from the 1940s when Marjory Warren, in her seminal work, recognised that older people benefit from proper assessment and rehabilitation, and a new specialty was born. 'New' in that much of the evidence is relatively new and comprehensive geriatric assessment, for example, was not confirmed as a beneficial intervention by a meta-analysis until the 1990s. Geriatric medicine has long had a passionate beating 'heart', attracting doctors, nurses and therapists with tremendous enthusiasm to improve the care for older people, but only relatively recently has the specialty developed a definite 'soul' of a sound evidence base to ensure this enthusiasm is targeted to achieve better outcomes for older people. This book eloquently describes the knowledge and evidence base essential for practitioners of geriatric medicine.

Although the book is written primarily for doctors starting in the specialty, it will also be valuable for all members of the multidisciplinary team and also established geriatricians who wish to update themselves. Hopefully, it will encourage research into the many areas in which our evidence base is still uncertain. There are four parts covering the 'geriatric giants' (falls, confusion, immobility and incontinence) and three parts on therapeutics, cardiovascular topics and end of life issues. Each part can be read in under an hour, but also can be dipped into when particular queries arise, for example during and after ward rounds. The evidence base for treatment and intervention in older people is clearly described, evaluated and referenced. Older people are particularly vulnerable in two ways. First, they may sometimes be denied treatment that is clearly of benefit to them simply because of their age. Second, and no less importantly, they may sometimes be offered treatment simply because it is feasible rather than being necessarily beneficial, especially as older people are likely to have multiple symptoms and diseases. Fortunately, older patients are often wiser than their doctors and when given the alternative options for their individual situation will make the right decision for themselves. The book gives geriatricians the information to inform and to share difficult decisions with our older patients.

Dr Woodford is to be congratulated for his practical approach and critical review of the literature. Enthusiasm and passion for the specialty are important but no longer enough as we enter a new era for geriatrics. Hopefully, this book will inspire the new generation of geriatricians to improve their clinical care of older patients and improve clinical outcomes.

It is a tribute to the popularity of this book, and to the growing interest in geriatrics as a specialty, that it is now into its third edition in only eight years. Since the first edition, the number of doctors, nurses and therapists training in the specialty has increased. The 'Future Hospital' 2013 report from the Royal College of Physicians has given the specialty a welcome boost by emphasising its contribution to high quality of care for older people and by espousing the value of generalist physicians for older people. Furthermore, the specialty has broadened its scope by becoming more involved in older patients pre- and post-surgery and also very acutely at the very front door of the hospital. This new third edition recognises these recent developments with extra sections on pre- and post-surgery, and also by increasing the number of self-assessment questions for trainees. There has never been a better time for the specialty and to learn from this book.

Essential Geriatrics neatly fills the gap between the expensive multi-author texts and the very basic handbooks on geriatrics. Unlike many textbooks, it has been kept up to date with rapidly developing modern day practice. It is essential reading for doctors, students and other healthcare professionals already working in the specialty or embarking on a career or training programme in caring for older people. I look forward to multiple further editions as our evidence base expands. Read, learn and enjoy.

James George
Consultant Geriatrician, Carlisle
March 2015

About the author

Henry Woodford was born in York and went to school in Yorkshire. He then went to medical school at King's College London. During this time he undertook an intercalated degree incorporating physiology. His elective period was spent in British Columbia, Canada. He did his house jobs in the south-east of England but then moved to the north-east for further training. He did his specialist registrar rotation based around Newcastle upon Tyne. One year was taken out of the programme to work at Westmead Hospital in Sydney, Australia. He worked as a consultant geriatrician in Carlisle from 2006 until 2012, when he moved to take up a post in North Tyneside, UK. He is married and has two daughters.

List of figures

Introduction

The population is getting older and those who specialise in the treatment of older people will be needed more than ever. Coupled to rising demand, the specialty is becoming more evidence-based with increasing research into the care of this important section of the community.

Is it still appropriate to use the word 'geriatrics'? It is not infrequent for people aged in their eighties to object to attending the 'geriatric' clinic or being cared for on the 'geriatric' ward. This has led to the suggestion that terms such as 'health and ageing' should be used instead. The word 'geriatric' is derived from the Greek words 'geron' (which means 'old man') and 'iatros' (which means 'healer'). The problem does not seem to lie in the word that simply describes what we do (unless objection is taken to the possible sexism of 'old man' rather than 'old person'). The problem is with the public perception of the term due to social stigma attached to advanced age. While those caring for older people could spend their time debating what we call ourselves, we would probably be best utilised in challenging the stigma that surrounds old age. Incidentally, the words 'senile' and 'senescence' are derived from the Latin word 'senex', which also means 'old man'. While 'senescence' appears to be an acceptable term in modern use, the term 'senile' carries particular stigma of decrepitude, and is usually avoided.

When I first became a specialist registrar in geriatric medicine I looked for a suitable textbook to introduce me to the finer points of the specialty. Those available seemed to be either extremely long or short, but above all not meeting the criteria of being both evidence-based and practical. As I progressed through my training I found that I was searching through textbooks, journal articles and web resources to cover the key subjects. I came to the conclusion that I may be able to prevent other people doing the same – this idea forms the basis for this book.

The text specifically focuses on key aspects of elderly care, aiming to be a bridge between general medicine and the particular problems that are encountered in geriatrics (targeted at the 'geriatric giants'[1]). It is envisaged that it will help the reader have a stepping-stone into this peculiar specialty. The subjects covered are chosen because they are not, traditionally, covered well in medical texts or have different characteristics in older people. At the end of each part there is often an attempt to convert the available evidence into a practical guide for the management of the covered conditions. Trying to practice evidence-based, elderly medicine can be a frustrating thing as there are so many gaps in our knowledge. Some of the guidance in this book reflects this – it tries to represent a reasonable approach but not everyone will agree. For clarity it is necessary to divide the text into differing topics, but the reader is reminded that elderly patients often present with multiple problems.

This third edition has not only been updated, but has also been extended in its coverage. In particular, there is a new chapter on perioperative care to reflect the growing involvement of geriatricians in this field. In addition there are now 200 questions throughout the text, divided into groups at the end of the relevant part of the book. These are in the 'best of five' format that is popular in modern knowledge-based assessments. The reader simply selects the one of the five possibilities that is most correct. Answers are provided in Appendix C.

The geriatrician should never forget that our aim is not simply to prolong life or extend the dying process. We are charged with reducing illness and suffering in older people. It appears to be possible that we may achieve the apparent paradox of increased lifespan with reduced lifetime morbidity.[2] We should consider this as one of humanity's greatest successes.

REFERENCES

1 Isaacs B. *The Challenge of Geriatric Medicine*. Oxford, Oxford University Press; 1992.
2 Tallis R. *Hippocratic Oaths: medicine and its discontents*. London: Atlantic Books; 2004.

PART A

Medicine and old age

CHAPTER 1

Age-related changes

Ageing is the accumulation of cellular damage over time that leads to a generalised decline in function and an increased probability of death. It is a complex multifactorial process, which happens to all of us, although there is much inter-individual variation in the manner and timing of its presentation (seen as differences in 'biological' and 'chronological' age). So, don't judge an age by its number. Gerontology is the study of the ageing process. It is sometimes further divided into 'biogerontology' (the cellular changes) and 'social gerontology' (the impact on demographics and society).

BIOGERONTOLOGY

Cellular damage may be as a result of both internal and external factors. External factors include solar radiation and damage secondary to smoking. Internal factors include the formation of harmful molecules during oxidative respiration. Many of the cellular changes are thought to be due to this oxidative damage. Free radicals contain an unpaired electron in their outer shell (also termed 'reactive oxygen species'), which makes them likely to interact with other molecules and cause harm. They are typically formed during mitochondrial electron transport process in the mitochondria. One example is superoxide (O_2^-), which can be converted to hydrogen peroxide (H_2O_2) by superoxide dismutase. Hydrogen peroxide is metabolised by the enzyme catalase. This may lead to the production of hydroxyl radicals (OH•) that may also cause intracellular damage, but can be neutralised by the naturally occurring compound glutathione.

Proteins may be affected by oxidation and glycation (binding of carbohydrates). This may lead to reduced enzyme activity and the accumulation of protein aggregates (including amyloid plaques). Lipid peroxidation is a process harmful to bodily membranes. Nucleic acids can also be damaged. This may be particularly likely to occur with mitochondrial DNA due to its proximity to the free radical production and the limited repair capacity of the DNA here. Damage to mitochondria can reduce energy availability within the cell. Natural repair mechanisms exist and greatly limit the damage done, but they are imperfect and are highly energy-dependent. Thus mitochondrial damage may reduce energy availability for cellular repair, further promoting the ageing process.

THEORIES OF AGEING

Many theories of ageing have been proposed. The following text outlines some of the more popular in recent years. The biologist Leonard Hayflick discovered in the 1960s that cells in culture can only divide about 50 times before they stop. This became known as the 'Hayflick Limit'. It was proposed that this might play a role in the ageing process. However, there is little evidence of non-dividing cells accumulating in older adults and it does not explain ageing of cells that don't divide in adult life – i.e. neurons. Telomeres are non-functional areas that protect the end of each chromosome. Telomerase is an enzyme needed to replicate these areas, but many cells do not express it. This leads to progressive shortening of the telomeres with cell divisions. Very short telomeres can trigger a mechanism that leads to cell death. Short telomeres have been associated with a higher risk of cognitive impairment, vascular disease and death, but also with risk factors for these conditions (i.e. smoking, obesity and physical inactivity).[1] This suggests that shorter telomeres are simply a marker of increased cell turnover. It has been suggested that telomeres may play a role in ageing. Again, it would not explain the senescence of non-dividing cells, and short-lived animals (e.g. rodents) have longer telomeres than humans.

Calorie restriction of around 30–40% of normal dietary intake in laboratory conditions has been shown to result in around a 30–40% increase in rodent lifespan. It has been speculated that this could be due to less free radical formation, but to date there is no evidence of the same effect in humans. Undoubtedly obesity will reduce the lifespan of many people over the coming decades. However, the increase in human longevity seen in the last century has been attributed in part to better nutritional intake. It seems ironic to talk of calorie restriction in the developed world to extend life when starvation continues to kill many in the developing world.

There has been much debate about the existence of genes that control ageing. In the wild, animals die of starvation, predation, hypothermia or accidents prior to growing old enough to show the signs of ageing. For this reason it is not a physical trait that is naturally expressed, and so is not subject to natural selection and could not have evolved. Some have questioned whether a gene that later results in ageing could evolve due to providing an early life advantage. This is termed 'antagonistic pleiotropy'. Examples could include a gene that promotes calcification of bone in youth but leads to increased calcification of arteries in older age, or a gene that suppresses cancerous cell division also inhibiting cellular repair mechanisms. But, all vertebrates are observed to age similarly, making the existence of a genetic variation unlikely. However, monozygotic twins do have more similar lifespans than other people, suggesting at least some role of genes in longevity. Overall they are thought to account for only around 25% of variance between individuals, probably due to a complex accumulative effect of interaction of several genes rather than a single allele.

However, several single gene defects in mice have been described that do prolong lifespan between 20 and 40%. These appear to be related to genes that are either important for the production of growth hormone, insulin-like growth factor, or the receptors important to their cellular actions. This finding is at odds with the observed fall in these hormones associated with normal ageing. Indeed, this fall in growth factors has been proposed to lead to frailty, and research has been directed towards replacement of such hormones to delay or reverse ageing.[2,3] Whether such rodent research will lead to significant therapeutic discoveries in humans is yet to be seen.

The decline in many hormonal levels in the body with advanced age has been identified as a potential therapeutic target. However, results of interventions have been non-beneficial. The supplementation of dehydroepiandrosterone (DHEA) in older women and DHEA or testosterone in older men over a two-year period did not result in any significant physiological benefits.[4] Nor did the use of megestrol,[5] or oestrogen replacement in women (*see* p. 273). Growth hormone supplementation has also not been found to be useful.[3] Ageing is likely to be a much more complex process than could be reversed by such simple interventions.

The 'disposable soma' theory of ageing suggests that it is due to a balance between energy spent on reproduction and cellular repair.[6] Both are heavily energy dependent processes. As animals rarely grow old in the wild it is seldom a disadvantage to age. The cellular repair mechanisms of somatic (non-reproductive) tissues are not perfect. It appears that our ancestors had a survival advantage for the population from investing more resources into reproduction and less into cellular repair. The germ (reproductive) cell DNA is better maintained and is able to be preserved unaltered across generations.

EPIDEMIOLOGY OF AGEING

The average age of the world's population is rising. According the World Health Organization (WHO) there were 600 million people worldwide aged 60 and above in the year 2000, and this will increase to 1.2 billion by 2025, and 2 billion by 2050.[7] The over-eighties are proportionally the fastest growing age group. In the UK 16% of population was aged 65 or over in 2006 and this is predicted to rise to between 20 and 25% by 2030. In the US this proportion is estimated to rise from 13% in 1995 to 20% in 2030. Figure 1.1 shows these estimated changes over time.[8]

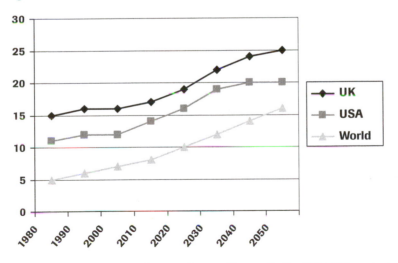

FIGURE 1.1 Percentage of population aged over 65 years in the UK, USA and whole world over time, with future estimates.

We are also seeing declining mortality rates in older adults, which is leading to rising average life expectancies. In developed countries life expectancy has risen in women from around 45 years in 1840 to around 80 years in 2000, and from 42 years to 76 years for men over the same period. This increase has been almost linear at a rate of approximately 0.25 years per year, and still shows no sign of slowing down. In 2015 the approximate life expectancy at birth for females in the UK was 84 years and for males 80 years. Figure 1.2 shows the changes in life expectancy over time for people at differing ages in developed countries. The gap between life expectancy in the developed and less developed world is narrowing. Global life expectancy at birth has risen from 48 years in 1955 to 65 years in 1995, 70 years in 2012 and is estimated to reach 73 years in 2025. The causes of this increase are thought mainly related to improved nutrition, sanitation and healthcare.

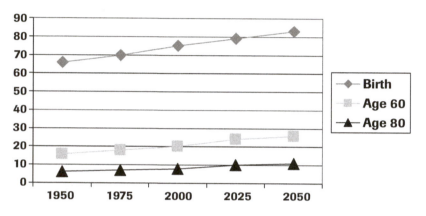

FIGURE 1.2 The changes over time in life expectancy (years) in developed countries at birth, age 60 and age 80 (male and female combined average).

In the UK the population aged over 100 years has risen fivefold in the 30 years from 1980 to 2010, going from 2500 to 12 640 (or around 0.2% of the population, with 84% being female).[9] Jeanne Louise Calment is the longest known survived person to date, having reached an age of 122 years and 164 days at her death in 1997.

FRAILTY

Homeostasis refers to the collection of physiological processes that attempt to maintain a constant bodily environment in response to external stressors. It includes maintaining a constant body temperature, pH level, blood pressure, and intracellular ion concentrations. These are heavily energy-dependent processes. As we age our body becomes less good at maintaining the consistency. More minor external stressors can cause imbalance. This narrowing of the physiological reserve plays a role in disease susceptibility for older adults. This is the essence of frailty, and caring for the frail is the essence of geriatric medicine.

For example, as we age the maintenance of body temperature becomes impaired. A reduced ability to vasoconstrict or dilate peripheral vessels can lead to hypo- or hyperthermia respectively. There is a reduced pituitary secretion of and renal response to vasopressin, leading to a reduced urine concentrating ability. This may increase 24-hour urine volumes. Thirst sensation is typically reduced in response to increased serum osmolality. These changes make dehydration more likely to occur. This may be made worse by increased fluid loss (e.g. diuretics, laxatives, and febrile illness) and reduced fluid intake (e.g. cognitive impairment, swallowing problems, access to fluids and fear of incontinence).

Frailty itself is not a disease and does not necessarily result in disability. In general the frail are more vulnerable to illness and recover more slowly. It is associated with a greater probability of death.[10] Its prevalence increases with advancing age. Sarcopenia (age-related muscle loss) is an important underlying physiological process (*see* later). In addition, end organs appear to become less responsive to stimuli, and feedback mechanisms become blunted. Disease itself may further enhance frailty. For example, illness may lead to reduced levels of physical activity, which may increase muscle loss (*see* Figure 1.3).

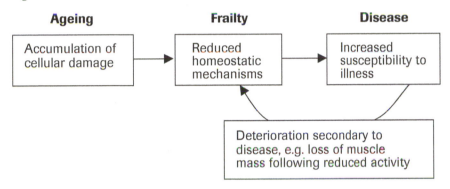

FIGURE 1.3 A simple scheme to show the relationship between ageing, frailty and disease.

Unfortunately an accurate definition of frailty is lacking.[11] Usually it is considered to cause a combination of problems with mobility (often defined by walking speed), strength (e.g. grip strength measured on a dynamometer), fatigue (often subjective), weight loss and reduced activity (together termed the 'frailty phenotype').[12] It may also be composed of cognitive elements and possibly even changes in social support structures. Although not all of these components need to be present, it is typically a multisystem impairment. Some argue that it is a condition of wasting and therefore weight loss, but it seems unlikely that obese people with muscle wasting due to inactivity ('sarcopenic obesity') are immune from being frail. One assessment method is to simply measure gait speed with velocities below 1 metre per second suggestive of frailty.[13] Some authors have proposed a 'frailty index' based on the number of physical impairments an individual possesses.[14] In reality there is much variation between individuals in the way that it manifests and this is probably why a practical definition is so elusive. Given the lack of a standardised definition, prevalence is difficult to calculate. It is estimated to affect 25–50% of people aged over 85 years.[15]

THE PRESENTATION OF ILLNESS IN THE OLD

Immobility, instability, incontinence and intellectual impairment have been termed the 'geriatric giants'.[16] These are not diagnoses but ways that illness tends to present in the frail. A minor nudge from pathology causes failure of homeostatic mechanisms. Walking, continence and cognition are complex actions that take years to learn in our youth. These complex actions are particularly likely to become impaired. Problems with performing activities of daily living (ADLs) may wrongly be labelled as 'social admissions' (sometimes referred to as 'acopia'). This form of presentation still requires a diagnosis to be made. Those with confusion may simply be labelled as a 'poor historian' (given the historian is the person who records history this statement may actually be quite accurate). If the patient is unable to give the history, the physician needs to find someone who can (e.g. a relative, carer, general practitioner or member of care home staff). The use of poorly descriptive terms such as 'collapse query cause' is unhelpful and cannot be justified.

'Atypical' presentations (in that they differ from 'typical' descriptions in medical textbooks) of disease are common in the elderly.[17,18] Where a urinary tract infection is likely to cause dysuria in a younger adult, it may present in a non-specific way in an older adult. Cognitive impairment (acute or chronic) may result in reduced or inaccurate symptom reporting. The classical febrile response to infection may be diminished.

Many hospital services are designed for people with just one problem. Medicine is tending to move away from generalists and towards increasingly organ-specific specialisation. For these reasons health services are often poorly suited to the elderly with complex needs.[19] This is not the patient's fault. Given the large, and rising, number of older patients being admitted to hospital services, it is the systems, and not the patients, that need to change. Attitudes of some medical staff are also inappropriate; most doctors can expect to be looking after an increasing proportion of frail patients as the population ages.[20] Older people are more likely to attend emergency departments than younger people and are more likely to be subsequently admitted.[21] A common solution is for healthcare systems to look to move complex frail patients out of the acute hospital sector – often to community-based settings. Yet there is little evidence that this is effective.

Some of the problems may be driven by financial reasons – there is often little reimbursement for non-procedural activities like rehabilitation and little private practice to be had in geriatrics. This is not a morally defensible basis from which to provide suboptimal care, and would not be tolerated if the discrimination were due to sex, race or religion rather than age. Other problems may arise from ignorance – geriatric medicine has been, at best, sporadically taught in medical schools.[22] For all of these reasons the geriatrician's task can be complex, but equally very rewarding when done well.

COMPREHENSIVE GERIATRIC ASSESSMENT

Comprehensive geriatric assessment (CGA) is a term for a systematic and thorough evaluation of an older adult's problems. It aims to assess medical (comorbidities), psychological (especially cognition and mood disorders), social (e.g. support systems and home environment) and functional (gait, balance and activities of daily living) issues. A multidisciplinary team is usually required to undertake it. This would typically include a geriatrician, a specialist nurse, a physiotherapist, an occupational therapist and a social worker (although other team members are frequently required). From this process a complete list of problems and appropriate management plan can be formulated. As older adults tend to present with multiple problems, assessments of multiple systems are necessary.

A meta-analysis of studies comparing CGA to standard assessment has shown it to be effective at promoting independent survival (3 more patients per 100 alive and in their own home, 95% confidence interval (CI) 1–6) especially when performed within a specialised ward environment.[23] A more recent analysis found that specialist geriatric units offering multidisciplinary assessment were associated with a lower risk of functional decline at discharge (combined odds ratio 0.82, 95% CI 0.68–0.99), a higher rate of discharge back to the patient's own home (1.30, 95% CI 1.11–1.52) without significant difference in mortality rates.[24]

ELDER ABUSE

Older people may be subjected to neglect and physical, financial, psychological or sexual abuse. The abuse can be deliberate or accidental (e.g. due to lack of knowledge) and may be a sign of carer stress. It can be hard to detect, as no clear definition or pathognomonic sign exists. It is estimated to affect around 6% of older people in the community, which equates to around a quarter of vulnerable adults.[25] Much of this, perhaps 84%,[26] usually goes unnoticed. A study in Spain found suspected abuse in 29% of people over the age of 75 (mean age 82 years) who lived in their own home.[27] A study in older adults (mean age 79 years) admitted to hospital in Israel found that 6% of people disclosed experiencing abuse, 21% had signs of abuse, and 33% were judged to be at high risk of abuse.[28]

Victims are more likely to be socially isolated and cognitively impaired. A report from the UK found that psychological abuse was commonest (34%), followed by financial (20%), physical (19%), neglect (12%), and sexual (3%).[29] Many suffered more than one type of abuse. Abusers are most commonly family members (46%), but may be paid carers (34%). Male family members are more likely to be the perpetrators, and women more likely to be the victims. Most abuse occurs within the person's own home (64%), with care homes (23%) and hospitals (5%) being the next most frequent settings. Carer depression or alcohol abuse increase the risk.[30–32]

Clues to diagnosis may include: delays to seeking medical help, multiple admissions, inconsistent stories, emotional withdrawal, medication overuse or underuse, multiple injuries (of varying age), malnutrition, pressure ulcers, occult fractures or poor hygiene. The potential victim should be assessed in the absence of their suspected abuser. Non-threatening questions such as 'do you feel safe where you live?' should be asked first.[33] When suspected, documentation of injuries, appropriate medical attention, and gathering of collateral information are the first steps. The patient and carer(s) should be separately asked about the origin of any injuries, with any inconsistencies noted. A vulnerable adult meeting coordinated by social services may be appropriate. The police may need to be involved if a crime has been committed.

PHYSIOLOGICAL CHANGES CAUSED BY AGEING
Nutritional status

The average proportion of weight composed of body fat increases from 18% to 36% in men and from 33% to 44% in women between the ages 18 to 85.[34] Fat also becomes more centrally distributed with a resulting increase in waist circumference. There is a reduction in fat-free mass, mainly due to sarcopenia. Muscle mass reduces by approximately 10% from age 50 to age 70 in men and women. This is probably multifactorial in nature. Older adults tend to be less active (leading to disuse atrophy), there is a reduction in some hormones (e.g. growth hormone and testosterone), and there may also be some neuronal degeneration and impairment of protein synthesis. For this reason weight may remain stable despite an increase in body fat. Total body water reduces in both sexes, in men aged 67 to 89 years the fall is around 14% compared to the amount in those aged 18 to 33.[35] Most of this reduction is in intracellular fluid. Peak bone mass occurs in the third decade, with a progressive reduction thereafter (*see* Chapter 16). Weight generally increases after age 30 up to age 60, secondary to increased body fat, and declines afterwards.

Basal metabolic rate (BMR) is reduced due to the reduction in muscle mass. Total energy needs are further reduced due to a decline in activity levels (partly due to chronic disease such as osteoarthritis). Overall energy requirements reduce by approximately 30% from age 30 to age 90. Therefore less food is required to meet energy needs. However, protein and micronutrient requirements remain almost constant, which means a diet high in protein and micronutrients is required to maintain health. Recommended daily requirements for water are around 30 mL/kg/day, and fibre intake of around 30 g/day. Both are necessary to prevent constipation (*see* p. 290). Vitamin deficiencies are associated with disease in older adults (*see* pp. 101, 331, 355 and 407). A, D, E and K are fat soluble.

Unintentional weight loss of 5% or more over a one-year period is associated with an increased risk of death.[36] An accurate prevalence for malnutrition is hard to calculate due to variations in definition, but it is estimated to affect 5 to 10% of elderly adults in the community.[37] It also affects 13–40% of patients acutely admitted to hospital, but goes unrecognised in around 75% of these cases.[38,39] Malnutrition risk is increased in older people by social isolation, poverty, chronic disease (cachexia – inflammation, catabolic state, altered protein metabolism), depression, reduced cognition, poor mobility, poor swallow, and reduced senses (smell, taste). Disease itself may lead to reduced appetite, self-feeding, and swallow ability. Drugs can also cause reduced appetite, nausea, and a dry mouth (*see* Figure 1.4). But up to 25% of cases have no identifiable cause despite extensive investigation.[36] Weight loss during a hospital stay is also very common.[39] Reduced exercise, even if normal nutritional intake is maintained, will result in a reduction in muscle mass. In this situation an increase in food intake is likely to result in a rise in body fat only. Exercise is necessary to promote muscle formation. It is also needed to maintain bone health and mineral density. A negative energy balance will result in protein breakdown (and muscle loss).

Assessment

The body mass index (BMI) is calculated by dividing the patient's weight in kilograms by their height in metres squared (kg/m^2). According to WHO criteria, those with a BMI <$18.5\,kg/m^2$ are defined as underweight. Limitations of this assessment method include the presence of oedema or ascites, loss of height due to osteoporotic fractures, and it takes no account of recent weight loss (unless serial measurements are taken). If height cannot be attained (e.g. patients who cannot stand), it can be estimated by measuring ulna length.[40] The usefulness of anthropometrics, such as skin fold thickness, is unclear. The Malnutrition Universal Screening Tool (MUST) aims to improve the sensitivity of the BMI by adding to it estimations of recent unintentional weight loss (over the past few months) and likelihood of poor oral intake in those who are acutely unwell over the coming five-day period (leading to a total score between 0 and 6).[40] Serum albumin concentration has a poor sensitivity and specificity to measure nutritional status.

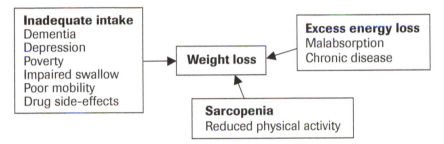

FIGURE 1.4 Factors that lead to weight loss in the elderly.

Treatment

Oral supplements are often given between meals to try to reduce a resultant reduction in food intake. The latest update of a Cochrane review of oral supplements in the elderly found that they were associated with significant weight gain (2.2%, 95% CI 1.8–2.5), no overall benefit in mortality – but a benefit in mortality when limited to those groups defined as malnourished (RR 0.79, 95% CI 0.64 to 0.97).[37] No significant gain in functional outcomes or length of stay was found, but complication rates were reduced (RR 0.86, 95% CI 0.75 to 0.99). Similarly, oral nutritional supplements given to patients following hip fracture were not found to reduce mortality rates but may reduce some complications.[41]

Non-oral enteral feeding is sometimes appropriate. Small bore and soft nasogastric tubes are usually better tolerated. Reducing the flow rate or changing feed formulation can diminish the incidence of diarrhoea. There is a risk of refeeding syndrome (*see* p. 221). Percutaneous endoscopic gastrostomy (PEG) tubes are discussed on pp. 115 and 220. Total parenteral nutrition is a possible alternative. However, there is little evidence of a benefit when used in the elderly. It has potential harms, and high costs. The hypertonic solution used needs to be given via a large calibre vein (usually via central venous access). In general terms enteral nutrition is preferable to the parenteral route whenever possible.[42]

Immune system and infection

B cell numbers are relatively preserved in older age. However, there is reduced specific antibody production, and increased low-affinity antibody production. Monoclonal gammopathies are more prevalent and autoantibody production is increased. Older adults are more likely to have a positive rheumatoid factor without clinical evidence of disease than younger adults. T cell numbers become reduced, causing a reduction in reactivity to antigens and immunological memory. This results in an increased susceptibility to infection, and a reduced efficacy of vaccines. Infection susceptibility may also be increased in older adults due to factors other than immune senescence; for example, comorbidities (e.g. COPD and diabetes), frailty and malnutrition, and poor quality housing.

The febrile response to infection may be absent or diminished in 20–30% of elderly patients with underlying serious infection.[43] This may be due to both a reduced reaction to pathogens and a lower baseline temperature. Some authors suggest that a temperature rise >1°C above baseline should raise suspicion of infection in the frail. Tests may be hard to interpret, e.g. chest X-rays due to poor positioning, kyphosis and poor inspiration, or normal changes with ageing (e.g. CT brain scans and white matter lesions). Antibiotics may be hard to select. Inappropriate agents often include nitrofurantoin and gentamicin (*see* p. 28), quinolones are linked with MRSA (*see* p. 434) and may cause confusion, *C. difficile* infection is associated with cephalosporins, clindamycin and penicillins (*see* p. 296).

Renal system

Renal mass peaks in the fourth decade of life, and then progressively declines. Most of the loss is from the cortex, not the medulla. Ageing is associated with a progressive decline in renal function, although the degree of this varies between individuals. The basement membrane becomes thickened. There is focal glomerulosclerosis scattered across the cortex, which eventually results in the loss of nephrons. Renal blood flow declines by around 10% per decade from the fourth decade onwards (from around 600 mL/min down to 300 mL/min). Renal arterial resistance progressively increases. Glomerular filtration rate (GFR) declines by around 10% per decade from the fourth decade onwards. This is mainly due to the nephron loss and reduced blood flow. Coexisting elevated systemic blood pressure or diabetes may accelerate the functional loss. A reduction in muscle mass means that serum creatinine concentration may change little despite the decline in function, which may make it hard to estimate GFR. The decreased renal reserve and concentrating ability lead to a reduced capacity to compensate for fluid or electrolyte imbalances. There is an increased risk of nephrotoxicity from drugs or radiocontrast agents. Proteinuria is not a feature of normal ageing. A larger proportion of urine is formed at night. The bladder becomes less elastic due to increased collagen deposition that leads to reduced distension and impaired emptying abilities.

Gastrointestinal system

Older age is associated with an accumulation of tooth decay and subsequent poor dentition. This may be made worse by a reduction in saliva, which may be due to an age-related decline in production, higher prevalence of comorbidities associated with the sicca syndrome (e.g. rheumatoid arthritis), or medication effects (e.g. anticholinergics). A lack of saliva may impair normal swallowing. Senses of taste and smell typically decline with age. This may remove some of the pleasurable sensation of eating.

Oesophageal motility is lessened. Upper and lower oesophageal sphincter pressures are reduced. Atrophic gastritis may develop due to either autoimmune disease or chronic *H. pylori* infection. This can lead to vitamin B_{12} deficiency due to reduced intrinsic factor production. The secretion of prostaglandins that are protective to the gastric wall is impaired. Hepatic mass and blood flow decrease by 30–40% at age 80 years compared to young adults. This change affects drug pharmacokinetics (*see* p. 24). Liver enzymes are unchanged in healthy elders. Gallstones rise in prevalence, being found in around 30% of men and 40% of women aged over 80 years,[44] although only 30% of these will cause symptoms.

Colonic transit time is increased, which may predispose to constipation (*see* p. 290). Bowel diverticula (diverticulosis) are more likely to develop due to reduced colonic wall tensile strength and increased evacuation pressure (e.g. secondary to constipation). They are found in more than half of people aged over 80 in developed countries but only a small proportion of these are symptomatic.[45] They are the most common cause of large volume lower gastrointestinal bleeds.[46]

Cardiovascular system

Ageing is associated with a reduction in the amount of elastin in the arterial walls and myocardium, and an increase in collagen deposition and cross-linkage. There is also calcium deposition in the vessel media. These changes cause increased stiffness. In blood vessels this leads to systolic hypertension and an increased pulse wave velocity (PWV). In the heart it leads to reduced diastolic relaxation and heart failure (*see* Chapter 17). An increased PWV has been found to be an independent risk factor for adverse cardiovascular events in the old.[47]

The endothelium, which helps regulate smooth muscle tone in the vessel walls, typically becomes less responsive to vasoactive substances such as nitric oxide and endothelin-1. There is also reduced baroreflex sensitivity, which may lead to a labile BP.[48] Protein glycation may further increase vessel stiffness, especially in people with diabetes. Endothelial permeability becomes increased.

Atherosclerosis is more common in older age. It may be promoted by the lipid peroxidation seen in ageing. Its formation is accelerated by associated comorbidities that are more common in the elderly (e.g. hypertension, diabetes and renal disease). Additional factors may include reduced physical activity and obesity. Large blood vessels become dilated and their walls become thickened. Amyloid deposition occurs in the walls of cerebral vessels (cerebral amyloid angiopathy, *see* p. 214) and is associated with an increased risk of intracerebral haemorrhage.

The left ventricle typically becomes enlarged. This may be exaggerated by some backwards conduction of the increased PWV. There is an increase in myocyte size, but a reduction in their number. Stiffening of the left ventricle leads to increased diastolic filling pressure and enlargement of the left atrium, which increases the risk of developing atrial fibrillation (AF). The is little change in the resting heart rate and cardiac output with normal ageing. However, peak heart rate (estimated by the 220–age formula in men), cardiac output and ejection fraction all tend to decline. Heart valves undergo degenerative changes and calcification. The conduction system of the heart undergoes fatty and fibrotic changes, which increase the chance of conduction abnormalities.[49] Common ECG changes include prolongation of the PR interval, QRS and QT durations, left axis deviation, and an increased incidence of ectopic beats.

Respiratory system

In older adults there is a reduction in lung elastic recoil (making the lungs more stretchy), but also a reduction in chest wall compliance (making the chest wall less easy to expand). Associated with frailty, muscles of respiration (including the diaphragm) become less strong. The combined effect of these changes is that total lung capacity (TLC) remains constant, but the reduced elastic recoil results in an increase in residual volume (RV). Vital capacity (VC) can be calculated by subtracting RV from TLC. Therefore VC becomes reduced (*see* Figure 1.5). Forced expiratory volume in one second (FEV_1) is lower in older adults, as is diffusing capacity. Partial pressure of oxygen (pO_2) is reduced but that of carbon dioxide (pCO_2) is unchanged. Respiratory drive in response to hypoxia or hypercapnia is impaired.

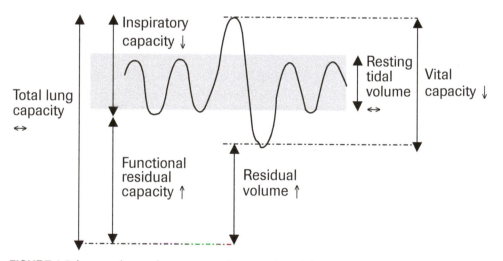

FIGURE 1.5 Lung volume changes seen in normal ageing.
(↓ = reduced, ↑ = increased, ↔ = unchanged)

Nervous system

Cognitive changes with normal ageing are likely to be minor.[50] Some studies have suggested reduced new memory learning, new problem solving and psychomotor speed, with relative preservation of remote memory. Vocabulary and comprehension of language appear largely unaffected but verbal fluency can be reduced. The performance of complex visuospatial tasks may be diminished. There may be a degree of slowing of cognition (bradyphrenia) and a more cautious pattern of behaviour. Other faculties are typically unaffected.

Pathological changes seen in older brains include beta-amyloid plaque accumulation and neurofibrillary tangles (tau protein filamentous aggregates found in degenerating neurons). Cerebral atrophy is associated with older age in asymptomatic individuals, but is more severe in those with dementia (especially Alzheimer's dementia).[51] In those without dementia, it appears to be more marked in hypertensive individuals.[52] Cerebral white matter lesions (or leukoaraiosis) are a common incidental finding on brain scans of older adults. In a sample of 822 randomly selected people over the age of 65 (mean age 73 years), 66% had either focal (17%) or diffuse (49%) white matter lesions on magnetic resonance imaging (MRI).[53] They are thought to be due to chronic ischaemic changes and are associated with vascular risk factors and an increased risk of vascular death.[54,55] White matter lesions are associated with an increased risk of falls, hip fracture, urinary dysfunction, physical functional decline and cognitive impairment.[53,56,57] Their origin may be due to small vessel strokes or to episodes of hypoperfusion related to loss of cerebral blood flow auto-regulation. Diffuse lesions are found more commonly in those with high blood pressure, who are also more likely to have both strokes and impaired cerebral auto-regulation.

Neurological examination of older people often reveals abnormalities even in those without a diagnosis of neurological disease.[50] Common examples include anosmia, reduced up-gaze, increased limb tone, tremor, reduced ankle reflexes and reduced vibration sense in the distal legs. But these abnormalities should not be considered benign and are associated with functional and cognitive decline plus higher mortality rates.

Eye and ear

Around 13% of people aged over 75 are visually impaired (defined as scoring <6/18 on Snellen acuity).[58] Changes due to the process of ageing include: reduced lens flexibility and altered light refraction, cataract formation, reduced ciliary muscle contractility, macular degeneration, reduced eye movements and slower visual processing. Presbyopia is a term for the loss of accommodation seen with advancing age. It is caused by changes in the lens and ciliary muscle, and can usually be corrected with glasses. In around 32% of patients with binocular visual loss the cause is related to refractive errors.[58] The commonest eye diseases affecting vision in older age are macular degeneration (36% of those with visual impairment), cataracts (25%), glaucoma (8%) and diabetic retinopathy (2%).

Age-related macular degeneration (AMD) is the commonest cause of irreversible visual loss in the elderly. It usually affects central vision, leading to a reduction in reading ability. Patients may also notice reduced ability to drive at night and impaired ability to adjust from bright daylight to dimmer indoor lighting. Peripheral vision is typically preserved, allowing patients to safely mobilise. Risk factors include smoking, Caucasian race and having a family history of AMD. Around 10% of sufferers have the 'wet' form, which is more likely to cause more severe and faster progressing impairment. It is associated with new retinal vessel formation. Recently treatment with drugs that inhibit vascular endothelial growth factor has been found to be helpful in those with wet variant.[59] Ongoing studies are evaluating the usefulness of laser therapy to treat the commoner dry form of AMD.

Cataracts can cause blurred vision, increased susceptibility to glare, and difficulty seeing in low light conditions. Surgery is only appropriate when they are causing significant symptoms. The lens is then extracted under local anaesthetic. Serious complications are rare. Glaucoma typically causes a loss of peripheral vision or visual field defects (scotomas). It is related to reduced aqueous humour outflow that results in an increased intraocular pressure (>21 mmHg). Primary open angle glaucoma is an insidious disease caused by a blockage of flow in the trabecular meshwork, which results in gradual damage to the optic nerve. A large cup to disc ratio is seen on ophthalmoscopy. Up to 40% of patients may have normal intraocular pressures.[60] It is usually managed initially with eye drops, such as prostaglandin analogues (e.g. latanoprost) or beta-blockers (e.g. timolol). Secondary treatments include acetazolamide, sympathomimetics (e.g. brimonidine eye drops) and surgical iridectomy. Primary angle closure glaucoma is caused by blockage of flow into the anterior chamber. It causes an acute red eye and should be urgently referred to an ophthalmologist.

Age-related hearing loss has been called presbyacusis, although more recently termed 'age-related sensorineural hearing impairment'. It typically affects men earlier in life than women. It tends to cause bilateral, high frequency hearing loss. The prevalence of bilateral hearing loss has been found to be around 28–43% in men, and 17–20% in women aged 60 to 69 years.[61] It is thought to be due to neuronal degeneration. Factors such as exposure to loud noises at work may accelerate the process.

Endocrine

Changes in endocrine system function may be concealed (i.e. normal serum hormone concentrations) when well, but then become apparent at times of stress (i.e. impaired homeostasis). Testosterone levels gradually decline with age. Oestrogen levels in women fall dramatically after the menopause. Aldosterone, DHEA, renin, angiotensin, growth hormone and insulin-like growth factor 1 levels all decline with advanced age. Thyroxine levels are typically unchanged. Atrial natriuretic peptide (ANP) levels increase in older age. The usual circadian rhythm of anti-diuretic hormone secretion is lost in old age.[62] This coupled to reduced renin-angiotensin-aldosterone activity and increased ANP results in increased nocturnal urine production in the elderly. This may cause nocturia and possibly urinary incontinence.

Cancer

In the UK, 36% of cancer is diagnosed in people aged over 75 years.[63] Whereas the age-specific mortality from cancer continues to increase as people age, the age-specific incidence of cancer appears to level out beyond the age of 75. In older people, the commonest non-cutaneous cancer sites are prostate then lung and bowel in men, and breast then bowel and lung in women. Around 80% of bone metastases originate from the breast, lung and prostate. These sites plus renal cancer cause the majority of cases of cord compression. Bone scans do not detect all metastases, especially lytic lesions (e.g. myeloma, thyroid and renal tumours). Bisphosphonates may reduce fracture rates and need for radiotherapy but may need over six months for a beneficial effect to be seen. Brain tumours are discussed on p. 228.

Mobility

Changes seen in healthy older people compared to younger individuals include a generalised slowing of gait speed and a reduction in stride length, increased postural sway while standing still, and a greater degree of deviation from the straight line when walking.[50] There may be forward flexion of the upper body and reduced arm swing. Higher level gait disorders are associated with frontal lobe dysfunction and may lead to periods of hesitation and freezing. In this situation, cerebral white matter lesions are typically seen on brain imaging. Capacity to perform exercise is reduced in older age and reaction times are increased.

DELIVERING HIGH QUALITY CARE TO OLDER PEOPLE

High quality care has elements of efficacy and safety, but also a positive patient experience. It is extremely important to show compassion and treat older people with dignity. Good communication is a key element. This not only applies to the patient, but also to their relatives or carers (with the patient's consent when possible). A 'hello my name is ...' brief introduction can pave the way for more detailed discussions when time allows.[64] A collateral history is very helpful in establishing baseline functional ability and a crucial component of assessing cognitive impairment. Someone who knows the patient well can also be asked to complete a 'this is me' document, which will inform the ward team of the patient's likes and dislikes, improving their overall experience.[65] If an informant is not seen on the ward, try to call them to ask if they can come in or speak over the phone. Another important but simple step in hospital is to ensure that all patients are in easy reach of their call bell and a drink of water every time you leave their bedside.

When looking for the cause of the patient's illness remember that presentations can be atypical, such as a heart attack presenting as 'off legs'. Commonly there is complexity. Performing a comprehensive geriatric assessment is vital to detect all of the relevant issues. A key element that is often overlooked is cognitive assessment (*see* p. 89). If this is not done, many issues will be missed that will impact on patient safety in hospital and hinder a safe discharge. Examination should include looking in concealed areas such as under bandages and at the common sites of pressure ulcers (preferably at the time of arrival at your department). Also, if there is hearing impairment look for ear wax and, when relevant, check hearing aid batteries. Test for visual impairment and ensure the correct (and clean) glasses are available. Always consider medications as part of the differential diagnosis and review drug lists to see if they can be optimised (ideally simplified) (*see* p. 32). High quality geriatric medicine is delivered by a range of members of a multidisciplinary team. It is important to work as a member of this team with good communication that can allow everyone to benefit from others' experience.

Older people are at a greater risk of adverse events while in hospital than younger people, particularly medication-related events and through poor knowledge application from their clinical team.[66] In healthcare we should all strive to avoid harm. This includes promoting mobilisation and independence, only inserting urinary catheters when necessary and removing them as soon as possible, and reducing the risk of falling (e.g. review medications, the patient's position on ward (proximity to the nurses' station), their footwear, toenails, vision and hearing). Beware of over-diagnosing urinary tract infections. Urine dipsticks are rarely helpful and asymptomatic bacteriuria can make urine cultures hard to interpret (*see* p. 258). Always consider if your patient is constipated and check their nutritional status. These can be helped by completing bowel charts, food charts and regular weighing. Pain can go undetected, especially in those with cognitive impairment. Be vigilant and consider the use of specialised assessment tools such as the Abbey Pain Scale (*see* Appendix A).

Frequently there are multiple small problems in combination rather than one larger issue. For example, poor vision, constipation and anticholinergic medications may make a frail elderly person profoundly delirious. Given the complex nature of our patient group, it is often helpful to make a problem list and then develop a plan to tackle each element with priority given to the most important. Try to be accurate with diagnosis and avoid vague terms such as 'collapse' or 'dizziness'. A 'mechanical fall' is not a diagnosis (*see* p. 326). 'Social' admissions are very rare and usually indicate that the true cause of the patient's presentation has not yet been identified. 'Acopia' is a nonsense term that should not be used. If a younger person develops cardiogenic shock they would not be able to 'cope' at home, but we do not belittle their problems. The nature of frailty is that a smaller nudge from pathology is enough to knock someone off their perch. But there is usually a treatable condition to be found, which can make a big difference for the person.

REFERENCES

1 von Zglinicki T. Will your telomeres tell your future? Not any time soon. *BMJ*, 2012; **344**: e1727.
2 Nass R, Pezzoli SS, Oliveri NC, *et al.* Effects of an oral ghrelin mimetic on body composition and clinical outcomes in healthy older adults: a randomized trial. *Ann Intern Med*, 2008; **149**(9): 601–11.
3 Liu H, Bravata DM, Olkin I, *et al.* Systematic review: the safety and efficacy of growth hormone in the healthy elderly. *Ann Intern Med*, 2007; **146**: 104–15.
4 Nair KS, Rizza RA, O'Brien P, *et al.* DHEA in elderly women and DHEA or testosterone in elderly men. *N Engl J Med*, 2006; **355**(16): 1647–59.
5 Sullivan DH. Megestrol. *J Am Geriatr Soc*, 2007; **55**: 20–8.
6 Kirkwood T. *Time of Our Lives*. London: Phoenix; 2000.
7 World Health Organization. *Ageing and Life Course*. Available at: www.who.int/ageing/en/ (accessed 5 August 2014)
8 United Nations. *World Population Ageing 2013*. Available at: www.un.org/en/development/desa/population/publications/pdf/ageing/WorldPopulationAgeing2013.pdf (accessed 5 August 2014).
9 Office of National Statistics. 2011. *Estimates of Centenarians in the UK, 2010*. Available at: www.ons.gov.uk/ons/dcp171780_233627.pdf (accessed 6 August 2014).

10 Cawthon PM, Marshall LM, Michael Y, *et al.* Frailty in older men: prevalence, progression, and relationship with mortality. *J Am Geriatr Soc*, 2007; **55**(8): 1216–23.

11 Rockwood K. Frailty and its definition: a worthy challenge. *J Am Geriatr Soc*, 2005; **53**(6): 1069–79.

12 Fried LP, Tangen CM, Walston J, *et al.* Frailty in older adults: evidence for a phenotype. *J Gerontol*, 2001; **56A**: M146–56.

13 van Kan GA, Rolland Y, Houles M, *et al.* The assessment of frailty in older adults. *Clin Geriatr Med*, 2010; **26**: 275–86.

14 Mitnitski AB, Graham JE, Mogilner AJ, *et al.* Frailty, fitness and late-life mortality in relation to chronological and biological age. *BMC Geriatrics*, 2002; **2**(1): 1–8.

15 Clegg A, Young J, Iliffe S, *et al.* Frailty in elderly people. *Lancet*, 2013; **381**: 752–62.

16 Isaacs B. *The Challenge of Geriatric Medicine.* Oxford: Oxford University Press; 1992.

17 Berman P, Hogan DB, Fox RA. The atypical presentation of infection in old age. *Age Ageing*, 1987; **16**(4): 201–7.

18 Jarrett PG, Rockwood K, Carver D, *et al.* Illness presentation in elderly patients. *Arch Intern Med*, 1995; **155**: 1060–4.

19 Rockwood K, Hubbard R. Frailty and the geriatrician. *Age Ageing*, 2004; **33**: 429–30.

20 Oliver D. 'Acopia' and 'social admission' are not diagnoses: why older people deserve better. *J R Soc Med*, 2008; **101**: 168–74.

21 Downing A, Wilson R. Older people's use of Accident and Emergency services. *Age Ageing*, 2005; **34**(1): 24–30.

22 Lally F, Crome P. Undergraduate training in geriatric medicine: getting it right. *Age Ageing*, 2007; **36**: 366–8.

23 Ellis G, Langhorne P. Comprehensive geriatric assessment for older hospital patients. *Br Med Bull*, 2005; **71**: 45–59.

24 Baztan JJ, Suarez-Garcia FM, Lopez-Arrieta J, *et al.* Effectiveness of acute geriatric units on functional decline, living at home, and case fatality among older patients admitted to hospital for acute medical disorders: metaanalysis. *BMJ*, 2009; **338**: 334–6.

25 Cooper C, Selwood A, Livingston G. The prevalence of elder abuse and neglect: a systematic review. *Age Ageing*, 2008; **37**: 151–60.

26 Levine JM. Elder neglect and abuse: a primer for primary care physicians. *Geriatrics*, 2003; **58**(10): 37–44.

27 Garre-Olmo J Planas-Pujol X, Lopez-Pousa S, *et al.* Prevalence and risk factors of suspected elder abuse subtypes in people aged 75 and older. *J Am Geriatr Soc*, 2009; **57**(5): 815–22.

28 Cohen M, Levin SH, Gagin R, *et al.* Elder abuse: disparities between older people's disclosure of abuse, evident signs of abuse, and high risk of abuse. *J Am Geriatr Soc*, 2007; **55**(8): 1224–30.

29 Action on Elder Abuse. *Hidden Voices: Older People's Experience of Abuse,* 2004. Available at: www.elderabuse.org.uk/Documents/AEA%20documents/AEA%20Report%20-%20 Hidden%20Voices%20Report.pdf (accessed 6 August 2014).

30 Jones J, Dougherty J, Schelble D, *et al.* Emergency department protocol for the diagnosis and evaluation of geriatric abuse. *Ann Emerg Med*, 1988; **17**: 1006–15.

31 Homer AC, Gilleard C. Abuse of elderly people by their carers. *BMJ*, 1990; **301**: 1359–62.

32 Lachs MS, Pillemer K. Elder abuse. *Lancet*, 2004; **364**: 1263–72.

33 Clarke ME, Pierson W. Management of elder abuse in the emergency department. *Emerg Clin N Am*, 1999; **17**: 631–44.

34 Evans WJ, Campbell WW. Sarcopenia and age-related changes in body composition and functional capacity. *J Nutr*, 1993; **123**: 465–8.

35 Fukagawa NK, Bandini LG, Dietz WH, *et al.* Effect of age on body water and resting metabolic rate. *J Gerontol*, 1996; **51A**(2): M71–M73.

36 Alibhai S, Greenwood C, Payette H. An approach to the management of unintentional weight loss in elderly people. *CMAJ*, 2005; **172**(6): 773–80.

37 Milne AC, Potter J, Vivanti A, *et al.* Protein and energy supplementation in elderly people at risk from malnutrition. *Cochrane Database Syst Rev.* 2009, Issue 2. Art. No.: CD003288.

38 McWhirter JP, Pennington CR. Incidence and recognition of malnutrition in hospital. *BMJ*, 1994; **308**: 945–8.

39 Kelly IE, Tessier S, Cahill A, *et al.* Still hungry in hospital: identifying malnutrition in acute hospital admissions. *Q J Med*, 2000; **93**: 93–8.

40 Malnutrition Advisory Group. *Malnutrition Universal Screening Tool (MUST)*. 2003. www. bapen.org.uk/musttoolkit.html (accessed 6 August 2014).

41 Avenell A, Handoll HHG. Nutritional supplementation for hip fracture aftercare in older people. *Cochrane Database Syst Rev.* 2006, Issue 4. Art. No.: CD001880.

42 Zaloga GP. Parenteral nutrition in adult inpatients with functioning gastrointestinal tracts: assessment of outcomes. *Lancet*, 2006; **367**: 1101–11.

43 Norman DC, Yoshikawa TT. Fever in the elderly. *Infect Dis Clin N Am*, 1996; **10**(1): 93–9.

44 Arthur JDR, Edwards PR, Chagla LS. Management of gallstone disease in the elderly. *Ann R Coll Surg Engl*, 2003; **85**: 91–6.

45 Jeyarajah S, Faiz O, Bottle A, *et al.* Diverticular disease hospital admissions are increasing, with poor outcomes in the elderly and emergency admissions. *Aliment Pharmacol Ther*, 2009; **30**: 1171–82.

46 Chait MM. Lower gastrointestinal bleeding in the elderly. *World J Gastrointest Endosc*, 2010; **2**: 147–54.

47 Sutton-Tyrrell K, Najjar SS, Boudreau RM, *et al.* Elevated aortic pulse wave velocity, a marker of arterial stiffness, predicts cardiovascular events in well-functioning older adults. *Circulation*, 2005; **111**: 3384–90.

48 Ford G. Ageing and the baroreflex. *Age Ageing*, 1999; **28**: 337–8.

49 Bharati S, Lev M. The pathologic changes in the conduction system beyond the age of ninety. *Am Heart J*, 1992; **124**(2): 486–96.

50 Woodford HJ, George J. Neurological and cognitive impairments detected in older people without a diagnosis of neurological or cognitive disease. *Postgrad Med J*, 2011; **86**: 199–206.

51 Kawamura J, Meyer JS, Ichijo M, *et al.* Correlations of leuko-araiosis with cerebral atrophy and perfusion in elderly normal subjects and demented patients. *J Neurol Neurosurg Psychiatry*, 1993; **56**: 182–7.

52 Wiseman RM, Saxby BK, Burton EJ, *et al.* Hippocampal atrophy, whole brain volume, and white matter lesions in older hypertensive subjects. *Neurology*, 2004; **63**: 1892–7.

53 Corti M, Baggio G, Sartori L, *et al.* White matter lesions and the risk of incident hip fracture in older persons. *Arch Intern Med*, 2007; **167**(16): 1745–51.

54 Inzitari D, Cadelo M, Marranci ML, *et al.* Vascular deaths in elderly neurological patients with leukoaraiosis. *J Neurol Neurosurg Psychiatry*, 1997; **62**: 177–81.

55 Fernando MS, Simpson JE, Matthews F, *et al.* White matter lesions in an unselected cohort of the elderly: molecular pathology suggests origin from chronic hypoperfusion injury. *Stroke*, 2006; **37**: 1391–8.

56 Sakakibara R, Hattori T, Uchiyama T, *et al.* Urinary function in elderly people with and without leukoaraiosis: relation to cognitive and gait function. *J Neurol Neurosurg Psychiatry*, 1999; **67**: 658–60.

57 Pantoni L, Poggesi A, Basile AM, *et al.* Leukoaraiosis predicts hidden global functioning impairment in nondisabled older people: The LADIS (Leukoaraiosis and Disability in the Elderly) Study. *J Am Geriatr Soc*, 2006; **54**: 1095–101.

58 Evans JR, Fletcher AE, Wormald RP. Causes of visual impairment in people aged 75 years and older in Britain: an add-on study to the MRC Trial of Assessment and Management of Older People in the Community. *Br J Ophthalmol*, 2004; **88**(3): 365–70.

59 Kauffman SR. Developments in age-related macular degeneration: diagnosis and treatment. *Geriatrics*, 2009; **64**(3): 16–19.

60 Pelletier AL, Thomas J, Shaw FR. Visual loss in older persons. *Am Fam Physician*, 2009; **79**(11): 963–70.

61 Gopinath B, Rochtchina E, Wang JJ, *et al.* Prevalence of age-related hearing loss in older adults: Blue Mountains Study. *Arch Intern Med*, 2009; **169**(4): 415–16.

62 Miller M. Nocturnal polyuria in older people: pathophysiology and clinical implications. *J Am Geriatr Soc*, 2000; **48**(10): 1321–9.

63 Cancer Research UK. *Cancer Incidence by Age.* www.cancerresearchuk.org/cancer-info/cancer stats/incidence/age/ (accessed 6 August 2014).

64 *See* http://hellomynameis.org.uk (accessed 26 November 2014).

65 Alzheimer's Society. *This is me.* Available at: http://alzheimers.org.uk/thisisme (accessed 18 November 2014).

66 Merten H, Zegers M, de Bruijne MC, *et al.* Scale, nature, preventability and causes of adverse events in hospitalised older patients. *Age Ageing*, 2013; **42**: 87–93.

CHAPTER 2

Medications

Medical research does not always answer physicians' dilemmas. Subgroups of patients, such as the elderly, are often not adequately represented in trials to be sure that results are also applicable to them. Trials may even specifically exclude this age group,[1] so evidence-based medicine may not support some common prescribing practices in the elderly. The other side to this is that by not prescribing certain treatments, elderly people may be unfairly denied therapies that work at least as well within their age group. There is evidence to suggest that many older people are not on treatments that are of proven benefit, such as anti-platelets for ischaemic heart disease and angiotensin-converting enzyme (ACE) inhibitors in heart failure.[2] Therefore, the geriatrician has to tread a careful path between the potential negative effects of both polypharmacy and unreasonable under-treatment. Perhaps what we are practising should be termed 'evidence-extrapolated medicine'.

There is a further difficulty that confronts all physicians. The design and reporting of many drug trials is influenced by the drug company that will benefit from subsequent marketing. The potential conflict of interest is quite obvious. Perhaps more disturbingly, a number of authors of clinical guidelines are in receipt of grants from, or hold shares in, pharmaceutical companies.[3] In addition, clinical trials are usually designed to test drug efficacy, and they do not necessarily give accurate information regarding long-term safety.

BASIC STATISTICS

To be able to evaluate the true benefits of medications as reported in clinical trials it is useful to have some basic knowledge of statistics. Drugs trials typically report results as relative risk reductions (RRR) because these numbers usually are larger, and sound more impressive, than absolute risk reductions (ARR). The RRR is the proportional change whereas the ARR is the observed change in incidence. For example, a new drug is developed that reduces the risk of having a myocardial infarction (MI). The incidence of MI within the population taking the new drugs is 3.2% over a one-year period, compared to 4.0% in those given a placebo.

$$\text{RRR} = \frac{4.0 - 3.2}{4.0} \times 100 = 20\%$$

$$ARR \ = \ 4.0 - 3.2 \ = \ 0.8\%$$

The ARR can be used to calculate the number needed to treat (NNT). This can give a number that is easier to understand when assessing the risks and benefits of prescribing a medication. For the example given above:

$$NNT \ = \ \frac{100}{ARR} \ = \ \frac{100}{0.8} \ = \ 125$$

So, we can say that 125 people would need to take the new drug for one year to prevent one MI. This does not sound anywhere near as favourable as saying there will be a 20% RRR.

Relative risk (RR) is the chance of having an adverse event in a group of people exposed to a risk factor compared to people who were not exposed to that risk factor. When RR > 1 the risk is increased, when RR < 1 the risk is reduced. Hazard ratios and odds ratios are conceptually similar but a more in-depth comparison is beyond the scope of this text.

$$RR \ = \ \frac{\text{Adverse event incidence in exposed group}}{\text{Adverse event incidence in non-exposed group}}$$

When we calculate the mean from a sample of values we are only getting an approximation of what the true mean is for the entire population. A 95% confidence interval (CI) is often used to give the range of values that we are 95% sure that the true mean lies within. In order to do this we need to know the standard error (SE), which can be obtained from the standard deviation (SD) and sample size (n). Imagine we counted the number of prescribed medications for 100 care home residents and came up with a mean number of 5.2 with a standard deviation of 1.4. The 95% CI can be calculated by the formulas below.

$$SE \ = \ \frac{SD}{\sqrt{n}} \ = \ \frac{1.4}{10} \ = \ 0.14$$

$$95\% \ CI \ = \ \text{mean} +/- (1.96 \times SE) \ = \ 5.2 +/- (0.27)$$
$$= \ 4.93 - 5.47$$

Many drug trials report the RR of adverse events with a calculated 95% CI for the true value. When the CI does not cross 1.0 then the effect can be described as significant. For example:

RR 1.20 (95% CI 1.04 – 1.36)   suggests a significant increased risk
RR 0.68 (95% CI 0.56 – 0.81)   suggests a significant risk reduction
RR 1.04 (95% CI 0.87 – 1.21)   suggests no significant effect.

PHARMACOKINETICS

Generally speaking, elderly patients absorb medications similarly to younger individuals. The main differences in the pharmacokinetics occur with drug distribution and elimination. The concentration of albumin in the blood does not change significantly with ageing in the absence of severe illness. Therefore, protein binding is not usually altered. But the body composition does change as people age. Older individuals have a higher proportion of body fat and a lower proportion of body water than younger people (*see* p. 10). This affects the volume of distribution (Vd) of drugs (the theoretical volume of fluid that would account for the observed plasma concentration). It is increased for lipophilic drugs and reduced for hydrophilic ones. Sarcopenia may also result in a reduced Vd for drugs that bind to muscle. As the half-life of a drug is proportional to its Vd divided by clearance, a larger Vd can increase a drug's half-life. Examples of drugs with longer half-lives in the elderly for this reason include benzodiazepines and barbiturates.[4] Similarly, a reduced clearance may have an additional effect. Permeability of the blood–brain barrier also appears to increase with advanced age, potentially increasing the risk of cognitive effects of medications.

The two main mechanisms of drug elimination are metabolism in the liver and excretion via the kidneys. Both of these are impaired in older age. The reduced hepatic metabolic capacity may be related to several processes, including reduced blood flow or enzyme activity. However, an age-related reduction in liver mass appears to be the most important factor.[5] The liver mass has been found to reduce by 20% to 50% by the time people reach 80 years of age.[6]

The glomerular filtration rate (GFR) also progressively declines with advancing age. On average this is in the order of a 10% reduction per decade after the age of 30, due to a number of physiological changes (*see* p. 12). This is taken into account in calculations to estimate GFR such as the Cockcroft–Gault formula:[7]

$$\frac{(140 - \text{age}) \times (\text{body weight in kg}) \ (\text{multiply by 0.85 for females})}{72 \times (\text{serum creatinine (mg/dL)})}$$

or the Modification of Diet in Renal Disease (MDRD) equation.[8] Digoxin is an example of a drug with a reduced renal clearance and increased risk of toxicity in the elderly.[6] Some drugs are eliminated by active excretion into the renal tubules, which also appears to be diminished in older adults.

Additionally, there may be changes in the sensitivity of target organs to certain concentrations of drugs compared to younger counterparts (pharmacodynamics). This causes either increased or decreased drug efficacies at similar plasma concentrations compared to younger people. One example is the apparent increased sensitivity of older people to psychoactive medications.[6]

So, the elderly are prone to variation in drug peak concentrations and half-lives. Altering the size of drug doses or their frequency can compensate for this.

INAPPROPRIATE MEDICATION USE

A number of medications have been judged inappropriate for use in the majority of older people due to inefficacy, unacceptable side-effects or the availability of more suitable alternatives. The Beers criteria were derived in 1993 by expert consensus and initially developed for use in nursing facilities. They have since been updated, with the most recent version published in 2012.[9] They contain a list of medications that are deemed inappropriate for use in older adults due to either unacceptable side-effects or the existence of more appropriate alternatives. Of course, there may be situations in some individuals where these drugs are appropriate, but they should always be given careful consideration before commencement. Table 2.1 contains a short list of commonly used medications derived from the Beers recommendations. Criticisms of the Beers criteria include the fact they contain a large number of drugs rarely prescribed these days (e.g. thioridazine), lack ability to detect drug–drug interactions or duplicate prescriptions, and do not provide an exhaustive list of potentially inappropriate drugs in older people.[10]

TABLE 2.1 Examples of medications potentially inappropriate for use in older adults

		Notes
Benzodiazepines	Chlordiazepoxide	*See* p. 26
	Diazepam	
	Lorazepam	
	Oxazepam	
	Temazepam	
Anticholinergics	Amitriptyline	*See* p. 27
TCAs	Doxepin	
	Orphenadrine	
	Oxybutynin	
NSAIDs	Indomethacin	Heart failure, renal failure, hypertension and GI bleeding
	Ketorolac	
	Naproxen	
	Piroxicam	
Cardiovascular	Amiodarone	Multiple side-effects
	Digoxin	Increased risk of toxicity
	Doxazosin	Orthostatic hypotension
	Methyldopa	Sedation, orthostatic hypotension
	Nifedipine (short-acting)	Orthostatic hypotension
Others	Chlorpheniramine	Confusion and sedation
	Cimetidine	Confusion
	Nitrofurantoin	*See* p. 28
	Oestrogens	*See* pp. 105 and 273

Despite these recommendations, there is evidence that elderly people are commonly prescribed such agents. One study found that 24% of people of 65 years or older were on at least one drug that was deemed unsuitable according to expert guidelines and 20% of these people were on two or more.[11] This appears to be worse among nursing home residents where 40% have been found to be on inappropriate drugs.[12] This value represented 7% of all prescriptions in this group. In the UK around 25% of nursing home residents are on antipsychotic medications, and around 85% of these prescriptions are inappropriate according to expert guidelines.[13,14] Many people are on higher than recommended doses or even multiple agents. A study of older patients (n=597, mean age 77 years) being acutely admitted to hospital found that 32% were on at least one inappropriate medication, and in 49% of these patients the medications were felt to be contributing to their presenting symptoms.[15]

Another issue is that some drugs become inappropriate due to a change in the clinical situation. A good example is the shifting focus from disease prevention to symptom control in the very frail elderly who are approaching end of life.[16] Such a consideration may be appropriate when life expectancy is less than two years but individuals vary and other factors including quality of life are also relevant. The ongoing risks and benefits of drugs such as statins and antiplatelets should be reviewed (especially if used for primary prevention). Medications like oral bisphosphonates may no longer be able to be taken safely due to an impaired swallow mechanism. Bisphosphonates may have a less clear indication in people who are no longer mobile (as less likely to fall). Also their antifracture benefits may persist for up to 18 months after discontinuation, which may exceed life expectancy (*see* p. 363). Antihypertensive medications do not improve mortality rates in very frail people – probably due to increasing falls risk (*see* Chapter 14). In this situation they may be another example of an inappropriate medication.

The following section discusses a number of classes of drug that are frequently prescribed inappropriately in frail older people.

Sedative drugs

Sedative hypnotics are associated with a small increase in sleep duration (mean 25 minutes) with an NNT of 13, but have many adverse effects (e.g. cognitive impairment and falls) with a number needed to harm of just six.[17] Benzodiazepines have few indications for use in the elderly, yet are one of the most commonly prescribed psychotropic drugs in this population. A study found that 30% of the over 85s are on such agents.[18] They are associated with an increased risk of falls (*see* p. 327), functional decline, cognitive impairment and fracture-related mortality.[17-20] If their use is judged absolutely necessary then drugs with shorter half-lives and lower lipid solubility are probably safer (e.g. lorazepam or oxazepam).[4]

Older patients are at risk of insomnia, especially when in hospital environments, which leads doctors to be asked to prescribe sedative medications. Not only are these potentially hazardous but there is also a risk they will be continued after discharge, leading to long-term dependency. Studies suggest that around 30% of patients receive a sedative drug for insomnia during hospital stays.[21,22] One found that around 1–2%

of elderly patients who were not previously on benzodiazepines became chronic users after discharge from hospital.[23]

There are also a number of non-benzodiazepine sedating drugs available. These include zopiclone and zolpidem (the 'Z drugs'). It had been suggested that these are less harmful due in part to shorter half-lives. However, a study of elderly people (mean age 82 years) found an adjusted odds ratio of hip fracture of 1.95 (95% CI 1.09–3.51) with these medications compared to non-users, which was similar to the risk with either benzodiazepines or antipsychotics.[24]

Our sleeping patterns change as we age. Older people tend to sleep for shorter time periods and complain of more fragmented and less satisfying sleep.[25] This can be mistaken for insomnia. The causes of insomnia can be described as intrinsic or extrinsic to the patient.[26] Possible intrinsic causes include delirium (reversal of normal diurnal variation), anxiety/depression, pain, nocturia, paroxysmal nocturnal dyspnoea, medications (e.g. theophylline, some antidepressants and withdrawal from alcohol or benzodiazepines) and daytime sleeping. Extrinsic causes relate to the ward environment (e.g. noise and light levels). Caffeinated drinks should be avoided in the evenings.

Evaluation of insomnia requires consideration of all potential intrinsic and extrinsic factors. It can be helpful to reduce noise on the ward at night (e.g. staff conversations or the volume of alarms), move the patient to a quieter room, or possibly use ear plugs. Warm, milky, non-caffeinated drinks can be beneficial. The use of sedative medication should be considered a last resort. They do not provide equivalent sleep quality to natural sleep.

Melatonin is an endogenous hormone produced at night by the pineal gland and plays a role in maintaining the normal circadian rhythm. Its production may be reduced in older people. Melatonin has been licensed for use in people over the age of 55 years with primary insomnia for periods of up to 13 weeks.[27] There is some evidence that it can be effective and has a lower risk of side-effects than traditional sedative drugs.

Anticholinergics

Anticholinergic drugs are associated with physical and cognitive functional decline and an increased risk of death in older adults.[28–31] Older people may be particularly susceptible due to polypharmacy (multiple drugs with anticholinergic effects), lower levels of intracerebral acetylcholine, reduced drug elimination or increased permeability of the blood–brain barrier.

The use of anticholinergic drugs for urinary incontinence is discussed on p. 274. Tricyclic antidepressants have significant anticholinergic properties and are discussed on p. 141. Anticholinergic drugs have also been used in Parkinson's disease (*see* p. 165). In addition, a number of drugs not considered primarily anticholinergic in mechanism of action have also been found to have anticholinergic side-effects. When these are taken in combination they can have a cumulative effect that has been termed 'anticholinergic burden'.[32,33] Examples include antipsychotic drugs (*see* p. 110), antihistamines, baclofen, codeine, diazepam, digoxin, nifedipine, prednisolone and theophylline.[32,34,35] It is good practice to minimise anticholinergic drug exposure in frail older people.

TABLE 2.2 Anticholinergic side-effects

System	Effects
Central nervous system	Sedation
	Cognitive impairment (*see* p. 274)
	Delirium (*see* p. 129)
Gastrointestinal	↓ Saliva production (which increases the risk of dental decay and swallow problems)
	Constipation (which can worsen urinary retention)
Ophthalmic	Mydriasis (which may precipitate glaucoma)
	Impaired accommodation (which may cause blurred vision)
Cardiovascular	Arrhythmias (especially if underlying cardiac disease)
	Tachycardia
	Orthostatic hypotension
Urinary	Retention (which may lead to overflow incontinence and catheterisation)

Antipsychotics

Antipsychotic (or 'neuroleptic') drugs are associated with an increased risk of falls, cognitive decline, stroke and death.[36-38] They are also associated with neuroleptic malignant syndrome (*see* p. 174). Their use in dementia is discussed on p. 110 – here their role is limited to the short-term control of psychosis and aggression. It is always worth considering whether these drugs should be discontinued.

Non-steroidal anti-inflammatory drugs (NSAIDs)

NSAIDs inhibit prostaglandin production, which can lead to numerous side-effects – peptic ulceration, hypertension, heart failure and renal impairment. They are not recommended for routine use in the management of pain in frail older pople.[39] Their role should be limited to patients whose pain is uncontrolled by other means or who are intolerant of alternative agents. They should be used at the lowest effective dose for the shortest possible duration.

Antibiotics

Antibiotic resistance is rising, yet the development of new antibiotic drugs is declining.[40] It is ever more imperative that these drugs are prescribed appropriately. This need must be weighed against the potential harm of giving an ineffective treatment.[41] Some antibiotics are less effective in the elderly (e.g. nitrofurantoin in those with renal impairment) and some cause more harm (e.g. aminoglycosides and nephrotoxicity). The risks of developing MRSA and *C. difficile* are also higher with some drugs (*see* pp. 434 and 296). As a general rule, when an empiric antibiotic is chosen prior to culture results, outside life-threatening infections, an agent with the narrowest possible spectrum of activity that is likely to be beneficial should be selected. When broad-spectrum antibiotics are thought initially necessary, if subsequent cultures show that a narrower spectrum agent would be equally effective, treatment should be changed. Antibiotic selection will frequently require a balance between potential benefits and harms to be made.

Over-diagnosis of urinary tract infection is a significant problem in frail older people (*see* p. 255). Also, there is very little evidence that antibiotic prophylaxis can prevent urinary tract infection in this group and reasons to believe that they can be harmful.

Other notable drugs

Digoxin is used in the management of atrial fibrillation (*see* p. 412) and heart failure (*see* p. 391). Studies have suggested only limited efficacy in either condition. Given its anticholinergic effects and the higher risk of toxicity in older people (due to declining renal function), its role is very limited and consideration should be given to switching to an alternative drug such as a beta-blocker. Iron tablets cause constipation. They are sometimes started in cases of anaemia without demonstrated iron deficiency and often given for long-term prophylaxis at higher than required doses (i.e. more than once per day). It is worthwhile reviewing their indication and ongoing need. Quinine tablets are used for the prevention of nocturnal leg cramps but the beneficial effect is small.[42] They can cause serious side-effects including thrombocytopenia, pancytopenia, vertigo, tinnitus, vomiting, visual disturbance and confusion. It is worth considering whether the benefits for a particular patient outweigh the risks. Calcium channel blockers can precipitate leg oedema and constipation in frail older people. This can lead to prescription cascades – *see* below. Alpha-blockers are associated with a high risk of orthostatic hypotension, may precipitate stress urinary incontinence in older women, and are not a first line drug for managing hypertension (*see* p. 399). Vestibular sedative medications (e.g. betahistine – *see* p. 321) may have a role in the short-term management of acute vertigo but are often prescribed over long periods of time for poorly defined 'dizziness' without beneficial effect. Sodium docusate is commonly prescribed but has only weak evidence of efficacy for constipation (*see* p. 294). Bulk-forming laxatives (e.g. ispaghula husk) can increase the risk of faecal impaction in frail people who do not drink sufficient fluids. Similarly, people with limited oral intake may not be able to take large volume laxatives such as macrogols (or possibly at the expense of nutritional intake). Theophylline has a high rate of adverse effects when used in older people (*see* p. 428). It is worth considering whether a change would be beneficial when any of these drugs are encountered.

Under-prescription

The under-prescription of appropriate medications to some older people is also a problem. In a review of 196 outpatients (mean age 75) who took an average of 8.1 drugs each (range 5 to 17), 65% were on one or more inappropriate agents.[43] However, 64% were not prescribed medicines of known benefit (most commonly antihypertensives, antiplatelets and statins). In total 87% were either on inappropriate or not on appropriate drugs, with 42% of people in both categories.

ADVERSE DRUG REACTIONS

Adverse drug reactions may account for around 12–16% of admissions to hospital in the over-seventies and should always be considered in a differential diagnosis.[15,44] These may be unrelated to drug doses (termed 'idiosyncratic' – e.g. penicillin allergy) but most are dose-dependent (e.g. hypoglycaemia while on insulin), and therefore potentially preventable. For this reason it is generally preferable to use the lowest possible effective dose of a drug. Some adverse reactions may develop after a prolonged exposure, for example tardive dyskinesia with neuroleptic agents (*see* p. 173). Therefore medications should be reviewed and withdrawn, when possible, at periodic intervals. Adverse drug reactions may be due to drug–drug interactions (e.g. clarithromycin inhibits the breakdown of phenytoin) or drug–disease interactions (e.g. NSAIDs may worsen heart failure).

Adverse drug reactions appear to occur commonly in the elderly,[6] especially among those residing in nursing homes.[45] This probably represents the fact that elderly people are on many different agents simultaneously due to multiple comorbidities, and the changes seen in pharmacokinetics and pharmacodynamics. Studies have found that the use of three or more medications significantly increases the chance of an adverse reaction.[44,46] Of the adverse events that are potentially preventable, many are related to the use of psychoactive medications with antipsychotics being the most common offenders.[46] An analysis of surveillance data found that the drugs warfarin, insulin and digoxin accounted for 33% of hospital emergency department visits for adverse drug events in the over-sixty-fives.[47] Careful consideration of the risks and benefits is needed when prescribing these classes of medication.

It has been proposed that pharmacists could be used to review medications, which may lead to a reduction in adverse events due to inappropriate prescribing or drug interactions. A study randomised 368 older hospitalised patients (mean age 87 years) to pharmacist review or standard care.[48] The pharmacists communicated recommendations to the treating physicians (75% of which were actioned). Over a 12-month follow-up period there were nine admissions related to adverse drug events in the intervention group compared to 45 in the controls (i.e. an 80% reduction). The scheme was associated with lower overall healthcare costs.

POLYPHARMACY

Polypharmacy is a term to describe large numbers of medications given to patients. Precise definitions vary but it is often taken as being on four or more regular medications. As people age they accumulate diagnoses and, subsequently, medications. Many conditions require two or more agents to control them, for example osteoporosis, heart failure, hypertension and ischaemic heart disease. A study found that a sample of people over the age of 72 (mean age 81 years) were on a mean number of 2.2 medications (range 0–15).[49] In a random sample of community-dwelling people over the age of 65, 19% of men and 23% of women regularly took five or more prescription drugs.[50] When a group of nursing home residents (mean age 84 years) was assessed, they were receiving an average number of 4.8 regular medications each.[51] A further sample of people aged 65 years or over who resided in residential care or assisted living settings averaged 5.8 regular medications per person.[52] A recent UK survey found that approximately 40% of people aged 85 or over reported taking six or more prescribed medications with the previous week.[53]

Polypharmacy may become exacerbated by the addition of more drugs to treat adverse effects of current agents, for example the addition of a diuretic agent to reduce the leg oedema caused by a calcium channel blocker. This process is what is called the 'prescribing cascade'.[54] To try to prevent this cycle, new symptoms should always be evaluated as possible drug adverse effects and alteration of prescriptions considered.

> *There was an old lady who swallowed a spider,*
> *That wriggled and jiggled and tickled inside her,*
> *She swallowed the spider to catch the fly,*
> *I don't know why she swallowed a fly – perhaps she'll die …*

It is not uncommon to find the co-prescription of agents that have directly opposing mechanisms of action, for example beta-blockers and salbutamol, dopamine agonists and antagonists, or furosemide and fludrocortisone. Also, a recent trend of prescribing anticholinergic agents with cholinesterase inhibitors appears to have developed. This may be true for as many as 35% of those on cholinesterase inhibitors.[55] This may sometimes be caused by the commencement of anticholinergic agents to treat urinary incontinence precipitated by the cholinesterase inhibitors.[56] Yet there is evidence that this is a harmful combination.[57]

The use of multiple agents increases the risks of side-effects and interactions; also, patients' adherence to their medication regimen reduces as the number of drugs increases. A regular review of medications and their ongoing justification and safety should be undertaken whenever possible. People should be asked about their understanding of the indication for each medication and their desire to continue taking it. It is very common to hear older people complain about the number of medications they are taking and to express a desire to be taking fewer. Agents without clear benefit should be withdrawn. This often occurs at the time of hospital admission when the results of medication adjustments can be closely monitored. There is little available data regarding the effects of medication discontinuation. It appears that the majority of drugs can be safely discontinued in older people but caution is sometimes needed (e.g. some cardiovascular drugs and benzodiazepines).[58] There is evidence that reducing the use of psychotropic drugs and reducing polypharmacy burden overall can lead to reductions in falls risk and cognitive improvements.[59]

MEDICATION CONCORDANCE

The old term 'compliance' is being replaced by the term 'concordance' to describe a patient's adherence to prescribed therapies. This is based on the philosophy that doctors and patients are entering into an alliance and good communication between these parties is essential to its proper functioning. The patient should not merely comply with instructions but should agree with the reasoning and be a willing participant in any treatment. An alternative term is 'medication adherence'.

Estimates of concordance rates depend on what definition is applied. The value falls among patients who are being treated for illnesses of long compared to short duration and figures between 40% and 80% have been found in clinical trials of chronic conditions.[60] There is also a reduction with increasing medication regimen complexity.

Patients on once-daily medications will take them around 80% of the time, whereas those on four times daily dosing will take only 50% of their medication.[60] Other factors that have been associated with reduced concordance include the presence of psychiatric disorders (e.g. depression and dementia), medications for conditions that cause no symptoms (e.g. hypertension) and the side-effects of drugs.

The identification of patients who are not taking their medications is not always easy. Sometimes drug levels (e.g. phenytoin), physiological parameters (e.g. blood pressure) or pill counts provide a clue. Usually patient self-reporting is relied upon. It is important not to be confrontational when enquiring about concordance, as this will tend to cause patients to over-report their taking of medications. Accepting that all patients will lapse from time to time, questions should focus on how often this occurs.

Patient education on the value of their various drugs may improve the situation but is unlikely to solve the problem altogether. A logical first step is to try to reduce the number of medications and limit the number of times they are to be taken each day. For example, a once-daily formulation could be used in place of one taken twice daily. Medication aids, as discussed below, may be beneficial in selected patients. Periodic telephone counselling by a pharmacist has been shown to increase adherence in patients on multiple drugs for chronic conditions, and reduce associated mortality.[61]

MEDICATION AIDS

Various devices and methods of drug packaging have been designed to try to improve the concordance of elderly patients with their medications. They include multi-compartment and blister packs. They usually have individual slots for tablets to be taken in the morning, lunch, afternoon, and night-time and span over a one-week period. Accepted wisdom is that they are of benefit; however, this is not evidence-based. Trials that have utilised them have not shown clear benefits in improved medication concordance.[62] That said, large-sized trials assessing their use in the frail elderly have not been performed. They are often started without adequate patient assessment and as many as half of these patients may do as well without them.[63] They may disassociate the patient from their medications as they become all mixed together. They are also only suitable for some drugs. Liquids or inhaled medications cannot be dispensed this way. Other medications, such as bisphosphonates or levodopa, may need to be taken at specific times or in specific ways.

MEDICATION REVIEW

Patients' medications should be periodically reviewed. This may be part of an annual programme or in response to an illness event (e.g. at the time of admission to hospital). The process can be complex for the many reasons discussed in this chapter. A reasonable balance often has to be reached between polypharmacy and inappropriate under-prescription. This is likely to be tailored according to individual patient characteristics and preferences. Some guidance of things to consider is given in Table 2.3.

TABLE 2.3 Guidance for performing a medication review.

Problem	Example
Is the medicine still indicated?	Some medications are only suitable for short-term use – e.g. antipsychotics for agitation in dementia.
	Has the focus of care shifted from disease prevention to symptom control?
Inappropriate medications	*See* Table 2.1
Drug–drug interactions	Warfarin and clarithromycin
Drug–disease interactions	NSAIDs worsen heart failure
Antagonising medications	Beta-blockers and beta-agonists
Co-prescription of the same class	Codeine and tramadol
Prescription cascades	Furosemide to treat leg oedema caused by diltiazem
Inappropriate dose or formulation	Minimal effective dose, preferably once daily.
	Can the patient take the medication as prescribed (e.g. swallowing disorders and oral bisphosphonates)? Consider liquid or transdermal formulations
Concordance	Does the patient want to, and are they able to, take their medication as prescribed (e.g. cognitive impairment and inhalers)?
	Consider education and medication aids
Polypharmacy	Consider limiting medication burden to a small number of the most beneficial agents
Inappropriate under-prescription	Are all comorbidities being treated in accordance with good practice guidance? If not, are there good reasons why (e.g. side-effects, life-expectancy, patient preference, difficulty taking as prescribed, or unacceptable polypharmacy)?

REFERENCES

1 Gurwitz JH. Polypharmacy: a new paradigm for quality drug therapy in the elderly? *Arch Intern Med*, 2004; **164**: 1957–9.
2 Sloane PD, Gruber-Baldini AL, Zimmerman S, *et al.* Medication undertreatment in assisted living settings. *Arch Intern Med*, 2004; **164**: 2031–7.
3 Taylor R, Giles J. Cash interests taint drug advice. *Nature*, 2005; **437**: 1070–1.
4 Chutka DS, Takahashi PY and Hoel RW. Inappropriate medications for elderly patients. *Mayo Clin Proc*, 2004; **79**: 122–39.
5 Wynne HA, Cope LH, James OFW, *et al.* The effect of age and frailty upon acetanilide clearance in man. *Age Ageing*, 1989; **18**: 415–18.
6 Vestal RE. Aging and pharmacology. *Cancer*, 1997; **80**: 1302–10.
7 Friedman JR, Norman DC, Yoshikawa TT. Correlation of estimated renal function parameters versus 24-hour creatinine clearance in ambulatory elderly. *J Am Geriatr Soc*, 1989; **37**: 145–9.
8 Department of Health. *Estimating Glomerular Filtration Rate (GFR): information for laboratories.* 2006. Available at: http://dh.gov.uk/en/Publicationsandstatistics/Publications/Publications PolicyAndGuidance/DH_4133024 (accessed 13 November 2014).

9 American Geriatrics Society. 2012 Beers Criteria Update Expert Panel. American Geriatrics Society updated Beers Criteria for potentially inappropriate medication use in older adults. *J Am Geriatr Soc*, 2012; **60**: 616–31.

10 O'Mahony D, Gallagher PF. Inappropriate prescribing in the older population: need for new criteria. *Age Ageing*, 2008; **37**: 138–41.

11 Wilcox SM, Himmelstein DU, Woolhandler S. Inappropriate drug prescribing for the community-dwelling elderly. *JAMA*, 1994; **272**(4): 292–6.

12 Beers MH, Ouslander JG, Fingold SF, *et al.* Inappropriate medication prescribing in skilled-nursing facilities. *Ann Intern Med*, 1992; **117**(8): 684–9.

13 McGrath AM, Jackson GA. Survey of neuroleptic prescribing in residents of nursing homes in Glasgow. *BMJ*, 1996; **312**: 611–12.

14 Oborne CA, Hooper R, Chi Li K, *et al.* An indicator of appropriate neuroleptic prescribing in nursing homes. *Age Ageing*, 2002; **31**: 435–9.

15 Gallagher PF, Barry PJ, Ryan C, *et al.* Inappropriate prescribing in an acutely ill population of elderly patients as determined by Beers' Criteria. *Age Ageing*, 2008; **37**: 96–101.

16 Holmes HM. Rational prescribing for patients with a reduced life expectancy. *Clin Pharmacol Ther*, 2009; **85**: 103–7.

17 Glass J, Lanctot KL, Herrmann N, *et al.* Sedative hypnotics in older people with insomnia: meta-analysis of risks and benefits. *BMJ*, 2005; **331**: 1169–73.

18 Vinkers DJ, Gussekloo J, van der Mast RC, *et al.* Benzodiazepine use and risk of mortality in individuals aged 85 years or over. *JAMA*, 2003; **290**(22): 2942–3.

19 Hilmer SN, Mager DE, Simonsick EM, *et al.* A drug burden index to define the functional burden of medications in older people. *Arch Intern Med*, 2007; **167**: 781–7.

20 Billioti de Gage S, Moride Y, Ducruet T, *et al.* Benzodiazepine use and risk of Alzheimer's disease: case-control study. *BMJ*, 2014; **349**: g5205.

21 Perry SW, Wu A. Rationale for the use of hypnotic agents in a general hospital. *Ann Intern Med*, 1984; **100**: 441–6.

22 O'Reilly R, Rusnak C. The use of sedative-hypnotic drugs in a university teaching hospital. *CMAJ*, 1990; **142**: 585–9.

23 Bell CM, Fischer HD, Gill SS, *et al.* Initiation of benzodiazepines in the elderly after hospitalization. *J Gen Intern Med*, 2007; **22**: 1024–9.

24 Wang PS, Bohn RL, Glynn RJ, *et al.* Zolpidem use and hip fractures in older people. *J Am Geriatr Soc*, 2001; **49**: 1685–90.

25 Kryger M, Monjan A, Bliwise D, *et al.* Sleep, health, and aging: bridging the gap between science and clinical practice. *Geriatrics*, 2004; **59**: 24–30.

26 Flaherty JH. Insomnia among hospitalized older persons. *Clin Geriatr Med*, 2008; **24**: 51–67.

27 Lyseng-Williamson KA. Melatonin prolonged release in the treatment of insomnia in patients aged ≥ 55 years. *Drugs Aging*, 2012; **29**: 911–23.

28 Hilmer SN, Mager DE, Simonsick EM, *et al.* A drug burden index to define the functional burden of medications in older people. *Arch Intern Med*, 2007; **167**: 781–7.

29 Campbell N, Boustani M, Limbil T, *et al.* The cognitive impact of anticholinergics: a clinical review. *Clin Interv Aging*, 2009; **4**: 225–33.

30 Carriere I, Fourrier-Reglat A, Dartigues J, *et al.* Drugs with anticholinergic properties, cognitive decline, and dementia in an elderly general population: The 3-City Study. *Arch Intern Med*, 2009; **169**: 1317–24.

31 Fox C, Richardson K, Maidment ID, *et al.* Anticholinergic medication use and cognitive impairment in the older population: the Medical Research Council Cognitive Function and Ageing Study. *J Am Geriatr Soc*, 2011; **59**: 1477–83.

32 Rudolph JL, Salow MJ, Angelini MC, *et al.* The anticholinergic risk scale and anticholinergic adverse effects in older persons. *Arch Intern Med*, 2008; **168**(5): 508–13.

33 Han L, Agostini JV, Allore HG. Cumulative anticholinergic exposure is associated with poor memory and executive function in older men. *J Am Geriatr Soc*, 2008; **56**(12): 2203–10.

34 Boustani MA, Campbell NL, Munger S, *et al.* Impact of anticholinergics on the aging brain: a review and practical application. *Aging Health*, 2008; **4**: 311–20.

35 Cancelli I, Beltrame M, Gigli GL, *et al.* Drugs with anticholinergic properties: cognitive and neuropsychiatric side-effects in elderly patients. *Neurol Sci*, 2009; **30**: 87–92.

36 Hien LTT, Cummings RG, Cameron ID, *et al.* Atypical antipsychotic medications and risk of falls in residents of aged care facilities. *J Am Geriatr Soc*, 2005; **53**: 1290–5.

37 Schneider LS, Dagerman KS, Insel P. Risk of death with atypical antipsychotic drug treatment for dementia: meta-analysis of randomized placebo-controlled trials. *JAMA*, 2005; **294**: 1934–43.

38 Ellul J, Archer N, Foy CML, *et al.* The effects of commonly prescribed drugs in patients with Alzheimer's disease on the rate of deterioration. *J Neurol Neurosurg Psychiatry*, 2007; **78**: 233–9.

39 American Geriatrics Society. Pharmacological management of persistent pain in older persons. *J Am Geriatr Soc*, 2009; **57**: 1331–47.

40 Cars O, Hogberg LD, Murray M, *et al.* Meeting the challenge of antibiotic resistance. *BMJ*, 2008; **337**: 726–8.

41 Leibovici L, Shraga I, Andreassen S. How do you choose antibiotic treatment? *BMJ*, 1999; 318: 1614–16.

42 Butler JV, Mulkerrin EC, O'Keeffe ST. Nocturnal leg cramps in older people. *Postgrad Med J*, 2002; **78**: 596–8.

43 Steinman MA, Landefeld CS, Rosenthal GE, *et al.* Polypharmacy and prescribing quality in older people. *J Am Geriatr Soc*, 2006; **54**(10): 1516–23.

44 Mannesse CK, Derkx FHM, de Ridder MAJ, *et al.* Contribution of adverse drug reactions to hospital admission of older patients. *Age Ageing*, 2000; **29**: 35–9.

45 Gurwitz JH, Field TS, Avorn J, *et al.* Incidence and preventability of adverse drug events in nursing homes. *Am J Med*, 2000; **109**: 87–94.

46 von Renteln-Kruse W, Thiesemann N, Thiesemann R, *et al.* Does frailty predispose to adverse drug reactions in older patients? *Age Ageing*, 2000; **29**: 461–2.

47 Budnitz DS, Shehab N, Kegler SR, *et al.* Medication use leading to emergency department visits for adverse drug events in older adults. *Ann Intern Med*, 2007; **147**(11): 755–65.

48 Gillespie U, Alassaad A, Henrohn D, *et al.* A comprehensive pharmacist intervention to reduce morbidity in patients 80 years or older: a randomized controlled trial. *Arch Intern Med*, 2009; **169**(9): 894–900.

49 Agostini JV, Han L, Tinetti ME. The relationships between number of medications and weight loss or impaired balance in older adults. *J Am Geriatr Soc*, 2004; **52**(10): 1719–23.

50 Kaufman DW, Kelly JP, Rosenberg L, *et al.* Recent patterns of medication use in the ambulatory adult population of the United States: the Sloane Survey. *JAMA*, 2002; **287**(3): 337–44.

51 Roberts MS, King M, Stokes JA, *et al.* Medication prescribing and administration in nursing homes. *Age Ageing*, 1998; **27**: 385–92.

52 Sloane PD, Zimmerman S, Brown LC, *et al.* Inappropriate medication prescribing in residential care/assisted living facilities. *J Am Geriatr Soc*, 2002; **50**: 1001–11.

53 Scholes S, Faulding S, Mindell J on behalf of the Health and Social Care Information Centre. *Use of Prescribed Medicines.* 2014. Available at: www.hscic.gov.uk/catalogue/PUB16076/HSE2013-Ch5-pres-meds.pdf (accessed 17 December 2014).

54 Rochon PA, Gurwitz JH. Optimising drug treatment for elderly people: the prescribing cascade. *BMJ*, 1997; **315**: 1096–9.

55 Carnaham RM, Lund BC, Perry PJ, *et al.* The concurrent use of anticholinergics and cholinesterase inhibitors: rare event or common practice? *J Am Geriatr Soc*, 2004; **52**: 2082–7.

56 Gill SS, Mamdani M, Naglie G, *et al.* A prescribing cascade involving cholinesterase inhibitors and anticholinergic drugs. *Arch Int Med*, 2005; **165**: 808–13.

57 Sink KM, Thomas J, Xu H, *et al.* Dual use of bladder anticholinergics and cholinesterase inhibitors: long-term functional and cognitive outcomes. *J Am Geriatr Soc*, 2008; **56**(5): 847–53.

58 Garfinkel D, Mangin D. Feasibility study of a systematic approach for discontinuation of multiple medications in older adults. *Arch Intern Med*, 2010; **170**: 1648–54.

59 van der Cammen TJM, Rajkumar C, Onder G, *et al.* Drug cessation in complex older adults: time for action. *Age Ageing*, 2014; **43**: 20–5.

60 Osterberg L, Blaschkle T. Adherence to medication. *N Engl J Med*, 2005; **353**(5): 487–97.

61 Wu JYFU, Leung WYS, Chang S, *et al.* Effectiveness of telephone counselling by a pharmacist in reducing mortality in patients receiving polypharmacy: randomised controlled trial. *BMJ*, 2006; **333**: 522–5.

62 Huang H, Maguire MG, Miller ER, *et al.* Impact of pill organizers and blister packs on adherence to pill taking in two vitamin supplementation trials. *Am J Epidemiol*, 2000; **152**: 780–7.

63 Raynor DK, Nunney JM. Medicine compliance aids are a partial solution, not panacea. *BMJ*, 2002; **324**: 1338.

CHAPTER 3

Rehabilitation

The terminology used in rehabilitation is undergoing change. 'Impairments' are the physical problems caused by illness, such as weakness secondary to a stroke. Traditionally, these caused 'disabilities' such as a reduced ability to mobilise, which led to 'handicap' – the loss of ability to perform functions such as gardening, dancing or playing golf. In an attempt to use more positive terminology the World Health Organization has advised that the latter two terms be changed to 'activity' and 'participation'.

Rehabilitation is performed by teams of people. These usually include doctors, nurses, physiotherapists, social workers and occupational therapists. Other specialties may also be involved, for example speech and language therapy, and dietetics. In some centres the traditional distinctions between professions are becoming blurred with individuals taking on multiple roles.

The standard aim of rehabilitation is to reduce the impact of physical or cognitive illness. This will mean different things to different individuals. Ideally, the patient will regain their usual level of activity. If this cannot be done, new techniques or strategies may be adopted to circumvent the problems. This may include adaptation of the person's living environment. Common sense and lateral thinking are often more important than scientific knowledge to solve problems for an individual patient. Rehabilitation should begin as soon as possible in the course of an illness to prevent further physical deterioration (e.g. muscle loss due to reduced activity or the development of contractures or pressure sores). For this reason rehabilitation services should be integrated with acute care but may continue beyond hospital discharge. It is an active process and not a period of 'bed rest' or 'convalescence'. In just a few days immobility can lead to significant amounts of muscle and bone loss. Hospital is not always a helpful environment. A study found that previously mobile older people spent 83% of their time in hospital lying in bed, 13% sitting in a chair and just 4% walking.[1] Promoting early mobilisation and participation in self-care is crucial.

Given the individualised nature of future aims, it is right that patients should be involved in the setting of appropriate and realistic goals with the help of medical personnel. Goals may be divided into an overall, long-term aim and a series of more easily achieved short-term ones. The acronym 'SMART' has been proposed to help set suitable goals:

S   specific
M   measurable
A   achievable
R   relevant
T   time-limited

For example, having a goal of walking the length of the ward within one minute is both specific and measurable. If this goal could realistically be attained within four weeks, it may be defined as both achievable and time-limited. If it would make going home a possibility, it is clearly relevant to the individual. It may be broken down into a series of smaller stages, for example standing unaided, walking several steps, walking several metres, and so on. This can make it easier to monitor the patient's progress towards the longer-term goal and help maintain morale.

Activities of daily living (ADLs) are tasks that we perform to maintain a normal existence. In their most basic form they include walking, eating, washing and dressing. More complex tasks are referred to as instrumental activities of daily living (IADLs), which often require the use of objects or tools. These include shopping, preparing meals, using transport, using the telephone and handling finances. Numerous assessment scales have been developed to measure these activities. An example for ADLs is the Barthel index, and for IADLs the Nottingham Extended Activities of Daily Living scale (*see* Appendix A).

Performing clinical trials in the field of rehabilitation is fraught with problems. There have been few large-scale controlled trials in any aspect of it. For this reason the evidence basis behind practice is often weak, but there is some proof of benefit.[2,3]

STROKE

Stroke is a major cause of disability in the adult population. After six months, around one-third of survivors are dependent on others for their activities of daily living.[4] Attempts at rehabilitation may be hindered by associated cognitive deficits, especially receptive dysphasia, making it harder for the patient to comply with interventions. There may also be components of apraxia, visuospatial impairment, or neglect (*see* Chapter 10), which should be specifically looked for in these patients. When such problems are detected, rehabilitation therapy sessions and ward environments should be adapted to lessen disability and promote recovery.[5]

Following a stroke, patients usually have some degree of recovery, and this improvement process can continue for periods of over a year. However, it is hard to predict in which patients and to what degree significant improvements will occur. The recovery process is thought to initially be due to the return of normal neuronal functioning around the infarcted area, but in the longer term is dependent on the formation of new inter-neuronal connections, similar to the normal process of learning new information.[6]

Inpatient rehabilitation is usual for those patients who are unable to safely return home. Its duration varies according to patient response. Typically a period of six to eight weeks will demonstrate the likely long-term functional need of the patient, and enable future care plans to be formulated. Early hospital discharge is sometimes appropriate with the continuation of rehabilitation in the community through specialised teams. Evidence suggests that selected patients may benefit from reduced death or dependency (6 patients per 100 treated), less time in hospital (an average of eight days), and improved functioning and satisfaction through the use of such services.[7] The typical minimal functional requirement for patients who live alone to manage is to be able to independently transfer from bed to chair. The provision of hoist equipment (available in various designs, e.g. overhead or standing) may enable more disabled patients with carers to safely be at home. Discharge often requires the provision, and education in the use of, equipment and the implementation of home adaptations (e.g. the provision of rails). Barriers to early discharge include the lack of wheelchair access or downstairs bathroom facilities (for downstairs living) in the home of the patient.

A study has compared additional educational sessions for carers of stroke patients just prior to discharge to standard care.[8] These sessions included both factual and practical aspects involving topics such as handling, transfers, continence and communication. The carers attended between three and five sessions of around 40 minutes' duration. They found improved psychosocial scores in both patients and carers after one year within the treatment group, although there was no resultant improvement in mortality, disability scores or institutionalisation rates.

Correct patient positioning is important to prevent contractures, spasticity and pressure ulcers. Severe and persistent shoulder pain is thought to occur in around 5% of patients.[5] Its aetiology is probably a combination of subluxation and spasticity. Prevention involves correct patient positioning, the use of supports and careful handling of hemiplegic limbs by carers.[4] Pain can usually be controlled with simple analgesia (e.g. paracetamol).

The initial aims of rehabilitation are usually modest, such as enabling a patient to transfer from bed to chair rather than to walk independently. For those with hemiplegia, one-handed techniques of self-care can be taught in the immediate phase. Once the affected limb has regained sufficient power to overcome gravity it may be incorporated into the performance functional tasks. The best evidence for a benefit of physiotherapy after stroke is for task-orientated exercise training, especially if intensive and performed in the early phase.[9] Team members other than the physiotherapist should then encourage the patient to incorporate the techniques into their usual daily routine.[5] An ankle–foot orthosis (AFO) may prevent footdrop hindering attempts at walking.[10] Foot inversion while walking can be prevented by a lateral ankle support.

Trials have demonstrated a small benefit of speech and language therapy for the treatment of dysphasia.[6] Patients with expressive dysphasia may be helped by the provision of communication aids. These include simple boards containing pictures or letters to which the patient points. More complex computerised speech-generation devices are also available.

SPASTICITY

'Spasticity' is a term for inappropriate increases in muscular tone. Not only can this cause reduced function of the affected area but also it may result in contracture formation and pain. Additionally, it may make dressing and personal hygiene more difficult (e.g. adequate cleaning of the palmar skin fold of a hand closed by spasticity). Appropriate joint positioning, movement and exercise, and splints or orthoses, can reduce its development. It may be made worse by intercurrent illness, stress/anxiety or medication effects.[11]

Various oral antispasmodic agents have been tried. Benzodiazepines have some efficacy but are rarely used due to associated side-effects. Baclofen is a gamma-aminobutyric acid (GABA) agonist. It has a short half-life of around four hours. Side-effects include sedation, confusion and muscle weakness. Tizanidine appears to be as effective as baclofen but may cause less muscle weakness.[11,12] Its mechanism of action is not well understood but probably involves a norepinephrine alpha-2 agonist action within the spinal cord. It may take up to one week to have its maximal effect.[13] Observed side-effects include somnolence (62%), dizziness (32%), dry mouth (21%) and hypotension (13%).[14] Abnormalities on liver function tests and occasional hallucinations have also been reported.[12]

Non-oral techniques include phenol nerve blocks and botulinum toxin injections. This latter agent blocks the release of acetylcholine at nerve synapses. The toxin is injected directly into the target muscle. The effects last for around three months. It is expensive and may be associated with a flu-like illness immediately after injections. When used in stroke patients to treat wrist and finger spasticity, 62% of the treatment group compared to 27% of the placebo arm reported at least some degree of improvement in severity of spasticity.[15] However, it is unlikely to provide significant functional improvements. Phenol nerve blocks involve the percutaneous injection of phenol into the target nerve. If a nerve that has mixed motor and sensory components is blocked, an area of dysaethesia may develop.[11] The duration of effect is variable.

SWALLOWING
There are four phases described in the process of swallowing.
➤ *Oral preparation*: chewing and mixing with saliva.
➤ *Oral phase*: the bolus of food is moved backwards in the mouth by the tongue.
➤ *Pharyngeal phase*: there is closure of the velopharynx (to block off the nasal cavity) and the larynx (by an upward and anterior movement). There is pharyngeal peristalsis to aid the transit. The food passes the cricopharyngeal muscle to enter the oesophagus.
➤ *Oesophageal phase*: transport to the stomach.

A simple bedside evaluation can be obtained by observing a patient swallowing a teaspoon of water and then asking the patient to give a cough or speak while listening for the moist sound of fluid in the airways or coughing/choking. More descriptive information can be obtained by the use of a videofluoroscopy test. This uses a swallowed radio-opaque substance under X-ray screening to watch the movement of food matter. In this way, a suitable food consistency for patients may also be identified during the test. The presence of a gag reflex is a poor predictor of swallowing ability. It is also absent in a number of normal individuals and can be unpleasant to elicit. For all of these reasons it has no place in the assessment of swallowing.

Parkinson's disease

Various swallowing problems have been associated with Parkinson's disease. They include abnormal tongue control or festination, delayed swallowing reflex and impaired pharyngeal peristalsis.[16] Aspiration may occur without preceding reports of dysphagia. Swallowing improvements do not closely correlate with other motor benefits observed with levodopa. Techniques may be used that allowing mechanical modification of the swallow process. There is some evidence of a benefit.[3]

Stroke

Around 50% of patients have been found to have swallowing abnormalities by clinical testing immediately after admission to hospital because of a stroke, and this value is around 60% when videofluoroscopy testing is used.[17] Screening for swallowing disorders is recommended in all patients following a stroke, and those with impairments should have specialist input.[5] Patients who have difficulty with swallowing on admission should be initially made nil by mouth and started on intravenous fluids. The use of thickened fluids, puréed/soft foods, and techniques such as using a chin tuck during swallowing can reduce the risk of aspiration in vulnerable patients. Around 90% of stroke survivors will return to a normal diet by six months.[17] The management of those patients who are unable to take sufficient oral nutrition is discussed on p. 219.

MOBILITY AIDS

A range of mobility aids has been developed. They typically aim to improve a patient's gait pattern by allowing the support of some body weight through the arms rather than the legs. This may protect a painful, weakened or unstable joint. Balance and confidence may also be benefited. The choice of which aid is most appropriate is usually based on individual patient preferences, ability and lifestyle, plus environmental factors within their discharge destination. Physiotherapists often help in selecting the most appropriate walking aid. Patients may decline, or never use, aids that they feel stigmatise them as disabled.

Sticks

The use of a walking stick provides a wider, and therefore more stable, base. For this purpose two sticks are better than one. They may also allow less weight to be transferred through a limb, so reducing pain. For patients with an antalgic gait (e.g. due to unilateral hip pain) using a single stick there is controversy as to which hand should hold the stick – ipsilateral or contralateral to the painful side. Contralateral usage is less disruptive to the normal gait pattern (the patient tends not to lean over the stick) and provides a wider, more stable, base. But it does not allow as much weight to be transmitted through the stick (and so not through the painful limb) as ipsilateral use.

A stick of correct length should have its handle at the level of the proximal wrist crease when the arm is hanging down at the patient's side. This should create around a 15-degree angle of flexion in the arm when standing still and allow the arm to be straight when planting the stick ahead when walking (to prevent the need to lean forwards). The loss of arm swing seen in patients with Parkinson's disease often means that they are not able to use a walking stick effectively.

Sticks with three or four feet (tri- or tetrapods) are also available. These have wider bases, which can increase stability when walking on the flat. The disadvantage is having a larger stick that can be clumsy in narrow spaces such as doorways, plus they are less stable on uneven surfaces and unsuitable for use on stairs. A Fischer stick has a moulded handle designed to spread weight more evenly. Such a stick is suitable for those with painful hands – e.g. due to arthritis.

A rubber tip on the end can reduce slipping of the stick, but this is less effective in wet or icy conditions. When using a stick on the stairs the free hand should be holding the stair rail. It is advised that the user leads with the good leg when going up and the bad leg when coming down (it might be remembered as 'good up to heaven, bad down to hell').

Crutches

Crutches are usually only for short-term use. They come in three main varieties. Axillary crutches are fitted under the arm. Elbow crutches have retaining cuffs around the forearm, which gives the advantage of making them easier to use on stairs and allows easier door opening by the user. Gutter crutches have supports that allow weight to be transferred through the forearms rather than the hands. They are for use by patients with reduced grip strength. Crutches provide little assistance with balance and so are not usually suitable for frail elderly people.

Frames

Frames have wider bases than either sticks or crutches and so provide the most stable base. The standard 'Zimmer' frame has four feet. The patient lifts the frame forwards and then walks into it. This creates an unnatural stop–start gait pattern. Gutter or pulpit frames provide support for the patient's forearms, which makes them more suitable for those with weakened or painful grips.

An alternative is to have a frame with two wheels replacing the two front feet – a 'rollator' frame. This allows the frame to be pushed forwards over even surfaces, which produces a more natural gait. It also does not have to be lifted, which can help the very frail. Disadvantages include a mild reduction in stability and it tends to be less manoeuvrable in tight spaces. Less stop–start gait is produced, which is particularly helpful for those with Parkinson's disease.

Three- and four-wheeled frames without feet are suitable for patients requiring less support but requiring help with balance (often called delta frames). They promote a more natural, unbroken gait pattern than standard frames. They may come with brakes, shopping baskets and seats (for resting between walking) attached. Larger wheels make them easier to get over outdoor obstacles. They may be foldable to allow easier transport and storage. Such frames may be too bulky for indoor use.

No frames are suitable for use on stairs and patients should not attempt to carry them up and down. Having a frame for upstairs and another for downstairs is an option. The correct height for a frame is such that a patient's elbows are flexed at approximately

15 degrees when holding the handgrips at rest. This should allow the patient to maintain an upright stance while walking.

Wheelchairs

Wheelchairs come in a wide variety according to their planned usage. Factors that need to be considered include indoor, outdoor or mixed use, and self-propelled, pushed or motorised. A folding chair may be necessary for transportation in a car. Chairs with removable armrests allow sideways transfers. Cushioning and support can usually be tailored to the individual patient.

Hoists

There are two main types of hoist: full body hoists where the user's entire weight is taken by the hoist, and standing hoists where the user still transfers some weight through their own legs.

Mobile full body hoists are moved around on wheels and can be used to transfer people in a range of situations. The user is placed within a correctly sized sling. They require two people to be safely operated. They also need adequate storage space and need to be plugged in to maintain charge when not in use. If used within a person's own home, there needs to be sufficient ceiling clearance to allow lifting out of bed (especially if a pressure mattress is being used) plus enough space to get the supporting legs under the bed. They can be fitted with scales to weigh immobile people.

Ceiling hoists are fitted to tracks that run along the ceiling. They require less strength to move the person and less storage space, but obviously they cannot be moved easily to different locations and are more expensive to install.

Standing hoists are used to transfer the user from one seated location to another, for example from chair to toilet. The user stands on a foot rest, a belt sling is placed around their trunk and their knees rest against a specialised support block. They are suitable for people who are able to support the majority of their weight while standing. They are only suitable for transferring short distances. One advantage over full body hoists is the ability to access the patient's clothing such as when toileting. They are usually operated by one person.

A turntable is a non-motorised device to assist transfers. The user stands on the foot rest and pulls themselves up from sitting to standing. The knees rest against specialised pads. Turntables are used for moving from one seat to another (e.g. on to the toilet or in and out of a wheelchair).

HOME ADAPTATIONS

A wide range of simple home environment modifications is available to help older people continue to live safely in their own home. Occupational therapists often advise which would be appropriate – this may follow a visit to the person's home to assess the living environment or accompanied by the patient to assess their function within their own home. Some of the more common examples are discussed below.

Handrails can be fitted next to steps and to both sides of stairways to improve balance. They can also be placed next to toilets and baths to aid getting on/off or in/out.

A raised toilet seat (essentially a plastic ring that sits on top of the normal toilet seat) and a specialised toilet surround (a support frame that is placed around the toilet) can also assist toilet access. Another option is a bedside commode to help at night or a down-stairs commode for during the day if the property lacks a downstairs toilet. Stair lifts can be fitted to properties but they can take time to order and are expensive (although they can be hired). They may not be an option for people in rented properties. Some properties can be adapted to allow downstairs living. However, this does reduce the useful size of a property and is unacceptable to some people.

Ramps may need to be fitted to steps in and out of a property for people who use a wheelchair or frame to mobilise outdoors. A key safe is a locked cupboard fitted near the entrance to a property. Carers can access the key stored within via a coded keypad and then let themselves into the user's home. This is helpful when the person has lim-ited mobility to get up and open the door (e.g. when the carer is coming to help get the person out of bed).

Telecare is a term for systems that connect the user's home to a remote service. This can include alarms (e.g. to warn if gas has been left on) or sensors (e.g. to remotely monitor room temperature to ensure it is not too cold in the winter). A falls alarm is used to summon help when a person has fallen and is unable to get up. They can be activated by pulling fixed cords or from user worn devices (e.g. a button attached like a watch around the wrist or a necklace around the neck). Typically they are linked to a care agency or family member's telephone. Sensors can be used to detect lack of move-ment (e.g. following a fall) or location (e.g. to check if someone is in bed or to detect if someone has wandered out of their home at night).

DISCHARGE
Discharge planning

Discharge from hospital is a major event for a frail elderly person. It requires not only a return of medical stability but also functional and environmental factors. The planning of a discharge should start well in advance of the discharge date and preferably near the start of the hospital admission. It typically involves multiple disciplines within the hospital and several teams in the community. Good communication and co-ordination of services are crucial.

The usual aim is for the patient to return to their previous residence. If there already was a package of care, this will need to be restarted. Depending on the type of care and the care agency involved this may take 48 hours or longer. The organisation of a new care package or a change in the type and frequency of care previously provided may take longer to arrange. Patients who need a change in residence (e.g. going into 24-hour care) will need to have funding decisions made (e.g. privately or state-funded) and will need time to choose an appropriate home (possibly delegating this to a friend or relative).

If a person has stairs at home, they will need to be able to safely practise doing these while in hospital (unless a stairlift is being fitted or downstairs living has been planned). An occupational therapist may need to provide equipment before the discharge date. Medications need to be ordered. The patient should have any changes explained to them and it should be ensured they are able to take the drugs correctly (e.g. inhaler technique). Consideration should be given to the need for medication aids (*see* p. 32) or assistance from others (this could include carers supervising administration or a district nurse attending to give insulin). If unable to go to the shops themselves, it may be necessary to ensure a friend or relative has arranged for food in the person's cupboards and fridge. They may require transportation to get home – either a lift from a friend/relative or hospital transport. Any required follow-up needs to be organised. It is important that all relevant information is passed on to the services that will be taking on caring for the person once back at home.

There may be a need for further rehabilitation in the community. In some circumstances, specialised early discharge teams (including nurses, physiotherapists and occupational therapists) are able to provide rehabilitation to patients within their own homes. This may have the advantage of freeing up hospital beds and allowing patients to be in a preferred environment. The disadvantage may be a reduced access to therapists – typically three times a week or less, rather than daily. Available evidence suggests that they can result in similar outcomes to standard hospital care, but may not have any financial advantage.[18]

COMMUNITY SUPPORT

Packages of care can help people remain in their own homes. In the UK this typically involves one or two carers attending from a care agency between one and four times a day. Examples of the type of support they can give include helping the person get up and dressed, assistance with personal hygiene and prompting to take medications. Some people do not like having strangers visiting their home. Another difficulty can be the periods between visits (e.g. can the client get to the toilet between calls?) and the absence of assistance overnight (e.g. for those with cognitive impairment who tend to wander).

Care homes in the UK are categorised as residential homes (RH) or nursing homes (NH). These are further subdivided into those that do or do not provide specialist care for people with cognitive impairment (termed 'elderly mentally infirm' or EMI). The key difference between RH and NH is that NH have the 24-hour provision of qualified nursing staff on site. RH generally house less disabled residents than NH. Typical criteria for RH care would include the ability to mobilise with the assistance of one person (plus walking aid) or better. NH are able to care for immobile residents and those with greater functional needs such as faecal incontinence. Currently in the UK around 59% of care home residents are aged 85 years or over.[19] The probability of residing in a care home increases with advancing age – around 0.7% of the population aged 65–74, 3% of those aged 75–84, 12% of those aged 85–89 and 25% of those aged 90 and over.[20]

In the UK 'sheltered accommodation' is a form of independent living typically within a group of purpose-built flats or bungalows. They may have communal areas such as laundry facilities and lounge rooms. A scheme manager or warden will live on site or be available through working hours. They can be a reassuring and friendly presence and help arrange appropriate support or help in emergencies but do not provide day-to-day care. Out of hours help may be accessed by a care alarm system. 'Extra care sheltered housing' is a form of sheltered accommodation that also provides carers to assist with personal care.

Intermediate care is a term for services that lie between traditional hospital settings and usual care within the patient's own home. Examples include community hospitals and 'hospital at home' services. They can be used to aid hospital discharge (termed 'step down') or to try to avoid a hospital admission (termed 'step up'). In the UK there is insufficient data to say that these services are either able to reduce length of stay or reduce healthcare costs.[21-23] However, the services do tend to be popular with patients and may have benefits in selected groups.

'Day hospital' is a term for a form of outpatient service that includes multidisciplinary assessment and elements of a day centre environment (e.g. company, activities and lunch provided). There is little trial evidence to support the efficacy of day hospital care.[24] One advantage for patients is the ability to see various disciplines in one visit, for example a doctor, physiotherapist and occupational therapist.

REFERENCES

1 Brown CJ, Redden DT, Flood KL, *et al*. The underrecognized epidemic of low mobility during hospitalization of older adults. *J Am Geriatr Soc*, 2009; **57**: 1660–5.
2 Rice-Oxley M. Effectiveness of brain injury rehabilitation. *Clin Rehabil*, 1999; **13**(Suppl. 1): S7–24.
3 Gage H, Storey L. Rehabilitation for Parkinson's disease: a systematic review of available evidence. *Clin Rehabil*, 2004; **18**: 463–82.
4 Warlow CP. Epidemiology of stroke. *Lancet*, 1998; **352**(Suppl. III): S1–4.
5 Intercollegiate Stroke Working Party. *National Clinical Guideline for Stroke*, 3rd ed. 2008. Available at: www.rcplondon.ac.uk/pubs/contents/6ad05aab-8400-494c-8cf4-9772d1d5301b.pdf
6 Dobkin BH. Rehabilitation after stroke. *N Engl J Med*, 2005; **352**(16): 1677–84.
7 Langhorne P, Taylor G, Murray G, *et al*. Early supported discharge services for stroke patients: a meta-analysis of individual patients' data. *Lancet*, 2005; **365**: 501–6.
8 Kalra L, Evans A, Perez I, *et al*. Training care givers of stroke patients: randomised controlled trial. *BMJ*, 2004; **328**: 1099–1101.
9 Van Peppen RPS, Kwakkel G, Wood-Dauphine S, *et al*. The impact of physical therapy on functional outcomes after stroke: what's the evidence? *Clin Rehabil*, 2004; **18**: 833–62.
10 de Wit DCM, Buurke JH, Nijlant JMM, *et al*. The effect of an ankle-foot orthosis on walking ability in chronic stroke patients: a randomized controlled trial. *Clin Rehabil*, 2004; **18**: 550–7.
11 Barnes MP. Management of spasticity. *Age Ageing*, 1998; **27**: 239–45.
12 Wallace JD. Summary of combined clinical analysis of controlled clinical trials with tizanidine. *Neurology*, 1994; **44**(Suppl. 9): S60–9.
13 The United Kingdom Tizanidine Trial Group. A double-blind, placebo-controlled trial of tizanidine in the treatment of spasticity caused by multiple sclerosis. *Neurology*, 1994; **44**(Suppl. 9): S70–8.
14 Gelber DA, Good DC, Dromerick A, *et al*. Open-label dose-titration safety and efficacy study of tizanidine hydrochloride in the treatment of spasticity associated with chronic stroke. *Stroke*, 2001; **32**: 1841–6.
15 Brashear A, Gordon MF, Elovic E, *et al*. Intramuscular injection of botulinum toxin for the treatment of wrist and finger spasticity after a stroke. *N Engl J Med*, 2002; **347**(6): 395–400.
16 Bushmann M, Dobmeyer SM, Leeker L, *et al*. Swallowing abnormalities and their responses to treatment in Parkinson's disease. *Neurology*, 1989; **39**: 1309–14.

17 Mann G, Dip PG, Hankey GJ, *et al.* Swallowing function after stroke: prognosis and prognostic factors at 6 months. *Stroke*, 1999; **30**(4): 744–8.

18 Shepperd S, Doll H, Broad J, *et al.* Early discharge hospital at home. *Cochrane Database Syst Rev* 2009, Issue 1. Art. No.: CD000356. DOI: 10.1002/14651858.CD000356.pub3.

19 Office for National Statistics. *Changes in the Older Resident Care Home Population between 2001 and 2011.* August 2014. Available at: www.ons.gov.uk/ons/dcp171776_373040.pdf (accessed 11 December 2014).

20 Office of Fair Trading. *Care Homes For Older People in the UK: a market study.* 2005. Available at: www.oft.gov.uk/shared_oft/reports/consumer_protection/oft780.pdf (accessed 11 December 2014).

21 Woodford HJ, George J. Intermediate care for older people in the UK. *Clin Med*, 2010; **10**: 119–23.

22 Purdy S. Avoiding Hospital Admissions: what does the research evidence say? The King's Fund 2010. Available at: www.kingsfund.org.uk/publications/avoiding-hospital-admissions (accessed 19 September 2014).

23 Steventon A, Bardsley M, Billings J, *et al.* An Evaluation of the Impact of Community-based Interventions on Hospital Use. 2011. Available at: www.nuffieldtrust.org.uk/publications/evaluation-impact-community-based-interventions-hospital-use (accessed 19 September 2014).

24 Black DA. The geriatric day hospital. *Age Ageing*, 2005; **34**: 427–9.

CHAPTER 4

Perioperative care

It is increasingly being recognised that frail older people need perioperative care that is tailored to meet their needs. Orthogeriatric services predominantly aimed at improving care following fractured neck of femur have been around for many years and are typically embedded in modern practice (*see* p. 356). More recently it has been accepted that such multidisciplinary care also benefits older people undergoing other types of operation.

Presentations of surgical conditions in older patients are frequently vague (e.g. diarrhoea, vomiting, constipation or wrongly labelled as 'urinary tract infection'), sometimes resulting in patients erroneously being admitted initially to medical wards, which reduces the chance of being assessed by a consultant surgeon and can delay effective treatment.[1,2] Just as frailty limits the ability of an individual to function in times of acute illness, this also applies to the perioperative period. In addition, changes in the skin increase the risk of postoperative infections and can impair wound healing.[3] Patients with poorer functional status are more likely to develop multidrug-resistant surgical wound infections.[4] The frail elderly have a higher risk of adverse postoperative events such as falls and delirium.

Unfortunately there is evidence that surgical care currently provided to frail older people often falls below acceptable standards. In a series of older people (age 80 plus) who died within 30 days of surgery, just 36% were judged by an expert panel to have received good quality care (83% having emergency surgery, 38% following fractured neck of femur and 31% having an abdominal operation).[2] Problems identified included lack of surgical consultant review, delays to operation, suboptimal pain management, lack of nutritional assessment and no geriatrician input prior to discharge.

PREOPERATIVE

Preoperative assessment provides the opportunity to optimise health prior to the stresses of surgery. Clearly this opportunity is greater in those having elective, rather than emergency, procedures. In this latter group, people are acutely ill and limited things can be achieved in the short optimisation period (e.g. fluid resuscitation).

Comprehensive geriatric assessment (CGA)

Given the complex nature of frail older people it is essential to perform a CGA to evaluate their combination of problems (*see* p. 8). Baseline cognitive assessment can provide an insight into the risk and aid early detection of postoperative delirium.

There is evidence that improved implementation of CGA can result in better outcomes. The 'Proactive care of Older People undergoing Surgery' (POPS) system evaluated people aged 65 and over who were within three months of having elective surgery with at least one risk factor (e.g. heart failure, poorly controlled diabetes, on warfarin or evidence of frailty (i.e. cognitive impairment, falls or functional impairment)).[5] The aim was to optimise detected health problems, give advice on exercise and nutrition, do therapy assessments including early discharge planning and provision of relevant equipment in advance. Also there was postoperative review to promote delirium detection, early mobilisation, pain management, nutrition, bowel and bladder function, and discharge planning. Before and after implementation cohorts suggested that POPS was associated with lower rates of postoperative pneumonia (20% before vs 4% after), delirium (19% vs 6%) and pressure ulcers (19% vs 4%). In addition, episodes of poor pain control, inappropriate catheterisation, delays in mobilisation and length of stay all appeared to be reduced.

Basic investigations such as blood tests and an ECG should be performed. Detected abnormalities such as electrolyte disturbances or anaemia can be further evaluated and corrected in advance of the operation. Further investigations may be required to explore health status; for example, echocardiography is usually recommended if clinical examination reveals a murmur suggestive of aortic stenosis.[6]

Health optimisation

For elective surgery it is recommended to provide a medication review (including anticoagulants), exercise plan, and dietary and smoking cessation advice.[7] There is a window of opportunity to review the control of chronic medical conditions, but the time taken to achieve optimal health needs to be weighed against the disadvantages of delaying surgery.[8]

Pre-operative beta-blockade has been suggested as potentially beneficial to those at risk of cardiovascular events. The use of metoprolol compared to placebo in patients with vascular risk factors (e.g. previous vascular disease or diabetes) having non-cardiac surgery has been shown to reduce the incidence of perioperative myocardial infarction (4.2% vs 5.7%), but the overall mortality rate was higher (3.1% vs 2.3%).[9]

Risks vs benefits

In frail older people the risks and benefits of any surgical procedure will need to be explored, with the patient (and/or their next of kin) being provided with all of the available relevant information. There is a need for the assessment and documentation of mental capacity to consent to the procedure.

Evaluation of operative risk can include cardiopulmonary exercise testing. Those with impaired cardiac or respiratory function are more likely to develop complications.[10] A low albumin level is also associated with a worse prognosis.[11] A number of scoring systems have been developed to try to predict risk for undertaking a surgical procedure. The American Society of Anesthesiologists (ASA) developed such a classification system. This ASA five-category scheme is as below.

1. A normal healthy person.
2. A person with mild systemic disease.
3. A person with severe systemic disease.
4. A person with severe systemic disease that is a constant threat to life.
5. A moribund person who is not expected to survive without the operation.

Other, more complex, schemes are available but the ASA scale has the advantage of being simple and quick to calculate. One criticism is the subjective distinction between categories 2, 3 and 4 (that make up the majority of cases) – especially in those with multiple comorbidities of varying severity. There is also a distinction to be made between what is classified as a systemic disease (e.g. diabetes) compared to a local disease (e.g. myocardial infarction), when both are likely to be relevant to risk.

Clearly the mortality risk is also proportional to the operation being proposed, e.g. cataract vs abdominal surgery. Generally it also increases in older age. For example, the operative mortality (deaths within 30 days of surgery or death during the same hospital admission) is shown below for coronary artery bypass graft and colectomy elective procedures.[12]

Age	65–69	75–79	85–99
Coronary artery bypass graft	2.8%	5.1%	8.6%
Colectomy	1.8%	3.2%	7.2%

Regarding emergency surgery in the elderly, no pre-operative risk assessment score has been found to be sufficiently accurate to act as a surrogate for clinical judgement.[13]

Planning the procedure

The pre-operative period also allows for planning of the procedure. There should be early input from anaesthetics and critical care teams. The likely need for a higher level of postoperative care (e.g. high dependency unit 'level 2 care' or intensive therapy unit 'level 3 care') can be judged to ensure that such a bed is available after the operation.

INTRA-OPERATIVE

The risk of dehydration can be reduced by allowing clear fluids to be taken usually up to two hours before surgery.[8] Patients with diabetes or Parkinson's disease (*see* p. 168) need a management plan for while they are nil by mouth (typically in accordance with local protocols). People on warfarin will need to have the anticoagulant effect reversed (i.e. vitamin K) and novel anticoagulants will need to be withheld (*see* p. 408). Depending on the indication, some people will require alternative anticoagulation in the interim (e.g. low molecular weight heparin). A decision also needs to be made on whether to discontinue antiplatelet agents (the elevated bleeding risk of aspirin and clopidogrel typically takes 7 to 10 days to fully reverse). Glasses, hearing aids and dentures should remain in place until just before the procedure to preserve patient dignity.[8] Operative positioning can be made difficult by kyphoscoliosis. Older people have an increased risk of pressure ulcers.

Laryngoscopy may be difficult due to loose dentition, an inflexible cervical spine (osteoarthritis or atlantoaxial subluxation) or temporomandibular joint disease.[14] Movements of the neck can trigger carotid sinus hypersensitivity causing bradycardia or syncope (*see* p. 342). Older patients may have loss of airway protective reflexes, which increases the risk of aspiration.[15]

The doses of any anaesthetic drugs need to be adjusted for the frail elderly. An anaesthetic agent should be chosen that has a higher chance of rapid recovery with minimal adverse effects. As these drugs affect the central nervous system and given changes in pharmacokinetics in older people, there can be a great degree of heterogeneity in their effective dose. The monitoring of depth of anaesthesia can assist. There is uncertainty about whether regional or general anaesthesia is the best option. People with significant cognitive impairment may require large doses of sedation during regional anaesthesia, which can offset any benefit on cognition status from not giving a general anaesthetic. Both techniques are associated with a risk of hypotension.

The use of laparoscopic procedures may lower the risk of complications. A review of 129 patients aged 71 and over (mean age 76 years) found lower morbidity rates with laparoscopic compared to open surgery (24% vs 51%), but 6% of laparoscopic patients required conversion to open procedures.[16] Laparoscopic operations may take longer and this has to be balanced against the possible shorter recovery time.

Intra-operative monitoring can aid decision making. Intra-arterial blood pressure monitoring can more rapidly detect hypotension (aim for no more than a 20% drop from baseline and not below 90 mmHg). Central venous pressure monitoring can also be helpful. Cardiac output monitoring (e.g. oesophageal Doppler) may be less accurate in older people.[8] It is possible to monitor cerebral oxygen saturation. Bispectral index monitors or entropy monitors can gauge depth of anaesthesia, which is used to judge the correct dose of anaesthetic agents and reduce the risk of adverse events. Alternatively a Lerou nomogram can be used to calculate the dose of inhalation anaesthetic agent. Peripheral nerve stimulation can be used to monitor neuromuscular function when neuromuscular blocking drugs are being used. A urinary catheter is likely to be required perioperatively to carefully monitor fluid balance.

Hypotension

Frail older people are at increased risk of organ ischaemia during surgery (particularly the heart and brain). It is imperative to ensure appropriate oxygenation and avoid hypotension. Frailty is associated with a reduced maximal heart rate and so tachycardia may not be such a helpful guide. Intra-arterial blood pressure monitoring should be considered. The treatment of hypotension is with a combination of intravenous fluids, inotropes and vasoconstrictor drugs. Avoiding dehydration also reduces the risk of thromboembolism.

Hypothermia

Perioperative hypothermia is common and is associated with delirium, cardiac dysfunction and impaired wound healing.[8] Frail older people are at an increased risk due to reduced muscle mass (i.e. shivering is less effective) and impaired thermoregulation (e.g. reduced vasoconstriction ability in the peripheral circulation).

Its prevention requires regular temperature measurement and correction (e.g. forced air warming or warmed intravenous fluids). This will need to be continued in the postoperative period.

The systematic approach term 'Enhanced Recovery After Surgery' (ERAS) may improve outcomes (see www.erassociety.org, accessed December 2014). It has four key elements: comprehensive preoperative evaluation, optimal anaesthesia and minimally invasive techniques, postoperative care (pain control and early mobilisation), and rapid resumption of normal diet. This is very intensive and requires significant nursing and therapy input and typically also involves the regular input of geriatricians on surgical units.

POSTOPERATIVE

Older frail patients often survive major operations only to die from a complication which could have been prevented by high quality shared postoperative care. It is recommended that daily input from geriatricians should be available to elderly people undergoing surgery.[2]

Postoperative acute kidney injury can be avoided by appropriate perioperative fluids. But excessive administration of fluids leading to water, sodium and chloride overload is also a recognised cause of increased postoperative morbidity and mortality. The prescription of fluids is often delegated to the most junior member of the clinical team. Postoperative oliguria is a common phenomenon and should not alone be used to judge fluid status, which is best assessed by a combination of factors including trends in pulse and blood pressure, capillary refill and jugular venous pressure. It is recommended that physiologically balanced solutions (e.g. Hartmann's or Ringer's) should be used in preference to normal saline in most situations. The exception to this is where excess chloride loss is anticipated (e.g. vomiting or gastric drainage). Dextrose saline or 5% dextrose pose a risk of hyponatraemia in the elderly.[17] The aim is to return to normal oral food and fluid intake as soon as possible following the surgery.

Vigilance is required to detect delirium as soon as possible following surgery. This should begin in the recovery room. Pain has been described as the 'fifth vital sign' to emphasise the importance of its effective detection and management.[2] Paracetamol is generally considered a first-line drug given its lack of side-effects. NSAIDs are associated with multiple problems in frail older people (see p. 28) and opiates are usually considered a safer option.[18] There is evidence that pain is less well managed in older people (see p. 357). Early ambulation is vital to minimise the risk of pressure ulcers, hypostatic pneumonia and muscle loss.

Outcomes

The postoperative mortality rate for non-cardiac surgery in patients aged over 80 years is around 5%, with a morbidity rate around 25%.[19] Surgery has a higher risk for those with comorbidities (especially cardiac disease) and those requiring major emergency procedures. This group has a mortality rate around 12% and they account for 84% of all surgical deaths.[20] Predictors of postoperative complications other than older age include high body mass index (>25), chronic obstructive pulmonary disease and longer operation times.[21] Frailty is also a risk factor for postoperative complications, as is longer length of stay and discharge to a care home.[22]

The risk of postoperative cognitive adverse effects is higher in the frail and those with baseline cognitive dysfunction. Postoperative delirium has been detected in 13% of those aged over 65 years undergoing surgery (emergency or elective), but this study excluded those with pre-existing dementia so the true incidence may have been higher.[23] Another group has reported that around 55% of patients aged over 65 undergoing non-cardiac surgery develop delirium in the first two days after their operation.[24] Older age (>75 years), multiple comorbidities, cognitive impairment, depression and abnormal glycaemic control are linked with greater risk. Delirium is associated with longer lengths of stay and increased mortality rates. Higher rates of delirium have been detected in those following surgery for fractured neck of femur (*see* p. 128). Route of anaesthesia does not seem to be an important factor.[25] Avoiding hypoxia, correcting fluid and electrolyte imbalances, controlling pain, rationalising medications and the early restoration of nutritional intake and mobility can reduce the incidence of postoperative delirium.[26] The diagnosis and management of delirium is discussed in Chapter 7.

Postoperative cognitive decline (POCD) is a reported sub-acute to chronic hazard of surgery that differs from delirium, possibly induced by perioperative cerebral hypoxia. Cognitive decline following coronary artery bypass graft surgery of one standard deviation or more in any cognitive domain has been detected in 53% of patients at discharge, and 24% at six months.[27] A study had estimated it to have a prevalence of around 10% three months after major non-cardiac surgery in people aged over 60 years.[28] However, more recent data that assessed pre-operative cognitive function and compared to controls did not find a significant association.[29] So uncertainty surrounds the phenomenon of POCD at the current time.[30]

ABDOMINAL PAIN

Abdominal pain accounts for approximately 3–6% of emergency department visits in people aged over 65 years.[31,32] Around 10–37% of these patients require acute surgical intervention.[32-36] Older patients have higher rates of surgery and mortality than younger cases.[37] They can be a challenging group to assess.[2,38] It should be remembered that abdominal pain can occasionally be the presenting complaint of patients with non-abdominal disorders (e.g. myocardial infarction). Urinary retention should also be considered, especially in elderly men.

Diagnosis

Surgical problems, like many other conditions in frail older people, are likely to present in an atypical way (i.e. not the textbook description seen in younger people). The initial diagnostic accuracy is lower in older adults compared to younger, falling from around 45–55% in young adults, to 29–44% in those aged 80 and over.[39,40] Inaccurate initial diagnosis puts patients at greater risk of morbidity.[41] Serious problems that are frequently initially misdiagnosed include ischaemic bowel, malignancy and pancreatitis.[42]

Presenting temperature and serum white blood cell counts have been found to be poor markers to detect the patients that required surgical intervention.[34] In a group of patients aged 80 and over (mean age 85 years) with acute abdominal pain requiring operation, 30% had a temperature <37.5°C and a serum white cell count (WCC) $<10.5 \times 10^9/L$.[43] Compared to those aged 64 and under, patients aged 80 and above who required surgical intervention were less likely to been found to have rebound tenderness (29 vs 62%), rectal tenderness (18 vs 32%) or abdominal rigidity (34 vs 43%).[40] Guarding and rebound tenderness sometimes only present late in the disease and may herald perforation or gangrene.[44] The reduced association with muscular guarding could also be explained by reduced muscle size and strength secondary to sarcopenia.

Atypical presentations

A review reported the presenting clinical features of 168 patients aged over 65 (mean age 74 years) with acute cholecystitis who required urgent cholecystectomy.[45] Overall 65% had right upper quadrant pain, 5% had no pain, 56% were apyrexial (<37.0°C) and 41% had a normal serum WCC. Nausea and vomiting are less commonly reported by older patients and Murphy's sign has a lower sensitivity.[46,47]

Large bowel obstruction is most commonly due to malignancy, diverticulitis or volvulus.[44,48,49] In the frail elderly it may also be caused by faecal impaction. The onset can be gradual over several days with non-specific initial symptoms. Volvulae cause around 15% of large bowel obstructions in older patients. They are more likely to occur in people taking laxatives, sedatives, anticholinergics or anti-Parkinsonian medications. Another possibility is acute pseudo-obstruction of the colon (also known as 'Ogilvie's syndrome'), which is characterised by massive dilatation of the large bowel in the absence of a true blockage. It is due to impairment of the autonomic nervous system. Overall it is a rare condition, but more common in the elderly.[50] It is associated with neurodegenerative conditions (e.g. Parkinson's disease and Alzheimer's dementia), electrolyte disturbances (e.g. hypokalaemia and hypomagnesaemia), postoperative patients and some medications (e.g. anticholinergics and opiates).[51]

Bowel perforation due to peptic ulcers has fallen in incidence following the widespread use of medications such as proton pump inhibitors. Compared to people aged below 65 years, those 65 and over are less likely to have classic epigastric pain (59% vs 85%), less likely to have a history of peptic ulcer disease (55% vs 68%), less likely to have epigastric tenderness and guarding (24% vs 70%), but more likely to be shocked (BP<90 mmHg) (21% vs 2%).[1] Mortality rates for those requiring emergency surgery following perforated peptic ulcers is around 27% for those aged 70–79, and 45% for those aged 80 and over.[52]

The classic presentation of appendicitis is a combination of right lower abdominal pain, fever (>37.6°C), raised serum WCC (>10 ×10⁹/L), nausea and vomiting. Among elderly patients this occurs in only around 15–30% of cases.[53,54] Right lower quadrant pain is present in 70–75%, fever (>37.6°C) in 23–37%, and a raised WCC (>10 ×10⁹/L) in 74–78%.

Another study found that 30% of patients (n=152, mean age 70 years) presenting with a ruptured abdominal aortic aneurysm were initially misdiagnosed.[55] Only 9% of this group of patients had all three symptoms of abdominal pain, back pain and a pulsatile mass.

Prognosis

Mortality rates for patients admitted with acute abdominal pain are higher in older than younger patients, reaching 5–7% in those aged 80 and over.[39,40] The prognosis is worse in those who require surgery. Around 10–20% of gastrointestinal surgery is performed on patients over the age of 75.[56] Compared to people age 55 and below, mortality rates are higher (4–5% vs <1%) and complications are more frequent (including pulmonary emboli, pneumonia, acute kidney injury, myocardial infarction and stroke). This is particularly true for patients requiring emergency rather than elective surgery. The reasons for this include a lack of time for thorough evaluation and to correct physiological abnormalities (e.g. shock, electrolyte disorders and acidosis).

In a group of patients aged over 80 (n=215, mean age 84 years) having surgery, morbidity and mortality rates of 49% and 14% were described overall.[11] Mortality was 19% in those having emergency procedures, compared to 8% in the elective group. Another study found a mortality rate after emergency abdominal surgery in patients aged 65 and over (n=92, mean age 73) of 15%.[57] One series of patients aged 80 and over (n=132, mean age 85 years) who were admitted to hospital with acute abdominal disorders found a perioperative mortality rate of 34%.[41] However, another series of patients aged 85 and over (n=179, mean age 89 years) having abdominal surgery (64% emergency procedures) found a mortality rate of 17%.[58] And a review of 32 patients aged 90+ who underwent surgery found an overall mortality rate of 9% (elective cases 0%, emergency 14%).[59] These data show quite wide variation, suggesting that appropriate patient selection is of key importance.

REFERENCES

1 Kum CK, Chong YS, Koo CC, *et al.* Elderly patients with perforated peptic ulcers: factors affecting morbidity and mortality. *J R Coll Surg Edinb*, 1993; **38**: 344–7.

2 Wilkinson K, Martin IC, Gough MJ, *et al. An Age Old Problem: a review of the care received by elderly patients undergoing surgery.* NCEPOD, November 2010. Available at: www.ncepod.org.uk/2010eese.htm (accessed 14 December 2014).

3 Aschkenasy MT, Rothenhaus TC. Trauma and falls in the elderly. *Emerg Med Clin N Am*, 2006; **24**: 413–32.

4 Chen T, Anderson DJ, Chopra T, *et al.* Poor functional status is an independent predictor of surgical site infections due to Methicillin-Resistant *Staphylococcus aureus* in older adults. *J Am Geriatr Soc*, 2010; **58**: 527–32.

5 Harari D, Hopper A, Dhesi J, *et al.* Proactive care of older people undergoing surgery ('POPS'): designing, embedding, evaluating and funding a comprehensive geriatric assessment service for older elective surgical patients. *Age Ageing*, 2007; **36**: 190–6.

6 Scottish Intercollegiate Guidelines Network. *Management of Hip Fracture in Older People.* June 2009. Available at: www.sign.ac.uk/pdf/sign111.pdf (accessed 14 December 2014).

7 Dodds C, Foo I, Jones K, *et al.* Peri-operative care of elderly patients – an urgent need for change: a consensus statement to provide guidance for specialist and non-specialist anaesthetists. *Perioperative Med*, 2013; **2**: 6.

8 Association of Anaesthetists of Great Britain and Ireland. Peri-operative care of the elderly 2014. *Anaesthesia*, 2014; **69**(Suppl.): S81–98.

9 POISE Study Group. Effects of extended-release metoprolol succinate in patients undergoing non-cardiac surgery (POISE trial): a randomised-controlled trial. *Lancet*, 2008; **371**: 1839–47.

10 Gerson MC, Hurst JM, Hertzberg VS, *et al.* Prediction of cardiac and pulmonary complications related to elective abdominal and noncardiac thoracic surgery in geriatric patients. *Am J Med*, 1990; **88**: 101–7.

11 Huang T, Hu F, Fan C, *et al.* A simple novel model to predict hospital mortality, surgical site infection, and pneumonia in elderly patients undergoing operation. *Dig Surg*, 2010; **27**: 224–31.

12 Finlayson EVA, Birkmeyer JD. Operative mortality with elective surgery in older adults. *Eff Clin Pract*, 2001; **4**: 172–7.

13 Rix TE, Bates TE. Pre-operative risk scores for the prediction of outcome in elderly people who require emergency surgery. *World J Emerg Surg*, 2006; **2**: 16.

14 Marang AT, Sikka R. Resuscitation of the elderly. *Emerg Med Clin N Am*, 2006; **24**: 261–72.

15 Buxbaum JL, Schwartz AJ. Perianaesthetic considerations for the elderly patient. *Surg Clin N Am*, 1994; **74**: 41–58.

16 Tei M, Ikeda M, Haraguchi N, *et al.* Postoperative complications in elderly patients with colorectal cancer: comparison of open and laparoscopic surgical procedures. *Surg Laparosc Endosc Percutan Tech*, 2009; **19**: 488–92.

17 Lane N, Allen K. Hyponatraemia after orthopaedic surgery. *BMJ*, 1999; **318**: 1363–4.

18 Abdulla A, Adams N, Bone M, *et al.* on behalf of the British Geriatrics Society. Guidance on the management of pain in older people. *Age Ageing*, 2013; **42**(Suppl. 1): S1–42.

19 Liu LL, Leung JM. Predicting adverse postoperative outcomes in patients aged 80 years or older. *J Am Geriatr Soc*, 2000; **48**: 405–12.

20 Pearse RM, Harrison DA, James P, *et al.* Identification and characterisation of the high-risk surgical population in the United Kingdom. *Critical Care*, 2006, **10**: R81 (doi:10.1186/cc4928).

21 Kennedy GD, Rajamanickam V, O'Connor ES, *et al.* Optimizing surgical care of colon cancer in the older adult population. *Ann Surg*, 2011; **253**: 508–14.

22 Makary MA, Segev DL, Pronovost PJ, *et al.* Frailty as a predictor of surgical outcomes in older patients. *J Am Coll Surg*, 2010; **210**: 901–8.

23 Ansaloni L, Catena F, Chattat R, *et al.* Risk factors and incidence of postoperative delirium in elderly patients after elective and emergency surgery. *Br J Surg*, 2010; **97**: 273–80.

24 Leung JM, Sands LP, Paul S, *et al.* Does postoperative delirium limit the use of patient-controlled analgesia in older surgical patients? *Anesthesiol*, 2009; **111**: 625–31.

25 Marcantonio ER, Goldman L, Orav EJ, *et al.* The association of intraoperative factors with the development of postoperative delirium. *Am J Med*, 1998; **105**: 380–4.

26 Marcantonio ER, Flacker JM, Wright RJ, *et al.* Reducing delirium after hip fracture: a randomized trial. *J Am Geriatr Soc*, 2001; **49**: 516–22.

27 Newman MF, Kirchner JL, Phillips-Bute B, *et al.* Longitudinal assessment of neurocognitive function after coronary-artery bypass surgery. *N Engl J Med*, 2001; **344**: 395–402.

28 Moller JT, Cluitmans P, Rasmussen LS, *et al.* Long-term postoperative cognitive dysfunction in the elderly: ISPOCD1 study. Lancet, 1998; **351**: 857–61.

29 Avidan MS, Searleman AC, Storandt M, *et al.* Long-term cognitive decline in older subjects was not attributable to noncardiac surgery or major illness. *Anesthesiol*, 2009; **111**: 964–70.

30 Avidan MS, Evers AS. Review of clinical evidence for persistent cognitive decline or incident dementia attributable to surgery or general anesthesia. *J Alzheimers Dis*, 2011; **24**: 201–16.

31 Wofford JL, Schwartz E, Timerding BL, *et al.* Emergency department utilization by the elderly: analysis of the National Hospital Ambulatory Medical Care Survey. *Acad Emerg Med*, 1996; **3**: 694–9.

32 Marco CA, Schoenfeld CN, Keyl PM, *et al.* Abdominal pain in geriatric emergency patients: variables associated with adverse outcomes. *Acad Emerg Med*, 1998; **5**: 1163–8.

33 Bugliosi TF, Meloy TD, Vukov LF. Acute abdominal pain in the elderly. *Ann Emerg Med*, 1990; **19**: 1383–6.

34 Parker JS, Vukov LF, Wollan PC. Abdominal pain in the elderly: use of temperature and laboratory testing to screen for surgical disease. *Fam Med*, 1996; **28**: 193–7.

35 Kizer KW, Vassar MJ. Emergency department diagnosis of abdominal disorders in the elderly. *Am J Emerg Med*, 1998; **7**: 357–62.

36 Lewis LM, Banet GA, Blanda M, *et al.* Etiology and clinical course of abdominal pain in senior patients: a prospective, multicenter study. *J Gerontol*, 2005; **60A**: 1071–6.

37 Hustey FM, Meldon SW, Banet GA, *et al.* The use of abdominal computed tomography in older ED patients with acute abdominal pain. *Am J Emerg Med*, 2005; **23**: 259–65.

38 Kamin RA, Nowicki TA, Courtney DS, *et al.* Pearls and pitfalls in the emergency department evaluation of abdominal pain. *Emerg Med Clin N Am*, 2003; **21**: 61–72.

39 de Dombal FT. Acute abdominal pain in the elderly. *J Clin Gastroenterol*, 1994; **19**: 331–5.

40 Laurell H, Hansson LE, Gunnarsson U. Acute abdominal pain among elderly patients. *Gerontol*, 2006; **52**: 339–44.

41 van Geloven AAW, Biesheuvel TH, Luitse JSK, *et al.* Hospital admissions of patients aged over 80 with acute abdominal complaints. *Eur J Surg*, 2000; **166**: 866–71.

42 Abi-Hanna P, Gleckman R. Acute abdominal pain: a medical emergency in older patients. *Geriatrics*, 1997; **52**: 72–4.

43 Potts FE, Vukov LF. Utility of fever and leukocytosis in acute surgical abdomens in octogenarians and beyond. *J Gerontol*, 1999; **54A**: M55–8.

44 Sanson TG, O'Keefe KP. Evaluation of abdominal pain in the elderly. *Emerg Med Clin N Am*, 1996; **14**: 615–27.

45 Parker LJ, Vukov LF, Wollan PC. Emergency department evaluation of geriatric patients with acute cholecystitis. *Acad Emerg Med*, 1997; **4**: 51–5.

46 Hendrickson M, Naparst TR. Abdominal emergencies in the elderly. *Emerg Med Clin N Am*, 2003; **21**: 937–69.

47 Martinez JP, Mattu A. Abdominal pain in the elderly. *Emerg Med Clin N Am*, 2006; **24**: 371–8.

48 Lyon C, Clark DC. Diagnosis of acute abdominal pain in older patients. *Am Fam Physician*, 2006; **74**: 1537–44.

49 Martinez JP, Mattu A. Abdominal pain in the elderly. *Emerg Clin N Am*, 2006; **24**: 371–88.

50 Tack J. Acute colonic pseudo-obstruction (Ogilvie's syndrome). *Curr Treat Options Gastroenterol*, 2006; **9**: 361–8.

51 De Giorgio R, Knowles CH. Acute colonic pseudo-obstruction. *Br J Surg*, 2009; **96**: 229–39.

52 Su Y, Yeh C, Lee C, *et al.* Acute surgical treatment of perforated peptic ulcer in the elderly patients. *Hepato-gastroenterol*, 2010; **57**: 1608–13.

53 Storm-Dickerson TL, Horattas MC. What have we learned over the past 20 years about appendicitis in the elderly? *Am J Surgery*, 2003; **185**: 198–201.

54 Paranjape C, Dalia S, Pan J, *et al.* Appendicitis in the elderly: a change in the laparoscopic era. *Surg Endosc*, 2007; **21**: 777–81.

55 Marston WA, Ahlquist R, Johnson G, *et al.* Misdiagnosis of ruptured abdominal aortic aneurysms. *J Vasc Surg*, 1992; **16**: 17–22.

56 Bentrem DJ, Cohen ME, Hynes DM, *et al.* Identification of specific quality improvement opportunities for the elderly undergoing gastrointestinal surgery. *Arch Surg*, 2009; **144**: 1013–20.

57 Ozkan E, Fersahoglu MM, Dulundu E, *et al.* Factors affecting mortality and morbidity in emergency abdominal surgery in geriatric patients. *Turkish J Trauma Emerg Surg*, 2010; **16**: 439–44.

58 Mirbagheri N, Dark JG, Watters DAK. How do patients aged 85 and older fare with abdominal surgery? *J Am Geriatr Soc*, 2010; **58**: 104–8.

59 Rigberg D, Cole M, Hiyama D, *et al.* Surgery in the nineties. *Am Surg*, 2000; **66**: 813–6.

CHAPTER 5

Palliative care

Palliative care is the treatment of advanced, incurable disease. This includes planning for death and may extend to bereavement support. Its main aims are excellent symptom control coupled with excellent communication with patients and their carers to maximise quality of life. Its purpose is neither to shorten life nor to prolong the dying process. A thorough review of all aspects of the specialty is beyond the scope of this book. Here a brief review of the management of some of the specific problems of palliative care is presented. For those in search of further information, a useful, free online resource is available at: learning.hospiceuk.org (accessed December 2014).

Traditionally the focus for this specialty has been on cancer care, but more recently this has extended into other conditions, such as heart failure, dementia and Parkinson's disease. There are many similarities with standard geriatric management, including the involvement of team members from different disciplines, the implementation of goal setting and the use of intermediary care facilities (day centre, respite and rehabilitation units). Currently, around two-thirds of deaths in the UK occur within standard hospitals[1] and the majority of these are older people. The care of dying patients should be inherent to our practice. Palliative care services augment this role by providing expert assistance with difficult symptom control and additional resources, such as community teams, enabling patients to die at home.

Many barriers to effective management of dying patients within hospitals exist. These include the fundamental hospital culture of investigating until a definitive diagnosis has been made, and persevering with interventions even when they are likely to be futile.[1] In the past, healthcare professionals, often in conjunction with families' wishes, have avoided revealing the true facts during discussions with the terminally ill. However, studies suggest that openness and honesty are the best strategies in the longer term.[2] It is, of course, unethical to withhold or give dishonest information to patients when asked.

A 'GOOD' DEATH

Recognising that a patient is dying and communicating this to them and their relatives is a key step towards achieving optimal care.[1] This can be relatively easy in some conditions with a more predictable trajectory (e.g. cancer) but harder in conditions with periods of exacerbation and remission (e.g. heart failure) or a prolonged period of gradual deterioration (e.g. frailty and dementia).[3]

Recognising the dying process allows appropriate planning to be made – both medical and social. Several processes should take place, including the discontinuation of unnecessary medications (e.g. statins for long-term cardiovascular risk reduction) and investigations (e.g. blood tests and vital signs). Essential drugs may need to be given via the subcutaneous route (e.g. in the presence of poor swallowing or vomiting). Anticipatory medications to cover common symptoms in the dying process should be prescribed on an 'as required' basis for all patients (e.g. analgesic, anxiolytic, antiemetic and secretion-reducing drugs).[3]

A plan of care that respects religious and spiritual needs can also be formulated in conjunction with the patient and their relatives. Issues regarding nutrition, hydration and resuscitation can be discussed (*see* later). Good mouth care is an important component, and can also be a process in which family members can be involved. All of this should occur in conjunction with optimal symptom control.

PAIN

'Pain' is a broad term for an unpleasant sensation that may have many different causations and mechanisms. The various subgroups respond to differing degrees to treatment modalities, for example bone pain, neuropathic pain and the pain of muscular spasm do not always improve with opiate therapy. A patient may have many different pains with different causes, and a careful history to elucidate all of the components is required. Emotional factors such as anger, depression or anxiety may also be involved.[4] Dying in pain is a significant fear for many patients. Yet it has commonly been found that relatives judge their loved one to be in discomfort in their final days of life despite palliative care input.[5]

Regular medication to prevent pain is far superior to allowing a patient to suffer pain prior to receiving 'as required' medication. 'Breakthrough' analgesia is additional medication that is given on top of the background analgesia at times when pain intensity increases. A common method of dose titration is to start with a low dose of four-hourly short-acting agents (such as morphine liquid) plus breakthrough doses.[4] After a period on this regimen, the total medication used can be converted to an equivalent dose of a regular longer-acting drug plus breakthrough short-acting doses. The assessment of symptoms is then repeated and doses titrated until pain control is achieved.

Analgesic agents are often used in combination. They are increased in a step-wise fashion as outlined in the World Health Organization analgesic ladder (*see* Figure 5.1) until pain control is achieved.[6] Adjuvant agents may be used in some circumstances. These include steroids for raised intracranial pressure and nerve compression, bisphosphonates for bone pain and antidepressants or anticonvulsants for neuropathic pain (*see* below).[4]

Opiates act at receptors at the terminal end of pain fibres within the dorsal columns of the spinal cord. The medium strength opiate agent tramadol also has non-opiate, mainly serotonergically mediated, properties (it may precipitate the serotonin syndrome when combined with other drugs – *see* p. 144). NSAIDs act by preventing the

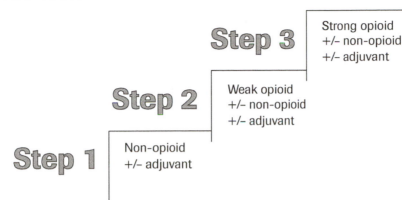

FIGURE 5.1 The World Health Organization analgesic ladder: reach the maximum dose of each agent before moving to the next step.

formation of prostaglandins at sites of inflammation. The mechanism of action of paracetamol is poorly understood.

Opiates

Standard-release morphine is usually started orally at low doses (2.5 mg to 5 mg) given four-hourly and 'breakthrough' doses are also given as required (typically at dose of approximately a sixth to a tenth of the total daily morphine dose). According to the requirements for additional medication, the regular doses can be adjusted. Once a stable dose has been reached, it can be converted to the equivalent amount as a slow-release formulation (given twice daily).

There is no pharmacological logic in combining weak (e.g. codeine) and strong opioid (e.g. morphine) agents. Side-effects include sedation, nausea/vomiting and constipation. The nausea and vomiting may settle after several days of therapy, but anti-emetics may be initially required. There is some evidence that different opiates may cause differing degrees of constipation. In a non-randomised study, transdermal fentanyl use was associated with lesser requirement for aperients than oral morphine.[7] When constipation is opiate-induced, there is some evidence from studies in younger people that orally taken inhibitors of opiate receptors (e.g. naloxone) that have poor systemic absorption may be beneficial without significantly affecting pain control.[8,9] In frail older people consideration should be given to co-prescribing laxative medications when starting opiates due to the high risk of developing constipation. Oxycodone and hydromorphone are alternative strong opioid drugs that may have different side-effect profiles in selected patients.

Tolerance and addiction are not seen in the context of acute pain. Toxicity can cause a delirium and myoclonic jerks.[4] Warning signs of toxicity include pinpoint pupils and oversedation.[10] The risk is increased in those with renal impairment and smaller, less frequent doses are usually required in such patients.

Subcutaneous administration is suitable for patients unable to take oral morphine. Diamorphine has the advantage of being extremely soluble in small volumes of liquid and is therefore ideal for use with a subcutaneous infusion pump. The required dose is estimated by dividing the total daily morphine dose by three.[10] As required break-through doses should also be prescribed.

Transdermal fentanyl (patch changed every 72 hours) and transdermal buprenor-phine (patch changed every four to seven days depending on preparation) are alternative options for those unable to take oral medication. Disadvantages of this approach are that it takes up to 24 hours to reach a steady plasma drug level and drug levels will take a while to fall after patch removal in those who experience adverse effects.[10] The available doses of the patches is also limited, making titration more difficult. Drug absorption can be increased in febrile patients who have increased blood flow to the skin.

Table 5.1 shows an approximate dose conversion chart to aid the switching between differing opiate medications.

TABLE 5.1 Approximate equivalent opiate drug doses for comparison to total oral morphine dose over 24 hours.

Drug	Conversion factor	Example
Oral morphine	Total dose over 24 hours	30 mg modified release morphine bd = 60 mg
Subcutaneous morphine	Divide 24 hour oral morphine dose by 2	60 mg oral morphine = 30 mg subcutaneous morphine over 24 hours
Subcutaneous diamorphine	Divide 24 hour oral morphine dose by 3	60 mg oral morphine = 20 mg subcutaneous diamorphine over 24 hours
Codeine or tramadol	Multiply 24 hour oral morphine dose by 10	60 mg qds codeine = 24 mg oral morphine over 24 hours
		100 mg qds tramadol = 40 mg oral morphine over 24 hours
Oxycodone	Multiply 24 hour oral morphine dose by 2/3	60 mg oral morphine = 40 mg oxycodone over 24 hours
Hydromorphone	Divide 24 hour oral morphine dose by 5	60 mg oral morphine = 12 mg hydromorphone over 24 hours
Buprenorphine 5 patch (releasing 5 mcg/hour for seven days)	–	Buprenorphine 5 patch = 12 mg morphine per day
Fentanyl 12 patch (releasing 12 mcg/hour for three days)	–	Fentanyl 12 patch = 30 mg morphine per day

Neuropathic pain

Neuropathic pain is caused by damage to nerves, resulting in their abnormal function. Figure 5.2 outlines the key differences between nociceptive and this type of pain. It may be attributed to a wide range of aetiologies and may be either peripheral (e.g. trigeminal neuralgia) or central (e.g. post-stroke pain). The pain may be provoked by a stimulus or may occur spontaneously. Stimuli causing pain may be normally non-noxious (allodynia) or may be an exaggerated response to a mildly noxious stimulus (hyperalgesia). The history may elucidate the particular characteristics of neuropathic pain, which is often described with terms such as 'burning', 'shooting' and 'tingling'.

The underlying cause may be identified (e.g. history of diabetes or shingles). The distribution of pain will guide towards the causative structures. Examination may reveal a region of altered sensation (either increased or reduced) in the region of the pain. Other neurological signs may suggest the underlying mechanism (e.g. stroke or Parkinson's disease).

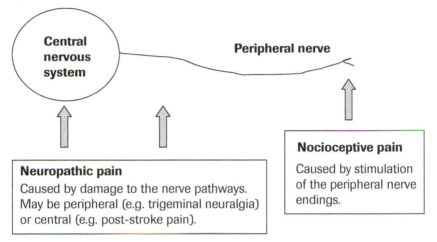

FIGURE 5.2 The sites of causation of nocioceptive and neuropathic pain.

Treatment

Control of the symptoms of neuropathic pain can be difficult and may take some time to achieve. An adequate trial of therapy will take at least two weeks once a therapeutic dose is attained. Pharmacological management must be linked with patient education and reassurance. Non-pharmacological strategies may also play a role. Given the diverse nature of neuropathic pain and the multiple possible treatment combinations, the best management strategy for all situations is not well established. What works well in one patient may be ineffective in another. The approaches most likely to be beneficial are listed in Table 5.2.

TABLE 5.2 Techniques for controlling neuropathic pain.

Method	Comments
Tricyclic antidepressants (TCAs)	Usually as a low dose given at night (*see* p. 141)
Anticonvulsants (e.g. gabapentin and carbamazepine)	Action probably due to glutamate inhibition within the central nervous system (CNS)
Capsaicin cream	Useful for localised pain in people intolerant of, or wanting to avoid, oral treatments. May cause initial burning sensation
Lidocaine gel or patches	May have a role in peripherally caused pains
Opiates	Not usually effective alone for this type of pain; may be used in combination with other agents
Tramadol	Has some additional serotonergic-type action similar to TCAs

(continued)

Method	Comments
Ketamine	Originally an anaesthetic agent. *N*-methyl-D-aspartate (NMDA) blocking action; used in low doses for pain control, under specialist supervision
Spinal analgesia	For severe pains unresponsive to less invasive measures; patients may be able to be managed in the community with spinal catheters connected to syringe-driver infusions for periods of several months
Nerve blocks	When a single causative, peripheral nerve can be identified
Transcutaneous electrical nerve stimulation (TENS)	Not effective in all patients, but non-invasive and with few side-effects

A recent NICE guideline recommends starting with one of amitriptyline, duloxetine, gabapentin or pregabalin as initial treatment for neuropathic pain (except trigeminal neuralgia where carbamazepine is recommended).[11] If the first drug is either ineffective or not tolerated, one of the other three drugs should be tried, and so on. More than one modality may be needed to control symptoms. A trial has suggested that the combination of gabapentin and morphine might be superior to either agent alone.[12]

The assessment of response to treatment may be helped by using a standard 0–10 scale (0 = no pain, 10 = worst pain ever experienced). Specific scales for the assessment of neuropathic pain have also been developed.[13]

NAUSEA AND VOMITING

Nausea and vomiting are common symptoms encountered in palliative care caused by a variety of mechanisms. Constipation may be a reversible underlying element (*see*

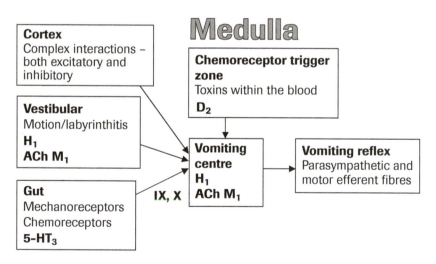

FIGURE 5.3 Pathways involved in the vomiting reflex.
H1 = histamine type 1 receptor, ACh M1 = acetylcholine muscarinic receptor type 1, 5-HT3 = serotonin type 3 receptor, D2 = dopamine type 2 receptor, IX = glossopharyngeal nerve, X = vagus nerve.

Chapter 12). Components of the vomiting pathway and the most important associated receptors are shown in Figure 5.3. Anti-emetic drugs should be targeted towards the most likely receptor group involved in symptom genesis. Steroids (e.g. dexamethasone) may be beneficial if the nausea/vomiting is caused by intracranial oedema secondary to a cerebral tumour or metastases. Listed below are some example drugs with actions at the associated receptor type:

➤ histamine – cyclizine
➤ acetylcholine – hyoscine
➤ serotonin – ondansetron
➤ dopamine – haloperidol, metoclopramide and domperidone (peripheral action only).

BREATHLESSNESS

Breathlessness at the end of life can be alleviated by opiates (typically in doses smaller than those required to control pain).[3] This is possibly medicated by an anxiolytic effect. Benzodiazepines are an alternative option. Oxygen may be useful in the presence of hypoxia.

AGITATION

Delirium is common towards the end of life (termed 'terminal agitation'). Reversible causes should be identified and treated accordingly (*see* Chapter 7). Persisting symptoms can be controlled with benzodiazepines, such as midazolam.[3]

DEATH RATTLE

'Death rattle' is a term coined for the gurgling sounds caused by air passing over secretions within the oropharynx in patients in a terminal phase of their condition. It occurs in around 50% of the dying, with a mean duration of around two days.[14] It is not clear whether this causes patients any distress but it is a source of concern for attending relatives.[5] The best treatment may simply be reassurance for the family members. When it is felt necessary, several therapeutic options are available. Non-pharmacological measures that may help include more upright positioning of the patient and suctioning of the upper airways. Anticholinergic drugs that act at muscarinic receptors have been shown to be effective. These include hyoscine hydrobromide and butylbromide, and glycopyrronium.

Available evidence suggests a similar efficacy for all of these agents. A significant reduction in death rattle is observed in around 80% of treated patients.[14] When these medications are given intravenously (IV) they have a more rapid onset but shorter duration of action than intramuscular dosing (IM). A 24-hour subcutaneous infusion is probably preferable in most patients. Hyoscine butylbromide is able to cross the blood–brain barrier and may cause confusion. Glycopyrronium and hyoscine hydrobromide may cause bradycardia, whereas hyoscine butylbromide may cause tachycardia. All of these agents may induce urinary retention. Hyoscine is also available as a transdermal patch.

ARTIFICIAL NUTRITION AND HYDRATION

The terminal stages of illness are often accompanied by a reduced oral intake. This often leads carers to be concerned about associated suffering due to hunger or thirst. When 32 patients (mean age 75 years, most with advanced cancer) in a palliative care setting, who were able to express themselves, were given food only when asked for, 63% experienced no hunger despite only a small oral intake of nutrition.[15] Thirty-four per cent experienced only initial hunger and only one patient had hunger up to the time of death. It therefore seems likely that comfort can be achieved in the dying despite minimal oral intake.

The General Medical Council guidance on good practice in withholding and withdrawing treatment (including artificial nutrition and hydration) is available on their website:

> www.gmc-uk.org/guidance/current/library/witholding_lifeprolonging_
> guidance.asp#2 (accessed 7 October 2014). Links to ethical information for those outside the UK are contained in Box 6.3.

CARDIOPULMONARY RESUSCITATION

The outcomes of cardiopulmonary resuscitation (CPR) attempts have been suboptimal and when considering elderly populations, these data become even less impressive. Older studies of people aged over 70 found survival rates to hospital discharge between 0 and 10%.[16-18] However, more recent studies have suggested that survival rates have improved to around 19% for patients aged 70 to 79 years, 15% for those aged 80 to 89 and 12% for those aged over 90.[19,20] The reasons for this may be that resuscitation procedures have improved or may reflect more widespread implementation of 'do not attempt resuscitation' orders. Outcomes tend to be worse for people who sustain a cardiac arrest within their own home rather than in hospital.[16,21]

In comparison to people who arrest in their own home, those who reside in nursing homes have worse outcomes. A study found that 11% of community-dwelling people over the age of 65 survived to discharge compared to only 2% of those from nursing homes.[22] Another study found that none of 14 nursing home residents survived CPR.[23] The outcomes of cardiac arrests within a long-term care facility, which had a resident advanced cardiac life support trained team, has also been evaluated.[24] Despite an initial 20% response to CPR, none of 57 residents survived to hospital discharge.

The initial rhythm is associated with the probability of successful outcome. Those in ventricular fibrillation (VF) or ventricular tachycardia (VT) generally do better than those in asystole or pulseless electrical activity (PEA).[21] We may also expect that complications such as fractured ribs and cerebral hypoxic damage may be more pronounced in this age group due to more prevalent comorbidities such as osteoporosis and dementia. In those who do survive resuscitation, a significant number will be left with a neurological impairment that limits function.

The majority of patients, when asked, appear to express an interest in being involved in the decision-making process regarding the receipt of CPR.[25] For CPR to occur it is clear that patients should be informed of the process and likely outcomes as their decisions may be influenced by unrealistic expectations. A large number of patients appear to gain their knowledge of CPR from watching television programmes, where outcomes are generally overly optimistic.[25] Around 70% of older patients rate themselves as having little or no knowledge of the procedure involved. A study found that 41% of 287 elderly patients (mean age 77, range 60–99 years) initially expressed a wish to receive CPR in the event of a cardiac arrest.[26] This figure fell to 22% once the subjects were informed of only a 10–17% estimated chance of survival to discharge after such an event.

In summary, CPR can be effective within selected elderly people but is less likely to be successful in the frail, especially those who reside in nursing homes. The public is, generally, unaware of the chances of recovery. If patients and relatives are to be involved in such decisions, it is right that they should be informed of the chances of success and the potential harms that it could cause. In settings where a treatment is highly unlikely to provide a benefit it may be inappropriate to provide a general assumption (unless stated otherwise) that all patients are for attempted resuscitation in the event of a cardiac arrest.[27] However, all decisions should be discussed with the relevant person and/ or their next of kin. Of course, it should be made clear that a decision to not attempt resuscitation in the event of a cardiac arrest still means that high-quality care is provided up to the time of any such event.

REFERENCES

1 Ellershaw J, Ward C. Care of the dying patient: the last hours or days of life. *BMJ*, 2003; **326**: 30–4.
2 Fallowfield LJ, Jenkins VA, Beveridge HA. Truth may hurt but deceit hurts more: communication in palliative care. *Palliative Med*, 2002; **16**: 297–303.
3 Sleeman KE, Collis E. Caring for a dying patient in hospital. *BMJ*, 2013; **346**: f2174.
4 O'Neill B, Fallon M. ABC of palliative care: principles of palliative care and pain control. *BMJ*, 1997; **315**: 801–4.
5 Hallenbeck J. Palliative care in the final days of life: "They were expecting it at any time." *JAMA*, 2005; **293**(18): 2265–71.
6 World Health Organization. *WHO Guidelines: cancer pain relief*, 2nd ed. Geneva: WHO; 1996.
7 Radbruch L, Sabatowski R, Loick G, *et al.* Constipation and the use of laxatives: a comparison between transdermal fentanyl and oral morphine. *Palliative Med*, 2000; **14**: 111–19.
8 Yuan C, Foss JF, O'Connor M, *et al.* Methylnaltrexone for reversal of constipation due to chronic methadone use: a randomized controlled trial. *JAMA*, 2000; **283**(3): 367–72.
9 Meissner W, Schmidt U, Hartmann M, *et al.* Oral naloxone reverses opioid-associated constipation. *Pain*, 2000; **84**: 105–9.
10 Quigley C. The role of opioids in cancer pain. *BMJ*, 2005; **331**: 825–9.
11 National Institute of Health and Care Excellence. Neuropathic Pain – pharmacological management: the pharmacological management of neuropathic pain in adults in non-specialist settings. CG173, 2013. Available at: www.nice.org.uk/guidance/cg173 (accessed 7 October 2014).
12 Gilron MD, Bailey JM, Tu D, *et al.* Morphine, gabapentin, or their combination for neuropathic pain. *N Engl J Med*, 2005; **352**(13): 1324–34.
13 Galer BS, Jensen MP. Development and preliminary validation of a pain measure specific to neuropathic pain: the Neuropathic Pain Scale. *Neurology*, 1997; **48**: 332–8.

14 Bennett M, Lucas V, Brennan M, *et al.* Using anti-muscarinic drugs in the management of death rattle: evidence-based guidelines for palliative care. *Palliative Med*, 2002; **16**: 369–74.

15 McCann RM, Hall WJ, Groth-Juncker A. Comfort care for terminally ill patients: the appropriate use of nutrition and hydration. *JAMA*, 1994; **272**(16): 1263–6.

16 Murphy DJ, Murray AM, Robinson BE, *et al.* Outcomes of cardiopulmonary resuscitation in the elderly. *Ann Int Med*, 1989; **111**: 199–205.

17 Taffet GE, Teasdale TA, Luchi RJ. In-hospital cardiopulmonary resuscitation. *JAMA*, 1988; **260**(14): 2069–72.

18 Longstreth WT, Cobb LA, Fahrenbruch CE, *et al.* Does age affect outcomes of out-of-hospital cardiopulmonary resuscitation? *JAMA*, 1990; **264**: 2109–10.

19 Ehlenbach WJ, Barnato AE, Curtis JR, *et al.* Epidemiologic study of in-hospital cardiopulmonary resuscitation in the elderly. *N Engl J Med*, 2009; **361**(1): 22–31.

20 van Gijn MS, Frijns D, van de Glind EMM, *et al.* The chance of survival and the functional outcome alter in-hospital cardiopulmonary resuscitation in older people: a systematic review. *Age Ageing*, 2014; **43**: 456–63.

21 Nolan JP, Soar J, Perkins GD. Cardiopulmonary resuscitation. *BMJ*, 2012; **345**: 34–40.

22 Applebaum GE, King JE and Finucane TE. The outcomes of CPR initiated in nursing homes. *J Am Geriatr Soc*, 1990; **38**: 197–200.

23 Ackermann RJ, Kemle KA, Vogel RL, *et al.* Emergency department use by nursing home residents. *Ann Emerg Med*, 1998; **31**: 749–57.

24 Awoke S, Mouton CP, Parrott M. Outcomes of skilled cardiopulmonary resuscitation in a long-term-care facility: futile therapy? *J Am Geriatr Soc*, 1992; **40**: 593–5.

25 Godkin MD, Toth EL. Cardiopulmonary resuscitation and older adults' expectations. *Gerontologist*, 1994; **34**(6): 797–802.

26 Murphy DJ, Burrows D, Santilli S, *et al.* The influence of the probability of survival on patients' preferences regarding cardiopulmonary resuscitation. *N Engl J Med*, 1994; **330**: 545–9.

27 Conroy S, Luxton T, Dingwall R, *et al.* Cardiopulmonary resuscitation in continuing care settings: time for a rethink? *BMJ*, 2006; **332**: 479–82.

QUESTIONS FOR PART A

1 Which of the following terms is associated with a genetic trait that has advantages in an organism's youth, but harmful effects in older age?
   A. Disposable soma
   B. Antagonistic pleiotropy
   C. Genetic anticipation
   D. Hayflick limit
   E. Shortened telomeres

2 What was the approximate predicted life expectancy at birth of a man in the UK born in 2015?
   A. 77
   B. 80
   C. 83
   D. 86
   E. 89

3 What was the approximate predicted life expectancy of an average person aged 60 years in the UK in 2015?
   A. 9 years
   B. 13 years
   C. 17 years
   D. 21 years
   E. 25 years

4 What was the approximate predicted life expectancy of an average person aged 80 years in the UK in 2015?
   A. 3 years
   B. 6 years
   C. 9 years
   D. 12 years
   E. 15 years

5 By 2050 the proportion of the world's population aged 65 years and older is expected to grow to what level?
   A. 8%
   B. 13%
   C. 16%
   D. 20%
   E. 24%

6 Regarding telomeres, which part of the cell are they associated with?
   A. Cell membrane
   B. Golgi apparatus
   C. Ribosomes
   D. Mitochondria
   E. Chromosomes

7 Which of the following changes is most likely to occur in normal ageing?
A. An increase in resting heart rate
B. A reduction in the diameter of large blood vessels
C. A rise in diastolic blood pressure
D. A fall in maximal cardiac output
E. A reduction in pulse wave velocity

8 Regarding lung volumes in older adults, compared to younger adults, which of the following statements is most likely to be correct?
A. Residual volume is reduced
B. Total lung capacity is unchanged
C. Resting tidal volume is reduced
D. Vital capacity is unchanged
E. Functional residual capacity is reduced

9 A 78-year-old man presents with a two-week history of shortness of breath. The results of his arterial blood gas are as listed below.

pH	7.33	(7.35 to 7.46)
pO_2	10.4	(12.0 to 14.6 kPa)
pCO_2	6.1	(4.6 to 6.0 kPa)
Oxygen saturation	92%	(94 to 100)
Bicarbonate	29	(22 to 26 mmol/L)
Base excess	−5	(−3 to 3 mmol/L)

Which of the following findings is most likely to be due to normal ageing?
A. His low pH
B. His low pO_2
C. His high pCO_2
D. His high bicarbonate
E. His low base excess

10 Which of the following is most commonly considered part of the frailty phenotype?
A. Osteoporosis
B. Hypotension
C. Cachexia
D. Falls
E. Fatigue

11 Which of the following changes in gait pattern is most commonly associated with normal ageing?
A. Greater path deviation from a straight line
B. Wide-based gait
C. Start hesitation
D. Small-stepping gait
E. Loss of arm swing

12 Which of the following hormones has a serum concentration that is typically elevated in healthy older adults compared to younger people?
   A. Thyroxine
   B. Aldosterone
   C. Atrial natriuretic peptide
   D. Renin
   E. Testosterone

13 According to the disposable soma theory of ageing, the following statement is most correct?
   A. Calorie restriction reduces free radical damage to cells
   B. Ageing is programmed by our genes
   C. Ageing occurs as a consequence of balancing energy used in reproduction to that used in cellular repair
   D. Ageing has a role in preventing genetic cross-contamination that would delay evolution
   E. Ageing is an inevitable consequence of oxidative metabolism

14 Age-related hearing loss (presbyacusis) is most suggested by which of the following patterns of deficit?
   A. Unilateral sensorineural hearing loss mainly affecting the lower frequency range
   B. Unilateral conductive loss
   C. Bilateral conductive hearing loss mainly affecting the lower frequency range
   D. Bilateral sensorineural hearing loss mainly affecting the higher frequency range
   E. Unilateral sensorineural hearing loss mainly affecting the higher frequency range

15 A 73-year-old man presents with visual loss. He has no significant past medical history. His intraocular pressures are measured as 35 mmHg in the right eye and 24 mmHg in the left. He is diagnosed as having primary open-angle glaucoma. What initial treatment would be most appropriate?
   A. Bilateral peripheral iridectomy
   B. Latanoprost drops to the left eye
   C. Timolol drops to both eyes
   D. Oral acetazolamide
   E. Brimonidine drops to the right eye

16 In the UK, what proportion of cancers are diagnosed in people over the age of 75 years?
   A. 6%
   B. 12%
   C. 24%
   D. 36%
   E. 52%

17 Which statement is most correct about the calorie requirements of healthy adults aged over 75 years?
   A. They require around 125% of that of people aged 30–50 years
   B. They require around 50% of that of people aged 30–50 years
   C. Requirements are proportional to muscle mass
   D. Basic metabolic rate is unchanged
   E. A larger proportion should be supplied by dietary fat

18 Which of the following statements regarding comprehensive geriatric assessment (CGA) is most correct?
   A. There have been no randomised controlled trials comparing CGA to standard care
   B. Nurse-led teams are equally effective as those involving specialist physicians
   C. A significant beneficial effect in reducing mortality has been shown
   D. A significant beneficial effect in increasing the chance of living at home has been shown
   E. Inpatient consultation services are similarly effect to those delivered on a dedicated ward

19 The main reason for the increase in the proportion of older persons in the UK population is:
   A. An increase in the proportion of ethnic minority elders
   B. Declining mortality rates in older people
   C. The post-war baby boom
   D. A decrease in birth rates in inner cities
   E. Emigration of young people out of the UK

20 The progressive reduction in glomerular filtration rate seen with advancing age is best explained by which of the following physiological changes?
   A. A reduction in renal vascular resistance
   B. Thickening of the basement membrane
   C. Glomerulosclerosis
   D. Increased nephrotoxicity of medications
   E. Tubular interstitial fibrosis

21 Which of the following is most likely to be seen during the normal ageing process?
   A. Increased nocturnal urine formation
   B. A reduction in linguistic and visuospatial abilities
   C. A gradual increase in weight from the age of 60 onwards
   D. A fall in left ventricular ejection fraction
   E. In the lungs: a rise in residual volume and a fall in functional residual capacity

22 Which of the following statements regarding spasticity is most likely to be correct?
   A. Botulinum toxin injections into spastic muscles improve motor function
   B. Baclofen is a gamma-aminobutyric acid (GABA) agonist
   C. Tizanidine causes less somnolence than baclofen
   D. Benzodiazepines are highly effective, but their use is limited by side-effects
   E. Phenol nerve blocks cause permanent effects

23 Digoxin is more likely to have toxic effects when taken by older people compared to younger individuals mainly due to the following reason:
    A. Altered glomerular filtration rate
    B. Changed body fat composition
    C. Reduced protein binding
    D. Variable rate of systemic absorption
    E. Reduced hepatic mass

24 Estimated creatinine clearance is unreliable in older people due to which of the following reasons?
    A. Increased body fat
    B. Lower glomerular filtration rate
    C. Drug interactions
    D. Reduced relative muscle mass
    E. Reduced intravascular volume

25 Gallstones are detected in approximately what percentage of women aged over 80 years?
    A. 5%
    B. 10%
    C. 25%
    D. 40%
    E. 60%

26 According to current WHO definitions, which of these is an 'impairment' in someone who has sustained a stroke?
    A. Unable to play golf
    B. Inability to drive
    C. Not able to walk beyond 5 m unaided
    D. Requiring hoist transfers
    E. Homonymous hemianopia

27 Which of the following is an example of an instrumental activity of daily living?
    A. Transferring from bed to chair
    B. Getting dressed
    C. Using the telephone
    D. Eating a meal
    E. Holding a conversation

28 Regarding the Nottingham Extended Activities of Daily Living scale, which of the following statements is most accurate?
    A. A score of 20 suggests full independence
    B. It evaluates mobility, including ability to climb stairs
    C. Points are awarded for continence
    D. A score of zero suggests no disability
    E. It evaluates ability with personal hygiene

29 Which of the following statements regarding the use of a walking stick to improve ambulation is most likely to be correct?
  A. A three-footed (tripod) stick improves stability when walking on uneven surfaces
  B. When of a correct length the top of the stick should be at the level of the patient's wrist while their arms are hanging down by their side
  C. Holding the stick in the hand ipsilateral to a leg with severe knee osteoarthritis causes less disruption to the normal gait pattern than contralateral use
  D. Elbow crutches are a less suitable alternative for people with reduced grip strength
  E. A walking stick tends to be more disruptive to a normal gait pattern than a Zimmer frame

30 Which of the following statements regarding white matter lesions (leukoaraiosis) seen on brain MRI scans in older adults is most likely to be correct?
  A. They are found in a third of unselected people over the age of 65 years
  B. Their presence is unrelated to arterial blood pressure
  C. They are of no functional significance
  D. They are mainly composed of tau protein filamentous aggregates
  E. They are associated with urinary dysfunction

31 Which statement regarding elder abuse is most likely to be correct?
  A. It is more likely to affect women than men
  B. It is most commonly perpetrated by paid carers
  C. It is most commonly financial in nature
  D. It most frequently occurs in care home settings
  E. Pathognomonic clinical signs can be used to detect it

32 Regarding medication use in the elderly, which statement is most likely to be correct?
  A. Adverse drug reactions are thought to contribute to around 5% of admissions to hospital in those aged over 70
  B. The co-administration of furosemide and fludrocortisone is an example of a prescription cascade
  C. Cognitively unimpaired patients taking medications four times a day can be expected to take only around 80% of their tablets consistently as prescribed
  D. Around 60% of adults over the age of 65 are on one or more inappropriate medications
  E. There is little evidence that blister packs improve medication concordance in the elderly

33 Which of the following conditions is the commonest cause of irreversible sight loss in the elderly?
  A. Diabetic retinopathy
  B. Cataracts
  C. Glaucoma
  D. Presbyopia
  E. Age-related macular degeneration

34 An 89-year-old woman had a fall at home and fractured both wrists. Following initial management of her fractures she is transferred to a rehabilitation ward. Which walking aid would be most suitable for use at this time?
    A. Elbow crutches
    B. Gutter frame
    C. Zimmer frame
    D. Delta frame
    E. Walking stick

35 Which of the following walking aids would be most suitable to improve the gait stability of a patient with rheumatoid arthritis?
    A. Tripod stick
    B. Elbow crutches
    C. Curved handled walking stick
    D. Fischer stick
    E. Tetrapod stick

36 Which of the following is true of a walking stick of the correct length?
    A. With the patient's arms hanging by their sides, its length is the same as the distance from the proximal wrist crease to the ground
    B. The elbow is not flexed when the stick is held straight down to the ground
    C. The elbow should maintain 15-degree flexion when the stick is placed ahead during walking
    D. The elbow is flexed 25 degrees when standing still with the stick resting on the ground
    E. The stick is the same length as the distance from the greater trochanter to the ground

37 A patient who has had Parkinson's disease for four years has developed an unsteady gait and has fallen twice in his bungalow. He no longer goes outdoors unaccompanied. He is keen to try a walking aid; what would you give him?
    A. Normal Zimmer frame
    B. Wheeled Zimmer frame
    C. Walking stick
    D. Delta frame
    E. Elbow crutches

38 Which of these is required for a maximal score on the Barthel index?
    A. Walks with no aids
    B. Normal sitting balance
    C. Continent
    D. Requiring only verbal assistance to manage stairs
    E. No cognitive impairment

39 Which method is best for assessing the correct height for a Zimmer frame for an elderly patient?
  A. Top of the frame comes to the level of the iliac crest
  B. Patient is leaning forwards 20 degrees when holding frame
  C. Frame measures 50% of the patient's total height
  D. Top of the frame is at the level of the patient's radial head when standing upright with their arms by their side
  E. Patient's elbows are flexed 15 degrees at rest

40 Which of the following drug combinations is the best example of a prescription cascade?
  A. Levodopa and quetiapine
  B. Furosemide and bendroflumethiazide
  C. Donepezil and tolterodine
  D. Amlodipine and lisinopril
  E. Tramadol and senna

41 Which of the following drugs is the current first line recommended medication for trigeminal neuralgia in the UK?
  A. Carbamazepine
  B. Gabapentin
  C. Amitriptyline
  D. Tramadol
  E. Pregabalin

42 A patient who is receiving oral morphine as part of palliative care for advanced oesophageal carcinoma now has an impaired swallow. How would you convert their total daily oral morphine to the equivalent subcutaneous diamorphine dose to be given over 24 hours?
  A. Divide by 2
  B. Divide by 3
  C. Same dose
  D. Multiply by 2
  E. Multiply by 3

43 Which of the following prescriptions is approximately equivalent to 30 mg of oral morphine over 24 hours?
  A. Tramadol 100 mg orally four times daily
  B. Codeine phosphate 15 mg orally four times daily
  C. Oxycodone 10 mg orally four times a day
  D. Fentanyl patch transdermally 12 mcg/hour
  E. Buprenorphine patch transdermally 5 mcg/hour

44 Which is the most likely estimate of the prevalence of frailty in people aged over 85 years?
   A. 5%
   B. 10%
   C. 15%
   D. 30%
   E. 65%

45 A 73-year-old man presents following a large rectal bleed. He denies any other symptoms. On examination his blood pressure in 95/68 mmHg and his pulse 114 beats per minute. What is the most likely underlying cause?
   A. Haemorrhoids
   B. Bowel neoplasia
   C. Inflammatory bowel disease
   D. Diverticular disease
   E. Angiodysplasia

46 What is the approximate proportion of people in the UK aged over 100 years at the present time?
   A. 0.1%
   B. 0.2%
   C. 0.5%
   D. 1.0%
   E. 1.5%

47 A 93-year-old woman has a diagnosis of metastatic lung cancer. Her functional ability has started to decline and following discussions with her and her next of kin it has been decided to adopt a palliative approach to her care. She lives alone with support from her family, continues to have a small oral intake and is mobile short distances with assistance. Her past history includes hypertension, osteoporosis, rheumatoid arthritis and a stroke five years ago. She has been on the same medications for several years but is now very keen to take fewer tablets. You plan to stop most of her drugs. Which one of the following medications would you choose to continue?
   A. Aspirin
   B. Simvastatin
   C. Bendroflumethiazide
   D. Alendronate
   E. Ibuprofen

48 Approximately which percentage of the UK population aged 90 and over reside within a care home?
   A. 1%
   B. 10%
   C. 15%
   D. 25%
   E. 35%

49 Which of the following statements regarding telomeres is most likely to be correct?
   A. They contain the gene required to produce telomerase
   B. Telomere shortening can trigger a mechanism that leads to cell death
   C. Shortened telomeres are found in the neurons of people with Alzheimer's dementia
   D. Longer telomeres are found in longer-living species
   E. Shortened telomeres are associated with an increased risk of vascular disease but not cognitive impairment

50 Approximately what percentage of people aged 90 years and over can be expected to survive attempted resuscitation to achieve hospital discharge following a cardiac arrest?
   A. 0%
   B. 3%
   C. 6%
   D. 12%
   E. 24%

51 Which of the following features is more likely to be present in frail older people presenting with a perforated peptic ulcer when compared to younger people?
   A. Hypotension
   B. Epigastric pain
   C. A history of peptic ulcer disease
   D. Abdominal guarding
   E. A raised serum amylase level

52 Which of the following statements regarding surgery in frail older people is most likely to be correct?
   A. Elective and emergency operations have similar mortality rates
   B. The American Society of Anesthesiologists (ASA) scale provides an objective assessment of surgical risk
   C. Regional anaesthesia has a significantly lower risk of inducing cognitive impairment and hypotension compared to general anaesthesia
   D. Smoking cessation advice is an important part of pre-operative assessment
   E. Pre-operative beta-blockade prior to non-cardiac surgery is associated with lower mortality rates

53 Which postoperative complication is most likely to have a reduced incidence following proactive comprehensive geriatric evaluation for older people prior to having elective surgical procedures?
   A. Pressure ulcers
   B. Hypotension
   C. Hypothermia
   D. Constipation
   E. Myocardial infarction

54 A new drug has been developed that has been shown to reduce the risk of stroke in a population of older people. Over a two-year treatment period stroke occurred in 4.6% of people taking the drug compared to 8.6% of people who were given a placebo. What is the number needed to treat with the new drug for one year to prevent one stroke?
   A. 25
   B. 50
   C. 75
   D. 100
   E. 125

55 You wish to calculate the average systolic blood pressure in older people who live in the local community. You take blood pressure readings from 100 people. Your measurements have provided a mean value of 160 mmHg with a standard deviation of 30. Which of the values below is the closest approximation to the 95% confidence interval for the mean?
   A. 158 to 162 mmHg
   B. 156 to 164 mmHg
   C. 154 to 166 mmHg
   D. 152 to 168 mmHg
   E. 150 to 170 mmHg

56 Which of the following medications is most likely to increase the duration of sleep in older adults with insomnia without significantly increasing the risk of hip fracture?
   A. Lorazepam
   B. Diazepam
   C. Melatonin
   D. Zopiclone
   E. Zolpidem

PART B

Brain

CHAPTER 6

Dementia

DEFINITION

Dementia is a syndrome attributed to disease of the brain, usually of a chronic or progressive nature, in which there is disturbance of multiple brain functions. These impairments may include calculation, learning capacity, language and judgement. It is usually only considered present when there is resultant impact on social or occupational function. Consciousness is usually unaltered. There may also be deterioration in emotional control, social behaviour or motivation. In other words, it is not simply memory loss but a complex condition that affects more than one aspect of cognition.

EPIDEMIOLOGY

Approximately 8–10% of people over the age of 65 years in the Western world have dementia. The prevalence rises from around 2% of those aged 65 to more than 35% of those over 85 years (Figure 6.1).[1-3] This figure represents, roughly, a doubling in prevalence for every five-year increase in age. A more positive thought is that around two-thirds of the very old do not have dementia. The number of people worldwide with dementia is predicted to double every 20 years.[4] The prevalence of dementia is higher

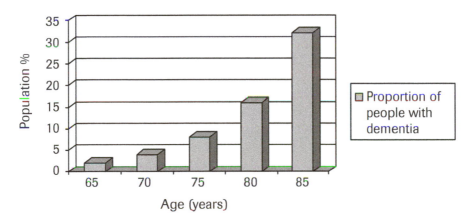

FIGURE 6.1 The rising prevalence of dementia with age.

among hospitalised older people – being present in around 48% of those aged 80–89 and 66% of those aged over 90.[5]

In addition, there is a significant population of individuals with some clinical evidence of cognitive impairment that is not severe enough to meet the criteria for a diagnosis of dementia ('mild cognitive impairment' – see p. 94). However, cognitive decline is not an inevitable feature of ageing and many older people continue to function at their baseline level (see p. 14).[6]

Mortality rates are increased in people with dementia compared to people without this condition. Survival time is heavily dependent on age at the time of diagnosis. A study found that people aged 65–69 years survived a median of 10.7 years, those aged 70–79 survived 5.4 years, those aged 80–89 survived 4.3 years, and those over 90 survived 3.8 years.[7] The overall median survival time was 4.5 years.

COGNITION

Attention

Attention is the ability to focus on a task and is determined by both concentration and arousal. It is mediated by the reticular activating system, which is a complex series of connections between the cerebral cortex, thalamus and the reticular formation (a 'net-like' collection of cells on the surface of the brainstem). In the presence of reduced attention other brain functions are also impaired.

Memory

Traditionally memory function has been loosely divided into short-term and long-term components. More recently, memory has been classified into four categories,[8] these are outlined below.

➤ **Episodic memory**: The memory of specific personal events and experiences, for example what you did on holiday last year. Predominantly mediated by the medial temporal lobes and limbic system (including the hippocampus – see Figure 6.7). Insults to this system tend to affect more recently learned memories more than older ones (i.e. short-term memory is more affected than long-term memory).

➤ **Semantic memory**: Knowledge of the world not related to personal experiences. This includes the names of objects, for example the names of animals. This is predominantly mediated by the inferolateral temporal lobes.

➤ **Procedural memory**: The memory of how to perform tasks, such as riding a bike. The basal ganglia and cerebellum predominantly mediate this. It occurs at a subconscious level. It may be particularly affected in movement disorders (see Chapter 9).

➤ **Working memory**: Short-term (seconds to minutes) 'keeping it in your head'. It can be phonologic (e.g. a phone number) or spatial (e.g. manipulating an object in your mind). The prefrontal cortex is important in this process along with other brain areas depending on the nature of the task. For an effective working memory, it is also necessary to be able to maintain attention/concentration.

Memories may be conscious (declarative) or non-conscious (non-declarative). Confabulation is the making-up of new 'memories' to replace those that have been lost. Memory impairment is common to many disorders, including dementia, delirium and depression.

Language

The dominant hemisphere encodes language. In all right-handed and most left-handed people this is the left side of the brain. The language centres are more diffuse and less well defined than traditionally thought. They include Broca's area in the frontal lobe and Wernicke's area at the margin of the temporal and parietal lobes. There is also a network of connections between these areas, called the arcuate fasciculus (*see* Figure 6.2). Paraphrasia is a term for the use of abnormal or incorrect words. These can be semantic (similar categories, e.g. 'dog' for 'cat'), phonemic (similar sounds, e.g. jar for car) or neologistic (made up words, e.g. strub for car). Prosody is a term for the melodic characteristics of speech including intonation, stress and cadence (rhythm). Anomia is a term for a naming deficit (e.g. cannot say the name for a pen). Anomic dysphasia is also called 'word block'. With this disorder people typically stop mid-sentence. Its presence is associated with space-occupying lesions within the dominant lobe. Progressive aphasia is a term for a slowly worsening non-fluent aphasia secondary to left frontotemporal degeneration (plus apraxia). Dysgraphia (impaired writing) and dyslexia (impaired reading) are usually associated with dysphasia.

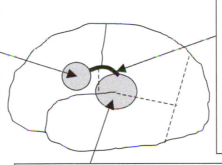

Broca's area (within the frontal lobe) A lesion here causes an expressive problem with relatively preserved comprehension. Reduced prosody, slow (word-finding pauses) and dysarthric speech. Short sentences (mainly nouns) and phonemic errors.

Arcuate fasciculus A lesion here causes conduction aphasia, which gives fluent, paraphrasic speech, with poor repetition but good comprehension.

Wernicke's area (exact boundaries poorly defined) A lesion here causes reduced comprehension and naming ability. Speech typically fluent with preserved prosody. Jargon speech with few nouns and many semantic errors.

FIGURE 6.2 The key language areas of the brain.

Visuospatial skills

Visuospatial deficits tend to be more severe with non-dominant hemisphere damage but are not unique to it. Constructional ability involves input from occipital (visual), parietal (association areas link visual and motor pathways) and frontal (motor) lobe functions.

Errors observed include perseveration (repetition of lines/shapes) and 'closing in' (merging objects together). Constructional 'apraxia' can occur with damage to either hemisphere. When affecting the left over-simplification of copied objects is seen, with the right an over-elaboration or 'explosion' of constituent parts is more typical. 'Neglect' is a term used for spatial inattention, which can cause visual or sensory extinction (stimuli are preferentially detected by one side of the body despite intact sensory systems).

Executive function

The frontal lobes perform executive functions, which relate to personality (drive, motivation, inhibition) and behaviour. Lesions here lead to failures with learning from errors, poor goal setting, intrusion of unwanted thoughts, perseveration (becoming fixed on one idea), the inability to switch tasks (also called 'set-shifting', leading to 'stimulus-bound' behaviour), reduced empathy, and poor sequencing of tasks. Affected individuals typically have reduced interest in their environment and poor social drive leading to impaired interpersonal relations and hygiene.

Apraxia

Apraxia is a high-level motor deficit. It is mainly seen with left hemisphere lesions, as the right hand is dominant in the majority of people, typically involving the parietal or frontal lobes. It can be described as 'ideomotor' (patients cannot mime simple tasks such as waving or combing their hair), 'orobuccal' (facial, e.g. mime blowing out a match), or ideational (can do individual items but cannot sequence them together (e.g. fold letter, put in envelope, seal, address and stamp envelope)). Dressing 'apraxia' is an inability to get dressed correctly. It is seen following parietal lobe lesions and is probably primarily a visuospatial disorder. It can also be secondary to frontal lesions causing poor sequencing of actions (e.g. putting underpants on over trousers).

ASSESSMENT
History

The history should incorporate all the features of a thorough medical history in other situations, for example past medical problems, current medication, and so on. In the presence of cognitive impairment this may be challenging. Getting a collateral history from someone who knows the patient well is essential. Those who love the patient may under-play their deficit, thinking that they are being protective. Or they may have been unaware of the degree of the problem as the patient was able to conceal it in their own home and usual routines. Questions relating to the patient's functional abilities are likely to be helpful, e.g. 'Do they still drive a car?', 'Do they do their own finances?', 'Can they get a bus in to town?' or 'Can they use the telephone?' Relatives or carers can be asked to fill in a 'This is me' document to give more information to ward staff about previous behaviours, care needs and personal preferences.[9] The following is a guide to the specific features required in cognitive assessment.

Onset and progression

The rate and nature of cognitive decline are helpful in distinguishing between different types of dementia. For example: Alzheimer's disease (AD) has an insidious, progressive nature; vascular dementia (VaD) may be stepwise; and a more rapid decline is seen in Creutzfeldt–Jakob disease (CJD). A fluctuating course may be associated with delirium (*see* Chapter 7) or dementia with Lewy bodies (DLB) (*see* p. 169). This is represented graphically in Figure 6.3. The initial presenting problem may be helpful in distinguishing subtypes when the presentation is late and deficits in multiple cognitive domains have developed.

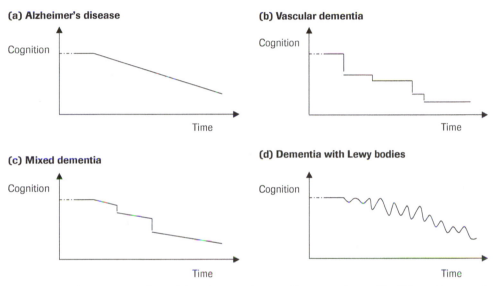

FIGURE 6.3 A representation of the changes in cognition over time with different types of dementia.

Cognitive deficits

It is important to explore different cognitive areas during the questioning in order to fully identify all the deficits. These functions will then be more formally tested during the mental state examination.

➤ *Memory loss*: both short and long-term aspects.
➤ *Language impairment*: problems including word-finding difficulties (dysphasia) and the use of inappropriate words (paraphrasias).
➤ *Calculation impairment*: may manifest as difficulty with financial matters.
➤ *Visuospatial problems*: such as getting lost in familiar environments.
➤ *Praxia*: the inability to perform learned movements despite intact motor function. This may present as difficulty with tasks, such as opening cans or turning on taps.
➤ *Executive functions*: complex tasks, goal-directed behaviour and insight.
➤ *Agnosia*: the inability to recognise objects despite intact sensory function.

Behavioural changes

➤ *Personality*: changes in social interaction and inappropriateness are common in frontotemporal dementia (FTD).

➤ *Sleep*: changes in diurnal variation. Early morning waking is associated with depression, which may coexist with, or mimic, dementia (*see* Chapter 8). REM disorders (vivid dreams, jerking or thrashing movements during sleep) are associated with DLB.

➤ *Food preferences*: a change in dietary preferences, especially a tendency to like more sweet foods, is associated with FTD.

➤ *Sexuality*: sexual drive may be increased or reduced.

➤ *Delusions and hallucinations*: early visual hallucinations are a feature of DLB, but may occur in other conditions, especially delirium.

➤ *Continence*: if urinary incontinence is an early feature, VaD or normal pressure hydrocephalus (NPH) (*see* p. 176) should be considered. Incontinence is important as a predictor of nursing home placement and survival.

Past medical history

A history of depression makes current depression more likely. Previous vascular disease or vascular risk factors may add weight to a diagnosis of vascular dementia.

Medication

Anticholinergic medication use is frequently associated with impaired cognition in the elderly (but not an increased risk of developing dementia).[10,11] (*See* pp. 27 and 274, and Table 2.2.)

Social and functional

A number of example questions to explore social and functional background are listed below.

➤ Who else is at home and what kind of residence is it?

➤ What help is required for mobility, self-care, cooking, cleaning, laundry, finances, etc. Are they still driving? If so how safe does the carer feel to be in the car with the patient?

➤ Do they have any external help – friends, family, Social Services? Are there any hazards and has there been an occupational therapist involved in home assessment?

➤ Are there any issues regarding carer well-being?

➤ Does the patient smoke or drink (important as risk factors for VaD and alcohol-related dementias)? If alcoholism is suspected, explore the patient's prior drinking habits and ask about specific problems, such as withdrawal seizures.

Sociocultural background

Neuropsychological assessment is interpreted in light of previous education. What age did the patient leave school and with what qualifications? What was their employment?

Familial history

Although not the norm, some dementing illnesses have a familial component. This is more likely with FTD when there is a history of onset before the age of 60 years.

Examination

This is divided into mental state and physical examinations.

Mental state

In clinical practice, time usually limits the depth and complexity of testing of the mental state. A wide range of assessment tools used both for screening and rating of disease severity has been developed.[12] Brief screening tools include the 10-point Abbreviated Mental Test (AMT) and Six-Item Screener (SIS) (*see* Appendix A). The 30-point Mini Mental State Examination (MMSE) offers a little more depth of assessment and is the most commonly used cognitive assessment tool. Here, the higher the score the better, with a score of 25 or below suggesting significant impairment (*see* Appendix A). It tests only limited cognitive domains (e.g. not executive function and little visuospatial ability). An alternative is the Montreal Cognitive Assessment (MOCA).[13] This test also gives a score out of 30 but requires a wider range of cognitive skills. It requires a specialised testing sheet, which includes animal pictures for identification.

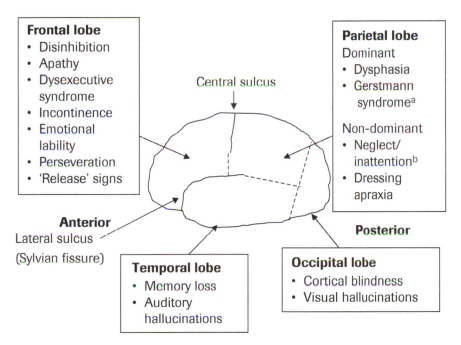

FIGURE 6.4 Cognitive functional neuro-anatomy of the brain: the basic features of damage to specific brain regions (*see also* Figure 10.5): a Gerstmann syndrome: difficulty with writing (dysgraphia) and calculation (dyscalculia), left–right indistinction and inability to identify fingers (finger agnosia); b dominant parietal lesions may also cause neglect and inattention, but tend to be less severe.

In the clock-drawing test the patient is asked to draw a circle, add numbers as though drawing a clock face and then place on the hands to indicate a specific time (e.g. 10 past 11). This requires both visuospatial skills and some executive function ability. There are differing score systems, but in the simplest of these one point is allocated for correctly completing each of the three elements just listed. It has also been found to be a reasonable screening test for dementia.[14]

Formal neuropsychological testing usually involves a series of tests that assess specific aspects of brain function. This process often takes far longer (typically two to three hours) than practical for a medical assessment, plus the results can only accurately be interpreted by a specialist with comparison to data on normal populations. A reasonable intermediate step between the MMSE or MOCA and formal neuropsychology is the Addenbrooke's Cognitive Examination third version (ACE-III).[15,16] This series of questions incorporates attention, memory and visuospatial tests along with more elaborate tests of a wider range of specific cognitive domains (including executive function) to give a score out of 100. The higher the score, the better the cognition, with a cut-off point suggesting significant impairment of below 87. Subtle deficits will only be detected with more complex testing. In late dementia all areas of cognition will become impaired and the discriminatory ability to diagnose specific dementia syndromes will become diminished.

Domains tested for include attention, memory, language, visuospatial skills and executive function. These are discussed in turn below. The process attempts to localise deficits within the brain. A simplified overview of the function of cortical regions is shown in Figure 6.4.

Attention

Patients with reduced attention are easily distracted. Simple tests of attention include digit span (the patient is asked to recall series of numbers), reverse sequences (e.g. recite the months of the year backwards or count down from 20 to 1), and 'serial sevens' (subtract sevens from 100). When attention is impaired the rest of the neuropsychological examination may be hard to interpret. It is typically impaired in patients with delirium.

Memory

Giving the patient a series of words to remember is a simple test of memory. A person who is able to recall words after clues are given is more likely to have a subcortical deficit that impairs memory retrieval rather than memory formation. Orientation questions (day, month, year, etc.) also tests the ability to form new memories. The non-dominant lobe predominantly determines visuospatial memory. Asking the patient to remember and then reproduce images can test this. Remote memory (e.g. recalling the dates of the Second World War) is more dependent on cortical processes than the limbic system (*see* p. 97).

Language

Spontaneous speech during the history may have given some clues to linguistic function. The assessment of speech is discussed in Chapter 10. Language disturbance is a common component of AD but rarely features in subcortical dementias. Verbal fluency can be assessed by asking the patient to name as many items as they can in a one-minute time period. This can be semantic lists (e.g. animals) or words beginning with specific letter (e.g. 'P'). Typical normal values for numbers of animals would be 18 or more. Acceptable values may be a little lower in older adults with 15 or more being reasonable over the age of 80. However, such verbal fluency tasks are not solely reliant on language skills, they also need a cognitive strategy to search for appropriate words. Frontal lobe impairment may lead to short lists and repetition of answers.

Visuospatial skills

Asking patients to copy figures can test visuospatial skills. Typically this would include interlocking pentagons, but more complex three-dimensional images may be used. This function is commonly impaired in dementia or delirium but rarely with primary psychiatric disorders. Deficits are more common and more severe when the non-dominant lobe is affected.

Executive function

Executive skills enable the performance of complex tasks or behaviours. They can be tested by asking patients to continue sequences, which can be alpha-numeric (e.g. 1A, 2B, 3C …) or drawn repetitive patterns. In the trail-making test the patient is asked to connect a series of numbers and/or letters in sequence while being timed (e.g. $1 \rightarrow 2 \rightarrow 3$… or $1 \rightarrow A \rightarrow 2 \rightarrow B \rightarrow 3$…). Alternative assessment methods include verbal fluency (*see* above), describe similarities between words (e.g. shirt and trousers) or to interpret the meanings of proverbs (e.g. people who live in glass houses shouldn't throw stones).

The Wisconsin card sort test assesses mental flexibility. Here the patient is asked to categorise specialised cards in response to changing criteria.

Gerstmann syndrome is caused by a lesion of the dominant lobe's angular gyrus (within the parietal lobe), which results in dyscalculia, dysgraphia, left–right disorientation and finger agnosia.

Physical

The physical examination should incorporate the features of a good general medical assessment, in particular looking for signs of neurological and vascular disease. Speech will have been assessed as part of the mental state examination. Cranial nerves may show reduced up and down gaze with progressive supranuclear palsy (PSP) (*see* p. 170). Impaired saccadic eye movements may provide more subtle signs of an underlying movement disorder (*see* Figure 9.5). Pyramidal tract or cerebellar signs may indicate VaD. Increased tone with cogwheeling and bradykinesia suggests an underlying movement disorder (*see* p. 150).

Frontal release signs

➤ *Grasp reflex*: the patient grasps an object that is stroked across the palm.
➤ *Pout (snout) reflex*: a pouting facial expression is produced when the area lateral to the upper lip is stroked.
➤ *Glabellar tap*: the area between the eyebrows is gently tapped (with the examiner's arm approaching from above/behind to prevent blinking to a threatening stimulus). A positive result is achieved when the patient continues to blink beyond the first three taps.

The frontal release signs are neurological phenomena that originate from the brainstem or below.[17] These signs are present in newborn children until subcortical myelination is completed. They may recur in later life in normal individuals or in association with cerebral damage.[6,18] They are then termed 'release' signs due to the loss of the cortical inhibition of the brainstem-mediated mechanisms. They have been detected in 55% of patients with AD (mean age 68 years) compared to 9% of normal control subjects (mean age 62).[19] In general their occurrence does not correlate well with cognitive function. The presence of grasp and pout reflexes appear to be the most suggestive of cognitive impairment.[17,20]

Test for dyspraxia by asking the patient to mime tasks with both hands individually and together, and to mime some tasks involving the face, such as combing hair, cutting bread, whistling. The Luria task is a test of executive function. It is a three-step hand sequence that the patient is asked to copy (*see* Figure 6.5). Hemiplegic or 'marche à petits pas' (small-stepping) gaits are associated with VaD. Parkinsonian gaits may signify an underlying movement disorder. The gait of NPH is broad-based with a 'foot stuck to the floor' appearance.

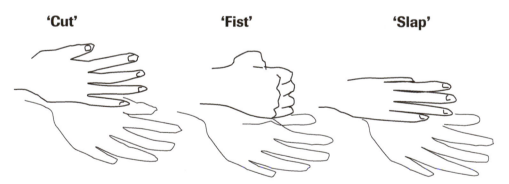

'Cut'   **'Fist'**   **'Slap'**

FIGURE 6.5 The Luria task. The patient is asked to copy the three-stage hand sequence shown above. A normal individual can correctly repeat this within several attempts.

Investigations

There are no laboratory tests to diagnose the common forms of dementia. Investigations may help to exclude potentially reversible causes. The standard 'dementia screen' bloods: ESR, vitamin B_{12} and TSH should be performed (to exclude vasculitis, combined degeneration and hypothyroidism). Syphilis serological testing (venereal disease research laboratory test; VDRL) may be considered – *see* Box 6.1. Brain imaging (CT or MRI) can exclude NPH or space-occupying lesions. Focal cerebral atrophy is rarely seen in early disease. Global cerebral atrophy is often seen in normal ageing and does not correlate with cognitive function. Vascular disease may be seen, lending weight to a diagnosis of VaD. Areas of leukoaraiosis (white matter lesions) are found in a third of those aged over 65 (*see* p. 15). More recently functional imaging using single-photon emission computed tomography (SPECT) has been proposed to assist in the diagnosis of dementia. It may be helpful in selected cases to distinguish between AD and VaD or to assist diagnosis of DLB.[21,22] However, the clinical role of this technology has yet to be defined and its current use is mainly limited to research settings.

Definitive diagnosis can only be achieved by correlation of clinical features with pathological specimens, usually post-mortem. Rarely a brain biopsy is undertaken. This typically involves obtaining a full-thickness frontal cortical section. One retrospective analysis found that diagnostic information was obtained in 57% of biopsies, and treatment decisions were affected in 11%.[23] Complications are seen in around 10% and include seizures, haemorrhage and infection. Biopsy should be considered when a reversible condition, such as inflammatory process, is suspected clinically but cannot be confirmed by an alternative method. More specific tests may be indicated in some individuals according to their clinical history, for example HIV serology. In a review of data from 5620 patients with dementia, a potentially reversible cause was identified in 9%, but just 0.6% of cases actually reversed (partially or completely).[24]

BOX 6.1 Note on syphilis

Syphilis serology is often performed as part of a dementia 'work-up'. It should be remembered that a VDRL stays positive after exposure to syphilis. There are also a number of conditions causing false positives (e.g. systemic lupus erythematosus (SLE)). A *Treponema pallidum* haemagglutinin antibody (TPHA) test is only positive at the time of acute infection. Neurosyphilis is a form of tertiary syphilis that occurs in about 10% of people who are untreated. The median age of onset has now fallen to 39 years and is mostly seen in relation to HIV infection.[25] The form of neurosyphilis associated with cognitive impairment is called 'general paresis'. This occurs between 3 and 40 years after exposure. The clinical features are reduced attention, memory and executive abilities. There may be associated delusions (classically grandiose), hallucinations and confabulation. Physical examination may reveal upper motor neuron signs in the limbs and possibly associated tabes dorsalis (demyelination of the dorsal columns). With adequate penicillin treatment 50% will improve.

In summary, neurosyphilis is an extremely rare presentation of cognitive impairment in the elderly. VDRL testing may well give a positive result in the absence of active syphilis. It should be considered when clinical suspicion is present but its value as a routine screening test in dementia is questionable.

DIFFERENTIAL DIAGNOSIS OF DEMENTIA

Mild cognitive impairment

Mild cognitive impairment (MCI) is a term for subtle cognitive decline that lies between normal ageing and a dementia process.[26] There are likely to be mild impairments on cognitive testing (e.g. ACE-III) but functional ability is mainly preserved. Its prevalence increases with advancing age – perhaps affecting 10–20% of people over the age of 65 years. It most commonly affects memory in isolation, but can affect other cognitive functions. People with MCI are a higher risk of developing dementia (typically AD) than people without MCI, with a conversion rate of 5–10% per year. Depression can present in a similar way and should be excluded. Cognitive enhancer drugs do not improve function in MCI but are associated with an increased risk of harm.[27]

Delirium and depression

Delirium and depression are the most important differential diagnoses of dementia in the elderly. These are discussed in Chapters 7 and 8, respectively. Core features that may help to distinguish them are outlined in Table 6.1.

TABLE 6.1 A comparison of the distinguishing features of dementia, delirium and depression*

	Dementia	Delirium	Depression
Onset	Insidious	Acute/subacute	Rapid
Course	Progressive	Fluctuating	Stable
Impaired consciousness	−	+	−
Reduced attention span	−	+	−
Impaired visuospatial skills	+	+	−
Hallucinations	−	+	−
Delusions	−	+	−
Psychomotor retardation	−	+	+
Psychomotor activation	−	+	−
Personal or family history of depression	−	−	+
Low mood	−	−	+
Poor appetite	−	−	+
Weight loss	−	−	+
Sleep disturbance	−	+	+
Insight preserved	−	−	+
Improves during the day	−	−	+
Response to antidepressants	−	−	+

* The purpose is to act as a guide rather than a rigid scheme. For example, hallucinations are most commonly seen with delirium, but may be associated with either dementia with Lewy bodies or psychotic depression. + = a characteristic feature; − = not usually a feature.

DISTINGUISHING DEMENTIA SUBTYPES

A broad division of the subtypes of dementia into cortical and subcortical has been proposed. This is not a perfect divide as much overlap exists[28] but it probably has some role as a simplistic model.

➤ *Cortical* (e.g. AD, FTD, asymmetric cortical atrophies): These dementias are characterised by deficits in specific cortical domains: memory problems, aphasia, apraxia, visuospatial impairment, reduced calculation and agnosia (perceptual difficulty).

➤ *Subcortical* (e.g. VaD, movement disorders (e.g. PSP), NPH, infections, toxins): These dementias are thought to affect circuits of the basal ganglia and thalamus (*see* Figure 9.1), which are thought to be important for information retrieval and storage. There is reduced speed of thought (bradyphrenia) and delayed access to information. There tend to be frontal-executive features, such as perseveration, sequencing problems and reduced verbal fluency (rather than aphasia). The use of clues may aid memory retrieval, whereas this is less likely to benefit those with a cortical deficit. There may be more prominent apathy and associated reduced speech quality, for example dysarthria, loss of prosody and hypophonia (reduced volume).

Table 6.2 outlines some of the distinguishing features of these two categories.

TABLE 6.2 Properties that may help to distinguish between cortical and subcortical patterns of dementia

	Cortical	Subcortical
Psychomotor speed	Normal	↓
Speech	Dysphasia or paraphrasia	Hypophonia or dysarthria
Executive function	Normal or ↓	↓↓
Verbal fluency	Normal or ↓	↓↓
Memory	Amnesia	↓ retrieval speed

Personality change

A change in personality suggests frontal lobe involvement and makes a diagnosis of FTD, VaD or CJD more likely.

Hallucinations and delusions

Visual hallucinations and cognitive impairment is suggestive of DLB. Alternative diagnoses include delirium, VaD and psychotic depression. Charles Bonnet syndrome is a condition in which cognitively normal people develop visual hallucinations, usually associated with chronic visual impairment. Auditory hallucinations are more compatible with schizophrenia. Delusions are common in advanced AD but may be an early feature of DLB.

Schizophrenia

The onset of schizophrenia is uncommon in old age. Approximately 4% present after the age of 60 years (termed 'very-late-onset schizophrenia-like psychosis').[29] Compared to those with a younger age of onset, hallucinations (including visual, tactile and olfactory) and delusions (including persecutory and third person) are more common. Thought disorder and negative symptoms (e.g. flat affect, and reduced spontaneous speech, socialisation, and personal hygiene) are less common. It appears to affect women more commonly than men. Compared to younger onset cases, a family history is less frequently associated.

Neurological signs

Focal neurological signs may help to diagnose VaD. Alternatively, a small-stepping gait ('marche à petits pas') may be detected. Movement disorders with associated dementia usually have characteristic physical signs; however, the cognitive features may predate the motor features by up to one year.

SPECIFIC CONDITIONS CAUSING DEMENTIA

In the Western world the most common diagnosis of cause of dementia is AD (50–60%).[30] The other common causes of dementia in the elderly are VaD, mixed dementia (mainly VaD–AD) and DLB (together accounting for around 40% in total). Alternative diagnoses represent less than 10% of cases in older people (*see* Figure 6.6). The estimates of actual prevalence vary quite widely between studies, in part due to differing diagnostic definitions and differing age groups studied. For example, FTD is a more common cause of dementia in younger people (<65 years) where it may represent as many as 20% of cases.

Mixed dementia is likely to be more common than traditionally thought. Pathological studies have found that the majority of people have more than one brain pathology (most commonly Alzheimer's and vascular).[31]

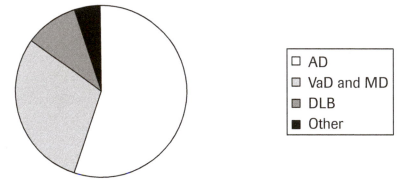

FIGURE 6.6 The approximate contribution of subtypes of dementia in the elderly.

Alzheimer's disease

➤ Percentage of all dementia: 50–60 (often as part of mixed pathology).
➤ Prevalence: 6% of people over 65 years.
➤ Key early features: memory loss, language deficits, visuospatial problems.

Alzheimer's disease most commonly presents as an initial loss of short-term memory. Usually procedural memory is retained in the early stages. Language problems present as word-finding difficulties and paraphrasias (using the wrong words). Verbal fluency may be reduced – particularly the generation of semantic lists (e.g. the names of animals). Visuospatial problems are prominent (e.g. a history of getting lost or difficulty with copying objects or clock drawing). Later in the disease comprehension is also reduced and there may also be repetition of other people's words (echolalia) or their own words (palilalia). Also, apraxia, agnosia and reduced executive functioning become more apparent. Patients usually continue to perform activities of daily living well until late in the disease.

Behavioural symptoms are not a significant presenting feature but may develop later. The most common early change is to become apathetic with reduced social interaction and participation in activities. Late changes may include disinhibition, wandering, psychosis and aggression. Delusions commonly develop in later disease and are often persecutory in nature. A study of 50 patients with AD of varying severity found that 80% had some form of behavioural change.[32] The most common were apathy (72%), agitation (60%) and anxiety (48%). The emergence of agitation, dysphoria, apathy and aberrant motor behaviour were significantly correlated with cognitive decline. Visual hallucinations may occur. They are more common in people with underlying visual impairment.[33] Neurovegetative changes (sleep, appetite and sexuality) are common. Neurological features, including extrapyramidal signs, gait disturbance and seizures, can occur in the late stages.

Familial forms also exist, which show an autosomal dominant pattern of inheritance.[34] These tend to have a younger age of onset and account for only a very small percentage of cases (<1%). There are a number of implicated genes: apolipoprotein

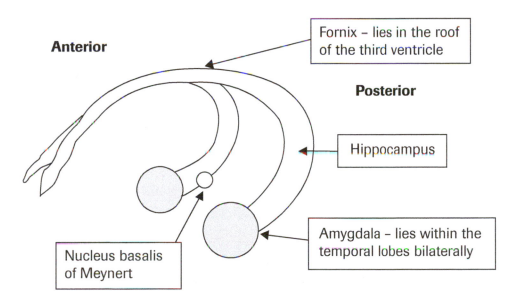

FIGURE 6.7 A three-dimensional representation of the limbic system.

E4 allele (APOE4) (on chromosome 19), presenilin 1 (chromosome 14), presenilin 2 (chromosome 1), amyloid precursor protein (APP) (chromosome 21), plus others. As yet the role of genetic analysis in clinical practice is not well established.

The accumulation of beta-amyloid plaques (also called neuritic plaques) within the brain appears to be the key mechanism in the pathogenesis of AD.[35] It has been termed the 'amyloid cascade'. The genetic links listed above all seem to enhance the accumulation of amyloid proteins. Secondary pathological changes include tau protein hyperphosphorylation (to form neurofibrillary tangles), inflammation, lipid peroxidation and excitotoxicity. The net result is neuronal cell death in specific brain areas. The parietal and temporal lobes are most frequently affected, although variants involving other brain areas have been described (e.g. the occipital lobes leading to visual disturbance). The limbic system, which lies predominantly within the medial temporal lobes, is thought to play a crucial role in the processing of memories (*see* Figure 6.7). Acetylcholine, norepinephrine and serotonin pathways are affected. The cholinergic neuronal projections of the nucleus basilis of Meynert within the limbic system to the cortex are particularly impaired.

The diagnosis is classified as definite only when confirmatory pathology is available (usually post-mortem). 'Probable AD' is based on a clinical diagnosis alone. More recent diagnostic criteria allow for findings from brain imaging, PET scanning and cerebrospinal fluid biomarkers to be used in diagnosis.[36] The rate of cognitive decline is around 3 points on the MMSE scale (out of 30) or 6–7 points on the ADAS-cog scale (out of 70) (*see* Appendix A) per year.

Vascular dementia

The prevalence of vascular dementia is hard to establish accurately due to a large proportion of patients with mixed pathology (*see* below). Estimates range from approximately 1% to 4% of people over the age of 65 years.

VaD encompasses a variety of clinical presentations. It can result from a range of vascular lesions, including a single cortical stroke, a number of subcortical events, cerebral haemorrhage or episodes of hypoperfusion. 'Binswanger disease' is a term for dementia in association with extensive peri-ventricular white matter lesions (leukoaraiosis) usually caused by atherosclerosis of deep penetrating end-arterioles. Diagnostic criteria for VaD usually require three factors:[30]

➤ dementia
➤ clinical and imaging evidence of cerebrovascular disease
➤ a temporal link between the above two components.

The nature of the cognitive impairment can be quite diverse. Small-vessel ischaemia appears to be the most common cause and this characteristically tends to result in a subcortical pattern of dementia. A clinical picture similar to either that of Parkinson's disease (PD) or NPH can occur. The onset is often abrupt and tends to deteriorate in a stepwise fashion. However, a gradually progressive dementia can occur. The history will usually reveal vascular risk factors. CT scanning may help to demonstrate vascular lesions but it is not, alone, diagnostic.

Patches of leukoaraiosis tend to be peri-ventricular in distribution and are seen as lucencies on CT scanning and areas of increased signal intensity on T2-weighted MRI scans. They are seen more commonly in patients with VaD, but are also seen in normal elderly people. Their role, if any, in the pathogenesis of dementia is unclear. They appear to be related to vascular insufficiency in the white matter, either through infarction or chronic hypoperfusion.[30] Pathological changes seen include loss of myelin and neurons. Identified risk factors for these lesions include hypertension, hypotension and having a labile blood pressure. Other conditions may mimic their MRI appearance (e.g. multiple sclerosis).

Around 20–30% of patients who have sustained an acute stroke will develop dementia in the following three-year period and about 10% will have dementia prior to the onset of this stroke.[37,38] Of those who develop post-stroke dementia, two-thirds seem to meet diagnostic criteria for VaD and one-third for AD.[37,39] These findings further suggest a large overlap between VaD and neurodegenerative changes. Features that make the development of dementia more likely include older age, pre-existing cognitive impairment, atrial fibrillation (AF) and severity of stroke.[38]

Treatment includes addressing vascular risk factors such as blood pressure control, cholesterol and antiplatelet agents where indicated (*see* p. 206).

Mixed aetiology

As already mentioned, there is a great deal of overlap between the dementia disorders. Many of the neurodegenerative diseases share common pathologic findings. Also, there is an association of AD with vascular lesions. So, it is not unexpected to find that some dementias are classified as being of mixed aetiology. The most common variant is a mixed AD–VaD condition, and most studies have defined mixed dementia as this combination of pathologies. Estimates of prevalence have varied considerably depending on diagnostic criteria. It is estimated that it accounts for around 20–40% of dementia.[40] Neuropathological studies have found that pure vascular dementia in the elderly is rare and is almost always associated with some AD-type changes.[30]

In patients with AD, the presence of vascular lesions appears to make the degree of dementia worse.[41] The neuropsychological deficits appear to resemble VaD more closely than AD.[40] A pattern of stepwise deterioration in combination with a progressive decline suggests a mixed aetiology (*see* Figure 6.3).[30]

Frontotemporal dementia

➤ Percentage of all dementias: 2–5%.
➤ Mean age of onset: 56–61 years.[42,43]
➤ Key early features: personality change, altered personal and interpersonal conduct, emotional blunting, loss of insight, behavioural disorder.

Frontotemporal dementia has several variants, including Pick disease. This latter condition is distinguished pathologically by the presence of Pick bodies, which are argentophilic intracellular inclusions. Tau protein is a normal cellular component of microtubules. FTD is associated with abnormal processing of this protein, often with hyperphosphorylation. Other conditions associated with tau abnormalities include AD, PSP and corticobasal degeneration (CBD) (*see* pp. 170 and 172) – together termed 'tauopathies'. As suggested by the name, FTD predominantly affects the frontal and anterior temporal lobes. Overall it represents around 2–5% of dementia, but it is a more common cause of younger-onset dementia. It presents uncommonly after the age of 65.[43]

FTD has an insidious onset and slow progression. Memory and visuospatial ability are relatively spared in the early stages. Patients tend to score adequately on the MMSE. There may be economy or stereotypy (patterns of repetition) of speech. Behavioural features may include reduced personal hygiene, dietary change and disinhibition.[44] Compulsive-like repetitive or stereotyped actions may occur. There may be perseveration of responses and utilisation behaviour. Some individuals become more impulsive and hyperactive; others become apathetic and less active. Urinary incontinence may occur early in the condition. Neurological examination may reveal primitive reflexes.

Obtaining a family history is important as around 40% will have an affected first-degree relative.[42,43] The majority of familial forms show an autosomal dominant pattern of inheritance.[43] Individuals with an affected first-degree relative have a 3.5 times increased risk of dementia before the age of 80 years compared to matched control subjects.[42]

Klüver–Bucy syndrome is a pattern of clinical features that results from bilateral anterior temporal lobe dysfunction. These features include dietary changes (e.g. eating only sweet things), emotional blunting, altered sexual behaviour, sensory agnosia and oral exploratory behaviour (e.g. putting inedible objects into the mouth). Neuroimaging may reveal focal atrophy of frontal and temporal lobes, but this is usually only detectable late in the disease course.

Involvement of the left frontotemporal region alone can lead to a presentation with progressive non-fluent aphasia. Semantic dementia is a variant where fluent speech is preserved but there are problems with naming and word comprehension. Other variants of FTD include overlap syndromes with features of PD, motor neuron disease or CBD. A familial form of FTD with PD features is linked to chromosome 17 (termed 'FTDP-17'), which has a younger age of onset and more rapid progression.

Dementia in movement disorders

The majority of movement disorders affecting older people are neurodegenerative in aetiology. It is not surprising to find that there is a great deal of overlap with the neurodegenerative dementias. Movement disorders presenting in the elderly and with associated cognitive changes include:

➤ Parkinson's disease
➤ progressive supranuclear palsy
➤ dementia with Lewy bodies
➤ corticobasal degeneration
➤ normal pressure hydrocephalus

These are discussed in Chapter 9. The pattern of dementia is generally of a subcortical type, as discussed on p. 95.

Other causes of dementia

Many causes of dementia have been identified, most of which are very rare in the elderly. These include HIV-associated dementia, Huntington disease, Wilson disease and neurosyphilis (*see* Box 6.1). Selected conditions are discussed below.

Alcohol-related dementia

Although mild to moderate alcohol intake may be protective against dementia (*see* p. 103), heavy intake appears to confer an increased risk. A study of 2873 people over the age of 65 found that 8.9% had a definite history of alcohol abuse (DSM criteria).[45] Of this subgroup (mean age 78 years) 48% had evidence of dementia compared to 35% of those with no history of abuse (mean age 82 years). It may be linked to around 10% of dementia in the elderly.[46]

There is more than one alcohol-related mechanism causing dementia. The first is simple alcohol dementia, which appears to be induced by a long history of excessive alcohol intake. It may be more common in binge drinkers and those with a low thiamine level. It presents with a subcortical pattern of cognitive impairment. Diagnostic criteria suggest alcohol intake of above 35 units per week for men and 28 units for women for a period of more than five years.[46]

Wernicke–Korsakoff syndrome is caused by thiamine (B$_1$) deficiency. The Wernicke stage is usually the precursor and has the clinical characteristics of ophthalmoplegia, ataxia and delirium. The Korsakoff stage usually, but not always, follows one or more episodes of Wernicke syndrome. This is a prolonged amnesic disorder affecting the ability to form new memories. It often causes the patient to confabulate. The pathological finding is of haemorrhagic necrosis of the mammillary bodies.

Marchiafava–Bignami disease is caused by acute demyelination of the corpus callosum. It was first described in middle-aged Italian men who drank excessive quantities of red wine. Associated with the dementia are seizures and inter-hemispheric disconnection.

In cases of alcohol-related dementia cognition may improve, or at least stabilise, with thiamine replacement and abstinence.

Hypothyroidism

Profound hypothyroidism has been associated with memory impairment, psychomotor slowing and visuospatial impairments.[47] Impairments such as these are probably only partially reversed by adequate treatment.

B$_{12}$ deficiency

The common cause of vitamin B$_{12}$ deficiency is pernicious anaemia that is attributed to reduced absorption secondary to insufficient gastric secretion of intrinsic factor.[48] It has been estimated to be present, yet undiagnosed, in around 2% of the population over the age of 60 and is more common in women than men (2:1).[49] But there are other possible causes of B_{12} deficiency (*see* p. 425). It can lead to neuronal lesions such as demyelination or even cell death. Rarely, cerebral involvement can present as progressive personality change or memory loss.[48] Advanced neurological complications may not be reversed by replacement therapy.

Creutzfeldt–Jakob disease

Creutzfeldt–Jakob disease (CJD) is medicated by a prion. In such disorders, a cellular prion protein (PrP^C) becomes pathogenic by misfolding into a harmful form (PrP^{SC}).[34] This is then capable of inducing change in other prion proteins with a resultant cascade and accumulation of protein aggregates (*see* Figure 6.8).[50] Pathological changes include spongiform degeneration and astrogliosis.[34] It is most commonly sporadic in nature (85%) but familial (10–15%) and infectious forms (<5%) also exist.[51] The infectious forms include new variant (nvCJD) that is related to the ingestion of infected animal products. The sporadic form has a mean age of onset of 62 years and runs a short course (mean survival five months).[51,52] Overall it has an incidence of around one per million per year but this figure rises to around five per million in those over the age of 60 years.[34] Key clinical features are:

➤ a rapidly progressive subcortical dementia
➤ myoclonus
➤ ataxia
➤ pyramidal or extrapyramidal signs.

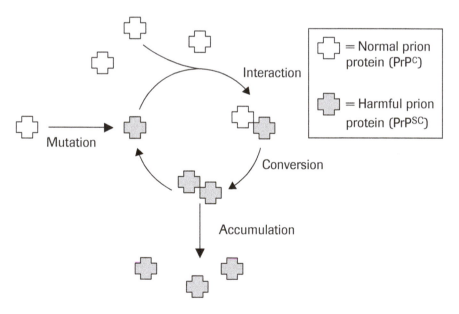

FIGURE 6.8 The proposed actions of harmful prion proteins.

In the sporadic form, around 60% will have periodic sharp wave complexes in their EEG (compared to 30% of people with AD),[53] around 90% will have 14-3-3 protein in their cerebrospinal fluid (CSF).[53–55] However, 14-3-3 protein is a normal cellular component and its presence in the CSF is merely a marker of cell turnover.[55] It may be present following cerebral insults such as a stroke. It has been detected in 10% of people with non-CJD dementia.[53–55] MRI scanning has demonstrated signal hyperintensity in the basal ganglia of 67% of patients with CJD compared to just 7% of non-CJD dementia control subjects.[56] The use of diffusion-weighted MRI may further increase diagnostic accuracy.[57] Autopsy studies have found the commonest misdiagnosis in older people is rapidly progressive AD.[58] The combination of clinical criteria and a CSF positive for 14-3-3 protein or a suggestive EEG has a high diagnostic sensitivity and specificity.[54,55] There is no effective treatment for this condition.

Motor neuron disease

Motor neuron disease (MND) is a disorder related to degeneration of anterior horn cell motor neurons (*see* p. 435). Onset is between the ages of 40 and 80 years. It is marginally more common in men than women. Ten per cent of cases are familial. There tends to be a mixed pattern of upper and lower motor lesions. There are no sensory signs or bladder or bowel neurological involvement. There is usually weakness with associated stiffness and fasciculations. The voice may become hoarse. Cognition is significantly affected in only one-third of patients.[59] A pattern of deficits similar to FTD is most commonly seen.

PREVENTING THE DEVELOPMENT OF DEMENTIA

Non-modifiable risk factors for the development of dementia include age, family history and Down syndrome. A wide range of strategies has been proposed to protect against the development of dementia. Some of these are discussed below.

Alcohol intake

The Rotterdam study is a prospective population-based cohort study of patients over the age of 55 years in a suburb of Rotterdam. Over a mean follow-up period of six years, dementia was diagnosed in 197 of 5395 participants (74% AD, 15% VaD, 11% other dementia).[60] There was a lower associated risk of dementia in those who consumed, on average, up to three alcoholic drinks per day compared to those who did not drink alcohol. The hazard ratio (HR) for people drinking one to three drinks per day for all types of dementia was 0.58 (95% CI 0.38–0.90). All subtypes of dementia appeared to be reduced with alcohol intake and all types of alcohol (beer, wine and spirits) appeared to offer a similar benefit. Similarly, a comparison of 373 individuals (mean age 78 years) who developed dementia with matched controls within the Cardiovascular Health Study (n=5888) found that mild to moderate alcohol intake appears to confer a lower risk of dementia.[61] The odds ratio (OR) compared to non-drinkers was lowest for those who reported drinking between one and six drinks per week (OR 0.46, 95% CI 0.27–0.77). Other studies seem to support these findings.[62–64] In terms of cardiovascular risk reduction, the benefit of alcohol appears to be mediated by changes in LDL and HDL cholesterol levels.[65] A similar mechanism may protect against cerebral small-vessel ischaemia. Conversely, alcohol abuse is associated with an increased risk of dementia (*see* p. 101).

Prevention of obesity

Over 10 000 men and women who were aged between 40 and 45 years when they were enrolled in the Kaiser Permanente programme between the years 1964 and 1973 have been assessed for the development of dementia on average 27 years later.[66] Some 713 people developed dementia at a mean age of onset of 74.5 years. The investigators found that increased weight in middle age was associated with an increased risk of developing dementia. Obese people (body mass index (BMI) $\geq 30\,kg/m^2$) had a 74% increased risk (HR 1.74, 95% CI 1.34–2.26) and overweight people (BMI 25.0–29.9) had a 35% increased risk (HR 1.35, 95% CI 1.14–1.60) compared to people of a normal weight. These differences were not explained by the presence of comorbid conditions. The mechanism of this apparent effect is not understood. It could be related to changes in vascular risk factors (including diabetes). One study has found that obesity is correlated with brain atrophy.[67] The onset of the clinical phase of dementia is usually accompanied by weight loss.

Vascular risk factors

Smoking, hypertension, high cholesterol and diabetes have all been found to be associated with an increased risk of dementia in later life.[68] This finding is clearly logical for VaD. The degree to which vascular factors are important in the genesis of AD is not known but they do appear to play some role.[69] The Syst-Eur trial randomised 2418 patients with hypertension but without dementia (mean age 70 years, mean blood pressure (BP) 173/86 mmHg) to placebo or BP control with a combination of agents.[70] BP fell in both groups, but significantly more in the treatment group. Mean values achieved were 160/83 mmHg for the placebo group compared to 152/80 mmHg in the treatment arm. After a median follow-up of two years, the incidence of dementia was significantly lower in the treatment group: 3.8 cases per 1000 patient-years vs 7.7 per 1000 patient-years in the placebo arm. Having a higher BP in middle age is also associated with an increased risk of cognitive impairment in later life.[71] Statin drugs appeared to have a protective action against the development of dementia in a non-controlled case series.[72] A further case series has suggested that patients with AD on either statins or ACE inhibitors have a slower rate of decline in function than those not on these drugs.[73] A study has found that diabetes in midlife is associated with a 19% greater cognitive decline over a 20-year period compared to people with no diabetes.[74]

Vitamins

It had been believed that the antioxidant properties of vitamin E might have a protective role against the development of dementia. A recent study of 769 people with mild cognitive impairment failed to demonstrate any benefit.[75] Further to this, there is some evidence that vitamin E may be harmful in high doses. A meta-analysis of studies comparing vitamin E supplementation to placebo in 136 000 people found an increase in all-cause mortality in the treatment arm.[76]

Folate and vitamins B_6 and B_{12} have been shown to reduce levels of potentially harmful homocysteine within the body. It has been speculated supplementation with these agents may reduce the risk of dementia. In a trial recruiting 409 patients (mean age

76 years) with mild to moderate AD (MMSE 14–26; mean 21/30) with an 18 month follow-up, despite a fall in serum homocysteine, no benefit was seen in cognitive scores.[77]

Ginkgo biloba

A trial that recruited over 3069 people aged 75 or over (mean age 79 years), with a median follow-up period of six years, compared *Ginkgo biloba* to placebo.[78] It had no beneficial effect in preventing dementia (HR 1.12, 95% CI 0.94–1.33).

Oestrogens

A series of small studies and meta-analyses had suggested a benefit of oestrogens in protecting against the development of dementia. The Women's Health Initiative Memory Study involved over 7000 women aged 65–79 years receiving either oestrogen alone or in combination with progesterone (depending on womb status) vs placebo.[79] Not only did these agents not protect against dementia but also there was a trend towards an increased incidence. Therefore, they should not be used to try to prevent dementia.

Other factors

Regular exercise and midlife physical fitness have been associated with lower incidence of dementia.[80,81] The mechanism of this apparent effect has not been defined. Living in a couple relationship in mid life has also been associated with a lower risk of cognitive impairment in later life.[82]

TREATMENT

Some simple measures such as installing safety devices, including smoke alarms and gas detectors, within the home may improve an individual's ability to live independently. Education, support and respite care can be helpful for caregivers and can delay nursing home placement.[83,84] A study of 206 people with dementia who lived at home and had a carer found that a series of six sessions (lasting around 1.5 hours each) of individual and family counselling plus support group involvement was able to delay the time of admission to nursing home by, on average, 329 days compared to a control group.[85] The sessions included education on AD and strategies to cope with problem behaviours. Patients with mild to moderate AD had more benefit from the intervention than those with advanced disease. There is some evidence that cognitive training may be beneficial in improving cognitive ability and physical functioning in older adults.[86]

Longer-term issues such as nursing home placement should be discussed. Advance directives, wills and power of attorney orders should be considered prior to cognitive decline to the point of mental incapacity (*see* p. 116). The discontinuation of potential harmful medications should also be considered. In particular medications with anticholinergic properties have been associated with cognitive decline in older adults (*see* p. 27).

Driving

In patients who currently drive, consideration needs to be given to stopping. Patients with early dementia of the Alzheimer type and VaD with mean MMSE scores of 23 and 25, respectively, have been found to perform significantly less well in driving test scores compared to age-matched control subjects.[87] This observed decline in function correlated with the degree of MMSE reduction. However, important factors such as impairments in judgement and visuospatial skills may not be detected if MMSE screening is used alone. It can be useful to ask relatives how they feel when in the car with the patient driving to help gauge the risk. For example, would they allow their mother or father to pick up the grandchildren from school? A formal driving assessment can also be arranged. Further details regarding regulations within the UK are available at the Driver and Vehicle Licensing Agency (DVLA) website (www.gov.uk/government/publications/at-a-glance – accessed November 2014). Links to information relating to countries outside the UK are given in Box 6.2.

BOX 6.2 International driving regulations

Useful web resources for driving regulations related to medical illnesses in some selected countries are given below (accessed October 2014).

Australia

Austroads has produced a guide, 'Assessing Fitness to Drive' available from its website (www.austroads.com.au/drivers-vehicles/assessing-fitness-to-drive/for-health-professionals). The Roads and Maritime Services Authority of New South Wales has produced a booklet for older drivers (www.rms.nsw.gov.au/documents/roads/licence/older-drivers-guide.pdf).

Canada

The Canadian Council of Motor Transport Administrators has produced a guide of medical standards for drivers (www.ccmta.ca/en/publications/resources-home/item/determing-driver-fitness-in-canada-september-2013).

USA

The physician's guide to assessing and counselling older drivers is available from the American Medical Association website (www.ama-assn.org/ama/pub/physician-resources/public-health/promoting-healthy-lifestyles/geriatric-health/older-driver-safety/assessing-counseling-older-drivers.shtml).

Cognition

Non-pharmacological interventions

Functioning can be maximised by maintaining daily routines and providing written down to-do lists. Orientation may be improved by providing readily visible clocks and calendars.[88]

A trial randomised 135 patients aged over 65 (mean age 78) with mild to moderate dementia (mean MMSE 19) to 10 sessions of occupational therapy over a five-week period or standard care.[89] At 12-week follow-up, the intervention group scored significantly higher on tests of functional ability and carer well-being. The NNT for a clinically relevant improvement was just 1.3 to 2.5 (depending on which outcome measure was used).

Cholinesterase inhibitors

The development of a treatment for dementia would be a major achievement and it is understandable why great excitement was initially expressed in relation to cholinesterase inhibitors. Early trials suggested a significant benefit in cognition in AD and possibly also VaD and DLB. Unfortunately more recent studies have been less favourable. Side-effects from this type of medication include nausea, vomiting, diarrhoea, weight loss, somnolence and syncope. They may also provoke bradycardia and heart block.

The AD2000 study randomised 565 patients with mild to moderate AD (mean age 76, range 46–93 years; mean MMSE score 19, range 10–27) to receive either donepezil (5 mg or 10 mg daily) or placebo over a three-year period.[90] There was a mean better MMSE score of 0.8 (out of 30) and a mean better Bristol Activities of Daily Living Scale (BADLS) score of 1.0 (out of 60) over the first two years in the donepezil group ($p<0.0001$ for both values). These suggest a minor cognitive and functional benefit with treatment; however, the clinical significance of such a minor change is questionable. Coupled to this, there were no significant differences in either the rate of institutionalisation or the progression of disability after three years. Also, no benefits in terms of behavioural symptoms or carer stress were demonstrated. The study concluded that the benefits were clinically insignificant and did not justify the high associated financial costs at that time.

Some people have argued that a subset of patients responds well to these medications. The AD2000 study found a normally distributed response to treatment curve (rather than a bimodal distribution), which would not favour this idea. Further, those patients who responded best initially were the ones who were more likely to score badly at the subsequent evaluation (i.e. demonstrating the phenomenon of regression to the mean[91]). Therefore, the practice of using a three-month MMSE score to predict those who will benefit from continued treatment is flawed.

Cholinesterase inhibitors have also been proposed for the slowing or prevention of development of AD. A trial of 769 patients with mild cognitive impairment (mean age 73 years, mean MMSE score 27/30) did not demonstrate a difference in rate of progression to AD over a three-year period compared to placebo.[75]

A meta-analysis of 22 trials looking at the use of the cholinesterase inhibitors donepezil, galantamine and rivastigmine in AD has been published.[92] The majority of trials used the Alzheimer's Disease Assessment Scale – cognitive subscale (ADAS-cog) as a primary outcome measure (see Appendix A). Values obtained showed a net improvement of between 1.5 and 3.9 points on this scale (out of 70). The trial lengths were variable, ranging from six weeks to three years. A number of methodological deficiencies were noted within most of the trials. These included incomplete or inaccurate data for patients who did not complete the trial, which, given that dementia is associated with a progressive cognitive decline, could artificially exaggerate the treatment effect.

The small benefit derived, coupled with the trial deficiencies, further question the use of these agents.

Rivastigmine is also available in a transdermal patch formulation. This may reduce the incidence of the gastrointestinal side-effects. It may also be useful for those with an impaired swallow or poor concordance with medications.

In conclusion, the cholinesterase inhibitors may have a small benefit in cognition but this is of questionable clinical significance, appears to be short-lived (less than three years) and must be offset against the risk of side-effects. Their main benefit has perhaps been the provocation of a new interest in dementia and the establishment of memory clinics. Currently they are licensed for use in mild to moderate Alzheimer's dementia (rivastigmine is also recommended for use in Parkinson's disease dementia and dementia with Lewy bodies – *see* p. 167).[93]

Memantine

Memantine is a glutamate antagonist that acts at *N*-methyl-D-aspartate (NMDA) receptors. It has been proposed that it may reduce excitatory neurotoxicity in dementia. A series of small trials of short duration (six months) has shown a possible mild benefit on cognition, function and behaviour in moderate to severe AD, but benefits are unclear in mild to moderate AD or VaD.[94] It is currently recommended for use in moderate to severe Alzheimer's dementia.[93] Generally memantine has few side-effects but may provoke constipation. There does not seem to be any additional benefit of combining memantine with a cholinesterase inhibitor.[95]

Non-cognitive symptoms
Agitation

The term 'agitation' is used to cover a number of behavioural disturbances in dementia. An alternative term 'behavioural and psychological symptoms of dementia' is also used (BPSD). It ranges from the more mild problems of apathy, fidgeting and wandering to the more alarming difficulties of verbal and physical aggression. Some such symptoms occur in the majority of people with advanced dementia. Consideration should be given to detecting any unmet physical or psychological needs. Getting to know your patient better by getting collateral history regarding their background is beneficial, e.g. by asking relatives to complete a 'This is me' document.[9] Agitation can be a sign of unhappiness, and associated reversible factors should be sought (e.g. depression). There may be misinterpretation of events (e.g. assistance with personal care being viewed as assault). Pain may present atypically in people with dementia. The Abbey Pain Scale may aid its detection (*see* Appendix A). A study found that a systematic approach to the management of pain can reduce agitation in residents of nursing homes with moderate to severe dementia.[96] A significant number of problem behaviours will spontaneously resolve and so, unless very severe, a policy of watching to see if it persists over a one-month period may be adopted.[97] A change in behaviour may represent the development of delirium – this should be assessed as discussed in Chapter 7.

Non-pharmacological management

Evidence for the efficacy of non-pharmacological interventions is, at best, minimal.[98] However, in the absence of a good alternative and given the lack of adverse effects, their implementation seems reasonable. In general, people with dementia respond better when they are in familiar, calm and quiet environments and in stable daily routines. Behavioural problems may become worse later in the day ('sun downing'). Confrontation of patients with problem behaviours may lead to escalation.

Identifying the trigger factors that are associated with problem behaviours can lead to being able to avoid their occurrence. One approach is for the carer to complete a diary, recording the antecedents, behaviour and consequences (ABC) each time a problem arises.[99] Typical data would include the people present and the activity being undertaken before the problem. Also, the outcome of the event should be noted to see if any reinforcement of negative behaviours is taking place.

Brief educational programmes and support groups for carers may have a small benefit but do not affect patient outcomes.[83] In episodes of aggression, the carer should be advised to remain calm and try to avoid contradicting, arguing or confrontation. The agitated patient should be approached from the front and addressed at eye level. Questions may be used to distract the person's attention and aim to refocus on something more pleasurable.[99] In patients who are resistant to their caregivers, setting more limited goals can be effective. For example, if showering is a particular problem, less frequent showering may help to reduce conflict. There is some evidence that a number of personalised psychosocial interventions may also help reduce agitation.[100]

In people who wander, increased daytime activity and exercise, preferably outdoors, can limit this tendency. Rooms might be labelled to reduce the chance of getting lost. Patients who wander at night may be less inclined to become lost if night-lights are fitted. Caffeine, alcohol and daytime naps may all affect sleep patterns and should be avoided. Alarms that are activated when a wandering person leaves a building or opens a door can be useful. Environmental adaptations such as putting stop signs or mirrors on doors can prevent persons from exiting through them. Alternatively, concealed or childproof locks may be fitted to external doors. A patient may be allowed to wander within a safe environment. Medications are usually ineffective for this problem.

A study that recruited 81 people with dementia who resided in a nursing home (mean age 82 years, mean MMSE score 9/30) compared an intervention consisting of an activity programme, medication review and educational sessions for staff to a control group over a six-month period.[101] It was found that behavioural disorders and antipsychotic drug use reduced in both groups, but the sizes of the reductions were greater in the treatment group (by 23% and 9%, respectively). However, this was achieved with additional staff usage and so financial costs were greater.

Aromatherapy has been suggested as an effective treatment to reduce behavioural symptoms in dementia. A study compared the use of an essential oil (lemon balm) mixed with a base lotion and applied to patients' arms and faces to a placebo lotion in 72 patients with dementia plus agitation over a four-week period.[102] Sixty per cent of the treatment group compared to 14% of the placebo group were judged to have had a significant improvement with this therapy. Sensory stimulation such as soft background music may cause a small reduction in problem behaviours.[83] Light therapy has been advocated to try to correct abnormal circadian rhythms in the institutionalised elderly with reduced sunlight exposure. Patients sit in front of a box that emits strong light for around two hours per day. Small initial studies suggest it may provide a minor benefit in behavioural control.[103] Pet therapy may also be tried.

Pharmacological management

Medications used to control problem behaviours may worsen a patient's cognitive function, leading to increased confusion and, paradoxically, worsened behaviour. Usually they are considered a last resort.

Antipsychotic medications

Antipsychotic drugs (also termed 'neuroleptics') are roughly divided into two categories: the older 'typical' and newer 'atypical' agents. Haloperidol is the most commonly used typical agent. Atypical agents include clozapine, risperidone, olanzapine and quetiapine. Comparing the groups, atypical agents tend to have lesser antagonism of dopamine receptors, but more anticholinergic, serotonergic and alpha-adrenergic effects.[104] In the UK risperidone is the only antipsychotic drug currently licensed for use in dementia, and this is for the treatment of severe aggression, not responding to other treatment, and for a time period limited to six weeks.

Adverse effects

Adverse events with all of these medications are considerable. Among these are drug-induced movement disorders (*see* p. 173) and an increased risk of falls (*see* p. 327). They have also been found to be associated with an increased rate of cognitive decline in patients with dementia compared to those not taking such medications.[73,105–107] This finding may be mediated by the anticholinergic properties of these drugs (*see* Table 2.2). Some of the atypical agents (olanzapine and clozapine) have been associated with increased weight gain and new onset of type 2 diabetes.[108] These problems may be mediated by serotonergic or histaminergic receptor actions.[109]

More recently, concerns have been generated that atypical antipsychotic medications may be associated with an increased risk of stroke.[110,111] This is based on results from trials comparing these agents to placebo where a two to three times increased relative risk for cerebrovascular events was observed. A retrospective review of the records of 32 710 people prescribed either typical (17 845) or atypical (14 865) antipsychotic agents failed to demonstrate a difference in hospitalisation rates for stroke between the medication groups (HR 1.01, 95% CI 0.81–1.26).[112] This suggests that either the association with stroke is artifactual or that both subgroups of antipsychotic agent are associated with an increased stroke risk. A more recent analysis of 6790 patients receiving antipsychotic drugs has suggested that this latter idea is most likely.[113] The risk of stroke was elevated with all antipsychotic drugs, but more so with atypicals (rate ratio 2.32, 95% CI 1.73–3.10) than typical (rate ratio 1.69, 95% CI 1.55–1.84) agents. Risks are highest in those with a diagnosis of dementia (rate ratio 3.50, 95% CI 2.97–4.12).

A meta-analysis of trials comparing atypical antipsychotic drug use to placebo in patients with dementia found an increased risk of death with these agents (OR 1.54, 95% CI 1.06–2.23, $p = 0.02$).[114] It is not known whether this also applies to conventional antipsychotic agents as similar safety data in dementia is not available. However, a recent retrospective analysis of mortality in elderly patients (mean age 83 years) found a higher risk of death with typical compared to atypical agents (within 180 days of commencement RR 1.37, 95% CI 1.27–1.49).[115] Of course, caution must be used when interpreting such data as there are significant differences between the medication groups, the subjects did not all have dementia (less than half), and prescriber bias cannot be analysed.

Efficacy

Risperidone and haloperidol have been compared to placebo in 344 people with advanced dementia and agitation within institutional care facilities (median age 81, range 56–97 years; mean MMSE score 8/30) over a 12-week period.[116] After dose titration, mean doses of 1.1 mg/day and 1.2 mg/day were attained for the risperidone and haloperidol groups, respectively. At the end of the trial there were no significant differences in total behavioural scores for the three groups. A subgroup analysis suggested that both risperidone and haloperidol were better than placebo for control of aggression. There was a 35% drop-out rate for this study (similar amounts of patients from each group). The majority of participants discontinued due to either adverse events (50%) or lack of efficacy (44%). Twenty-two per cent of patients on haloperidol had extrapyramidal side-effects compared to 15% on risperidone and 11% on placebo. Somnolence was more common in both treatment arms compared to placebo. Similarly, when other neuroleptics have been compared, they all appear to have a similar, mild efficacy.[117]

Haloperidol, trazodone, behavioural management techniques (BMT), and placebo have been compared in 149 community-dwelling people with AD and agitation (mean age 75 years, mean MMSE score 13/30) over a 16-week period.[118] Doses of the medications were gradually titrated up, achieving mean doses of 1.8 mg/day for haloperidol and 200 mg/day for trazodone. The BMT consisted of 11 sessions, including education and strategies to reduce agitation. There were no significant differences between the groups in primary outcome measures. There was a 38% discontinuation rate overall, with no significant differences between the groups. Extrapyramidal side-effects occurred more commonly in the haloperidol arm.

A dose of 2–3 mg per day of haloperidol has been found to be more effective than 0.5–0.75 mg per day in controlling disruptive behaviours (mainly psychosis and/or aggression) in 71 outpatients with dementia (mean age 72 years).[119] However, there was a 20% incidence of extrapyramidal side-effects rated as 'moderate to severe' at this higher dose. A Cochrane review of the use of haloperidol for agitation in dementia concluded that there was evidence to support the use of haloperidol to reduce aggression but not for any other behavioural problems.[120]

A trial randomised 345 people with dementia (mean age 83 years, mean MMSE score 5/30) plus aggressive behaviour, who lived in nursing homes, to receive either risperidone (mean dose 0.95 mg per day) or placebo over a 12-week period.[121] There was a significant reduction in aggression in the risperidone arm. Adverse effects occurring more commonly in the risperidone group included somnolence (37% vs 25%), cerebrovascular events (9% (including two deaths due to stroke) vs 2%) and extrapyramidal disorders (6% vs 3%). Similarly, another trial of 625 patients with dementia plus psychotic and behavioural symptoms (mean age 83 years, mean MMSE score 7/30) comparing risperidone to placebo over a 12-week period found a significantly lower rate of aggression and psychosis with risperidone.[122] Additionally, a study of 206 demented people (mean age 83 years, mean MMSE score 7/30) over a six-week period found that olanzapine (5–10 mg per day) was superior to placebo in the control of psychosis and behavioural disturbance (most of whom displayed aggression).[123] Patients in the treatment arm had a significantly higher incidence of somnolence and abnormal gait.

Yet, a recent randomised study compared olanzapine, quetiapine or risperidone to placebo in 421 patients (mean age 78 years, mean MMSE score 15/30) with AD plus aggression, psychosis or agitation over a 36-week period.[124] Overall they found similar discontinuation rates between the groups, with discontinuation due to inefficacy more common with placebo, but this was offset by higher discontinuation due to adverse effects with the active drugs (including Parkinsonism, sedation and cognitive changes). Also, quetiapine has been compared to placebo and rivastigmine treatment for the management of agitation in 93 demented individuals over the age of 60 years who live in institutional care over a 26-week period.[106] Not only did quetiapine not improve agitation but it also was associated with a significant cognitive decline compared to the other groups. A more recent study has also failed to show a benefit of quetiapine compared to placebo.[125]

When a programme of reduction of antipsychotic use in nursing homes was implemented, no worsening of behavioural features was encountered compared to a matched group of patients without a reduction in their medication.[126] Such a technique may be even more effective if coupled to nursing education programmes to teach alternative management strategies to medication use.[127] A study randomised 165 people with AD (mean age 85 years) who resided in care facilities and were taking an antipsychotic drug for a behavioural disturbance to either continue their current medication or switch to a placebo.[128] The discontinuation of antipsychotic medication had little effect on behavioural scores. However, after 12 months the survival rate was higher in those on placebo (77% vs 70%). This difference appeared to increase over time; at three-year follow-up survival was just 30% in those who continued antipsychotic drugs, compared to 59% in the placebo group. A more recent meta-analysis has also supported the safety of antipsychotic drug withdrawal.[129]

These studies emphasise the point that many nursing home residents are on medication that is either unjustified or ineffective. Investigators have found that 16–24% of nursing home residents are on antipsychotic medication.[130-133] Yet the majority of these prescriptions (up to 88%) are inappropriate according to expert guidelines.[132] The trigger to prescribe many of these medications appears to be nursing home admission and is associated with little, if any, specialist input.[131]

Summary

In summary, antipsychotic agents may have a role in controlling aggression in dementia but not other forms of agitation. They are generally overprescribed, especially within nursing home environments. Atypical antipsychotics are more expensive and no more effective. They have only been studied in a small number of trials with short durations.[134] They appear to cause fewer extrapyramidal side-effects but this may be at the expense of an increased risk of stroke and death. The clinical relevance of reduced extrapyramidal effects is unclear as all of the agents are associated with a similarly increased risk of falls (*see* p. 327). Antipsychotic drugs are likely to result in cognitive decline if taken over a prolonged time period. Regular review with attempts to withdraw antipsychotic agents should be undertaken at least six-monthly.[135] Most prescriptions should not exceed 12 weeks.

Cholinesterase inhibitors

Most studies assessing the effect of cholinesterase inhibitors were not primarily designed to assess non-cognitive symptoms. The AD2000 study did not demonstrate an improvement in behavioural symptoms in patients with mild to moderate AD on donepezil.[90]

A study of 134 patients with AD (mean age 81 years, mean MMSE score 20/30) and neuropsychiatric symptoms (Neuropsychiatric Inventory (NPI) score >11) (*see* Appendix A) compared the effect of continued donepezil therapy (10 mg/day) to medication replacement with placebo over a 12-week period.[136] The mean NPI score for both groups was 15.2 at randomisation, this fell to 12.3 in the continued donepezil group and rose to 18.5 in the placebo group ($p = 0.02$). However, only 60% of the participants completed the study. Most withdrawals were due to adverse events or inefficacy of the medication. It cannot be excluded that the difference between groups is due to drug withdrawal effects rather than a true benefit of continued donepezil. A more recent study randomised 272 patients (mean age 85 years, mean NPI score 24) with AD and agitation to receive donepezil or placebo over a 12-week period.[137] No significant benefit was observed with cholinesterase inhibitor use.

A trial of 120 people with dementia with Lewy bodies (mean age 74 years, mean MMSE score 17/30) compared rivastigmine to placebo in the control of behavioural features of the condition over 23 weeks.[138] NPI scores were used as the main outcome measure. A benefit was found with rivastigmine in the symptom domains of apathy, anxiety, delusions and hallucinations, but overall differences failed to reach statistical significance. Side-effects occurring more commonly in the treatment group included nausea (37%), vomiting (25%), anorexia (19%) and somnolence (9%). A worsening of Parkinsonian features with pro-cholinergic medication was not found in this study, but there have been a few case reports of this occurring.[139] Similarly, rivastigmine was not found to improve agitation in individuals with AD.[106]

In summary, there is little evidence to support the use of cholinesterase inhibitors for the control of non-cognitive symptoms in dementia. Available studies recruited only small numbers of patients and used short time periods. When a difference has been found, the magnitude has been small and of doubtful clinical significance.[140]

Anti-epileptic agents

Carbamazepine and valproate have been suggested as treatments for agitation in dementia. Carbamazepine (mean dose 304 mg/day) has been compared to placebo in 51 patients with dementia plus agitation (mean age 86 years, mean MMSE score 6/30) over a six-week period.[141] Previously used psychotropic agents were withdrawn prior to the study. Carbamazepine was started at 100 mg/day and increased by 50 mg every three to four days if no side-effects occurred. A significant reduction in behavioural scores was noted in the treatment group. Side-effects were significantly more common in the carbamazepine group (59% vs 29%). These included increased incidences of drowsiness, ataxia and disorientation. However, the behavioural efficacy of carbamazepine has not been demonstrated in a subsequent study.[140]

A number of small, short-duration studies have evaluated the use of valproate for agitation in dementia. A Cochrane review concluded that lower doses of valproate (from 480 mg per day) were ineffective and higher doses (up to 1 g per day) were associated with an unacceptably high rate of adverse effects, including sedation.[142]

Benzodiazepines

Benzodiazepines have also been tried in the management of behavioural disturbance in dementia. Alprazolam (a short to intermediate length half-life benzodiazepine given at a dose of 0.5 mg bd) has been compared to haloperidol (mean dose 0.64 mg) in the management of disruptive behaviours in 68 elderly people (mean age 83, range 65–98 years) with cognitive impairment, in a crossover design, over a 12-week period.[143] There were no significant differences between the groups for outcome measures. Alarmingly, there was a trend for a worsening of behaviour following commencement of either agent after the placebo pre-treatment phase. A further non-randomised case series has associated benzodiazepine use with an increased rate of functional decline in patients with AD.[73] It seems fair to assume that benzodiazepines are equally ineffective as neuroleptics in the control of agitation and are associated with their own range of significant adverse effects (e.g. sedation, confusion and falls).

Antidepressants

Various antidepressant drugs have been proposed for the management of agitation in dementia. Trazodone is a sedating antidepressant agent with serotonergic agonist and antagonist properties. It has been show to be no better than placebo in the control of agitation in AD.[118] A Cochrane review concluded that there was insufficient evidence to recommend the use of trazodone for the control of agitation in dementia.[144] A meta-analysis concluded that antidepressant agents have not been found to be effective in the management of symptoms other than depression in people with dementia.[140]

Depression

See Chapter 8. Non-pharmacological interventions that may be beneficial to depressed patients with dementia include increasing social activities, reminiscing about previous pleasurable life events and adapting formerly enjoyed activities to fit in with their current functional levels.[99]

Reduced oral intake

A reduction in oral intake and body weight are normal changes seen in older adults (*see* p. 10). These are partly related to reduced physical activity and reduced muscle mass. In patients with advanced dementia they may be aggravated by a concurrent depressive episode or the result of either the loss of desire to eat or the loss of cerebral coordination of the swallowing mechanism. These latter causes usually herald the terminal phase of dementia. Therefore it is important to try to exclude or treat a depressive illness (*see* Chapter 8). An antidepressant that may also cause stimulation of appetite, such as mirtazapine, could be tried.

Nasogastric and percutaneous endoscopic gastrostomy (PEG) tubes are used to bypass abnormal swallowing mechanisms to prevent malnutrition (*see* p. 220). Nasogastric tubes are usually only a temporary measure (days to weeks), with PEG tubes being more appropriate for long-term use. They have also been utilised in patients with end-stage dementia with reduced oral intakes.

The insertion is often justified by the notion that suffering will be alleviated, life will be prolonged or on grounds that not providing nutrition is morally wrong.[145] Evidence from available studies does not support tube feeding as beneficial in terms of quality of life, prolonging survival or nutritional status.[146,147] An improved survival following PEG insertion has only been demonstrated in patients with cerebrovascular disease or oropharyngeal cancer.[148] If the patient is physically able but choosing not to eat, and a reversible condition such as depression has been excluded, it is questionable how forcibly feeding them would improve their quality of life. At the most extreme, patients may actually be restrained to prevent them from pulling an irritating tube out.[145]

There is an argument that denying nutrition in the setting of palliative care is causing patients suffering. This is, obviously, hard to assess in advanced dementia but evidence from patients with other terminal conditions suggests that comfort can be achieved despite minimal oral intake (*see* p. 66).

Another common reason for PEG insertion is to prevent aspiration pneumonia.[149] However, PEG insertion has not been found to prevent aspiration pneumonia and may even make it more likely to occur.[150] This latter scenario could be due to a reduced lower oesophageal sphincter efficacy following gastrostomy insertion.[147] One study found that 57% of PEG-fed patients with dementia had had an episode of aspiration pneumonia in the preceding six months.[151]

Patients with dementia who have PEG tubes inserted have poorer survivals than age-matched controls without PEG tubes.[152,153] Feeding tube placement has not been associated with a survival advantage in patients with dementia compared to demented people without feeding tubes.[154,155] The mortality following PEG insertion is higher in patients with dementia than those without. The 30-day mortality rate for procedures within elderly hospitalised demented people is around 54% and the one-year mortality 90%[156] (compared to 24–28% and 63%, respectively (*see* p. 220)). There are also complication rates associated with tube feeding, including blockage of the tube and infection at the insertion site. Another harm that should be considered is the removal of the pleasurable sensation of the taste of food.

In summary, there is no convincing evidence that feeding tubes result in any beneficial effects in advanced dementia and there is good reason to think that they cause harm. Alternative techniques that may safely improve oral intake include ensuring an upright position when feeding, small and frequent meals, adjusted type and consistency of food, and protected feeding times with increased supervision.[147]

ETHICAL AND LEGAL ISSUES

The following text refers to law within the UK at the time of writing. This may be subject to change over time and will also vary in different countries (although general principles are likely to be very similar). The components are also relevant to conditions other than dementia (e.g. delirium). Box 6.3 provides links to some information relating to countries outside the UK.

BOX 6.3 Ethical guidance in countries outside the UK

Although principles remain similar, variance occurs in ethical issues between countries and sometimes between states. The information below is intended to act as a starting point for those seeking more information (accessed November 2014).

Australia

The website of the Office of the Public Advocate of South Australia contains some useful information on guardianship legislation (www.opa.sa.gov.au/what_we_do/guardianship). Information from the Medical Board of Australia is available on its website (www.medical board.gov.au/Codes-Guidelines-Policies.aspx).

Canada

The Canadian Medical Association code of ethics can be found at their website (http://policybase.cma.ca/dbtw-wpd/PolicyPDF/PD04-06.pdf).

USA

The American Medical Association website (www.ama-assn.org/ama/pub/physician-resources/medical-ethics/code-medical-ethics.shtml) contains ethical information. The University of Washington School of Medicine website contains information around end of life decisions including the assessment of mental capacity (depts.washington.edu/bioethx/topics/termlife.html#compquest).

Mental capacity

There comes a point when cognitive function becomes so impaired that individuals are no longer able to make reasonable decisions regarding their own care – this is termed 'lacking mental capacity'. Medical practitioners are commonly asked to make decisions as to whether this has occurred. This is often very difficult as we are asked to make a decision in a black and white manner about a process that represents shades of grey. Standard cognitive assessments, such as the MMSE, do not evaluate a person's mental capacity to make decisions about their welfare. A patient who makes what appear to be irrational decisions due to personal idiosyncrasy does not necessarily lack mental capacity.

Patients should be assumed to have mental capacity to make a decision until it is proved otherwise. Capacity assessments should be judged for each matter to be evaluated; that is, they are decision-specific. For example, if a patient is judged not to have the capacity to handle their finances, it does not automatically follow that they are incapable of choosing where they wish to live. The assessments should also be made when the patient is functioning at their best and with all appropriate support (e.g. an interpreter). This may be particularly relevant to people who have fluctuating conditions (e.g. DLB (*see* p. 169)), or conditions that may improve with time (e.g. delirium).

When a patient is judged to lack capacity to make a particular decision for him or herself, then a decision is made 'in their best interests'. This decision is usually made by agreement between different members of a multidisciplinary team. What constitutes 'best interests' is not exclusively based on medical evidence, and factors such as the person's previously expressed opinions regarding their healthcare and their religious beliefs should also be considered.[157] In some instances this may include the information contained in a living will. It is advised that the option chosen should be the least restrictive for the patient.[158]

Relatives or carers cannot make such decisions for an individual who lacks capacity (except in the case of a 'Lasting Power of Attorney' order (*see* p. 118). However, their opinions as to what the person would have chosen for themselves, if they were able, are clearly very relevant and important in deciding what represents 'best interests' for that individual. This would include information from a living will (*see* p. 118). Ideally, medical staff and family members are in agreement with regard to the appropriateness of any decision. When conflict occurs a second opinion may be sought, and occasionally a court judgment is required.

Patients who do not have an obvious relative or friend to help make choices may benefit from an independent person to act for them. In the UK, an Independent Mental Capacity Advocate is such a deputy appointed by court.

Assessing mental capacity

In situations where what the patient wishes to do and what would be in the patient's best interests are the same, assessing capacity is irrelevant. Capacity assessments can be performed by any doctor but are usually best done by the doctor who knows the patient best. In difficult cases the opinion of someone with more expertise in making these decisions, such as psychiatrist, may also be sought. In order to have mental capacity, a patient should comply with the following points:

➤ understand the information that they are being told
➤ believe that the information is true
➤ be able to retain the information long enough to 'weigh it in the balance'.

They must also have the ability to communicate their decision to others (this may be in spoken words, written language or some other means, e.g. for those with dysphasia). All of these things must occur in the absence of coercion from others.

In practical terms, when a specific decision is to be made then the patient's knowledge of this subject should be explored. For example, if this is a decision to return to their home, the patient should be asked to describe their home. If they provide grossly inaccurate information (such as living with their parents), they are unlikely to be able to base a decision on sound data. Next, the benefits and risks of each option should be discussed. Following this, the patient should be asked to repeat the information given so as to assess their ability to retain it. Information from other members of the medical team (e.g. nursing staff, physiotherapists and occupational therapists) may also be useful. As a general principle, when there is substantial doubt, it is best to assume that the patient does have mental capacity. It may well be that the least restrictive option (e.g. returning home) is the patient's preferred choice anyway, thereby making the establishment, or not, of mental capacity irrelevant.

Living wills/advance directives

Living wills or advance directives are oral or written instructions made by a person, at a time when they are well, in regard to their preferences for future care. These are only relevant if appropriate to the current clinical situation. If a patient has made a desire to refuse a particular treatment, this is legally binding. If the decision is in favour of receiving a specific treatment, this should be taken into consideration by the medical team but it is not legally binding that they must receive it.[147]

Power of attorney

➤ *Enduring power of attorney* is a legally binding appointment of another person to take responsibility for financial matters of an individual at some point in the future when they no longer have mental capacity to do this for themselves. It does not apply for non-financial matters. It cannot be set up for individuals who have already lost the capacity to make such a decision. In this instance they have to apply for 'Court of Protection' – a more difficult and costly procedure. For this reason it is advisable for all people to appoint someone with an Enduring Power of Attorney responsibility early in the course of a dementia illness.

➤ *Lasting power of attorney* is similar to Enduring Power of Attorney in most aspects, except that it allows the appointed person to also make decisions regarding social and health care.[159] Future treatment decisions should be specifically stated.

Guardianship

Guardianship refers to the legal allocation of another person to make decisions in an individual's best interests for the foreseeable future. This person may be a relative or a public appointed person. This procedure is usually unnecessary, but in some cases a guardian's input can help to enforce the 'best interests' upon the patient. For example, a person judged to lack capacity who repeatedly tries to leave a care home, which has been chosen to be the best living environment for them, can be returned against their will if the guardian is in agreement.

PROGNOSIS

Life expectancy is reduced in people with a diagnosis of dementia. Estimates of average survival from the time of symptom onset are typically in the range 3.3 to 11.7 years, and survival from diagnosis in the range 3.2 to 6.6 years.[160] Survival duration is influenced by the person's age at the time of diagnosis. It falls from an average of 6.7 years when aged 60 to 69 years, around 4.2 years when aged 70–79, around 3.0 years when aged 80–89 and 1.9 years when aged 90 or over.[161] Other factors are subtype of dementia (FTD and VaD seem to do worse), severity of dementia at diagnosis, degree of functional impairment and gender (males do a little worse).[162]

PALLIATIVE CARE

Dementia is a progressive disorder, and ultimately the palliation of symptoms will be the most appropriate intervention (*see* Chapter 5). Currently, palliative care services and medications are underutilised within this patient group.[163]

REFERENCES

1 Skoog I, Nilsson L, Palmertz B, *et al*. A population-based study of dementia in 85-year-olds. *N Engl J Med*, 1993; **328**: 153–8.

2 Lobo A, Launer LJ, Fratiglioni L, *et al*. Prevalence of dementia and major subtypes in Europe: a collaborative study of population-based cohorts. *Neurology*, 2000; **54**(Suppl 5): S4–9.

3 Rocca WA, Bonaiuto S, Lippi A, *et al*. Prevalence of clinically diagnosed Alzheimer's disease and other dementing disorders: a door-to-door survey in Appignano, Macerata Province, Italy. *Neurology*, 1990; **40**: 626–31.

4 Ferri CP, Prince M, Brayne C, *et al*. Global prevalence of dementia: a Delphi consensus study. *Lancet*, 2005; **366**: 2112–17.

5 Sampson EL, Blanchard MR, Jones L, *et al*. Dementia in the acute hospital: prospective cohort study of prevalence and mortality. *Br J Psychiatry*, 2009; **195**: 61–6.

6 Woodford HJ, George J. Neurological and cognitive impairments detected in older people without a diagnosis of neurological or cognitive disease. *Postgrad Med J*, 2011; **86**: 199–206.

7 Xie J, Brayne C, Matthews FE, *et al*. Survival times in people with dementia: analysis from population based cohort study with 14 year follow-up. *BMJ*, 2008; **336**: 258–62.

8 Budson AE, Price BH. Memory dysfunction. *N Engl J Med*, 2005; **352**(7): 692–9.

9 Alzheimer's Society. *This is Me*. Available at: alzheimers.org.uk/thisisme (accessed 18 November 2014).

10 Ancelin ML, Artero S, Portet F, *et al*. Non-degenerative mild cognitive impairment in elderly people and the use of anticholinergic drugs: longitudinal cohort study. *BMJ*, 2006; **332**: 455–8.

11 Fox C, Smith T, Maidment I, *et al*. Effect of medications with anti-cholinergic properties on cognitive function, delirium, physical function and mortality: a systematic review. *Age Ageing*, 2014; **43**: 604–15.

12 Woodford HJ, George J. Cognitive assessment in the elderly: a review of clinical methods. *Q J Med*, 2007; **100**(8): 469–84.

13 Available at: www.mocatest.org/pdf_files/test/MoCA-Test-English_7_1.pdf (accessed 14 October 2014).

14 Wolf-Klein GP, Silverstone FA, Levy AP, *et al*. Screening for Alzheimer's disease by clock drawing. *J Am Geriatr Soc*, 1989; **37**: 730–4.

15 Hsieh S, Schubert S, Hoon C, *et al*. Validation of the Addenbrooke's Cognitive Examination III in frontotemporal dementia and Alzheimer's disease. *Dementia Geriatr Cogn Disord*, 2013; **36**: 242–50.

16 Available at: www.dementia.ie/images/uploads/site-images/ACE-III_Administration_(UK).pdf (accessed 14 October 2014).

17 Tweedy J, Reding M, Garcia C, et al. Significance of cortical disinhibition signs. *Neurology*, 1982; **32**: 169–73.

18 Owen G, Mulley GP. The palmomental reflex: a useful clinical sign? *J Neurol Neurosurg Psychiatry*, 2002; **73**: 113–15.

19 Huff FJ, Boller F, Lucchelli F, et al. The neurologic examination in patients with probable Alzheimer's disease. *Arch Neurol*, 1987; **44**: 929–32.

20 Burns A, Jacoby R, Levy R. Neurological signs in Alzheimer's disease. *Age Ageing*, 1991; **20**: 45–51.

21 Dougall NJ, Bruggink S, Ebmeier KP. Systematic review of the diagnostic accuracy of 99mTc-HMPAO-SPECT in dementia. *Am J Geriatr Psych*, 2004; **12**: 554–70.

22 McKeith I, O'Brien J, Walker Z, et al. Sensitivity and specificity of dopamine transporter imaging with 123I-FP-CIT SPECT in dementia with Lewy bodies: a phase III, multicentre study. *Lancet Neurology*, 2007; **6**(4): 305–13.

23 Warren JD, Schott JM, Fox NC, et al. Brain biopsy in dementia. *Brain*, 2005; **128**: 2016–25.

24 Clarfield AM. The decreasing prevalence of reversible dementias: an updated meta-analysis. *Arch Intern Med*, 2003; **163**(18): 2219–29.

25 Flood JM, Weinstock HS, Guroy ME, et al. Neurosyphilis during the AIDS epidemic, San Francisco, 1985–1992. *J Inf Dis*, 1998; **177**: 931–40.

26 Petersen RC. Mild cognitive impairment. *N Engl J Med*, 2011; **364**: 2227–34.

27 Tricco A, Soobiah C, Berliner S, et al. Efficacy and safety of cognitive enhancers for patients with mild cognitive impairment: a systematic review and meta-analysis. *CMAJ*, 2013; **185**: 1393–401.

28 Kraybill ML, Larson EB, Tsuang W, et al. Cognitive differences in dementia patients with autopsy-verified AD, Lewy body pathology or both. *Neurology*, 2005; **64**: 2069–73.

29 Howard R, Rabins PV, Seeman MV, et al. Late-onset schizophrenia and very-late-onset schizophrenia-like psychosis: an international consensus. *Am J Psychiatry*, 2000; **157**: 172–8.

30 Nyenhuis DL, Gorelick PB. Vascular dementia: a contemporary review of epidemiology, diagnosis, prevention and treatment. *J Am Geriatr Soc*, 1998; **46**: 1437–48.

31 Schneider JA, Arvanitakis Z, Bang W, et al. Mixed brain pathologies account for most dementia cases in community dwelling older persons. *Neurology*, 2007; **69**: 2197–204.

32 Mega MS, Cummings JL, Fiorello T, et al. The spectrum of behavioral changes in Alzheimer's disease. *Neurology*, 1996; **46**: 130–5.

33 Assal F, Cummings JL. Neuropsychiatric symptoms in the dementias. *Curr Op Neurol*, 2002; **15**(4): 445–50.

34 Prusiner SB. Shattuck Lecture – neurodegenerative diseases and prions. *N Engl J Med*, 2001; **344**(20): 1516–26.

35 Cummings JL. Alzheimer's disease. *N Engl J Med*, 2004; **351**: 56–67.

36 Dubois B, Feldman HH, Jacova C, et al. Research criteria for the diagnosis of Alzheimer's disease: revising the NINCDS–ADRDA criteria. *Lancet Neurol*, 2007; **6**: 734–46.

37 Henon H, Durieu I, Guerouaou D, et al. Poststroke dementia: incidence and relationship to prestroke cognitive decline. *Neurology*, 2001; **57**: 1216–22.

38 Barba R, Martinez-Espinosa S, Rodriguez-Garcia E, et al. Poststroke dementia: clinical features and risk factors. *Stroke*, 2000; **31**: 1494–501.

39 Desmond DW, Moroney JT, Paik MC, et al. Frequency and clinical determinants of dementia after ischaemic stroke. *Neurology*, 2000; **54**: 1124–31.

40 Zekry D, Hauw J, Gold G. Mixed dementia: epidemiology, diagnosis and treatment. *J Am Geriatr Soc*, 2002; **50**: 1431–8.

41 Snowdon DA, Greiner LH, Mortimer JA, *et al.* Brain infarction and the clinical expression of Alzheimer disease. The Nun Study. *JAMA*, 1997; **277**(10): 813–17.

42 Stevens M, Van Duijn CM, Kamphorst W, *et al.* Familial aggregation in frontotemporal dementia. *Neurology*, 1998; **50**: 1541–5.

43 Chow TW, Miller BL, Hayashi VN, *et al.* Inheritance of frontotemporal dementia. *Arch Neurol*, 1999; **56**: 817–22.

44 The Lund and Manchester Groups. Clinical and neuropathological criteria for frontotemporal dementia. *J Neurol Neurosurg Psychiatry*, 1994; **57**: 416–18.

45 Thomas VC, Rockwood KJ. Alcohol abuse, cognitive impairment, and mortality among older people. *J Am Geriatr Soc*, 2001; **49**(4): 415–20.

46 Oslin DW, Cary MS. Alcohol-related dementia: validation of diagnostic criteria. *Am J Geriatr Psychiatry*, 2003; **11**(4): 441–7.

47 Dugbartey A. Neurocognitive aspects of hypothyroidism. *Arch Intern Med*, 1998; **158**: 1413–18.

48 Toh B, van Driel IR, Gleeson PA. Pernicious anaemia. *N Engl J Med*, 1997; **337**(20): 1441–8.

49 Carmel R. Prevalence of undiagnosed pernicious anaemia in the elderly. *Arch Intern Med*, 1996; **156**: 1097–100.

50 Glatzel M, Stoeck K, Seeger H, *et al.* Human prion diseases: molecular and clinical aspects. *Arch Neurol*, 2005; **62**: 545–52.

51 De Silva R, Findlay C, Awad I, *et al.* Creutzfeldt–Jakob disease in the elderly. *Postgrad Med J*, 1997; **73**: 557–9.

52 Johnson RT, Gibbs CJ. Creutzfeldt–Jakob disease and related transmissible spongiform encephalopathies. *N Engl J Med*, 1998; **339**(27): 1994–2004.

53 Tschampa HJ, Neumann M, Zerr I, *et al.* Patient's with Alzheimer's disease and dementia with Lewy bodies mistaken for Creutzfeldt–Jakob disease. *J Neurol Neurosurg Psychiatry*, 2001; **71**: 33–9.

54 Zerr I, Pocchiari M, Collins S, *et al.* Analysis of EEG and CSF 14-3-3 proteins as aids to the diagnosis of Creutzfeldt–Jakob disease. *Neurology*, 2000; **55**: 811–15.

55 Lemstra AW, van Meegen MT, Vreyling JP, *et al.* 14-3-3 testing in diagnosing Creutzfeldt–Jakob disease: a prospective study of 112 patients. *Neurology*, 2000; **55**: 51–6.

56 Schroter A, Zerr I, Henkel K, *et al.* Magnetic resonance imaging in the clinical diagnosis of Creutzfeldt–Jakob disease. *Arch Neurol*, 2000; **57**: 1751–7.

57 Shiga Y, Miyazawa K, Sato S, *et al.* Diffusion-weighted MRI abnormalities as an early diagnostic marker for Creutzfeldt–Jakob disease. *Neurology*, 2004; **63**: 443–9.

58 Poser S, Mollenhauer B, Kraub A, *et al.* How to improve the clinical diagnosis of Creutzfeldt–Jakob disease. *Brain*, 1999; **122**: 2345–51.

59 Massman PJ, Sims J, Cooke N, *et al.* Prevalence and correlates of neuropsychological deficits in amyotrophic lateral sclerosis. *J Neurol Neurosurg Psychiatry*, 1996; **61**: 450–5.

60 Ruitenberg A, van Swieten JC, Witteman JCM, *et al.* Alcohol consumption and risk of dementia: the Rotterdam study. *Lancet*, 2002; **359**: 281–6.

61 Mukamal KJ, Kuller LH, Fitzpatrick AL, *et al.* Prospective study of alcohol consumption and risk of dementia in older adults. *JAMA*, 2003; **289**(11): 1405–13.

62 Ganguli M, Vander Bilt J, Saxton JA, *et al.* Alcohol consumption and cognitive function in late life: a longitudinal community study. *Neurology*, 2005; **65**: 1210–17.

63 Truelsen T, Thudium D, Gronbaek M. Amount and type of alcohol and risk of dementia: the Copenhagen City Heart Study. *Neurology*, 2002; **59**: 131–9.

64 Stampfer MJ, Kang JH, Chen J, *et al.* Effects of moderate alcohol consumption on cognitive function in women. *N Engl J Med*, 2005; **352**(3): 245–53.

65 Hein HO, Suadicani P, Gyntelberg F. Alcohol consumption, serum low density lipoprotein cholesterol concentration, and risk of ischaemic heart disease: six year follow up in the Copenhagen male study. *BMJ*, 1996; **312**: 736–41.

66 Whitmer RA, Gunderson EP, Barrett-Connor E, *et al.* Obesity in middle age and future risk of dementia: a 27 year longitudinal population based study. *BMJ*, 2005; **330**: 1360–2.

67 Gustafson D, Lissner L, Bengtsson C, *et al.* A 24-year follow-up of body mass index and cerebral atrophy. *Neurology*, 2004; **63**: 1876–81.

68 Whitmer RA, Sidney S, Selby J, *et al.* Midlife cardiovascular risk factors and risk of dementia in late life. *Neurology*, 2005; **64**: 277–81.

69 Hofman A, Ott A, Breteler MMB, *et al.* Atherosclerosis, apolipoprotein E, and prevalence of dementia and Alzheimer's disease in the Rotterdam study. *Lancet*, 1997; **349**: 151–4.

70 Forette F, Seux M, Staessen JA, *et al.* Prevention of dementia in randomised double-blind placebo-controlled Systolic Hypertension in Europe (Syst-Eur) trial. *Lancet*, 1998; **352**: 1347–51.

71 Launer LJ, Masaki K, Petrovitch H, *et al.* The association between midlife blood pressure levels and late-life cognitive function: the Honolulu-Asia Aging Study. *JAMA*, 1995; **274**(23): 1846–51.

72 Cramer C, Haan MN, Galea S, *et al.* Use of statins and incidence of dementia and cognitive impairment without dementia in a cohort study. *Neurology*, 2008; **71**: 344–50.

73 Ellul J, Archer N, Foy CML, *et al.* The effects of commonly prescribed drugs in patients with Alzheimer's disease on the rate of deterioration. *J Neurol Neurosurg Psychiatry*, 2007; **78**: 233–9.

74 Rawlings AM, Sharrett AR, Schneider ALC, *et al.* Diabetes in midlife and cognitive change over 20 years: a cohort study. *Ann Intern Med*, 2014; **161**: 785–93.

75 Petersen RC, Thomas RG, Grundman M, *et al.* Vitamin E and donepezil for the treatment of mild cognitive impairment. *N Engl J Med*, 2005; **352**: 2379–88.

76 Miller ER, Pastor-Barriuso R, Dalal D, *et al.* Meta-analysis: high-dosage vitamin E supplementation may increase all-cause mortality. *Ann Intern Med*, 2005; **142**(1): 37–46.

77 Aisen PS, Schneider LS, Sano M, *et al.* High-dose B vitamin supplementation and cognitive decline in Alzheimer disease: a randomized controlled trial. *JAMA*, 2008, **300**(15): 1774–83.

78 DeKosky SA, Williamson JD, Fitzpatrick AL, *et al.* Ginkgo biloba for prevention of dementia: a randomized controlled trial. *JAMA*, 2008; **300**(19): 2253–62.

79 Shumaker SA, Legault C, Kuller L, *et al.* Conjugated equine estrogens and incidence of probable dementia and mild cognitive impairment in postmenopausal women: Women's Health Initiative Memory Study. *JAMA*, 2004; **291**(24): 2947–58.

80 Larson EB, Wang L, Bowen JD, *et al.* Exercise is associated with reduced risk for incident dementia among persons 65 years of age and older. *Ann Intern Med*, 2006; **144**(2): 73–81.

81 DeFina LF, Willis BL, Radford NB, *et al.* The association between midlife cardiorespiratory fitness levels and later-life dementia: a cohort study. *Ann Intern Med*, 2013; **158**(3): 162–8.

82 Hakansson K, Rovio S, Helkala E, *et al.* Association between mid-life marital status and cognitive function in later life: population based cohort study. *BMJ*, 2009; **339**: 99.

83 Doody RS, Stevens JC, Beck C, *et al.* Practice parameter: management of dementia (an evidence-based review). *Neurology*, 2001; **56**: 1154–66.

84 Brodaty H, Green A, Koschera A. Meta-analysis of psychosocial interventions for caregivers of people with dementia. *J Am Geriatr Soc*, 2003; **51**(5): 657–64.

85 Mittleman MS, Ferris SH, Shalman E, *et al.* A family intervention to delay nursing home placement of patients with Alzheimer disease: a randomized controlled trial. *JAMA*, 1996; **276**(21): 1725–31.

86 Willis SL, Tennstedt SL, Marsiske M, *et al.* Long-term effects of cognitive training on everyday functional outcomes in older adults. *JAMA*, 2006; **296**(23): 2805–14.

87 Fitten LJ, Perryman KM, Wilkinson CJ, *et al.* Alzheimer and vascular dementias and driving. *JAMA*, 1995; **273**(17): 1360–5.

88 Small GW, Rabins PV, Barry PP, *et al.* Diagnosis and treatment of Alzheimer disease and related disorders. *JAMA*, 1997; **278**: 1363–71.

89 Graff MJL, Vernooij-Dassen MJM, Thijssen M, *et al.* Community based occupational therapy for patients with dementia and their care givers: randomised controlled trial. *BMJ*, 2006; **333**: 1196–9.

90 AD2000 Collaborative Group. Long-term donepezil treatment in 565 patients with Alzheimer's disease (AD2000): randomised double-blind trial. *Lancet*, 2004; **363**: 2105–15.

91 Morton V, Torgerson DJ. Effect of regression to the mean on decision making in health care. *BMJ*, 2003; **326**: 1083–4.

92 Kaduszkiewicz H, Zimmermann T, Beck-Bornholdt H, *et al.* Cholinesterase inhibitors for patients with Alzheimer's disease: systematic review of randomised clinical trials. *BMJ*, 2005; **331**: 321–3.

93 National Institute for Health and Care Excellence. Donepezil, Galantamine, Rivastigmine and Memantine for the Treatment of Alzheimer's Disease. TA217, 2011. Available at: www.nice.org.uk/guidance/ta217 (accessed 8 October 2014).

94 Areosa Sastre A, Sherriff F, McShane R. Memantine for dementia. *Cochrane Database Syst Rev 2005*, Issue 3.

95 Rodda J, Carter J. Cholinesterase inhibitors and memantine for symptomatic treatment of dementia. *BMJ*, 2012: **344**: 43–7.

96 Husebo BS, Ballard C, Sandvik R, *et al.* Efficacy of treating pain to reduce behavioural disturbances in residents of nursing homes with dementia: cluster randomised clinical trial. *BMJ*, 2011; **343**: d4065.

97 Krishnamoorthy A, Anderson D. Managing challenging behaviour in older adults with dementia. *Prog Neurol Psychiatry*, 2011; **15**: 20–7.

98 Ayalon L, Gum AM, Feliciano L, *et al.* Effectiveness of nonpharmacological interventions for the management of neuropsychiatric symptoms in patients with dementia: a systematic review. *Arch Intern Med*, 2006; **166**: 2182–8.

99 Teri L, Logsdon RG, McCurry SM. Nonpharmacologic treatment of behavioral disturbance in dementia. *Med Clin N Am*, 2002; **86**: 641–56.

100 Testad I, Corbett A, Aarsland D, *et al.* The value of personalized psychosocial interventions to address behavioral and psychological symptoms in people with dementia living in care home settings: a systematic review. *Int Psychogeriatrics*, 2014; **26**: 1083–98.

101 Rovner BW, Steele CD, Shmuely Y, *et al.* A randomized trial of dementia care in nursing homes. *J Am Geriatr Soc*, 1996; **44**(1): 7–13.

102 Ballard CG, O'Brien JT, Reichelt K, *et al.* Aromatherapy as a safe and effective treatment for the management of agitation in severe dementia: the results of a double-blind, placebo-controlled trial with Melissa. *J Clin Psych*, 2002; **63**(7): 553–8.

103 Sutherland D, Woodward Y, Byrne J, *et al.* The use of light therapy to lower agitation in people with dementia. *Nurs Times*, 2004; **100**(45): 32–4.

104 Neil W, Curran S, Wattis J. Antipsychotic prescribing in older people. *Age Ageing* 2003; **32**: 475–83.

105 McShane R, Keene J, Gedling K, *et al.* Do neuroleptic drugs hasten cognitive decline in dementia? Prospective study with necropsy follow up. *BMJ*, 1997; **314**: 266–70.

106 Ballard C, Margallo-Lana M, Juszczak E, *et al.* Quetiapine and rivastigmine and cognitive decline in Alzheimer's disease: randomised double blind placebo controlled trial. *BMJ*, 2005; **330**: 874–7.

107 Devanand DP, Sackeim HA, Brown RP, *et al.* A pilot study of haloperidol treatment of psychosis and behavioural disturbance in Alzheimer's disease. *Arch Neurol*, 1989; **46**: 854–7.

108 Wirshing DA, Spellberg BJ, Erhart SM, *et al.* Novel antipsychotics and new onset diabetes. *Biol Psychiatry*, 1998; **44**: 778–83.

109 Wirshing DA. Adverse effects of atypical antipsychotics. *J Clin Psychiatry*, 2001; **62**(Suppl. 21): S7–10.

110 Wooltorton E. Risperidone (Risperdal): increased rate of cerebrovascular events in dementia trials. *CMAJ*, 2002; **167**(11): 1269–70.

111 Wooltorton E. Olanzapine (Zyprexa): increased incidence of cerebrovascular events in dementia trials. *CMAJ*, 2004; **170**(9): 1395.

112 Gill SS, Rochon PA, Herrmann N, *et al.* Atypical antipsychotic drugs and risk of ischaemic stroke: population based retrospective cohort study. *BMJ*, 2005; **330**: 445.

113 Douglas IJ, Smeeth L. Exposure to antipsychotics and risk of stroke: self controlled case series study. *BMJ*, 2008; **337**: 616–18.

114 Schneider LS, Dagerman KS, Insel P. Risk of death with atypical antipsychotic drug treatment for dementia: meta-analysis of randomized placebo-controlled trials. *JAMA*, 2005; **294**(15): 1934–43.

115 Wang PS, Schneeweiss S, Avorn J, *et al.* Risk of death in elderly users of conventional vs. atypical antipsychotic medications. *N Engl J Med*, 2005; **353**(22): 2335–41.

116 De Deyn PP, Rabheru K, Rasmussen A, *et al.* A randomized trial of risperidone, placebo, and haloperidol for behavioral symptoms of dementia. *Neurology*, 1999; **53**: 946–55.

117 Schneider LS, Pollock VE and Lyness SA. A metaanalysis of controlled trials of neuroleptic treatment in dementia. *J Am Geriatr Soc*, 1990; **38**(5): 553–63.

118 Teri L, Logsdon RG, Peskind E, *et al.* Treatment of agitation in AD: a randomised placebo-controlled clinical trial. *Neurology*, 2000; **55**: 1271–78.

119 Devanand DP, Marder K, Michaels KS, *et al.* A randomized, placebo-controlled dose-comparison trial of haloperidol for psychosis and disruptive behaviors in Alzheimer's disease. *Am J Psych*, 1998; **155**(11): 1512–20.

120 Lonergan E, Luxenberg J, Colford J. Haloperidol for agitation in dementia. *Cochrane Database Syst Rev* 2002, Issue 2. Art. No.: CD002852. DOI: 10.1002/14651858.CD002852.

121 Brodaty H, Ames D, Snowdon J, *et al.* A randomized placebo-controlled trial of risperidone for the treatment of aggression, agitation and psychosis of dementia. *J Clin Psychiatry*, 2003; **64**(2): 134–43.

122 Katz IR, Jeste DV, Mintzer JE, *et al.* Comparison of risperidone and placebo for psychosis and behavioural disturbances associated with dementia: a randomized, double-blind trial. *J Clin Psychiatry*, 1999; **60**(2): 107–15.

123 Street JS, Clark WS, Gannon KS, *et al.* Olanzapine treatment of psychotic and behavioral symptoms in patients with Alzheimer's disease in nursing care facilities. *Arch Gen Psychiatry*, 2000; **57**: 968–76.

124 Schneider LS, Tariot PN, Dagerman KS, *et al.* Effectiveness of atypical antipsychotic drugs in patients with Alzheimer's disease. *N Engl J Med*, 2006; **355**(15): 1525–38.

125 Paleacu D, Barak Y, Mirecky I, *et al.* Quetiapine treatment for behavioural and psychological symptoms of dementia in Alzheimer's disease patients: a 6-week, double-blind, placebo-controlled study. *Int J Geriatr Psychiatry*, 2008; **23**: 393–400.

126 Ray WA, Taylor JA, Meador KG, *et al.* Reducing antipsychotic drug use in nursing homes. *Arch Intern Med*, 1993; **153**: 713–21.

127 Fossey J, Ballard C, Juszczak E, *et al.* Effect of enhanced psychosocial care on antipsychotic use in nursing home residents with severe dementia: cluster randomised trial. *BMJ*, 2006; **332**: 756–61.

128 Ballard C, Hanney ML, Theodoulou M, *et al.* The dementia antipsychotic withdrawal trial (DART-AD): long-term follow-up of a randomised placebo-controlled trial. *Lancet Neurol*, 2009; **8**: 151–7.

129 Declercq T, Petrovic M, Azermai M, *et al.* Withdrawal versus continuation of chronic antipsychotic drugs for behavioural and psychological symptoms in older people with dementia. *Cochrane Database Syst Rev*, 2013; **3**: CD007726.

130 Gurwitz JH, Field TS, Avorn J, *et al.* Incidence and preventability of adverse drug events in nursing homes. *Am J Med*, 2000; **109**: 87–94.

131 Bronskill SE, Anderson GM, Sykora K, *et al.* Neuroleptic drug therapy in older adults newly admitted to nursing homes: incidence, dose, and specialist contact. *J Am Geriatr Soc*, 2004; **52**: 749–55.

132 McGrath AM, Jackson GA. Survey of neuroleptic prescribing in residents of nursing homes in Glasgow. *BMJ*, 1996; **312**: 611–12.

133 Barnes TR, Banerjee S, Collins N, *et al.* Antipsychotics in dementia: prevalence and quality of antipsychotic drug prescribing in UK mental health services. *Br J Psychiatry*, 2012; **201**(3): 221–6.

134 Lee PE, Gill SS, Freedman M, *et al.* Atypical antipsychotic drugs in the treatment of behavioural and psychological symptoms of dementia: systematic review. *BMJ*, 2004; **329**: 75–8.

135 American Geriatric Society and American Association for Geriatric Psychiatry. Consensus statement on improving the quality of mental health care in U.S. nursing homes: management of depression and behavioral symptoms associated with dementia. *J Am Geriatr Soc*, 2003; **51**: 1287–98.

136 Holmes C, Wilkinson D, Dean C, *et al.* The efficacy of donepezil in the treatment of neuropsychiatric symptoms in Alzheimer disease. *Neurology*, 2004; **63**: 214–19.

137 Howard RJ, Juszczak E, Ballard CG, *et al.* Donepezil for the treatment of agitation in Alzheimer's disease. *N Engl J Med*, 2007; **357**(14): 1382–92.

138 McKeith I, Del Ser T, Spano P, *et al.* Efficacy of rivastigmine in dementia with Lewy bodies: a randomised, double-blind, placebo-controlled international study. *Lancet*, 2000; **356**: 2031–6.

139 Onofrj M, Thomas A. Severe worsening of parkinsonism in Lewy body dementia due to donepezil. *Neurology*, 2003; **61**: 1452.

140 Sink KM, Holden KF, Yaffe K. Pharmacological treatment of neuropsychiatric symptoms of dementia: a review of the evidence. *JAMA*, 2005; **293**(5): 596–608.

141 Tariot PN, Erb R, Podgorski CA, *et al.* Efficacy and tolerability of carbamazepine for agitation and aggression in dementia. *Am J Psychiatry*, 1998; **155**(1): 54–61.

142 Lonergan ET, Luxenberg J. Valproate preparations for agitation in dementia. *Cochrane Database Syst Rev* 2005, Issue 3.

143 Christensen DB, Benfield WR. Alprazolam as an alternative to low-dose haloperidol in older, cognitively impaired nursing facility patients. *J Am Geriatr Soc*, 1998; **46**(5): 620–5.

144 Martinon-Torres G, Fioravanti M, Grimley Evans J. Trazodone for agitation in dementia. *Cochrane Database Syst Rev* 2005, Volume 3.

145 Gillick MR. Rethinking the role of tube feeding in patients with advanced dementia. *N Engl J Med*, 2000; **342**(3): 206–10.

146 Dharmarajan TS, Unnikrishnan D, Pitchumoni CS. Percutaneous endoscopic gastrostomy and outcome in dementia.*Am J Gastroent*, 2001; **96**(9): 2256–63.

147 Finucane TE, Christmas C, Travis K. Tube feeding in patients with advanced dementia: a review of the evidence. *JAMA*, 1999; **282**(14): 1365–70.

148 Sanders DS, Anderson AJ, Bardhan KD. Percutaneous endoscopic gastrostomy: an effective strategy for gastrostomy feeding in patients with dementia. *Clin Med*, 2004; **4**(3): 235–41.

149 Mitchell SL, Berkowitz RE, Lawson FME, *et al.* A cross-national survey of tube-feeding decisions in cognitively impaired older persons. *J Am Geriatr Soc*, 2000; **48**: 391–7.

150 Finucane TE, Bynum JPW. Use of tube feeding to prevent aspiration pneumonia. *Lancet*, 1996; **348**: 1421–4.

151 Peck A, Cohen CE, Mulvihill MN. Long-term enteral feeding of aged demented nursing home patients. *J Am Geriatr Soc*, 1990; **38**(11): 1195–8.

152 Nair S, Hertan H, Pitchumoni CS. Hypoalbuminemia is a poor predictor of survival after percutaneous endoscopic gastrostomy in elderly patients with dementia. *Am J Gastroent*, 2000; **95**(1): 133–6.

153 Abuksis G, Mor M, Segal N, *et al.* Percutaneous endoscopic gastrostomy: high mortality rates in hospitalised patients. *Am J Gastroent*, 2000; **95**(1): 128–32.

154 Meier DE, Ahronheim JC, Morris J, *et al.* High short-term mortality in hospitalized patients with advanced dementia. *Arch Intern Med*, 2001; **161**: 594–9.

155 Mitchell SL, Kiely DK, Lipsitz LA. The risk factors and impact on survival of feeding tube placement in nursing home residents with severe cognitive impairment. *Ann Intern Med*, 1997; **157**: 327–32.

156 Sanders DS, Carter MJ, D'Silva J, *et al.* Survival analysis in percutaneous endoscopic gastrostomy feeding: a worse outcome in patients with dementia. *Am J Gastroent*, 2000; **95**(6): 1472–5.

157 British Psychological Society. *Guidance on Determining the Best Interests of Adults who Lack the Capacity to Make a Decision (or Decisions) for Themselves.* 2007. Available at: www.mentalhealthcare.org.uk/media/downloads/Best_Interests_Guidance.pdf (accessed 15 October 2014).

158 Hotopf M. The assessment of mental capacity. *Clinical Med*, 2005; **5**(6): 580–4.

159 The Mental Capacity Act 2005. Available at: www.legislation.gov.uk/ukpga/2005/9/contents (accessed 15 October 2014).

160 Todd S, Barr S, Roberts M, *et al.* Survival in dementia and predictors of mortality: a review. *Int J Geriatr Psychiatry*, 2013; **28**: 1109–1124.

161 Rait G, Walters K, Bottomley C, *et al.* Survival of people with clinical diagnosis of dementia in primary care: cohort study. *BMJ*, 2010; **341**: 377.

162 Brodaty H, Seeher K, Gibson L. Dementia time to death: a systematic literature review on survival time and years of life lost in people with dementia. *Int Psychogeriatr*, 2012; **24**: 1034–45.

163 Sampson EL, Gould V, Lee D, *et al.* Differences in care received by patients with and without dementia who died during acute hospital admission: a retrospective case note study. *Age Ageing*, 2006; **35**(2): 187–9.

CHAPTER 7

Delirium

CLINICAL FEATURES

Delirium is an acute confusional state. Its key features are listed below:

➤ acute onset
➤ fluctuating course
➤ cognitive impairments: short-term memory, orientation, attention and consciousness.

It is characterised by an onset that is usually a matter of hours to days. There is also a fluctuation in severity that is typically worse in the evening or night-time ('sun downing'). Cognitive function most often shows a reduction in attention (97%), but impairments in short-term memory (88%), visuospatial skills (87%) and orientation (76%) are frequently detected.[1] Consciousness is impaired – in this context consciousness refers to awareness of one's surroundings rather than a Glasgow Coma Scale (GCS) score. Misinterpretation of events or objects is common. This may be associated with full-blown hallucinations – usually visual and involving animals such as spiders. There may also be delusions, often of persecution. Patients may continually pick at bed sheets, clothing or the air as though trying to grasp an object (termed 'carphology' or 'floccillation'). Disturbances in mood may also be associated.

Alterations in psychomotor activity commonly occur; these may result either in an agitated or a hypo-alert state.[2] Patients in this hypoactive variant are more likely to be missed and neglected than are those who have behavioural problems due to a hyperactive state (e.g. agitation or aggression). Accordingly, they are noted to have less favourable clinical outcomes (e.g. pressure ulcers and pneumonia) and so extra vigilance is required. Some patients will alternate between hypo- and hyperactive periods.

Differential diagnoses commonly include dementia and psychiatric disorders (mainly psychotic depression and schizophrenia). Patients with a hypoactive delirium have a high chance of being misdiagnosed as having depression.[3] (See Table 6.1 for a comparison of the core features of delirium, dementia and depression). In addition, dementia is a major risk factor for developing delirium and many patients will have delirium superimposed on background dementia.[4] This can be difficult to distinguish clinically. A collateral history from someone who knows the patient well is vital.

The cognitive impairment is traditionally thought of as fully reversible (*see* p. 134). The duration is variable from just one day to several months. Typical episodes last around 8 to 12 days but are often prolonged in the elderly.[2,5] In some patients delirium may cause lasting cognitive impairment, but this is hard to evaluate because of the possibility of preceding, undetected dementia. In a cohort of patients with Alzheimer's disease, a significant cognitive decline was detected following an episode of delirium.[6] It results in worse outcomes and longer lengths of stay. The worse outcomes include complications, such as falls and pressure sores, and a higher rate of institutionalisation. There is also an increased mortality rate.[7]

EPIDEMIOLOGY

Delirium is more common with advancing age. The mean age of acute medical patients with delirium is 75–82 years.[8–10] Estimates of prevalence among acutely hospitalised elderly patients vary widely due to differing diagnostic criteria used, but appear to be between 10% and 40%.[5,11–15] It is even more common among elderly people admitted with hip fractures (between 30% and 60%).[13] Lower figures are probably noted in clinical practice due to high rates of underdiagnosis as only around a third of cases are detected by the initial assessing doctor.[15,16] This is most likely to be explained by the low rate of performing cognitive assessment. Patients may be mislabelled as 'poor historians' without any thought as to the underlying cause.[17] In addition, a significant number of elderly patients (2–25%) develop delirium during a hospital stay.[14,18,19]

RISK FACTORS

Multiple risk factors for the development of delirium have been identified. Some of the more common ones are listed below.
➤ *Advanced age.*
➤ *Pre-existing dementia.*
➤ *Comorbidity*: one study found a mean of 6.3 medical diagnoses per person.[10]
➤ *Postoperative period*: in a cohort of patients (mean age 68 years) without a baseline deficit who underwent major surgery, 26% had cognitive dysfunction at one week after surgery, falling to 10% after three months.[20] Associated risk factors were older age, longer duration of anaesthesia and the occurrence of postoperative complications. It is also more likely if benzodiazepines are used in this period.[21]
➤ *Terminal illness.*
➤ *Sensory impairment*: visual and hearing deficits are significantly more prevalent in those with delirium.[9]
➤ *Polypharmacy*: one study found a mean of 6.9 medications per person.[10]

CAUSES

The cause of an episode of delirium in the elderly is usually multifactorial,[7] and the more frail the individual at baseline, the less noxious the insults that are required to induce it.[19] Often an acute illness is superimposed on potentially causative medication in a person with a low threshold, for example due to background cognitive impairment. Drug (e.g. benzodiazepine) and alcohol withdrawal are also aetiologically important.

Almost any illness can potentially precipitate delirium. A list of common causative factors is given in Table 7.1. Hospitalisation itself is associated with the induction of delirium.[22] Precipitating factors have been found to include commencing multiple medications, and bladder catheterisation.[19] Rarer causes that are easily missed include non-convulsive seizures and subdural haematomas.[17] Despite extensive investigation, the cause of delirium will remain undiagnosed in around 5–10% of patients.[5,10]

TABLE 7.1 Common causes of delirium in the elderly

Causative factor	Comments
Drugs: there are multiple potential agents; some of the more common offenders are listed here	*Anticholinergics* (e.g. tricyclic antidepressants (TCAs), oxybutynin and tolterodine); other agents or their metabolites have also been found to have some anticholinergic activity (e.g. other antidepressants, quinine, H_2-receptor antagonists, quinolones, prednisolone, theophylline and digoxin[23]); such drugs may increase the chance of toxicity when taken with other drugs with anticholinergic properties
	Sedatives: especially benzodiazepines – a meta-analysis found that cognitive adverse events were 4.8 (95% CI 1.5–15.5) times more likely with sedative hypnotics than placebo[24]
	Opioid analgesics
	Anti-Parkinsonian drugs: including levodopa, dopamine agonists, selegiline and amantadine
Alcohol and drug withdrawal	Benzodiazepines should not be discontinued abruptly in the elderly as this may induce delirium[25]
Medical illnesses	Especially infection (found to be the cause of delirium in 34% of cases in one study[9]) and stroke
Pain	Consider using the Abbey Pain Scale (*see* Appendix A)
Metabolic disturbances	For example, dehydration, hypercalcaemia, hypoglycaemia and hypoxia
Urinary catheterisation	
Urinary retention	May require a bladder scan to exclude
Constipation	
Malnutrition	
Environmental factors	Including the sudden change that occurs when patients are admitted to hospital

A simple mnemonic 'PINCH ME' can be a useful guide to help clinical teams seek for reversible causes of delirium:

P	Pain
I	Infection
N	Nutrition
C	Constipation
H	Hydration
M	Medications
E	Environment

PATHOPHYSIOLOGY

'Acute brain failure' is a term that has been used to describe delirium. There appears to be a relative reduction in acetylcholine (ACh) and an increase in dopamine activity. This idea is supported by the facts that anticholinergic and dopaminergic medications frequently cause delirium, whereas antidopaminergic agents (e.g. haloperidol) are sometimes used to reduce the clinical features. There may also be disturbances in other transmitter types, such as serotonergic. It is thought to be mediated by an acute stress response with resultant increased cortisol levels, sympathetic activation and elevated cytokines. Many brain regions are impaired by this disorder, but prefrontal, non-dominant parietal and anterior thalamic processes appear to be particularly affected.

ASSESSMENT

Obtaining an accurate history from the patient and performing a thorough examination is often not possible due to the confusion and agitation. A background history obtained from a friend or carer is highly valuable and should be specifically sought. This may confirm the acute nature of symptom onset and give an impression of background cognition and functional status. An assessment of cognition can be made with a screening tool such as the Six-Item Screener (SIS), Mini Mental State Examination (MMSE) or Abbreviated Mental Test (AMT) (*see* Appendix A). Tools such as the Confusion Assessment Method (CAM) (*see* Appendix A) have also been developed in order to improve the recognition of this condition by a wider range of healthcare workers. Attention deficits may be demonstrated by simple bedside tests such as listing the months of the year backwards (*see* p. 90).[17] Taking accurate medication and alcohol histories is also important. In practical terms it is usually appropriate to assume that new or worsened confusion is at least partly due to delirium in the first instance.

Once a diagnosis of the clinical syndrome of delirium has been made it is necessary to search for the underlying causes as outlined earlier.

Investigations

The basic tests that should be performed in all patients with suspected delirium are listed below.

➤ *Blood tests*: full blood count, electrolytes, urea, creatinine, calcium, glucose, liver function tests, C-reactive protein or erythrocyte sedimentation rate, thyroid function and blood cultures.
➤ *Oxygen saturation* ± arterial blood gas analysis
➤ *Chest X-ray*
➤ *Electrocardiogram.*

Although urinary tract infections (UTI) can trigger delirium, urinalysis is no longer recommended for use in the diagnosis of UTI (*see* p. 258). Urine culture can help with the selection of an appropriate antibiotic once a clinical diagnosis of UTI has been made. Other tests may be indicated according to the clinical situation. They include vitamin B_{12} and folate estimation, serum drug levels (e.g. digoxin), CT/MRI scanning, lumbar puncture and electroencephalogram (EEG) recording. EEGs often show generalised slowing, but the absence of an abnormality does not exclude delirium.[2] This test may be especially helpful in diagnosing suspected non-convulsive status epilepticus (*see* p. 430).

MANAGEMENT

Patients in an agitated state of delirium may be resistant to hospital admission and medical treatment. It is important to establish whether they have mental capacity to reliably make decisions about these issues (*see* p. 116). If the patient is judged not to have mental capacity at that time, treatment may be undertaken against his or her wishes under common law; that is, administering a treatment that a reasonable person would wish to receive. The use of 'sectioning' under the Mental Health Act is rarely applicable as delirium is not usually classified as a mental disorder. It is important to remember that as cognition characteristically fluctuates in delirium, so may a patient's mental capacity. Therefore, multiple assessments may need to be made during the course of an illness.

Guidelines have been developed to try to improve physicians' management of this problem (e.g. those of the Royal College of Physicians[26] and NICE[27]), but they do not appear to have a dramatic effect alone.[8] There are few controlled trials in the management of delirium. Accordingly the best clinical practice is not well defined. Surveys have demonstrated much variation in the practices of physicians.[11] Trials of multifactorial interventions have suggested a benefit.[12,13] These usually include components of improvement in the recognition of delirium, staff education, medication review and management in specialised units.

A study that assessed a total of 374 patients over the age of 75 years (mean age 81) before and then four and nine months after the inception of such a multifactorial intervention found that the in-hospital prevalence of delirium fell from 41% to 19% nine months later.[12] There was an associated reduction in the prescribing of benzodiazepines, opiates and antihistamines, and an increase in neuroleptic and antidepressant use.

Another study randomised 400 patients aged 70 years or above (mean age 80 years) to either an intervention or a control ward.[13] Components of the intervention were educational sessions for doctors and nurses, and reorganisation of the care and staffing of the ward (to include better continuity of care and interaction with patients). Both wards had a prevalence of delirium of around 31% in the 24 hours following admission. A smaller proportion of those people on the intervention ward remained delirious after seven days (30% vs 60%; $p = 0.001$). Both length of stay and mortality rates were lower in those with delirium on the intervention ward (11 vs 21 days; $p<0.001$, and 3% vs 15%; $p=0.03$, respectively). However, the assessors were not blinded to the allocation and there were significant differences in patient composition between the wards. For example, there were more patients who had been admitted due to stroke on the control ward.

The management of delirium can be divided into four basic components:
➤ identify and reverse any underlying causes
➤ environmental and supportive factors

➤ symptom control

➤ clinical review and follow-up.

Identify and reverse any underlying causes

The initial assessment is aimed at identifying underlying causes. Where possible these deficits should be corrected. In those whom alcoholism is suspected, thiamine supplementation is appropriate.[17] This should initially be given intravenously (e.g. two pairs of Pabrinex vials given three times daily for at least 48 hours).[28]

Environmental and supportive factors

Continuity of staff should be promoted whenever possible. Generally, a quiet and calm environment is best. This may be most reliably achieved in a side room. Low wattage night lighting can help to reduce confusion and misinterpretation of sounds and noises overnight. Orientation aids, such as clearly visible clocks and calendars, may help. Potentially dangerous objects should be removed. Sensory deficits should be corrected. This may simply be ensuring the patient has their glasses or hearing aid fitted. Familiar people such as family members help to calm an agitated patient. Multiple ward moves are counterproductive and should be avoided. However, these steps are often difficult to achieve at the time of acute hospitalisation due to the transitory nature of admission units.[7] Education of patients and their relatives about the condition is important.

Some physicians have suggested the development of specialised delirium units to improve management. Typically these have joint medical and psychiatric specialist input.[29] Given the pressures on resources it may not be feasible to set up such units in all hospitals. The components of good delirium care can usually be incorporated into standard acute geriatric wards.[30]

Bed rails (or cot sides) have been used to try to reduce the risk of falls. Evidence for their efficacy is lacking and they may be associated with increased harm (*see* p. 332). Despite this, they are used in around a third of delirious patients.[8] In those who are very agitated and at high risk of falls, a mattress placed directly on the floor is probably the safest option. Hospital beds that can be lowered to ground level may be a suitable alternative.

Symptom control

For mild to moderate delirium a non-pharmacological approach is preferable. Drugs should be used with caution. Paradoxically, they may worsen confusion and make the situation harder to manage. They also have other adverse effects, including an increased risk of falls (*see* p. 327). Additionally, there are no randomised controlled trials comparing medications to placebo in the treatment of delirium, and evidence of any benefit is mainly anecdotal.[31] In those in whom it is deemed necessary, it is preferable to give medication regularly rather than as required as this is more likely to prevent the development of problem behaviours. A response to oral medication may take three to four hours. It is important to remember the fluctuating nature of symptoms and that they tend to be worse overnight. A patient may be asleep during the ward round but then cause pandemonium for the staff on the night shift. It is also important to try to restore normal sleep patterns by non-pharmacological measures (e.g. avoid daytime napping and caffeinated drinks in the evening).

In those with associated hepatic impairment, some medications will not be metabolised effectively and will tend to accumulate within the patient. The antipsychotic agent, haloperidol, and the benzodiazepine, lorazepam, do not require much hepatic clearance and are therefore relatively safe to use in this situation.[2]

Oral medication

There is very little trial data on the pharmacological treatment of delirium. Thus the best management strategy is unclear. The one trial that has compared the use of antipsychotic agents to benzodiazepines (in 30 AIDS patients with a mean age of 39 years) found evidence of efficacy with haloperidol or chlorpromazine but no benefit from lorazepam.[32] Antipsychotic drugs may be better for treating psychosis and aggression, whereas benzodiazepines may be preferable if sedation is the main aim.

➤ *Antipsychotics*: haloperidol is the usual first choice. It has a high potency, few anticholinergic effects and no active metabolites.[2] Generally, cardiac safety with this medication is good but there is a possibility of QT prolongation and torsade de pointes. In older people low starting doses (0.25–0.5 mg once or twice a day) are necessary.[11] Atypical antipsychotics have been used in delirium and do appear to have a similar efficacy to typical agents.[33] They are more expensive but may cause fewer extrapyramidal side-effects, though with their short-term use in delirium this may not be relevant. The many potential side-effects of these agents are discussed on p. 110.

➤ *Benzodiazepines*: these agents are useful when the delirium is due to either alcohol or benzodiazepine withdrawal, or when there are associated seizures.[7] In other situations they are likely to be ineffective.[11,32] Shorter-acting agents without active metabolites, such as lorazepam, tend to be favoured.[2] Occasionally antipsychotic medications are inappropriate (e.g. patients with dementia with Lewy bodies (*see* p. 169)) and so benzodiazepines are then used in preference.

Parenteral medication

In emergency situations it is occasionally necessary to rapidly sedate a patient. This is associated with significant risks and should be considered a last resort when harm is otherwise likely to be caused to the patient or others. Options in this situation include intravenous (IV) or intramuscular (IM) haloperidol or IV lorazepam. The IM route has the benefit that a cannula is not required; however, it will have a slower onset of action (around 30 minutes). As with most medications in the elderly, lower doses are usually required than those for younger people. It is best to start small and gradually increase if necessary. Starting doses of 0.5 to 1 mg for both haloperidol and lorazepam are usually appropriate.[17] Any adverse effects are generally those seen with oral preparations. Lorazepam has a rapid onset of action and is more likely to cause respiratory depression than haloperidol. In this situation the antagonist flumazenil may be necessary.

Review and follow-up

Communication with the patient and the relatives is an important component of management. A significant number of patients will still have cognitive deficits at the time of discharge (*see* below). The patient's medication requirements should be reviewed before discharge. Alternative medications to replace those that precipitated a delirium episode may be appropriate. If medications were commenced to control symptoms, their discontinuation should now be considered. Multidisciplinary team assessment is useful for most patients. Referral to psychiatry of old age services should be considered for those who have residual cognitive deficits.

OUTCOME

The symptoms of delirium commonly take a long time to fully resolve in the elderly, and in some cases they do not resolve at all.[17] The actual numbers of patients who have some lasting impairment is hard to calculate because of the common association with background dementia. Typically, more than half of elderly delirious patients will have ongoing impairment at the time of discharge. In one study of such people (mean age 82 years), admission MMSE scores averaged 12 and rose to 17 at discharge.[5] A meta-analysis of studies found that one month after admission 47% of elderly patients were in institutions and only 55% had improved mentally.[34] Delirium also seems to accelerate the rate of cognitive decline in those with underlying dementia.[35]

During episodes of delirium the risk of medical complications, such as pressure ulcers (*see* p. 441), is increased.[2] Following an episode there is a higher chance of admission to institutional care.[9] Delirium is also associated with increased mortality: rates of 10–30% have been seen in the setting of acute medical patients with delirium.[8,9,34]

One study of older people admitted to general medical care (n=433, mean age 80 years) found that 13% developed delirium during their stay, and 6% were still delirious at discharge.[36] The rates of death or institutional care at one year were 83% for those with persisting delirium at discharge, 68% for those with resolved delirium, and 42% for those who never developed delirium. A review of studies found that on average 45% of older people who had delirium still had evidence of cognitive impairment at discharge and this figure fell to 21% at six months.[37]

PREVENTION

Ideally it would be possible to identify those patients at risk and take steps to prevent the occurrence of delirium. One trial stratified 852 patients over the age of 70 (mean age 80 years) into intervention and usual care groups.[38] The trial targeted interventions to try to improve or correct for six proposed risk factors: cognitive impairment; sleep disorders; immobility; dehydration; visual impairments; and hearing impairments. This resulted in a lower incidence of delirium in the intervention arm (10% vs 15%). A study using an educational intervention for acute admissions ward staff has also been shown to be associated with a lower prevalence of delirium.[39]

Another study randomised patients over the age of 65 (mean age 79 years) with a fractured hip, who had been admitted to an orthopaedic ward to receive either geriatrician consultation or usual care.[40] The geriatrician input involved making recommendations to enhance the patients' care based on a structured protocol. Interventions included actions to restore normal physiological values (e.g. oxygen saturation), appropriate medication use and care environment, and steps to improve the early detection of complications. The incidence of delirium was reduced to 32% in the intervention group compared to 50% among the control subjects (RR 0.64, 95% CI 0.37–0.98). Thus proactive specialist input to non-medical units may reduce the rate of development of delirium. However, a Cochrane review concluded that evidence of effectiveness in this field is sparse.[41]

Some authors have suggested that cholinesterase inhibitors may have a role in the management or prevention of delirium. However, a recent trial randomised 120 older patients (mean age 74 years) who were undergoing elective cardiac surgery to receive rivastigmine or placebo.[42] No significant difference in the incidence of delirium was observed.

REFERENCES

1 Meagher DJ, Moran M, Raju B, *et al.* Phenomenology of delirium: assessment of 100 adult cases using standardised measures. *Br J Psychiatry*, 2007; **190**: 135–41.
2 American Psychiatric Association. Practice guideline for the treatment of patients with delirium. *Am J Psychiatry*, 1999; **156**(5 Suppl.): S1–20.
3 Farrell KR, Ganzini L. Misdiagnosing delirium as depression in medically ill elderly patients. *Arch Intern Med*, 1995; **155**: 2459–64.
4 Meagher DJ, Leonard M, Donnelly S, *et al.* A comparison of neuropsychiatric and cognitive profiles in delirium, dementia, co-morbid delirium-dementia and cognitively intact controls. *J Neurol Neurosurg Psychiatry*, 2010; **81**: 876–81.
5 Rockwood K. The occurrence and duration of symptoms in elderly patients with delirium. *J Gerontol*, 1993; **48**(4): M162–6.
6 Fong TG, Jones RN, Shi P, *et al.* Delirium accelerates cognitive decline in Alzheimer disease. *Neurology*, 2009; **72**: 1570–5.
7 Meagher DJ. Delirium: optimising management. *BMJ*, 2001; **322**: 144–9.
8 Young LJ, George J. Do guidelines improve the process and outcomes of care in delirium? *Age Ageing*, 2003; **32**: 525–8.
9 George J, Bleasdale S, Singleton SJ. Causes and prognosis of delirium in elderly patients admitted to a district general hospital. *Age Ageing*, 1997; **26**: 423–7.
10 Rudberg MA, Pompei P, Foreman MD, *et al.* The natural history of delirium in older hospitalized patients: a syndrome of heterogeneity. *Age Ageing*, 1997; **26**: 169–74.
11 Carnes M, Howell T, Rosenberg M, *et al.* Physicians vary in approaches to the clinical management of delirium. *J Am Geriatr Soc*, 2003; **51**: 234–9.
12 Naughton BJ, Saltzman S, Ramadan F, *et al.* A multifactorial intervention to reduce the prevalence of delirium and shorten hospital length of stay. *J Am Geriatr Soc*, 2005; **53**: 18–23.
13 Lundstrom M, Edlund A, Karlsson S *et al.* A multifactorial intervention program reduces the duration of delirium, length of hospitalization, and mortality in delirious patients. *J Am Geriatr Soc*, 2005; **53**: 622–8.
14 Iseli RK, Brand C, Telford M, *et al.* Delirium in elderly general medical inpatients: a prospective study. *Int Med J*, 2007; **37**: 806–11.
15 Collins N, Blanchard MR, Tookman A, *et al.* Detection of delirium in the acute hospital. *Age Ageing*, 2010; **39**: 131–5.
16 Elie M, Rousseau F, Cole M, *et al.* Prevalence and detection of delirium in elderly emergency department patients. *CMAJ*, 2000; **163**: 977–81.

17 Nayeem K, O'Keeffe ST. Delirium. *Clin Med*, 2003; **3**: 412–15.

18 Inouye SK, Viscoli CM, Horwitz RI, *et al.* A predictive model for delirium in hospitalized elderly medical patients based on admission characteristics. *Ann Intern Med*, 1993; **119**: 474–81.

19 Inouye SK, Charpentier PA. Precipitating factors for delirium in hospitalized elderly patients: predictive model and interrelations with baseline vulnerability. *JAMA*, 1996; **275**(11): 852–7.

20 Moller JT, Cluitmans P, Rasmussen LS, *et al.* Long-term postoperative cognitive dysfunction in the elderly: ISPOCD1 study. *Lancet*, 1998; **351**: 857–61.

21 Marcantonio ER, Juarez G, Goldman L, *et al.* The relationship of postoperative delirium with psychoactive medications. *JAMA*, 1994; **272**: 1518–22.

22 McCusker J, Cole M, Abrahamowicz M, *et al.* Environmental risk factors for delirium in hospitalized older people. *J Am Geriatr Soc*, 2001; **49**: 1327–34.

23 Tune L, Carr S, Hoag E, *et al.* Anticholinergic effects of drugs commonly prescribed for the elderly: potential means for assessing risk of delirium. *Am J Psychiatry*, 1992; **149**: 1393–4.

24 Glass J, Lanctot KL, Herrmann N, *et al.* Sedative hypnotics in older people with insomnia: meta-analysis of risks and benefits. *BMJ*, 2005; **331**: 1169–73.

25 Foy A, Drinkwater V, March S, *et al.* Confusion after admission to hospital in elderly patients using benzodiazepines. *BMJ*, 1986; **293**: 1072.

26 Royal College of Physicians. *The Prevention, Diagnosis and Management of Delirium in Older People.* 2006. Available at: www.rcplondon.ac.uk/sites/default/files/concise-delirium-2006.pdf (accessed 12 November 2014).

27 National Institute for Health and Care Excellence. *Delirium: diagnosis, prevention and management.* CG103, 2010. Available at: www.nice.org.uk/guidance/cg103 (accessed 12 November 2014).

28 Thomson AD, Cook CCH, Touquet R, *et al.* The Royal College of Physicians report on alcohol: guidelines for managing Wernicke's encephalopathy in the accident and emergency department. *Alcohol Alcoholism*, 2002; **37**(6): 513–21.

29 George J, Adamson J, Woodford H. Joint geriatric and psychiatric wards: a review of the literature. *Age Ageing*, 2011; **40**: 453–8.

30 Rozzini R, Sabatini T, Trabucchi M, *et al.* Do we need delirium units? *J Am Geriatr Soc*, 2005; **53**(5): 914–15.

31 Ryan CS. Placebo controlled trials of pharmacological treatments are needed. *BMJ*, 2001; **322**: 1602.

32 Breitbart W, Marotta R, Platt MM, *et al.* A double-blind trial of haloperidol, chlorpromazine, and lorazepam in the treatment of delirium in hospitalized AIDS patients. *Am J Psychiatry*, 1996; **153**: 231–7.

33 Tune L. The role of antipsychotics in treating delirium. *Curr Psych Reports*, 2002; **4**: 209–12.

34 Cole MG, Primeau FJ. Prognosis of delirium in elderly hospital patients. *Can Med Assoc J*, 1993; **149**(1): 41–6.

35 Fong TG, Jones RN, Shi P, *et al.* Delirium accelerates cognitive decline in Alzheimer disease. *Neurology*, 2009; **72**: 1570–5.

36 McAvay GJ, van Ness PH, Bogardus ST, *et al.* Older adults discharged from hospital with delirium: one year outcomes. *J Am Geriatr Soc*, 2006; **54**(8): 1245–50.

37 Cole MG, Ciampi A, Belzile E, *et al.* Persistent delirium in older hospital patients: a systematic review of frequency and prognosis. *Age Ageing*, 2009; **38**: 19–26.

38 Inouye SK, Bogardus ST, Charpentier PA, *et al.* A multicomponent intervention to prevent delirium in hospitalized older patients. *N Engl J Med*, 1999; **340**(9): 669–76.

39 Tabet N, Hudson S, Sweeney V, *et al.* An educational intervention can prevent delirium on acute medical wards. *Age Ageing*, 2005; **34**: 152–6.

40 Marcantonio ER, Flacker JM, Wright RJ, *et al.* Reducing delirium after hip fracture: a randomized trial. *J Am Geriatr Soc*, 2001; **49**(5): 516–22.

41 Siddiqi N, Holt R, Britton AM, *et al.* Interventions for preventing delirium in hospitalised patients. *Cochrane Database Syst Rev* 2007, Issue 2. Art. No.: CD005563. DOI: 10.1002/14651858. CD005563.pub2.

42 Gamberini M, Bolliger D, Buse GAL, *et al.* Rivastigmine for the prevention of postoperative delirium in elderly patients undergoing elective cardiac surgery: a randomized controlled trial. *Crit Care Med*, 2009; **37**(5): 1762–8.

CHAPTER 8

Depression

EPIDEMIOLOGY

The term depression is used to cover a range of conditions from minor mood disturbance to major depression. Major depression has been estimated to have a prevalence of 2% to 4% in those aged over 65, and 5% to 9% in those aged over 75.[1-3] The figure rises to 15% of those in long-term care and 24–40% of those in acute hospital beds.[4,5] It is more common among people with chronic illnesses, especially neurodegenerative disorders. It has been estimated to occur in up to 50% of those with Parkinson's disease,[6] and 20–40% of those with Alzheimer's disease.[7,8] Post-stroke depression has been found to have a prevalence of about 30% in the first two years following an event.[9] 'Vascular depression' is a term for a mood disorder that accompanies generalised cerebrovascular disease. It is associated with subcortical hyperintensities and the theory is that such lesions disrupt the neural circuits that influence mood.

There is a genetic component in some depressive and bipolar disorders; however, this is more common in younger presentations. A prior history of psychiatric illness may be elicited. Major adverse life events, such as loss of spouse or onset of serious illness, are common precipitants. Untreated depression has been associated with increased risk of medical conditions such as heart attack and stroke.[4] Despite this, physicians generally appear to be undertreating depression.[10] Around 60% of depressed older adults in the community may not be receiving appropriate treatment.[11]

The median duration of depressive episodes in older adults is 18 months.[11] Around 35% recover within one year, 60% within two years, and 68% within three years. A worse prognosis is associated with more severe depression, a family history of depression, and poor physical functioning.

SUBTYPES OF DEPRESSION
Major depression

According to the DSM criteria,[12] major depression is defined as depressed mood or marked loss of interest experienced most of the time for more than two weeks' duration, plus four or more of the symptoms listed below.

➤ *Vegetative*: weight or appetite loss, insomnia/hypersomnia, loss of energy, psychomotor agitation/retardation, ↓ concentration.

➤ *Cognitive*: worthlessness/guilt, suicidal ideation, loss of interest.

Psychotic depression

Psychotic depression refers to the association of depression with delusions, paranoia and auditory hallucinations, or both. Delusions may be mood congruent (inadequacy, guilt, nihilism) or incongruent (non-depressive themes). This seems to occur more commonly in older people.[4] Such people are at an increased risk of self-harm. They should be managed by specialists and may require a combination of antidepressant and antipsychotic medications, or electroconvulsive therapy (ECT).

Bipolar disorder

Bipolar disorder is defined as depression plus one or more episodes of mania. It is less likely to present in older individuals. A manic episode is a period of abnormally elevated mood plus three or more of:[12]

➤ delusions of grandeur
➤ ↓ sleep
➤ pressured speech
➤ flight of ideas
➤ distractibility
➤ ↑ activity
➤ excessive involvement in pleasurable activities.

ASSESSMENT

The problem with the assessment of older adults with concomitant disease is that many of the vegetative symptoms are non-specific for depression. For example, slowing down is also a feature of Parkinson's disease, and fatigue may be caused by anaemia. Reports of reduced appetite, weight loss, reduced energy and insomnia are common in depression and this is especially true of older people.[13] There may be a coexistent anxiety disorder. Patients should be asked about alcohol intake – both as a cause and effect of low mood. Depression may be suspected when a patient is more functionally impaired or progressing more slowly than would otherwise be expected. Hypoactive delirium can resemble depression.

The gold standard of diagnosis is the psychiatric interview. A number of screening tools suitable for use by the non-specialist with limited time have been developed. These include the Hospital Anxiety and Depression Scale (HAD) and the Geriatric Depression Scale (GDS). They are discussed further in Appendix A. The use of a single question ('Are you depressed?') has also been found to have a reasonable efficacy in detecting depression in a cohort of terminally ill patients.[14]

Simple blood tests should be performed to exclude possible physical causes of depressive symptoms. These include the conditions listed below:

➤ hypothyroidism
➤ vitamin B_{12} deficiency
➤ hypercalcaemia.

DEPRESSION AND DEMENTIA

Depressive 'pseudo-dementia'

Depression may mimic dementia and therefore be a cause of a reversible cognitive impairment.[7] (*See* Table 6.1 for a comparison of the features of depression and dementia.) However, the conditions are associated and often occur together within individuals. Also, there is an increased risk of developing a dementia in the years following a depressive presentation with memory impairment. One study found that depressed people with a reversible cognitive deficit (an initial Mini Mental State Examination (MMSE) score of 19 rising to 26 after treatment for depression) had a 4.7 times higher risk of subsequent irreversible dementia in the following three years than similar-aged (mean 74 years) control subjects with depression alone (43% vs 12% developed dementia).[15] This raises the possibility that depression may be an aetiological factor in the development of some dementias.[7]

Compared to a genuine dementia, there are thought to be more 'I don't know' rather than incorrect answers during cognitive testing, but this feature may not be common in the elderly.[15] Patients usually retain awareness of their memory loss. Speech and response times tend to be slowed. There may be associated neuro-vegetative changes (e.g. altered sleep and eating patterns). Pseudo-dementia is more common in people with a prior history of depression.

Depression occurring in people with dementia

Depression occurs more commonly in people with dementia, perhaps affecting 20% of those with Alzheimer's disease.[16] This is probably due to the interruption of mood-related neural circuits. Alzheimer's disease often affects norepinephrinergic and serotonergic pathways of the locus ceruleus and dorsal raphe nuclei.

Screening for depression in patients with dementia is more challenging than that of cognitively normal populations. It is made harder by both the difficulty of reliable history from those with memory impairment and the overlap of physical symptoms such as apathy. There may be an increased tendency for delusions and agitation in depressed patients with dementias,[7] making it an important, treatable factor in such people. Patients with only mild dementia may be assessed with standard screening tests (e.g. the GDS). It has been estimated that these remain valid down to an MMSE score of 15.[7] Those with moderate or severe dementia are better assessed with the Cornell Scale for depression in dementia (a 19-item clinician administered test that incorporates information from carers).[17] The prevalence of depression appears to reduce with more advanced disease, but this may reflect the greater difficulty with diagnosis in this group.

It is generally accepted among clinicians that medications with more anticholinergic activity (e.g. tricyclic antidepressants (TCAs)) be avoided in favour of alternative agents (e.g. selective serotonin reuptake inhibitors (SSRIs)) in these patients.[18] But drug therapy may be ineffective.[19] Specialist psychiatry input is advised when there is associated suicidal ideation, psychotic features or a failure to respond after six weeks of treatment.

TREATMENT

The therapeutic options of psychotherapy, pharmacotherapy and ECT are discussed below. There is some evidence that, at least in primary care, an integrated approach involving a depression care manager, a general practitioner (GP) and a psychiatrist can lead to improvements in patients' symptoms and quality of life.[20] A system such as this may incorporate patient education, psychotherapy, antidepressant drugs and relapse prevention strategies.

Psychotherapy

Psychotherapy alone may be considered as a first-line management strategy in mild, but not severe, depression. It may be used in combination with other modalities for more serious mood disorders. It is thought to be most useful when background personality disorders, psychosocial factors or interpersonal stressors are prominent.[21] Cognitive therapy tries to identify and correct negative thought patterns. Behavioural therapy aims to promote the positive reinforcement of pleasurable activities and the negative reinforcement of harmful behaviours. It may have a role in reducing suicide rates among those who have made previous suicide attempts.[22] Meta-analyses suggest that they may have a similar efficacy to pharmacological agents.[23] However, a recent trial that compared the use of psychotherapy, paroxetine, or both, for the maintenance of remission in older adults (mean age 77 years) found a far lower rate with paroxetine (37%) compared to psychotherapy alone (68%).[24] Also, there was no significant benefit from adding psychotherapy to paroxetine. These treatment modalities have the advantage of avoiding the risk of side-effects and drug interactions but their use may be dictated by local access to such services.

Pharmacotherapy

The majority of antidepressant agents act by potentiating the effects of serotonin and/or norepinephrine within the brain. There is insufficient evidence to reliably compare all of the available antidepressant medications with one another. From meta-analyses, there appears to be little difference in either efficacy or number of adverse events between any of SSRIs, TCAs and atypical agents.[24,25] However, a review of studies performed in primary care patients has suggested that SSRIs are better tolerated than TCAs.[26] The decision on which agent to choose may be based on side-effect profiles (*see* Table 8.1) and financial costs. Those with more anticholinergic properties (e.g. TCAs) are usually best avoided in the elderly.[27]

A recent review of studies assessing newer antidepressant drugs for major depression in adults found that escitalopram and sertraline had the most favourable balance of efficacy and side-effects.[28] Given the lower price of sertraline, the authors suggested this would be the most appropriate first choice. A number of drugs, including paroxetine and duloxetine, scored badly both for efficacy and acceptability.

Another factor to be considered when choosing a drug is whether it would be beneficial to stimulate or sedate the patient, depending on their presenting symptoms. Those with insomnia may benefit from a sedating drug such as mirtazapine at night, whereas those with lethargy or withdrawal may be stimulated by a drug such as sertraline.

TABLE 8.1 Key properties of commonly used antidepressant agents

Drug class (examples)	Comments
TCAs (amitriptyline, dosulepin, nortriptyline)	Block the reuptake of norepinephrine and serotonin; antidepressants with the most anticholinergic effects (*see* Table 2.2); may cause cardiac arrhythmias (sinus tachycardias due to pro-adrenergic and anticholinergic effects, also ventricular tachycardia secondary to QT prolongation); may be lethal in overdose; sedating
SSRIs (citalopram, paroxetine, sertraline, fluoxetine)	Serotonergic mechanism of action (block reuptake); may cause gastrointestinal side-effects (e.g. nausea and diarrhoea), sexual dysfunction and gastrointestinal bleeding; less cardiac toxicity (but citalopram dose should not exceed 20 mg daily due to risk of QT prolongation)
Atypical agents	
trazodone	Serotonergic mechanism of action; sedating; may cause priapism; generally similar to TCAs but with perhaps less anticholinergic effects
mirtazapine	Possible appetite-stimulating property: may have a role in people with reduced dietary intake. Otherwise similar to TCAs
venlafaxine	Similar to SSRIs; best avoided in people with heart disease, electrolyte disturbance or hypertension
MAOIs (phenelzine)	Rarely used in the current treatment of depression; one of the reasons for this is the need for a low tyramine diet to avoid provoking the serotonin syndrome (*see* Box 8.1); another reason is the high potential for drug interactions; they may be lethal in overdose

TCA = tricyclic antidepressant; SSRI = selective serotonin reuptake inhibitor; MAOI = monoamine oxidase inhibitor.

A period of six to eight weeks on treatment is usually required to achieve maximal improvement,[21] but beneficial effects are seen in many people within two weeks.[29] Six months after the resolution of symptoms the drugs may be gradually withdrawn. If treatment is deemed to have been unsuccessful after a period of at least four weeks on a reasonable dose of the drug, an alternative class of agent may be considered. When switching between agents it is preferable to have a period of around two days off all antidepressant medications. This time period should be increased when switching to or from monoamine oxidase inhibitors (MAOIs) or fluoxetine due to the prolonged half-lives of these drugs or their metabolites. If there is still no improvement, specialist input is necessary to consider alternative strategies such as combinations of antidepressant agents or ECT.

A trial of 4041 younger adult patients with depression found that a remission rate of approximately 30% was seen after treatment with citalopram at a mean dose of 42 mg and mean duration of 47 days (Note: daily doses of citalopram in older people should not exceed 20 mg).[30] Two further trials were performed on patients from the initial cohort who failed to respond to or were intolerant of citalopram after up to 12 weeks of treatment. The first recruited 727 patients (mean age 42 years) who agreed to participate in a randomised change in therapeutic agent to either bupropion-MR, venlafaxine-XR, or an alternative SSRI (sertraline).[31] Bupropion is thought to act by blocking the neuronal reuptake of dopamine and norepinephrine. It has a tendency to lower seizure thresholds and so should be avoided in patients at risk. It is also used in smoking cessation (*see* p. 211). The study found that around 25% of patients had a remission of their depressive symptoms irrespective of which agent was used.

The second study enrolled patients willing to add a second agent to citalopram.[32] Here 565 patients (mean age 41 years) were randomised to citalopram plus either bupropion-MR or buspirone (a selective serotonin receptor agonist). Similar remission rates of around 30% were seen in both groups. Withdrawal rates due to intolerance were a little lower with bupropion (13% vs 21%). However, a placebo group was not used in either of the secondary studies and so true effect sizes cannot be calculated. Taken together these studies suggest that about 50% of younger patients with severe, recurrent depression will not achieve remission with pharmacotherapy.

Other drugs

St John's wort (hypericum extract WS 5570) is a herbal remedy that has been proposed to have antidepressant properties. It appears to be as effective as SSRIs in the management of moderate to severe depression.[33] It may have interactions with other medications. Mood stabilisers are additional agents used in the management of bipolar disorder. They include lithium and some anticonvulsant drugs (e.g. sodium valproate). Antipsychotic agents are occasionally used in the management of depression with psychotic features (which is usually best done by a specialist on an inpatient basis).

Side-effects

All antidepressants appear to be associated with an increased risk of falls (*see* p. 327). The elimination of TCAs is slowed in older people, leading to lower doses causing higher serum levels than those seen in younger people.[27] SSRIs have been associated with an increased risk of gastrointestinal haemorrhage and so caution should be taken when combining with other such agents, such as non-steroidal anti-inflammatory drugs (NSAIDs). The SSRIs, MAOIs and venlafaxine more commonly cause insomnia or agitation.[34] The TCAs, mirtazapine and trazodone are more likely to cause sedation.[21] Of the newer agents, venlafaxine appears to be associated with a higher rate of nausea (30%). Paroxetine, sertraline and mirtazapine appear to have a higher rate of sexual-type side-effects. Mirtazapine is associated with the greatest amount of weight gain (an average of 2 kg over an eight-week period).[25] This effect is probably mediated by a histamine receptor-blocking action. It may be a good choice for patients with reduced appetite. The TCAs appear to have the most anticholinergic effects (*see* p. 27). Of the SSRIs, paroxetine is thought to be more anticholinergic.

Other side-effects seen with antidepressants include hyponatraemia (probably secondary to syndrome of inappropriate secretion of antidiuretic hormone (SIADH)) and the serotonin syndrome[35] – *see* Box 8.1. A recent observational study found SSRIs were associated with the greatest risk of falls and hyponatraemia, and non-SSRI non-TCA drugs (mirtazapine, trazodone and venlafaxine) were associated with a higher risk of cerebrovascular events, fracture and seizures.[36] But these apparent differences may be due to prescriber bias. Some drugs can prolong the QT interval on electrocardiogram recordings, which increases the risk of ventricular arrhythmias. This effect seems to be most marked with citalopram, escitalopram and amitriptyline.[37]

Electroconvulsive therapy

Electroconvulsive therapy involves the passing of an electric current through the cerebrum of anaesthetised patients. It has been found to be an effective treatment for depression in the short term, probably more effective than drug therapy, but data on the elderly are limited.[38] ECT treatment, given by specialists, is suitable for either refractory depression or when severe symptoms need to be addressed rapidly. Examples of indications include high suicide risk, self-starving, catatonia and psychotic delusions.[21]

ECT usually involves two or three treatments per week with a total of 6 to 12 treatments. Response rates of between 30% and 55% have been reported in case series.[39,40] In those who do respond there is a high relapse rate, overall affecting around two-thirds of the patients treated this way.[39] The number relapsing can be reduced by maintenance pharmacological treatment. A study that compared such maintenance treatment with placebo found relapse rates of 39% in those receiving a combination of a TCA and lithium, 60% in those on a TCA alone and 84% in those on placebo medication over a 24-week period.[40]

The major side-effects following treatment are memory impairment and confusion. These usually improve over a period of days to weeks. Cognitive adverse effects are more common with higher electrical doses, bilateral application and more frequent sessions.[38] The risk of these may be reduced by less frequent or unilateral treatments in those with baseline cognitive impairment, which places them at a higher chance of problems.[7]

BOX 8.1 The serotonin syndrome

The serotonin syndrome occasionally occurs following the ingestion of pro-serotonergic agents. It has a rapid onset. Clinical features range from mild cases of tremor and diarrhoea to severe cases of potentially fatal neuromuscular rigidity, hyperthermia and delirium.[35] Metabolic changes that may occur include rhabdomyolysis, acidosis and disseminated intravascular coagulation (DIC).

The range of clinical manifestations of serotonergic syndrome:

Mild	Moderate	Severe
Tremor	Pyrexia (38–40°C)	Pyrexia (>40°C)
Tachycardia	Hypertension	Hypertension/hypotension
Mydriasis	Hyper-reflexia	Rigidity
Diarrhoea	Clonus	Delirium
Increased bowel sounds		
Agitation		

Causative agents include all antidepressants, but especially SSRIs and MAOIs, and some other agents with pro-serotonergic activity, such as tramadol, sumatriptan, ondansetron and 'ecstasy' (MDMA). It may be more likely to occur with combinations of serotonergic drugs or in the presence of agents that block the hepatic degradation of serotonergic agents, for example erythromycin or valproate. Tryptophan is the precursor to serotonin (5-HT) and the ingestion of large quantities can also provoke the syndrome.

The diagnosis is made by the combination of a history of recent serotonergic drug ingestion in tandem with characteristic clinical features. The differential diagnosis includes neuroleptic malignant syndrome (*see* p. 174), malignant hyperthermia (hypertonicity, hyperthermia and acidosis following inhalational anaesthetic agent administration) and anticholinergic toxicity (mydriasis, delirium, dry erythematous skin, urinary retention and reduced bowel sounds).

Treatment involves removing the causative agents, intravenous fluids and benzodiazepines. Severe cases may need sedation and ventilation. The 5-HT$_{2A}$ antagonist cyproheptadine has been utilised but no randomised controlled trial evidence of efficacy is available; an alternative is the atypical antipsychotic olanzapine.[35] Hypertension and tachycardia may be controlled with intravenous beta-blockers.

SUICIDE

The elderly are the group in society most at risk of completed suicide.[3,41] It is strongly associated with depression. Suicide is more common in males, in those with a history of previous mental illness, and in association with alcohol abuse. It is also more likely in those socially isolated, with a chronic illness, or having had a previous attempted suicide. It more commonly affects those who are widowed or divorced, and may be triggered by bereavement. Screening for suicidal ideation in high-risk groups may reduce suicide rates in the elderly.

ANXIETY

Anxiety is commonly seen in association with depression. There is a variety of clinical presentations, for example generalised anxiety disorder (GAD), obsessive-compulsive disorder, and post-traumatic stress disorder. It may be accompanied by physical symptoms such as shortness of breath, palpitations, dizziness, tingling and chest pain.

TABLE 8.2 Physical causes of anxiety disorders

Drugs
  antidepressants
  lithium toxicity
  digoxin toxicity
  anticholinergics
  steroids
  theophylline
  calcium channel blockers
  benzodiazepine withdrawal
  alcohol withdrawal
Hypoglycaemia
Thyroid disorders

Assessment should be aimed to try to exclude physical causes. The more common of these are listed in Table 8.2.

Management

SSRI antidepressants have been found to be effective in reducing anxiety. An analysis of studies of the SSRI-like agent venlafaxine found a 66% response rate in those aged over 60 years compared to 41% of those in the placebo group.[42] A trial of escitalopram in older adults (n=177, mean age 72 years) over a 12-week period showed a trend towards benefit compared to placebo, but this did not reach significance on an intention to treat analysis.[43] Benzodiazepines have also been used and may have a quicker onset of action; however, their multiple associated side-effects makes them unsuitable for most elderly people (*see* pp. 26 and 327). Pregabalin has also been used in GAD with some symptomatic benefit.[44] Behavioural therapies may be appropriate in some patients, depending on local availability. A trial randomised 134 patients (mean age 67 years) with GAD to cognitive behavioural therapy (CBT) or usual care.[45] Treatment was for three months with follow-up 12 months later. Worry severity was significantly reduced, but GAD severity was not.

REFERENCES

1 Copeland JR, Dewey ME, Wood N, *et al*. The range of mental illness among the elderly in the community: prevalence in Liverpool using the GMS-AGECAT package. *Br J Psychiatry*, 1987; **150**: 815–23.

2 Livingston G, Hawkins A, Graham N, *et al*. The Gospel Oak Study: prevalence rates of dementia, depression and activity limitation among elderly residents in inner London. *Psychol Med*, 1990; **20**: 137–46.

3 Rodda J, Walker Z, Carter J. Depression in older adults. *BMJ*, 2011; **343**: 683–7.

4 Raj A. Depression in the elderly: tailoring medical therapy to their special needs. *Postgrad Med*, 2004; **115**(6): 26–42.

5 Goldberg SE, Whittamore KH, Harwood RH, *et al*. The prevalence of mental health problems among older adults admitted as an emergency to a general hospital. *Age Ageing*, 2012; **41**: 80–6.

6 Dooneief G, Mirabello E, Bell K, *et al*. An estimate of the incidence of depression in idiopathic Parkinson's disease. *Arch Neurol*, 1992; **49**: 305–7.

7 Katz IR. Diagnosis and treatment of depression in patients with Alzheimer's disease and other dementias. *J Clin Psychiatry*, 1998; **59**(Suppl. 9): S38–44.

8 Lazarus LW, Newton N, Cohler B, *et al*. Frequency and presentation of depressive symptoms in patients with primary degenerative dementia. *Am J Psychiatry*, 1987; **144**(1): 41–5.

9 Robinson RG, Bolduc PL, Price TR. Two-year longitudinal study of poststroke mood disorders: diagnosis and outcome at one and two years. *Stroke*, 1987; **18**: 837–43.

10 Hirschfeld RMA, Keller MB, Panico S, *et al*. The National Depressive and Manic-Depressive Association consensus statement on the undertreatment of depression. *JAMA*, 1997; **277**: 333–40.

11 Licht-Strunk E, Van Marwijk HWJ, Hoekstra T, *et al*. Outcome of depression in later life in primary care: longitudinal cohort study with three years' follow up. *BMJ*, 2009; **338**: 463–6.

12 American Psychiatric Association. *Diagnostic and Statistical Manual of Mental Disorders*, 4th ed. Washington, DC: American Psychiatric Association; 1994.

13 Hegeman JM, Kok RM, van der Mast RC, *et al*. Phenomenology of depression in older compared with younger adults: meta-analysis. *Br J Psychiatry*, 2012; **200**: 275–81.

14 Chochinov HM, Wilson KG, Enns M, *et al.* 'Are you depressed?' Screening for depression in the terminally ill. *Am J Psychiatry*, 1997; **154**(5): 674–6.

15 Alexopoulos GS, Meyers BS, Young RC, *et al.* The course of geriatric depression with 'reversible dementia': a controlled study. *Am J Psychiatry*, 1993; **150**(11): 1693–9.

16 Gartlehner G. Hansen RA, Morgan CL, *et al.* Comparative benefits and harms of second-generation antidepressants for treating major depressive disorder. *Ann Intern Med*, 2011; **155**: 772–85.

17 Alexopoulos GS, Abrams RC, Young RC, *et al.* Cornell scale for depression in dementia. *Biological Psychiatry*, 1988; **23**(3): 271–84.

18 American Geriatric Society and American Association for Geriatric Psychiatry. Consensus statement on improving the quality of mental health care in U.S. nursing homes: management of depression and behavioral symptoms associated with dementia. *J Am Geriatr Soc*, 2003; **51**: 1287–98.

19 Banerjee S, Hellier J, Dewey D, *et al.* Sertraline or mirtazapine for depression in dementia (HTA-SADD): a randomised, multicentre, double-blind, placebo-controlled trial. *Lancet*, 2011; **378**: 403–11.

20 Hankeler EM, Katon W, Tang L, *et al.* Long term outcomes from the IMPACT randomised trial for depressed elderly patients in primary care. *BMJ*, 2006; **332**: 259–62.

21 Mann JJ. The medical management of depression. *N Engl J Med*, 2005; **353**: 1819–34.

22 Brown GK, Have TT, Henriques GR, *et al.* Cognitive therapy for the prevention of suicide attempts: a randomized controlled trial. 2005; **294**(5): 563–70.

23 Bartels SJ, Dums AR, Oxman TE, *et al.* Evidence-based practices in geriatric mental health care: an overview of systematic reviews and meta-analyses. *Psychiatr Clin N Am*, 2003; **26**: 971–90.

24 Reynolds CF, Dew MA, Pollock BG, *et al.* Maintenance treatment of major depression in old age. *N Engl J Med*, 2006; **354**(11): 1130–8.

25 Hausen RA, Gartlehner G, Lohr KN, *et al.* Efficacy and safety of second-generation antidepressants in the treatment of major depressive disorder. *Ann Int Med*, 2005; **143**: 415–26.

26 MacGillivray S, Arroll B, Hatcher S, *et al.* Efficacy and tolerability of selective serotonin reuptake inhibitors compared with tricyclic antidepressants in depression treated in primary care: systematic review and meta-analysis. *BMJ*, 2003; **326**: 1014–17.

27 Chutka DS, Takahashi PY, Hoel RW. Inappropriate medications for elderly patients. *Mayo Clin Proc*, 2004; **79**: 122–39.

28 Cipriani A, Furukawa TA, Salanti G, *et al.* Comparative efficacy and acceptability of 12 new-generation antidepressants: a multiple-treatments meta-analysis. *Lancet,* 2009; **373**: 746–58.

29 Tylee A, Walters P. Onset of action of antidepressants. *BMJ*, 2007; **334**: 911–12.

30 Trivedi MH, Rush AJ, Wisniewski SR, *et al.* Evaluation of outcomes with citalopram for depression using measurement-based care in STAR*D: implications for clinical practice. *Am J Psychiatry*, 2006; **163**: 28–40.

31 Rush AJ, Trivedi MH, Wisniewski SR, *et al.* Bupropion-SR, sertraline, or venlafaxine-XR after failure of SSRIs for depression. *N Eng J Med*, 2006; **354**(12): 1231–42.

32 Trivedi MH, Fava M, Wisniewski SR, *et al.* Medication augmentation after failure of SSRIs for depression. *N Engl J Med*, 2006; **354**(12): 1243–52.

33 Szegedi A, Kohnen R, Dienel A, *et al.* Acute treatment of moderate to severe depression with hypericum extract WS 5570 (St John's Wort): randomised controlled double-blind non-inferiority trial versus paroxetine. *BMJ*, 2005; **330**: 503–6.

34 Anonymous. Do SSRIs cause gastrointestinal bleeding? *Drug and Therapeutics Bulletin*, 2004; **42**(3): 17–18.

35 Boyer EW, Shannon M. The serotonin syndrome. *N Engl J Med*, 2005; **352**(11): 1112–20.

36 Coupland C, Dhiman P, Morriss R, *et al.* Antidepressant use and risk of adverse outcomes in older people: population based cohort study. *BMJ*, 2011; **343**: d4551.

37 Castro VM, Clements CC, Murphy SN, *et al.* QT interval and anti-depressant use: a cross sectional study of electronic health records. *BMJ*, 2013; **346**: f288.

38 UK ECT Review Group. Efficacy and safety of electroconvulsive therapy in depressive disorders: a systematic review and meta-analysis. *Lancet*, 2003; **361**: 799–808.

39 Prudic J, Olfson M, Marcus SC, *et al.* Effectiveness of electroconvulsive therapy in community settings. *Biol Psychiatry*, 2004; **55**: 301–12.

40 Sackeim HA, Haskett RF, Mulsant BH, *et al.* Continuation pharmacotherapy in the prevention of relapse following electroconvulsive therapy. *JAMA*, 2001; **285**(10): 1299–307.

41 O'Connell H, Chin A, Cunningham C, *et al.* Recent developments: suicide in older people. *BMJ*, 2004; **329**: 895–9.

42 Katz IR, Reynolds CF, Alexopoulos GS, *et al.* Venlafaxine ER as a treatment for generalized anxiety disorder in older adults: polled analysis of five randomized placebo-controlled clinical trials. *J Am Geriatr Soc*, 2002; **50**: 18–25.

43 Lenze EJ, Rollman BL, Shear MK, *et al.* Escitalopram for older adults with generalized anxiety disorder: a randomized controlled trial. *JAMA*, 2009; **301**(3): 295–303.

44 Boschen MJ. A meta-analysis of the efficacy of pregabalin in the treatment of generalized anxiety disorder. *Can J Psychiatry*, 2011; **56**: 558–66.

45 Stanley MA, Wilson NL, Novy DM, *et al.* Cognitive behavior therapy for generalized anxiety disorder among older adults in primary care: a randomised clinical trial. *JAMA*, 2009; **301**(14): 1460–7.

Movement disorders

This chapter does not include all movement disorders but instead specifically covers those conditions that more commonly present in the elderly. There is some overlap of clinical features with other diagnoses. For example, patients with advanced Alzheimer's disease often develop some extrapyramidal signs (*see* p. 91).

Movement disorders are predominantly caused by lesions affecting the basal ganglia. The main components of this system are shown in Figure 9.1. Complex interconnections, both excitatory and inhibitory, exist between the various ganglia. A review of these is beyond the scope of this book and is of questionable relevance to clinical practice. Their overall effect is modulation of the motor cortex output via connections from the ventrolateral thalamus.

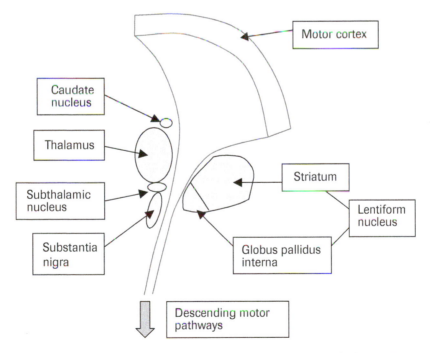

FIGURE 9.1 The basic anatomy of the basal ganglia (coronal view of left-sided structures from an anterior aspect).

ASSESSMENT

History

The assessment of patients with suspected movement disorders clearly requires a careful history plus a neurological and gait examination. A thorough medication history may reveal potentially causative agents. Previous stroke and vascular risk factors may suggest a vascular aetiology. Some conditions have a genetic basis and a family history should be sought. Movement disorders are commonly associated with depression and cognitive impairment and so screening for these problems is appropriate. Enquiry should be made about related complications, including constipation and urinary incontinence. These may be part of an autonomic disturbance, which could also include postural hypotension and male impotence. Disturbed sleep patterns, including rapid eye movement (REM) sleep disorder, may be associated with movement disorders. Hallucinations can be caused by some movement disorders or they may occur as secondary to prescribed medications. The timing of the occurrence of gait problems and falls within the illness can give clues to the diagnosis. Other symptoms and signs may be looked for according to the suspected condition, as discussed later.

Examination

In patients with Parkinson's disease (PD) the classic Parkinsonian tremor may not be present at rest. Distracting the patient can sometimes induce it. This can be achieved by asking the patient to rest their hands on their knees, palms facing upwards, and then recite the months of the year backwards. It may also become more apparent while the patient is walking during the gait assessment.

   Bradykinesia (slow movement) is a key clinical feature of Parkinsonism. Its detection is somewhat subjective. There are various techniques that have been proposed to test it. One of these is shown in Figure 9.2. In the feet it can be demonstrated by asking the patient to repeatedly tap the foot on the floor as fast as they can.

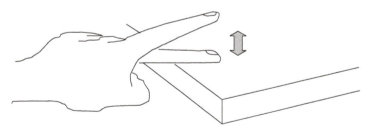

FIGURE 9.2 Testing for bradykinesia. The patient is asked to tap their index and middle fingers in turn onto a desk surface or the back of their other hand, as fast as they can.

Increased tone can be made more obvious by asking the patient to perform voluntary movements with the contralateral limb at the same time. This is termed 'reinforcement'. Increased tone in Parkinsonism is usually described as 'lead pipe' (present throughout the range of movement) or cog-wheeling (a tremor superimposed on underlying increased tone). The glabellar tap is one of the frontal release signs (*see* p. 92). It is not specific for any diagnosis and has limited value in the assessment of such patients.

A gait examination should be performed. The classic Parkinsonian 'festinating' gait is described in Figure 9.3. More subtle changes may be loss of arm swing or unsteadiness/difficulty turning around. A small-stepping gait ('marche à petits pas') without other characteristic abnormalities is suggestive of a vascular cause. A method for testing for postural instability is shown in Figure 9.4.

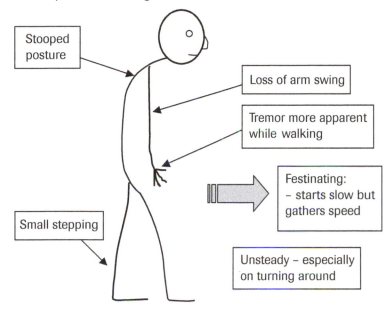

FIGURE 9.3 The classic Parkinsonian gait.

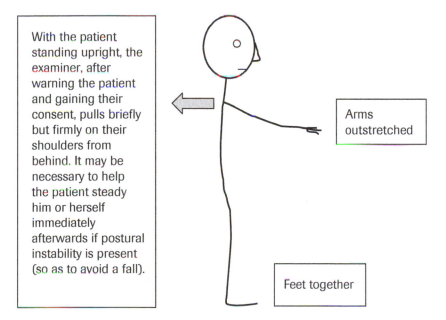

FIGURE 9.4 Testing for postural instability.

Eye signs may occur with movement disorders. Supranuclear palsy (caused by a lesion above the level of the cranial nerve nuclei) is a particular feature of progressive supranuclear palsy (PSP) (*see* p. 170), which characteristically leads to reduced up gaze. Subtler, and less specific, signs include abnormal saccades and square wave jerks. The assessment of saccades is shown in Figure 9.5. Square wave jerks are movements of the eyes (saccadic intrusions) while the patient is trying to maintain a fixed gaze on an object. They are deemed abnormal when they occur at a rate of more than 10 per minute. They are more commonly seen in people with PSP or multiple system atrophy (MSA) than those with PD.[1]

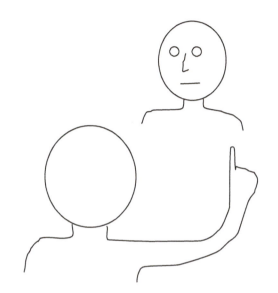

The patient is asked to look at the examiner's nose and then to look at the outstretched finger, while keeping their head still. The examiner watches for the speed and number of eye movements (saccades) taken by the patient. In normal individuals this occurs very rapidly in just one eye movement.

FIGURE 9.5 The assessment of visual saccades.

Investigations

Blood tests can occasionally exclude other causes of tremor (e.g. hyperthyroidism or hypoglycaemia). Computerised tomography (CT) and magnetic resonance imaging (MRI) scans may be suggestive of a vascular aetiology or hydrocephalus. They are not usually helpful in the diagnosis of other movement disorders. Regional cerebral atrophy is associated with some conditions but these changes are rare in early disease.

Functional imaging of the dopamine transporter (DAT) using single positron emission computerised tomography (SPECT) gives information regarding the integrity of the nigrostrial dopaminergic pathways. Scans are typically abnormal in PD, PSP, MSA and DLB.[2] This technique is currently most used to distinguish PD from other forms of tremor (e.g. essential tremor and drug-induced Parkinsonism). Scans may appear abnormal in vascular Parkinsonism if there is focal basal ganglia infarction. It may have a role in distinguishing DLB and AD (*see* later). The diagnostic accuracy of these scans is imperfect and their role in routine practice is not yet well defined.

PARKINSON'S DISEASE

➤ Prevalence: 100–190 per 100 000 people.

➤ Survival: approximately 13 years.[3]

➤ Mean age of onset: 62 years.[3,4]

➤ Key clinical features: bradykinesia, resting tremor, rigidity, postural instability.

The prevalence of PD rises with increasing age (*see* Figure 9.6).[5] It is the second most common neurodegenerative disorder after Alzheimer's disease. Parkinsonism refers to the presence of clinical features of PD, which may be due to other causes (e.g. drug-induced or vascular); these are discussed later in this chapter. The overall population prevalence is in the region of 100–190 cases per 100 000 in the Western world. It is probably marginally more common in men than women.

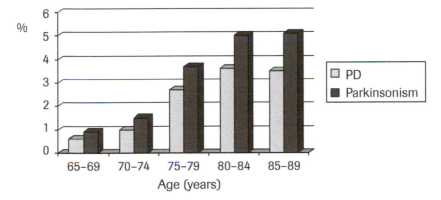

FIGURE 9.6 The rising prevalence of Parkinson's disease (PD) and Parkinsonism with age.

A non-specific prodromal illness such as depression or anxiety may precede the motor symptoms.[6] Initial onset is almost always unilateral and affects the arms first. The typical progression is next to affect the ipsilateral leg after around one year and then the contralateral arm two to three years later.[7]

The characteristic pill-rolling resting tremor is a common early sign but 25% of PD patients will never develop a tremor.[6] In some patients a tremor is the primary clinical sign – termed 'tremor predominant'. The tremor may be suppressed in some situations and can be induced by distraction or while the patient is walking. Hallucinations occur in 10–40% of patients treated for PD,[8] mainly secondary to dopaminergic medications, but other factors such as depression and cognitive or visual impairments increase the risk.[9] They are typically visual but may be auditory. Speech is affected with a tendency to develop a quiet, monotonous voice. Handwriting may become small and irregular. Early falls (occurring within the first two to three years from diagnosis) are very uncommon in PD and suggest an alternative diagnosis, for example PSP or MSA (*see* later).

The clinical accuracy of diagnosing PD is less than perfect. Experts in PD implementing standard diagnostic criteria and with a prolonged follow-up period can expect to have around a 90% accuracy.[4]

Several disease rating scales have been developed to try to assess severity of PD. These are used primarily in research trials and are of limited clinical value. They include the Hoehn and Yahr, and Unified Parkinson's Disease Rating Scale (UPDRS) (*see* Appendix A).

Pathogenesis

Pathological changes of PD include neuronal loss in the substantia nigra and Lewy body deposition. Inherited forms of PD have been identified but they account for less than 10% of all cases;[10] they are more frequently associated with younger-onset PD. However, they do provide some insight into the pathogenic mechanisms of PD. Implicated genes are multiple but include those that encode the proteins parkin and alpha-synuclein. Parkin is involved in assisting the action of the ubiquitin-proteasome system that degrades abnormal proteins. Alpha-synuclein is a major component of Lewy bodies. It is postulated that the accumulation of abnormal proteins is key to the development of PD (and many other neurodegenerative disorders). These proteins may affect mitochondrial function with resultant oxidative stress damage rather than be directly toxic to neurons.[10]

So far, no particular environmental agent has been strongly implicated in the development of typical PD. Extrinsic agents such as MPTP (a street drug contaminant) and following viral encephalitis (post-encephalitic Parkinsonism) can, rarely, result in conditions mimicking PD. Smoking and caffeine intake seem to confer a small protective advantage in epidemiological studies but the mechanism of these possible effects is unclear.[11-13] Rural living has also been associated with PD in some epidemiological studies.

Dementia associated with PD

Dementia occurs more commonly in people with PD than age-matched control subjects. It has been estimated that around 75% of people with PD will develop some degree of dementia.[14] However, a significant dementia appears to develop in around 30%.[15] Using a definition of a Mini Mental State Examination (MMSE) score <25, cognitive impairment was found to have a prevalence of 23% in a PD population (mean age 75 years).[16] A more recent study detected some degree of cognitive impairment in two-thirds of PD patients after a mean time of 3.5 years from diagnosis.[17] People with early hallucinations or an akinetic-rigid or symmetrical pattern at onset appear to be most at risk.[14] These latter features are often seen in dementia with Lewy bodies (DLB) and suggest a common mechanism. The major distinction between PD dementia (PDD) rather than DLB is the timing of onset of symptoms. In the latter condition, motor and cognitive features must occur with one year of each other to meet current diagnostic criteria (*see* p. 169). The pattern of cognitive deficit is very similar to that seen in DLB.[18] Both PDD and DLB are associated with Lewy bodies in the cerebral cortex. They appear to be differing presentations of the same process. Given the older age of most patients with PD and the prevalence of AD (*see* p. 83) in this age group, it is reasonable to assume that a number people diagnosed with PDD will have AD-type cerebral pathology. An autopsy study has found AD pathology in

33% of PD patients.[19] Conditions such as PSP (*see* p. 170) may also be misdiagnosed as PDD.

TREATMENT OF PARKINSON'S DISEASE

Motor symptoms

Symptomatic treatments for PD motor features are not believed to affect disease progression and so there is usually no rush to initiate them. The right time to commence therapy is arbitrary. It usually happens when symptoms begin to significantly affect the patient's life. This may occur earlier in the disease process if the dominant hand is the first involved. Ultimately, this decision will vary according to individual patients' preferences. Drug treatments are only mildly effective in reducing tremor and so delaying initiation may be appropriate for those with a tremor-predominant

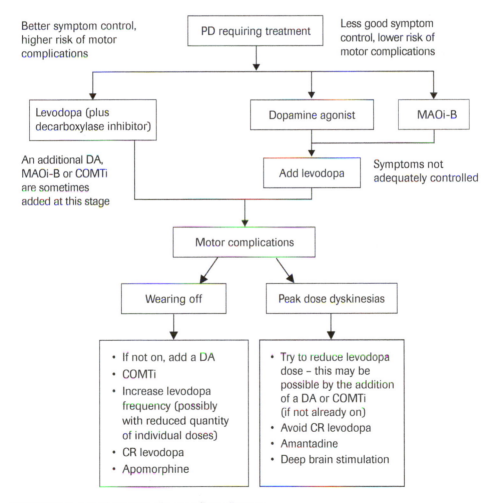

FIGURE 9.7 A Parkinson's disease flow diagram.

DA = dopamine agonist; MAOi-B = monoamine oxidase inhibitor type B; COMTi = catecholamine-o-methyltransferase (COMT) inhibitor; CR = controlled release

presentation. A number of agents have been proposed as neuroprotective but, to date, the evidence is unconvincing.[20] Early-stage disease is relatively easy to treat. As the condition progresses the response to pharmacologic agents diminishes and additional complications such as wearing-off phenomena and dyskinesias present. This aspect of PD management is very challenging. A range of agents is available for use in PD. Much uncertainty still exists regarding the optimal ones to use.[15] Many of the drug trials involved only small patient numbers and inadequate follow-up.[21] An additional dilemma for the geriatrician is the absence of data regarding the use of such agents in older people with comorbidities. A suggested scheme for choice of therapy as disease progresses is shown in Figure 9.7.

Levodopa

Levodopa remains the most effective anti-Parkinsonian treatment available. Almost all patients will have a marked response to this agent, so much so that this has become a supportive diagnostic feature of PD. Exactly what constitutes a reasonable trial of levodopa before declaring a failed response is unclear. Most physicians would advocate several weeks of therapy on at least 300 mg a day. No improvement after this time suggests an alternative diagnosis, but occasionally patients require higher doses of levodopa, up to 1500 mg per day.[15]

Pharmacology

The rationale for the use of levodopa is that it is converted to dopamine within the surviving neurons of the basal ganglia to help compensate for the causative loss of dopaminergic cells (giving dopamine would be ineffective as it cannot cross the blood–brain barrier). It is always given with a decarboxylase inhibitor (carbidopa or benzeraside) to prevent excessive peripheral conversion of levodopa to dopamine, which would reduce cerebral availability and produce excessive side-effects (mainly nausea, vomiting and orthostatic hypotension) (*see* Figure 9.8).

Levodopa is absorbed in the small intestine and reaches peak plasma concentrations after about 30 minutes. This onset is slower if gastric emptying is delayed, for example by food or anticholinergic drugs, or as a result of accompanying autonomic neuropathy. This may account for some variation in dose response in later-stage disease. Its absorption from the gut and movement across the blood–brain barrier is dependent on an amino acid transporter system. This system can become saturated after eating a meal containing protein, which can reduce drug availability in the central nervous tissues. Therefore, levodopa should be taken 30 minutes before or 60 minutes after meals.

Doses are titrated up slowly to avoid precipitating side-effects, namely nausea, vomiting and orthostatic hypotension. The dosage times of levodopa should also take into account the duration of action of the drug and the times of activity during the day. In early disease levodopa can be expected to work for four hours or more, but this time will reduce with disease progression (*see* below). The first dose should be taken immediately on waking and subsequent doses at four-hour intervals, for example 7 am, 11 am and 3 pm. The last dose should not be taken too late in the day as motor improvements are, generally, not beneficial while asleep.

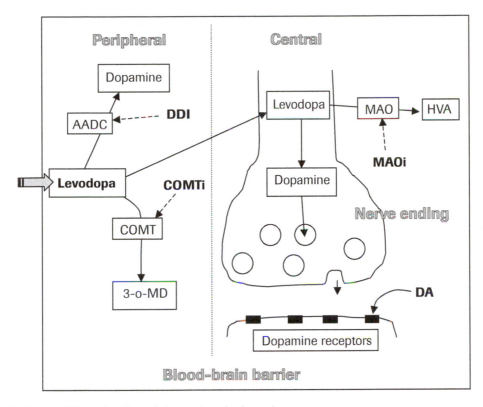

FIGURE 9.8 Sites of action of dopaminergic therapies.

DDI = dopa decarboxylase inhibitor; AADC = aromatic amino acid decarboxylase; COMT = catecholamine-o-methyltransferase; COMTi = COMT inhibitor; MAO = monoamine oxidase; MAOi = MAO inhibitor; HVA = homovanillic acid; 3-o-MD = 3-o-methyldopa; DA = dopamine agonist; broken arrows = inhibitory effects.

Usually levodopa is more effective at reducing bradykinesia and rigidity than tremor. It continues to be an effective treatment for PD for several decades in many individuals.[22] However, complications do develop – as discussed below. Non-oral formulations of levodopa, including intravenous and intraduodenal, have also been proposed but are associated with various practical difficulties.[23] There is a small amount of evidence that intraduodenal levodopa may be beneficial in selected patients.[24]

Controlled-release preparations

Specialised formulations of levodopa have been developed that give a slow, sustained release of the drug over a 12-hour period, but the onset of action is delayed. It is particularly useful for nocturnal problems – such as reduced mobility that limits getting out of bed to use the toilet. Other benefits may include reducing motor fluctuations. It is usually used in combination with rapid-acting preparations to prevent a delay in onset, especially first thing in the morning. Because of poorer absorption, around a 30% higher total dose equivalent is needed for controlled-release (CR) preparations compared to standard-release formulations.[15] They may be associated with more psychiatric adverse effects and prolonged dyskinesias compared to standard levodopa in advanced disease.[15]

Dispersible preparations

Dispersible levodopa has the advantage of a faster onset of action (20–30 minutes vs 30–60 minutes with standard formulations).[22] This may be useful to rapidly control Parkinsonism at key times, such as when first waking in the morning.

Side-effects
Non-motor complications

Combining levodopa with a peripheral decarboxylase inhibitor mainly prevents nausea caused by the peripheral conversion of levodopa to dopamine. When it does occur, it can be minimised by slow dose titration. Alternatively, the dopamine receptor antagonist domperidone can be used to block peripheral dopamine-induced adverse effects as it has a very poor penetration of the blood–brain barrier. It is usually possible to reduce this medication after a few weeks on levodopa therapy. Other potential complications include hallucinations, orthostatic hypotension (*see* p. 344), delirium and features of the dopamine dysregulation syndrome (*see* later).

Motor complications

Dose response variations to levodopa occur late in the disease. They affect around half of patients after five years of levodopa treatment and nearly all after 10 years.[24,25] They seem to be at least partly related to levodopa use rather than PD alone as animal model studies suggest that they can be induced in normal individuals following levodopa administration.[26] However, they do not tend to occur in other diseases treated with levodopa (e.g. some dystonias).[25] They have also been developed in a small number of patients receiving dopamine agonists alone, with no prior levodopa exposure.[27,28] They include motor fluctuations (wearing off and on–off phenomena) and dyskinesias. Their mechanisms are not well understood. Patients are described as being in the 'on' state when their Parkinsonism is controlled by medication and in the 'off' state when this is not the case. In general, the therapeutic window becomes narrower and the pharmacodynamics of levodopa within the brain tissue change as time progresses; *see* Figure 9.9.

One theory to explain this phenomenon is that therapeutic levodopa acts through being converted to dopamine within surviving nigrostriatal neurons and is stored pre-synaptically. It is then released as required. As the disease progresses there are less available neurons to store dopamine, leading to shorter treatment effects of levodopa doses.[25] Eventually there is almost no dopamine storage capacity and cerebral dopamine availability is directly related to peripheral levodopa concentrations. This leads to the need for very regular drug dosing or continuous infusions.

An alternative theory is that there are changes in the post-synaptic response to dopamine stimulation as the disease progresses. This concept is supported by an observed shortening of duration of action of a bolus infusion of apomorphine (a post-synaptic acting dopamine agonist) in advanced disease.[29] This may be partially

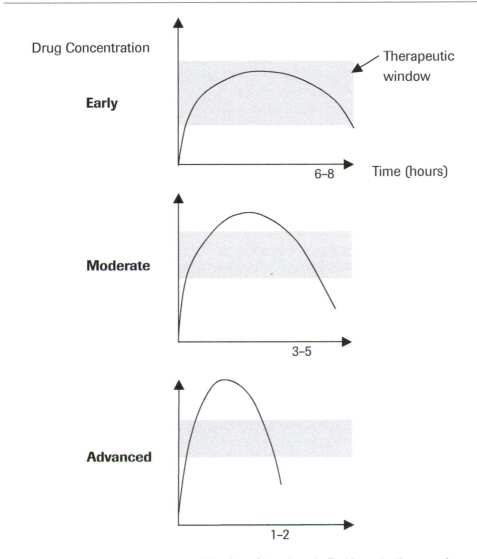

FIGURE 9.9 The changing pharmacokinetics of levodopa in Parkinson's disease after prolonged exposure.

mediated by changes in *N*-methyl-D-aspartate (NMDA) pathways – as supported by the apparent beneficial action of amantadine (an NMDA receptor blocker; *see* p. 165). The reality is probably a combination of both pre- and post-synaptic mechanisms.

There has been concern that the increased dopamine metabolism induced by giving exogenous levodopa may lead to oxidative stress within the remaining nigrostriatal neurons and thereby worsen the condition. However, available evidence does not strongly support this idea.[20] Some of the motor complications may be worsened by pulsatile stimulation of the neuronal pathways. There is evidence that they can be improved by continuous dopamine stimulation.[30] Therefore, there may be some logic in using CR preparations of levodopa in this population. However, a trial comparing the use of CR to standard-release levodopa did not find a difference in the development of motor complications after five years.[31] Alternative strategies include the use of more frequent doses of standard-release levodopa or the addition of a COMT inhibitor (*see* below). Lower doses of levodopa may reduce the tendency to develop dyskinesias. A maximum daily levodopa dose of 600 mg is probably appropriate.[22] Despite these side-effects levodopa remains an important and effective treatment for PD. Most patients would choose to accept some dyskinesia than be stuck in the 'off' state.

➤ *'Wearing off'* is a term for the re-emergence of Parkinsonian features as plasma levo-dopa levels fall. It occurs more frequently as the disease progresses and is caused by a shortening of the effective time of each dose of levodopa. It is usually defined as being present once levodopa doses are effective for less than four hours.[15]

➤ *'Freezing'* describes the sudden onset of the inability to initiate gait, which gives the appearance of being frozen in time. It may be provoked by actions such as turning round or by environmental factors such as doorways. The provision of visual cues such as a striped pattern on floors can sometimes reduce this phenomenon.[32] Occasionally, movements such as stamping of the feet or walking sideways can allow normal walking to resume. It is usually poorly responsive to pharmacologic manipulation.

➤ *'On–off'* is an expression for the pattern whereby patients suddenly change from the 'on' state to the 'off' state unrelated to medication doses or plasma levodopa concentrations. It is usually poorly responsive to pharmacologic manipulation.

Dyskinesia

There are several subtypes of dyskinesia associated with PD. The most common is a chorea (rapid, irregular movements) associated with peak dose drug levels, but diphasic and 'off' phase types have also been described.[33] These may present as dystonia (sustained contractions), stereotypy (repetitive movements) or myoclonus (muscular jerks). More than one of these may occur at the same time. The diphasic type causes dyskinesia when drug levels are either rising or falling – thereby occurring twice with each levodopa dose. 'Off' dystonia usually presents as early morning or nocturnal cramps that most commonly affect the distal legs, and may be painful. Most patients would rather accept a degree of dyskinesia than suffer immobility related to underdosing. They are more likely to develop in younger rather than older patients.[33]

Peak dose dyskinesias may be improved by smaller, more frequent levodopa doses. Diphasic ones may be improved by using dopamine agonists in preference to levodopa. Off dystonias may be reduced by using long-acting agents overnight (e.g. CR levodopa or dopamine agonists).

COMT inhibitors

COMT inhibitors (COMTi) act by blocking one of the degradation pathways of levo-dopa (to 3-o-methyldopa) (*see* Figure 9.8). Tolcapone has both central and peripheral actions but due to cases of hepatoxicity its use is limited.[34] Current guidance recommends it is only used in those who do not respond to entacapone and with monitoring of liver blood tests every two weeks.[35] Entacapone does not cross the blood–brain barrier. It has a half-life of just one hour and is taken with each dose of levodopa. It increases the half-life of levodopa without increasing the maximum concentration and so, in theory, it should not worsen dyskinesias. The benefit is in the order of an additional 30 minutes 'on' time with each levodopa dose.[36] It appears to be helpful in patients who are experiencing motor fluctuations.[37] A 15–30% reduction in levodopa dose is recommended at the initiation of entacapone therapy.[15] It has not been associated with hepatic toxicity. Patients should be warned that an orange discolouration of their urine could occur. It occasionally causes diarrhoea. Preparations containing levodopa, a decarboxylase inhibitor and entacapone in combination are available.

Dopamine agonists

Dopamine agonists act directly on post-synaptic dopamine receptors (*see* Figure 9.8), of which there are at least five subtypes (D_1–D_5). The agonists can be subdivided into two groups: those that are derived from ergot (e.g. bromocriptine, cabergoline and pergolide) and those that are not (e.g. ropinirole and pramipexole). Generally, there seems little to choose between the various dopamine agonists in terms of efficacy at any stage of the disease.[20,38–41] However, the ergot-derived drugs are not recommended as first-line treatment due to a greater risk of adverse effects (*see* below).[35]

Side-effects

Pulmonary, pericardial, heart valve and retroperitoneal fibrosis are infrequent side-effects associated with the ergot-derived agents, occurring, on average, two years after commencement.[42–44] For these reasons it has been suggested that all patients should undergo baseline investigations when starting these medications (e.g. ESR, urea and electrolytes and chest X-ray) and these should be repeated at least annually.[35,45] An echocardiogram prior to treatment should also be considered.[46] Problematic side-effects with all dopamine agonists include somnolence, hallucinations and leg oedema. Somnolence is a feature of advanced PD irrespective of treatment but does appear to be made worse by dopamine agonists.[47] Rarely, sudden episodes of sleep have resulted in motor vehicle accidents.[48] This should be considered when initiating treatment in patients who still drive. The leg oedema is characteristically poorly responsive to diuretic therapy but rapidly reversed by stopping the offending medication.[49] These drugs are also associated with the dopamine dysregulation syndrome (*see* below).

Dopamine dysregulation syndrome

A number of behavioural disorders have been described in advanced PD after prolonged exposure to dopaminergic medications. These include the dopamine dysregulation syndrome (DDS), punding and impulse control disorders (ICD). Dopamine agonists are most often implicated, but these disorders may occur following levodopa exposure. The prevalence of DDS is 3–4% among PD patients attending movement disorder services.[50] ICD may be present in 10–14% of PD patients.[51] However, these figures may be inaccurate given the wide range of potential behavioural problems and a reluctance to talk openly about some of them. They are more common in those with a younger age of onset (e.g. below 45 years).[52]

DDS is a term used to describe a situation where people with PD increase their medication doses on their own and can describe getting a 'kick' or 'high' from taking these drugs, a situation not dissimilar to other forms of drug abuse (also termed 'hedonistic homeostatic dysregulation').[53] Cases can be associated with stockpiling medication and requests for more from their doctors. Sufferers tend to take very large doses of dopaminergic drugs despite disabling dyskinesias and resist dose reduction. The commencement of subcutaneous apomorphine may trigger DDS, and some patients develop a rapid onset of a 'high' with this agent.

Dopamine appears to have a central role in the normal brain reward system. This mechanism can, rarely, be affected by dopaminergic therapies and result in the development of ICD. Example behaviours include gambling, stealing, excessive buying, compulsive eating and hypersexuality.[50,54] Potentially these can have disastrous personal, social and financial consequences. Problems seem to present within three months of maintaining a target dose and can resolve on drug withdrawal. The most commonly implicated agent is pramipexole but others include pergolide and ropinirole. Pramipexole is the most potent agonist of D_3 receptors, which may explain its stronger association with gambling behaviour.

Punding is a term for repeating tasks without purpose, such as sorting objects or continually digging in the garden. Performing the task does not seem to give the person pleasure but they are likely to be irritable if prevented from doing it. When intense it can lead to sleep deprivation and loss of sociable activity.

Management is difficult as withdrawal of dopaminergic drugs may lead to unacceptable motor symptoms. Typical advice is to stop rapid acting preparations (e.g. dispersible co-beneldopa and subcutaneous apomorphine) and switch dopamine agonists to equivalent doses of levodopa.[50] Consideration may be given to deep brain stimulation for selected patients to allow reduction in dopaminergic medications.[52]

Dopamine agonists in early PD

Dopamine agonists are often advocated for the initial treatment of PD due to concerns that levodopa use may be associated with increased neuronal toxicity. Additionally, they may reduce dopamine turnover and subsequent oxidative stress due to their direct postsynaptic action. However, these issues remain a matter of ongoing debate.[55,56] They are less effective than levodopa but may delay its introduction for several years. This is particularly important in patients with a younger age of onset, who are at a higher risk of motor complications due to the long duration of their illness.

A study randomised 268 patients (mean age 63 years) with early PD to receive either ropinirole or levodopa over a five-year period.[27] Both groups of patients were allowed additional open label levodopa doses as required. After five years, 20% of the ropinirole group had developed dyskinesia compared to 45% of the levodopa group. However, UPDRS scores were better in the levodopa arm. Around half of the patients in both groups withdrew prematurely (mainly due to adverse events). Side-effects occurring more commonly with ropinirole compared to levodopa included somnolence (27% vs 19%), hallucinations (17% vs 6%) and leg oedema (14% vs 6%).

A similar study has compared pramipexole to levodopa: 301 patients were randomised (mean age 61 years) and followed up for a two-year period.[28] After this time 28% of the pramipexole group had developed either motor fluctuations or dyskinesias compared to 51% of the levodopa group. This benefit was offset by better UPDRS and quality of life scores in the levodopa group. Side-effects more commonly seen with pramipexole also included somnolence (32% vs 17%), hallucinations (9% vs 3%) and leg oedema (15% vs 4%). Results for studies involving cabergoline and pergolide appear to show similar results.[57]

Studies of 10-year duration have failed to show a mortality benefit of initial dopamine agonist therapy compared to initial levodopa use.[58,59] Also, the evidence that dyskinesias are less severe with agonists after 10 years of treatment is less convincing. One study found that the numbers with moderate to severe dyskinesias were similar in both groups after this length of time despite early results in favour of the agonist arm.[59] Again the patients treated with levodopa had lower levels of disability. So, the use of these agents may not significantly reduce motor complication rates after prolonged treatment.[22]

The dilemma is whether the reduced risk of motor complications seen with dopamine agonists early in the disease justifies their use despite poorer efficacy and associated side-effects. The trials, so far, have recruited young cohorts of patients who are more likely to develop motor complications than older people. The occurrence of side-effects, particularly psychiatric ones, could be different in the elderly. Many physicians are currently advising the use of dopamine agonists as initial therapy in biologically younger patients and levodopa in the older, more frail.[15,57] This distinction is fairly arbitrary and the best practice may only be determined by the results of future clinical trials.

Dopamine agonists in advanced PD

Dopamine agonists have also been tried as supplementary therapy to levodopa in advanced PD. A study randomised 360 patients (mean age 63 years) with sub-optimally controlled advanced PD plus motor fluctuations to receive either pramipexole or placebo over a 32-week period.[60] There were significant improvements in UPDRS scores with pramipexole compared to placebo for motor scores (25% vs 12%) and reduction in 'off' time (31% vs 7%). Resting tremor, rigidity and bradykinesia were improved. Side-effects seen more commonly with pramipexole included dyskinesia (61%), hallucinations (19%) and confusion (11%). Similar results have been found with studies of both pergolide and ropinirole.[61,62] The addition of these agents to levodopa often allows a reduction in levodopa dose of around 30%. This levodopa-sparing effect may lower the incidence of future motor fluctuations.

Rotigotine patch

The dopamine agonist rotigotine is available in a transdermal patch. It has been found to be more effective than placebo, but probably a little less effective than oral dopamine agonists in the management of PD.[63] Side-effects are similar to other agents, but also include erythema and pruritis at the patch site. It may be of value in patients with advanced PD who have an impaired swallow.

Apomorphine

Apomorphine is a dopamine agonist that needs to be taken by a parenteral route. It appears to activate mainly D_1 and D_2 receptors. When given subcutaneously it has an onset of action after 5–15 minutes.[64] The initial concomitant use of domperidone limits (but may not remove) the associated nausea, vomiting and postural hypotension. It is indicated for use in patients with advanced PD plus motor fluctuations.

It is usually given as either a continuous subcutaneous infusion, via a portable infusion pump, or as intermittent subcutaneous injections that are self-administered. To select patients who are likely to benefit an 'apomorphine test' is given. This involves increasing bolus doses of apomorphine at 90-minute intervals, with careful monitoring, until either an anti-Parkinsonian effect or unacceptable side-effects occur.[64] The threshold dose that leads to benefit is recorded and is used to calculate a reasonable starting dose for individual patients. It may be possible to slowly reduce, and occasionally withdraw, levodopa therapy once a continuous infusion is established.[65]

With continuous infusions, patients appear to benefit in terms of reduction in the percentage of day spent in the 'off' state (from around 50% to around 25%) and in the incidence of dyskinesias.[64,65] Minor local reactions, including nodules, may occur at injection sites. Psychiatric side-effects, including psychosis and hallucinations, and sedation may limit the use of apomorphine in many older people.

A trial of intermittent apomorphine injections compared to placebo injections has demonstrated a benefit in UPDRS scores with this treatment when administered in the 'off' state (a 24 vs 0 point reduction – *see* Appendix A).[66] Side-effects occurring more commonly in the treatment group included yawning, dyskinesias, somnolence, nausea/vomiting, postural dizziness, rhinorrhoea (runny nose), hallucinations/confusion, and leg oedema. The benefit lasts for around one hour with each dose.

Monoamine oxidase inhibitors

The monoamine oxidase inhibitor (MAOI) selegiline (also known as deprenyl) has been used both as a putative neuroprotective agent and as a treatment for PD. The enzyme monoamine oxidase type B is involved in the degradation of dopamine (as compared to type A that degrades serotonin and norepinephrine, and is targeted in the treatment of depression – *see* p. 142). The theory is that blocking this enzyme will increase the available dopamine within the brain (*see* Figure 9.8). Selegiline has a specific action on the type B enzyme and so has a low risk of 'cheese reaction' or serotonin syndrome (*see* Box 8.1). However, there have been rare cases of serotonin syndrome with combination of selegiline and antidepressant drugs necessitating caution with this combination.[67] Given the high incidence of depression in PD, this is potentially very important.

It has been speculated that inhibition of this enzyme could prevent the formation of harmful free radicals from dopamine metabolism. Thus it could have a neuroprotective effect and this has been suggested by several trials.[68] However, there is controversy as to whether this apparent effect could be explained by a mild symptomatic benefit allowing a delay in the need for levodopa.

A meta-analysis of 17 randomised trials (involving 3525 patients) of selegiline use in early PD found evidence to support a small beneficial effect on disability, the need for levodopa and motor fluctuations.[69] Side-effects did not appear to be a significant problem. The DATATOP study did not demonstrate a survival benefit in 800 patients receiving either selegiline or placebo after 13 years of follow-up.[70] Unfortunately, there is very little data comparing MAOI with dopamine agonists, the main alternative levodopa-sparing therapy in early PD.

The drug has amphetamine metabolites that may cause insomnia. Data from the Parkinson's Disease Research Group study suggests that selegiline may be associated with an increased incidence of falls and dementia.[71] It seems logical to avoid this medication in patients with cognitive impairment, significant orthostatic hypotension or a history of falls.

A fast-absorbed sublingual preparation of this medication is available which may help patients with swallowing difficulties. There is some trial evidence of a symptomatic benefit when it is used in combination with levodopa therapy in patients with motor fluctuations.[72]

A newer MAOI called rasagiline is also available. It has been compared to placebo in 404 patients (mean age 61 years) with early PD over a 26-week period.[73] It was associated with significant benefits in UPDRS scores (−4.2 points for 1 mg dose; 95% CI −5.7 to −2.7). The benefits of early commencement of rasagiline appeared to persist in a subsequent open-label continuation of this trial, possibly suggesting a neuroprotective effect.[74] A trial has found a similar reduction in daily off time with this agent in people with advanced PD to that seen with entacapone.[75] Recent guidelines also recommend the consideration of MAOI for the treatment of motor complications in advanced PD.[46]

Amantadine

Amantadine was initially introduced as an anti-viral agent but was subsequently found to have anti-Parkinsonian properties. It has an NMDA receptor-blocking action, which leads to an anti-glutaminergic effect. In patients with PD this is thought to help by inhibiting excitatory pathways within the basal ganglia. It may also have dopaminergic and cholinergic effects. It has been found to lead to a modest improvement in Parkinsonism. Studies recruiting small numbers of patients (14–24) over short durations (six weeks) and using crossover designs have suggested a beneficial role in the control of dyskinesias and motor fluctuations when used in combination with levodopa in advanced PD.[76,77] This benefit is maintained to at least one year.[78] A six-week trial of amantadine may be tried in those patients with disabling dyskinesias.[22] It may also have some neuroprotective properties. Observational data has suggested an association between amantadine use and improved survival in PD.[79] This notion needs to be confirmed in a controlled trial setting. Side-effects include confusion, hallucinations and leg oedema. Cognitive side-effects often limit the use of this drug in the elderly.

Anticholinergic drugs

Anticholinergic agents (e.g. benzhexol, procyclidine and orphenadrine) are associated with cognitive impairment, particularly in the elderly (*see* p. 27), and are now very rarely used for the management of PD. There is evidence that they are associated with increased rates of Alzheimer-type pathology formation (amyloid plaques and neurofibrillary tangles).[80] These agents may have a place in the control of tremor-predominant PD in younger people.[22]

Surgical techniques

Surgical interventions for PD are usually performed with stereotactic techniques under local anaesthesia in order to assess motor response during the procedure. Due to the associated complications, they are usually reserved for those with advanced disease that causes significant disability and can no longer be controlled with medical therapy alone. This normally equates to patients with severe motor fluctuations and dyskinesias. Successful positioning requires intra-operative feedback from the patient and so significant cognitive impairment is a contraindication. Evaluation of these techniques in randomised controlled studies is difficult due to ethical considerations with placebo surgery. To date they have almost exclusively been performed in people under the age of 75 years. They are probably only suitable for a small number of highly selected, younger PD patients.

Deep brain stimulation

Deep brain stimulation (DBS) is a technique that involves the implantation of a device much like a cardiac pacemaker but with the electrode sited in the basal ganglia. This device then uses low-current, high-frequency electrical stimulation to inhibit local neuronal functioning. The effects are reversed if the device is switched off. The most common target sites are the subthalamic nucleus (STN) and globus pallidus interna (GPi). Both sites are associated with improvements in dyskinesias and both on and off period symptoms.

A crossover study of 143 patients (mean age 58 years) who had received DBS devices compared motor symptoms with the devices turned on and off.[81] It was found that stimulation of the STN or GPi was associated with median improvements of 49% and 37% in motor scores, respectively. Fifty-eight adverse events occurred in 143 patients (undergoing 277 procedures). These included haemorrhage, seizures and infection. Four patients (2.8%) had lasting neurological deficits. A randomised trial compared DBS to standard care (no blinding) in 156 patients with advanced PD (mean age 61 years, mean duration of levodopa treatment 13 years).[82] After six months they found that DBS was more effective at controlling Parkinsonian symptoms than medical management, but serious adverse events were more common (13% vs 4%, p<0.04), including one death related to surgery. A more recent study of PD patients with early motor complications (n=251, mean age 52 years, mean disease duration 7.5 years) found that STN stimulation was associated with improvements in both motor symptoms and quality of life compared to medial therapy alone.[83] This suggests that DBS may be appropriate for selected patients at an earlier stage of PD than previously thought.

After insertion it may be possible to reduce drug doses. A study found that 50% of patients were able to come off levodopa altogether and in these patients dyskinesias were markedly reduced.[84] The motor benefits appear be maintained, at least in part, to beyond five years from implantation.[85] Thalamic stimulation has been used to treat tremor associated with both PD and essential tremor with some success.[86] When the effects of DBS have been compared between patients over the age of 70 years and younger patients, the benefits are less clear.[87] Both groups had reduced dyskinesias but the older patients had a tendency towards worsening of axial signs (including gait impairment, which led to increased rates of falls).

DBS has been recommended for improving motor function, reducing off time and reducing dyskinesias in advanced PD.[88] Suitable candidates usually have minimal or no cognitive impairment at the time of surgery. Possible long-term neurological complications include cognitive impairment, motor disturbances and a range of emotional/psychiatric disorders.

Stereotactic surgery

Surgery for PD is usually performed using radiofrequency ablation. Thalamotomy has had some success in the treatment of tremor in the past but has now been outmoded by DBS, which has had similar success rates with fewer complications.[89] Pallidotomy, usually unilateral, appears to reduce the occurrence of dyskinesias (mainly contralateral). This benefit is maintained up to at least four years.[90] Side-effects are not inconsiderable. Around 14% will have an adverse event with 5% of these being rated as severe (e.g. persisting neurological deficit) and the mortality rate is around 0.4%.[91] Bilateral pallidotomy is associated with cognitive, behavioural and motor complications.[92]

Non-motor symptoms

Depression is a frequent component of PD, perhaps affecting as many as 50% of patients.[93] The clinical features of Parkinsonism (e.g. psychomotor retardation) can mimic depression and its diagnosis in these patients is not always easy. Sedating antidepressants, such as mirtazapine or tricyclic antidepressants (TCAs), taken at night may aid sleep pattern restoration. Their anticholinergic properties may reduce salivation (and so improve drooling) but may also worsen cognition, orthostatic hypotension (OH) and falls. SSRIs have occasionally been associated with worsening of tremor.[94] All these agents could potentially interact with selegiline and so caution is needed with such a combination. The management of depression is discussed further in Chapter 8.

Cognitive impairment and psychotic features are not easily treated. It is important to limit contributory drugs. It is suggested that sedating medications, then anticholinergics or amantadine, then selegiline, and then dopamine agonists are withdrawn in that order.[15] Lastly, it may be necessary to reduce levodopa doses. Hallucinations, if distressing to the patient, may be similarly reduced by the above medication changes. If this fails it is occasionally necessary to try a low dose of an antipsychotic agent in combination with levodopa. Of the available agents, quetiapine appears to have a lower incidence of worsened Parkinsonism than either risperidone or olanzapine.[95,96] This class of agent has many side-effects (*see* p. 28) and should only be used with caution. An alternative option is clozapine, but this requires specialist supervision and weekly blood monitoring.[46]

Cholinesterase inhibitors have been tried in the treatment of PDD. A group of 541 patients with PDD (mean age 73 years, mean MMSE score 19/30) received either rivastigmine or placebo over a 24-week period.[97] There was a small but statistically significant difference in ADAS-cog scores (*see* Appendix A) of 2.8 (out of 70) in favour of the rivastigmine group. However, the clinical significance of this degree of change is questionable and differential drop-out rates may have accounted for some of the difference. Also, there were significantly more side-effects observed in the treatment arm. Those occurring more commonly with rivastigmine compared to placebo included nausea (29% vs 11%), vomiting (17% vs 2%) and tremor (10% vs 4%). The cost–benefit ratio does not appear to justify the routine use of cholinesterase inhibitors in PDD.

Falls are more common in patients with PD due to the combination of a gait and balance disorder, postural instability and OH due to both autonomic and medication-induced neuropathy. They have been found to occur in 68% of a cohort of patients with PD over a one-year period.[98] A history of previous falls, the presence of cognitive impairment and loss of arm swing are associated with a higher risk. Adequate motor control is clearly important. The management of OH is discussed on p. 345. There is very little evidence from trials recruiting patients with PD.[46] Physiotherapy may help patients learn safer methods of mobilisation in difficult situations such as turning around. Gait and balance training is likely to be appropriate. Other causes of falls should also be considered (*see* Chapter 14).

Sleep disturbance is common in PD.[99] Excessive daytime sleepiness is a feature of the disease and is made worse by dopaminergic treatments, especially dopamine agonists. Nocturia, restless legs syndrome or the inability to turn over in bed may disturb night-time sleep. These latter two factors may improve with long-acting dopaminergic agents taken before bed. Depression may also be causative. Steps to improve nocturnal sleep may reduce daytime sleepiness. Simple measures include avoiding caffeine and alcohol, being active, getting exercise, and trying not to nap during the day.

Drooling (sialorrhoea) is caused by a reduction in swallowing frequency and efficacy, not by an increase in saliva production. It has been successfully improved by botulinum toxin injections to the salivary glands.[100] Constipation is a common manifestation in PD due to both autonomic neuropathy and levodopa. Its management is discussed in Chapter 12. Urinary frequency and incontinence may occur in advanced disease (*see* Chapter 11). Erectile dysfunction may be managed with sildenafil but this treatment can precipitate OH.[101]

Swallowing disorders (*see* Chapter 3) are common and can develop even in the early stages of PD.[102] They do not always respond to dopaminergic therapy and can be made worse by intercurrent illness. This may lead to an inability to take usual medications and a further functional impairment. The withdrawal of dopaminergic drugs can trigger a neuroleptic-like syndrome (*see* later). This is also an issue when PD patients are made 'nil by mouth' in the perioperative period.[103] Options include giving medications in a dispersible form via a nasogastric tube, using a transdermal rotigotine patch or a subcutaneous infusion of apomorphine. Equivalent doses of drugs can be calculated – *see* Table 9.1.

TABLE 9.1 Conversion scheme for dopaminergic drugs to the approximate equivalent dose of levodopa.

Drug	Adjustment – multiply dose in milligrams by ...
Levodopa	1
Levodopa controlled release	0.7
Levodopa plus COMTi	1.3
Pramipexole (base) Cabergoline Pergolide	100
Ropinirole Rotigotine	20
Bromocriptine Apomorphine	10

Specialties allied to medicine

PD nurse specialists are often employed in a variety of components of patient care, including education, counselling and monitoring of treatments. Their use has been found to improve patients' sense of well-being with no additional overall cost, but does not appear to effect patient outcomes.[104] Speech therapy may have a role in improving the quality of patients' speech and swallow ability.[105,106] Physiotherapy has been found to improve motor and activities of daily living (ADL) UPDRS scores but this effect was not maintained once therapy was discontinued.[107] It may well have a role in improving mobility and reducing falls as mentioned previously.

DEMENTIA WITH LEWY BODIES

➤ Percentage of all dementia: 10–15%.[108]
➤ Mean age of onset: 66 years.[109]
➤ Male:female ratio = 2:1.
➤ Key clinical features: Parkinsonism, fluctuating cognitive impairment, visual hallucinations.

Other suggestive features are early falls, episodes of reduced consciousness, neuroleptic sensitivity, REM sleep disorder and other hallucinations or delusions.[108] The cognitive impairment and Parkinsonism may not occur simultaneously at the onset; however, they should occur within 12 months of each other to meet standard diagnostic criteria.[110] Some autopsy-confirmed cases have been identified that did not develop Parkinsonism during the course of their illness.[108] The episodes of reduced consciousness are probably autonomically mediated due to Lewy body pathology within the autonomic centres of the brainstem. Three or more of daytime drowsiness, daytime sleeping >two hours, staring into space for long periods and episodes of disorganised speech occur in 63% of people with DLB compared to 12% of people with AD and only 0.5% of normal elderly people.[111]

The features of the cognitive impairment are generally those of other subcortical dementias (*see* p. 95) but typically it is fluctuating in severity (*see* Figure 6.3). In the early stages, patients may function at a near-normal level between fluctuations. The duration of these may vary from hours to weeks. Problems with frontal-executive functions, attention and visuospatial tests are characteristic. A study comparing clinical features with autopsy pathology in a cohort of people with cognitive impairment found that, in comparison to AD, DLB patients tend to perform worse in tests of executive function and attention but better in tests of memory and verbal skills.[112] However, they also found that a large percentage of patients have mixed cerebral pathology with a combination of the plaques and tangles of AD plus Lewy bodies in the substantia nigra or amygdala. This group of patients with mixed pathology tended to do similarly to the AD group in neuropsychological testing but had a worse prognosis with an average annual decline in MMSE score of 5.0 points compared to 3.5 and 3.4 for the AD and Lewy body pathology only groups, respectively. DAT scanning may reveal low striatal activity, and brain imaging may show relative preservation of the temporal lobes.[113] These findings would favour a diagnosis of DLB rather than AD.

Neuroleptic sensitivity occurs in around 60–80% of patients with DLB compared to <10% of those with AD, and about half of these reactions appear to be severe.[114] They usually present as a sudden onset of confusion, sedation and rigidity. A number will develop neuroleptic malignant syndrome (*see* p. 174) and some reactions are fatal. Visual hallucinations usually take the form of animals or people. Neuroleptic agents can reduce them, but given the risk of sensitivity, this should only be undertaken if they are distressing to the patient. Available observational evidence suggests that quetiapine may be the safest agent in this patient group.[95] The lowest effective dose should be used for the shortest possible length of time.

Pathologic findings include Lewy bodies. These are spherical, eosinophilic, intra-cytoplasmic inclusion bodies. They may be found throughout the brain but appear more commonly in the basal ganglia and limbic system. There are some pathological similarities with AD (*see* p. 98): beta amyloid plaques are commonly associated, but neurofibrillary tangles are infrequent.[110]

Treatment

Treatment of the cognitive and behavioural aspects of this condition is similar to that of other dementias and is discussed on p. 105. The treatment of the movement disorder aspects is similar to those of PD as discussed earlier. Dopaminergic agents may worsen hallucinations and cognitive impairment making it difficult to find the right therapeutic balance.

PROGRESSIVE SUPRANUCLEAR PALSY

➤ Prevalence: 5–6/100 000.[115,116]
➤ Mean survival: six years.[117,118]
➤ Mean age of onset: 63 years.[117]
➤ Male:female ratio = 2:1.
➤ Key clinical features: supranuclear gaze palsy, axial rigidity, pseudobulbar palsy, subcortical dementia, early gait abnormality, postural instability and falls.

PSP (formerly known as Steele–Richardson–Olszewski syndrome) is more common in men than women. Pathological features include atrophy of the upper brainstem with tau protein deposition and neurofibrillary tangles. The cause is unknown; however, some cases are inherited in an autosomal dominant manner and may be linked to mutations affecting the tau protein gene.[119] Diagnostic criteria have been published.[120]

The most common presenting complaint is of gait unsteadiness or falls.[118] When falls occur within the first year of diagnosis in patients with Parkinsonism, PSP is highly likely.[121] Classically the gaze palsy affects up and down gaze, which can present as problems negotiating flights of stairs. The earliest ophthalmic feature is usually impairment of saccadic movements. Commonly seen as slowing of vertical saccades.[6] A method for demonstrating this is shown in Figure 9.5. Other ophthalmic features that may be present include lid retraction, blepharospasm (abnormal eyelid contractions), reduced convergence and internuclear ophthalmoplegia.

The axial rigidity causes an extended posture with neck hyperextension commonly present. The pseudobulbar palsy manifests as dysarthria and dysphagia. Generalised hyper-reflexia, a positive jaw jerk and frontal release signs (*see* p. 92) may be present on examination. Cognitive signs are those of a subcortical dementia. There may also be palilalia (repetition of words) and emotional lability. There appears to be an increased incidence of hypertension in patients with PSP, possibly due to involvement of the brainstem adrenergic nuclei.[122] Urinary incontinence commonly develops. The onset of the condition is usually symmetric in distribution. It is often misdiagnosed before the development of characteristic signs such as gaze palsy. A non-specific prodromal illness may precede motor and cognitive impairment.

MRI scanning may demonstrate atrophy of the upper brainstem, temporal and frontal lobes. These changes are unlikely to occur in early disease and so are rarely helpful in the diagnosis. Falls occurring within the first year of presentation, absence of a tremor-predominant pattern and poor levodopa response all suggest PSP rather than PD.[109]

Treatment

Generally patients do not respond to levodopa. Around 20% will have a small benefit that is usually only short-lived.[6] Cholinesterase inhibitors have not produced significant cognitive benefits in PSP and also appear to impair mobility and functional status.[123] Botulinum toxin may help with rigidity.[124] Physiotherapy and falls prevention strategies (*see* p. 329) may be beneficial. Swallowing assessment and intervention may reduce the risk of aspiration pneumonia.

MULTIPLE SYSTEM ATROPHY

Multiple system atrophy (MSA) is a heterogeneous condition with a variety of clinical manifestations. It was initially classified as three separate conditions – striatonigral degeneration, olivopontocerebellar atrophy and Shy–Drager syndrome – depending on whether Parkinsonian, cerebellar or autonomic features predominated, respectively. More recently these have been considered as parts of the spectrum of this condition and much overlap, both clinically and pathologically, is observed.

The onset of motor symptoms is usually symmetrical. Autonomic dysfunction is seen in 97% of cases with male impotence, OH and urinary incontinence being the most commonly seen features.[125] Parkinsonism is present in around 90% of cases, pyramidal tract signs 60% and cerebellar signs in 50%.[125] The Parkinsonism is more commonly of an akinetic rigid type, but two-thirds of patients will have a tremor though not usually the classic pill-rolling variety. Dysarthria (95%), stridor (30%) and myoclonus (30%) may also be present.[125] Some patients develop obstructive sleep apnoea. There is an association between MSA and peripheral neuropathy. Cognition is usually not affected but a mild subcortical type dementia may develop. There is a high rate of misdiagnosis even among specialists. Early autonomic, cerebellar and gait disorders in the absence of marked cognitive impairment are suggestive of MSA.[126]

MRI scanning may demonstrate cerebellar and brainstem atrophy. The putamen may show relative signal hypointensity and atrophy with signal hyperintensity at its lateral margin. These changes are specific for MSA but are not very sensitive and may not be apparent until late in the disease.[127] Functional imaging studies may show reduced metabolism in the cerebellum and putamen. The role of these investigations in the diagnosis of MSA is not fully established.

Treatment

Around 30% of patients will have a significant response to levodopa therapy[125] so a trial of this is usually warranted. However, any response is often only short-lived and the majority are poorly responsive. The management of orthostatic hypotension and urinary incontinence are discussed in Chapters 15 and 11, respectively. Erectile dysfunction may be managed with sildenafil but this treatment can precipitate or aggravate OH.[101]

CORTICOBASAL DEGENERATION

➤ Prevalence: <1/100 000.
➤ Survival: eight years.[128]
➤ Mean age of onset: 63 years.[128]
➤ Key clinical features: asymmetric Parkinsonism, dystonia and myoclonus, ideomotor apraxia, subcortical dementia, alien limb phenomena.

Corticobasal degeneration (CBD) is a neurodegenerative condition of unknown aetiology. It shares pathological similarities with both PSP and frontotemporal dementia (FTD).[129] It is also associated with abnormal tau protein processing.

The most common presenting signs are unilateral limb clumsiness or rigidity, bradykinesia, ideomotor apraxia, postural imbalance and arm dystonia. The ideomotor apraxia can be demonstrated by asking the patient to mime activities such as combing their hair or cutting a piece of paper with a pair of scissors. The myoclonus can usually be induced ('stimulus-sensitive'). Around 50% will develop an 'alien limb'. This may present as spontaneous limb elevation, uncontrollable reaching for objects or intermanual conflict when performing tasks. This is not specific for CBD and may occur in other neurodegenerative disorders. Cortical sensory signs such as astereognosis (the inability to recognise objects by touch, e.g. keys placed in the hand), agraphaesthesia (the inability to distinguish numbers or letters 'drawn' on the palm) and reduced two-point discrimination may occur. Approximately one-third of patients will have early cognitive impairment.[130] There may also be clinical features similar to PSP, such as pseudobulbar palsy and ophthalmic signs. Clinical variants of this condition also exist. It can initially present as a focal cortical degenerative syndrome, for example primary progressive aphasia, or similarly to FTD.

Diagnostic accuracy is low (less than 50%) in comparison to autopsy pathology.[128] This is probably due to the clinical heterogeneity of CBD and the large degree of overlap both clinically and pathologically between all of the neurodegenerative disorders.[130] MRI scanning may demonstrate focal cortical atrophy or atrophy of the corpus callosum in later disease.[6]

Treatment

Around 25% of those with Parkinsonism will have a small response to levodopa. This medication should not be continued in the absence of a continued benefit due to potential adverse effects. Benzodiazepines may help reduce myoclonus in about 25%. Botulinum toxin may be useful for dystonia.

DRUG-INDUCED MOVEMENT DISORDERS

Drug-induced movement disorders include Parkinsonism, acute dystonia, neuroleptic malignant syndrome and tardive dyskinesia. Antipsychotic medications most commonly cause them. The indications for these medications, given their multiple harmful effects, should be carefully reviewed (*see* p. 28). The mainstay of diagnosis and treatment is to identify potentially causative agents and attempt to withdraw them where possible.

Parkinsonism

Drug-induced Parkinsonism accounts for around 9% of all Parkinsonism.[131] It usually presents as a rapid onset of symmetrical bradykinesia.[6] A Parkinsonian tremor can occur but is uncommon. It is usually reversible over weeks to months on discontinuation of the offending agent. Typical antipsychotic medications are more likely to induce Parkinsonism than atypical ones (*see* p. 110). A long list of other potentially causative agents has been produced. Most of these are very rare. Anti-dopaminergic anti-emetics (e.g. metoclopramide), monoamine depletors (e.g. reserpine) and some calcium channel blockers (e.g. cinnarizine) are occasionally implicated.

The use of levodopa in combination with the offending neuroleptic agent to treat drug-induced Parkinsonism is ineffective and illogical. Anticholinergic agents have been used previously to control such symptoms but they are associated with cognitive impairment in the elderly and should be avoided (*see* pp. 27 and 274).

Tardive dyskinesia

Tardive dyskinesia (TD) is a term for choreoathetoid movements that develop after a period of months to years on neuroleptic agents. The likelihood of its development appears to be related to cumulative exposure. Paradoxically, it is often precipitated or worsened by drug dose reductions or withdrawal. It is frequently permanent but may slowly improve once the causative agent has been discontinued. The most common manifestation is orofacial dyskinesia but athetosis or dystonia are possible.

The relative risk of the development of TD with typical or atypical agents is controversial. One study compared matched groups of 61 patients (mean age 66 years) on haloperidol or risperidone for the development of tardive dyskinesia over a nine-month period.[132] A higher rate was seen with haloperidol compared to risperidone (RR 4.1, 95% CI 2.5–5.7). However, the study included patients with a mixture of diagnoses and variable previous neuroleptic exposure. It cannot be excluded that some of the dyskinesias were induced by changes in medication or dose adjustments.

An open-label study of 330 patients with dementia (mean age 83 years) on various doses of risperidone (mean dose 0.96 mg/day) found an annual incidence of TD of 2.6%.[133] This figure is lower than the previous estimates of around 25% per year for those on typical agents. However, a retrospective review of 21 835 older adults with dementia (mean age 83 years) who had been started on neuroleptic medication found that there were 5.24 cases of drug-induced movement disorders other than Parkinsonism per 100 person-years with typical agents compared to 5.19 cases with atypical agents.[134] This difference was not statistically significant (RR 0.99, 95% CI 0.86–1.15).

Neuroleptic malignant syndrome

Key clinical features:

➤ muscle rigidity
➤ hyperthermia (>37.5°C)
➤ autonomic instability, for example tachycardia, hypertension or a labile blood pressure
➤ altered level of consciousness
➤ ↑ creatine kinase (CK).

Neuroleptic malignant syndrome (NMS) should be suspected in patients with a combination of the above clinical features while on a potentially causative medication. It has been seen most frequently with typical antipsychotic medications, especially haloperidol.[135,136] But, it has also been described in patients taking atypical antipsychotic agents,[137–139] and occasionally in patients taking metoclopramide.[135] Rarely, it is seen in patients with PD who have been rapidly withdrawn from their medication.[140] It may, very infrequently, be induced by antidepressants and pro-cholinergic medications (e.g. cholinesterase inhibitors).[141] Polypharmacy may be an important factor in many patients. It also appears to be more likely to occur in those who become dehydrated while on causative drugs.[142]

NMS is an idiosyncratic reaction (irrespective of drug dose or duration of therapy), which usually occurs within the first four weeks of commencement of the causative drug but occasionally only after several months of therapy. Estimates of incidence among those on antipsychotic medications vary between 0.1% and 2%,[142] probably reflecting differing populations studied. It is seen much more commonly in younger schizophrenic patients than older patients with dementia.[136] It is mostly likely caused by a relative deficit in dopamine within the brain but shares similarities with the serotonin syndrome (*see* Box 8.1) and so this neurotransmitter may also be involved. An important differential diagnosis is the neuroleptic sensitivity seen in DLB (*see* p. 169).

Investigations

Serum levels of CK and a full blood count (FBC) should be performed. An elevated CK is a common, but non-specific, finding. It may also be seen simply with sepsis or falls. An elevated white cell count (WCC) is supportive, but, obviously, not specific for a diagnosis of NMS. A urinary myoglobin will usually be elevated (this may give a false positive result for haemoglobin on standard urine dipsticks with an absence of red blood cells seen on urine microscopy). Tests to exclude alternative diagnoses may also be considered.

DSM-IV diagnostic criteria

A Rigidity and hyperthermia on neuroleptic medication.
B Two or more of: diaphoresis (excessive sweating), dysphagia, tremor, incontinence, confusion/coma, mutism, tachycardia, increased/labile blood pressure, increased WCC, increased CK.
C Not caused by other drug/condition.
D Not better accounted for by a mental disorder.

Complications

There are many potential complications of this condition and significant ones have been reported in around 30% of cases.[135] Some of the more common are:
➤ myoglobinuric renal failure (rhabdomyolysis)
➤ respiratory failure (± aspiration)
➤ thromboembolism
➤ dehydration.

Treatment

The first step is to stop the antipsychotic (or other suspected causative) medication, ensure adequate hydration and control pyrexia. As may be expected in such a rare and sporadic condition, large-scale randomised controlled trials of treatment modalities have not been performed.

Pro-dopaminergic medications bromocriptine and dantrolene have been proposed to reduce hyperthermia and rigidity in these patients, but this approach is controversial. Their use is usually unnecessary when the disorder is detected early and the offending agent is discontinued. There is also some evidence that bromocriptine or dantrolene may actually worsen or prolong the duration of episodes.[142] Mechanical ventilation is sometimes required for those with respiratory failure.

Outcome

The length of episodes varies widely, but they typically last around 7–10 days, and it has a mortality rate of around 20%.[142,143] Recommencement of causative medications, if thought absolutely necessary, should be delayed until at least two weeks after the event.[144] After this time, a low dose of a low-potency drug (e.g. an atypical rather than a typical antipsychotic agent) should be used and the patient should be carefully monitored for signs of recurrence.

Vascular Parkinsonism

Parkinsonism induced by vascular lesions is an important cause in the elderly, and accounts for around 8% of all Parkinsonism.[131] It more commonly affects the legs than the arms ('lower-body Parkinsonism') and rarely causes the characteristic 'pill-rolling' tremor of PD. The onset is usually rapid or step-wise, and clinical features are bilateral and symmetrical, with rigidity, a small-stepping gait ('marche à petits pas') and a mask-like face.[145] The history usually reveals vascular risk factors (especially hypertension and diabetes) or prior strokes. Non-Parkinsonian neurological signs may also be present (e.g. pyramidal tract). Any of dysarthria, dysphagia, emotional lability, incontinence and cognitive impairment may be early features. Table 9.2 compares some of the distinguishing features of vascular Parkinsonism and PD.

TABLE 9.2 Vascular Parkinsonism vs Parkinson's disease

	Vascular Parkinsonism	**Parkinson's disease**
Onset	Bilateral and symmetrical	Unilateral
Progression	Rapid or step-wise	Slow and insidious
'Pill-rolling' tremor	Rare	Frequent
Gait	Upright stance, broad-based and small-stepping	Stooped and festinating
Other features	History of strokes or vascular risk factors; pyramidal tract signs; early emotional lability; incontinence or cognitive impairment	Good response to levodopa therapy

Multiple lacunar strokes or basal ganglia infarction are thought to be causative. CT imaging may show vascular changes. The role of functional imaging is controversial. The response to levodopa is poor or non-existent (this feature often helps support a diagnosis). Other PD therapeutic strategies are not indicated. Treatment includes addressing vascular risk factors, and commencing antiplatelet agents and statins were indicated (*see* p. 206).

NORMAL PRESSURE HYDROCEPHALUS

Normal pressure hydrocephalus (NPH) is a rare but potentially reversible cause of cognitive impairment (<1 % of cases of dementia). It may be idiopathic or occur secondarily to intracerebral pathology, for example meningitis, subarachnoid haemorrhage or tumour. It is a clinical syndrome with a characteristic triad of features:

➤ gait disturbance
➤ cognitive impairment
➤ urinary incontinence.

The presenting feature is usually a gait disorder. Classically this is of a 'foot stuck to the floor' nature. Alternatively the gait may be simply unsteady and broad-based with small steps and low floor clearance. The legs and bladder are affected more than the upper limbs due the positioning of their fibres within the motor cortex. As they lie inferomedially, they are more stretched by the ventricular enlargement. The urinary incontinence is urge in nature (*see* p. 266). Cognitive deficits are usually of a subcortical type (*see* p. 95).

Examination may show upper motor neuron signs in the legs. The upper limbs may show reduced coordination and a fine action tremor. Classic Parkinsonism may be present. Papilloedema is absent.

CT scanning reveals enlarged ventricles usually with sulcal effacement. This latter feature helps to distinguish NHP from the ventricular enlargement seen with brain atrophy but this is not absolute (*see* Figure 9.10). Lumbar puncture opening pressure is not elevated. It is believed that the damage is caused by initial raised intracranial fluid pressure, which then normalises once the ventricles have become dilated.

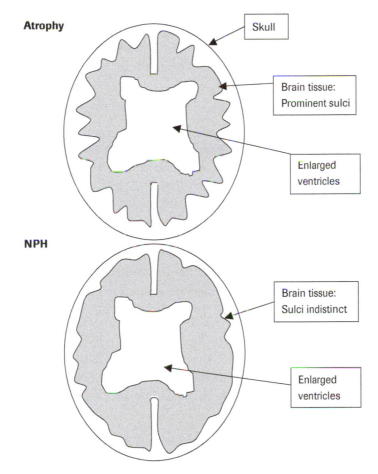

FIGURE 9.10 A comparison of the CT appearance of cerebral atrophy and that of normal-pressure hydrocephalus.

The removal of 40–50 mL of cerebrospinal fluid (CSF) followed by repeat assessment of walking speed or cognition has been used to identify those patients likely to respond to a shunting procedure. It is a fair predictor of those who will have cognitive improvement.[146] A better test appears to be external lumbar drainage (ELD). Here a drain is placed into the spinal canal and 10 mL of CSF is drained each hour through a valve over a three-day period. An improvement in walking or cognition following this test has a 92% sensitivity to detect those who will improve with a shunting procedure.[147] Such an improvement appears to occur in patients of all ages.

Treatment

Ventriculoperitoneal shunting is the usual treatment for this condition; however, there is no randomised controlled trial evidence demonstrating that shunting is effective.[148] Patients with idiopathic NPH do less well than those with an underlying disorder after shunting. Approximately 30% of patients with the idiopathic variant will improve following shunting at the expense of a 38% complication rate, with a 6% incidence of serious complications (permanent neurological deficit and death).[149] Patients with a known underlying cause have around a 70% response rate to shunting.[150] Predictors of shunt response include early gait disturbance, the presence of all three of the classic features and a recent onset of symptoms. Dementia is the least likely feature to improve post-shunting.[147]

ESSENTIAL TREMOR

Essential tremor (ET) is a very common movement disorder, affecting around 5% of people over the age of 65 years.[151] Characteristically it causes a tremor when maintaining a fixed body position (postural) or on movement (action). It does not usually cause a resting tremor and never causes the classic pill-rolling tremor of PD. Nor does it characteristically cause a tremor that worsens on approaching a target (intention), which is seen with cerebellar disorders. It may be confused with an exaggerated physiological tremor, which is seen with metabolic disorders (e.g. thyrotoxicosis and alcohol withdrawal) or medication-induced (e.g. sodium valproate, beta-agonists, lithium and antidepressants). Previously, the prefix 'benign' was attached to ET. This was misleading as some patients may become severely disabled due to this disorder.

Approximately 50% of patients have affected family members, and it is thought to be autosomal dominantly inherited.[151] The causative gene (or genes) has not been identified and the pathogenesis of ET is unknown. It causes a bilateral tremor in the hands of almost all patients. In smaller numbers the head (34%), legs (20%), and voice (12%) are affected.[151] There are no symptoms or neurological signs other than tremor. Patients usually give a history of having been tremulous for many years. They may improve following drinking alcohol.

Treatment

Not all patients with ET will require treatment and many will be asymptomatic. Some patients will self-medicate with alcohol, and alcoholism is a potential, but uncommon, association. When intervention is required, no treatment strategy has proven beneficial to all patients. Response rates are variable. The more commonly used techniques are discussed below.

Medications

➤ *Beta-blockers*: beta-blockers have been shown to reduce the severity of tremor in 40–50% of patients.[152] This is probably mediated by a peripheral mechanism. Fewer lipophilic drugs, that do not cross the blood–brain barrier (e.g. atenolol and metoprolol), appear to be as effective as ones that do (e.g. propranolol). They are contraindicated in some patients (e.g. those with asthma).

➤ *Primidone*: the mechanism of action of primidone is unclear. It may have a direct effect or it may be predominantly due to its barbiturate metabolites. It has been evaluated in several small randomised controlled trials mainly recruiting patients in their fifties and sixties. The mean tremor-reduction efficacy is in the region of 40–50%.[152] The main side-effects are sedation, dizziness and unsteadiness. It is likely to increase the risk of falls within the elderly. Similar to barbiturates, it is probably best avoided in older, frailer patients.

➤ *Anticonvulsants*: gabapentin has a GABA-mediated mechanism of action. Results of small trials have suggested a probable mild benefit.[153] Topiramate is an anticonvulsant medication believed to have a broad spectrum of actions. It was found to have a mild benefit in ET in a small crossover-designed trial.[154]

➤ *Botulinum toxin*: injections of botulinum toxin into the wrist flexors and extensors have been used in patients with ET of disabling severity.[155] This was associated with reductions in the tremor severity but induced some hand weakness and very little functional improvement.

Surgery

DBS of the thalamic nuclei has been used to successfully reduce tremor and improve functional disability in non-randomised studies using small numbers of patients.[156,157] The high associated complication rate is unlikely to make this a common treatment modality for this condition.

RESTLESS LEGS SYNDROME

Restless legs syndrome (RLS) causes an irresistible desire to move one's legs while sitting or lying down. There may be an associated 'crawling' or 'tingling' sensation in the thighs and calves, and there may be jerking movements in the legs. Symptoms may be more common overnight, and are typically relieved by walking about. This may lead to reduced sleep and quality of life. Typically it is a chronic and progressive disorder. It appears to be commoner in older age but an accurate prevalence is unknown. It is estimated to affect 4–10% of the adult population, although it may only be severe in a third of these cases.[158] It is more common in women than men.

It may be primary or secondary to underlying disease. Those with the primary condition are likely to have a family history. The aetiology is believed to involve reduced brain dopamine. Secondary causes include iron deficiency anaemia and uraemia. A full blood count, ferritin and urea level should be performed. Symptoms due to secondary causes should improve following treatment of the underlying problem. Drug treatment is probably only necessary for those with a primary disorder that is severe enough to disrupt lifestyle. Dopamine agonists have the best evidence for efficacy. Much lower doses than those required in PD are used (10–20%).[159] Alternative options for those with refractory symptoms include opiates and gabapentin.

REFERENCES

1 Rascol O, Sabatini U, Simonetta-Moreau M, *et al.* Square wave jerks in Parkinsonian syndrome. *J Neurol Neurosurg Psychiatry*, 1991; **54**: 599–602.

2 Marshall V, Grosset D. Role of dopamine transporter imaging in routine clinical practice. *Mov Disord*, 2003; **18**(12): 1415–23.

3 Hughes AJ, Daniel SE, Blankson S, *et al.* A clinicopathologic study of 100 cases of Parkinson's disease. *Arch Neurol*, 1993; **50**: 140–8.

4 Hughes AJ, Daniel SE, Lees AJ. Improved accuracy of clinical diagnosis of Lewy body Parkinson's disease. *Neurology*, 2001; **57**: 1497–9.

5 De Rijk MC, Tzourio C, Breteler MMB, *et al.* Prevalence of parkinsonism and Parkinson's disease in Europe: the EUROPARKINSON collaborative study. *J Neurol Neurosurg Psychiatry*, 1997; **62**: 10–15.

6 Chadwick WC, Aminoff MJ. Clinical differentiation of parkinsonian syndromes: prognostic and therapeutic relevance. *Am J Med*, 2004; **117**: 412–19.

7 Poewe WH, Wenning GK. The natural history of Parkinson's disease. *Ann Neurol*, 1998; **44**(Suppl. 1): S1–9.

8 Barnes J, David AS. Visual hallucinations in Parkinson's disease: a review and phenomenological survey. *J Neurol Neurosurg Psychiatry*, 2001; **70**: 727–33.

9 Holroyd S, Currie L, Wooten GF. Prospective study of hallucinations and delusions in Parkinson's disease. *J Neurol Neurosurg Psychiatry*, 2001; **70**: 734–8.

10 Eriksen JL, Wszolek Z, Petrucelli L. Molecular pathogenesis of Parkinson disease. *Arch Neurol*, 2005; **62**: 353–7.

11 Gorell JM, Rybicki BA, Johnson CC, *et al.* Smoking and Parkinson's disease: a dose-response relationship. *Neurology*, 1999; **52**: 115–19.

12 Beneditti MD, Bower JH, Maraganore DM. Smoking, alcohol, and coffee consumption preceding Parkinson's disease: a case-control study. *Neurology*, 2000; **55**: 1350–8.

13 Ross GW, Abbott RD, Petrovitch H, *et al.* Association of coffee and caffeine intake with the risk of Parkinson disease. *JAMA*, 2000; **283**: 2674–9.

14 Aarsland D, Andersen K, Larsen JP, *et al.* Prevalence and characteristics of dementia in Parkinson disease: an 8-year prospective study. *Arch Neurol*, 2003; **60**: 387–92.

15 Olanow CW, Watts RL, Koller WC. An algorithm (decision tree) for the management of Parkinson's disease (2001): treatment guidelines. *Neurology*, 2001; **56**(Suppl. 5): S1–88.

16 Athey RJ, Porter RW, Walker RW. Cognitive assessment of a representative community population with Parkinson's disease (PD) using the Cambridge Cognitive Assessment-Revised (CAMCOG-R). *Age Ageing*, 2005; **34**: 268–73.

17 Williams-Gray CH, Foltynie T, Brayne CEG, *et al.* Evolution of cognitive dysfunction in an incident Parkinson's disease cohort. *Brain*, 2007; **130**: 1787–98.

18 Press DZ. Parkinson's disease dementia – a first step? *N Engl J Med*, 2004; **351**(24): 2547–9.

19 Boller F, Mizutani T, Roessmann U, *et al.* Parkinson disease, dementia, and Alzheimer disease: clinicopathological correlations. *Ann Neurol*, 1980; **7**: 329–35.

20 Horn S, Stern MB. The comparative effects of medical therapies for Parkinson's disease. *Neurology*, 2004; **63**(Suppl. 2): S7–12.

21 Wheatley K, Stowe RL, Clarke CE, *et al.* Evaluating drug treatments for Parkinson's disease: how good are the trials? *BMJ*, 2002; **324**: 1508–11.

22 Lees AJ. Drugs for Parkinson's disease: oldies but goodies. *J Neurol Neurosurg Psychiatry*, 2002; **73**: 607–10.

23 Mouradian MM. Should levodopa be infused into the duodenum? *Neurology*, 2005; **64**: 182–3.

24 Riley D, Lang AE. The spectrum of levodopa-related fluctuations in Parkinson's disease. *Neurology*, 1993; **43**: 1459–63.

25 Thanvi BR, Lo TCN. Long term motor complications of levodopa: clinical features, mechanisms, and management strategies. *Postgrad Med J*, 2004; **80**: 452–8.

26 Togasaki DM, Tan L, Protell P, *et al.* Levodopa induces dyskinesias in normal squirrel monkeys. *Ann Neurol*, 2001; **50**: 254–7.

27 Rascol O, Brooks DJ, Korczyn AD, *et al.* A five-year study of the incidence of dyskinesia in patients with early Parkinson's disease who were treated with ropinirole or levodopa. *N Engl J Med*, 2000; **342**: 1484–91.

28 Parkinson Study Group. Pramipexole vs levodopa as initial treatment for Parkinson disease: a randomized controlled trial. *JAMA*, 2000; **284**(15): 1931–8.

29 Bravi D, Mouradian MM, Roberts JW, *et al.* Wearing-off fluctuations in Parkinson's disease: contribution of postsynaptic mechanisms. *Ann Neurol*, 1994; **36**(1): 27–31.

30 Mouradian MM, Heuser IJE, Baronti F, *et al.* Modification of central dopaminergic mechanisms by continuous levodopa therapy for advanced Parkinson's disease. *Ann Neurol*, 1990; **27**: 18–23.

31 Koller WC, Hutton JT, Tolosa E, *et al.* Immediate-release and controlled-release carbidopa/levodopa in PD: a 5-year randomized multicenter study. *Neurology*, 1999; **53**: 1012–19.

32 Jiang Y, Norman KE. Effects of visual and auditory cues on gait initiation in people with Parkinson's disease. *Clin Rehabil*, 2006; **20**: 36–45.

33 Fahn S. The spectrum of levodopa-induced dyskinesias. *Ann Neurol*, 2000; **47**(Suppl. 1): S2–11.

34 Assal F, Spahr L, Hadengue A, *et al.* Tolcapone and fulminant hepatitis. *Lancet*, 1998; **352**: 958.

35 National Institute of Health and Care Excellence. *Parkinson's Disease: diagnosis and management in primary and secondary care.* CG 35, 2006. Available at: www.nice.org.uk/guidance/cg35 (accessed 5 November 2014).

36 Merello M, Lees AJ, Webster R, *et al.* Effect of entacapone, a peripherally acting catechol-O-methyltransferase inhibitor, on the motor response to acute treatment with levodopa in patients with Parkinson's disease. *J Neurol Neurosurg Psychiatry*, 1994; **57**: 186–9.

37 Parkinson Study Group. Entacapone improves motor fluctuations in levodopa-treated Parkinson's disease patients. *Ann Neurol*, 1997; **42**: 747–55.

38 Inzelberg R, Nisipeanu P, Rabey JM, *et al.* Double-blind comparison of cabergoline and bromocriptine in Parkinson's disease patients with motor fluctuations. *Neurology*, 1996; **47**: 785–8.

39 Guttman M and the International Pramipexole-Bromocriptine Study Group. Double-blind comparison of Pramipexole and bromocriptine treatment with placebo in advanced Parkinson's disease. *Neurology*, 1997; **49**: 1060–5.

40 Korczyn AD, Brunt ER, Larsen JP, *et al.* A 3-year randomized trial of ropinirole and bromocriptine in early Parkinson's disease. *Neurology*, 1999; **53**: 364–70.

41 Bonuccelli U. Comparing dopamine agonists in Parkinson's disease. *Curr Op Neurol*, 2003; **16**(Suppl. 1): S13–19.

42 Shaunak S, Wilkins A, Pilling JB, *et al.* Pericardial, retroperitoneal, and pleural fibrosis induced by pergolide. *J Neurol Neurosurg Psychiatry*, 1999; **66**: 79–81.

43 Van Camp G, Flamez A, Cosyns B, *et al.* Treatment of Parkinson's disease with pergolide and relation to restrictive valvular heart disease. *Lancet*, 2004; **363**: 1179–83.

44 Pinero A, Marcos-Alberca P, Fortes J. Cabergoline-related severe restrictive mitral regurgitation. *N Engl J Med*, 2005; **353**(18): 1976–7.

45 Committee on Safety of Medicines. Fibrotic reactions with pergolide and other ergot-derived dopamine receptor agonists. *Curr Problems Pharmacovigilance*, 2002; **28**: 3.

46 Scottish Intercollegiate Guideline. *Diagnosis and Pharmacological Management of Parkinson's Disease: a national clinical guideline*. SIGN 113, 2010. Available at: www.sign.ac.uk/pdf/sign113.pdf (accessed 5 November 2014).

47 Ondo WG, Dat Vuong K, Khan H, *et al.* Daytime sleepiness and other sleep disorders in Parkinson's disease. *Neurology*, 2001; **57**: 1392–6.

48 Frucht S, Rogers JD, Greene PE, *et al.* Falling asleep at the wheel: motor vehicle mishaps in persons taking pramipexole and ropinirole. *Neurology*, 1999; **52**: 1908–10.

49 Tan E, Ondo W. Clinical characteristics of pramipexole-induced peripheral edema. *Arch Neurol*, 2000; **57**: 729–32.

50 O'Sullivan SS, Evans AH, Lees AJ. Dopamine dysregulation syndrome: an overview of its epidemiology, mechanisms and management. *CNS Drugs*, 2009; **23**: 157–70.

51 Ceravolo R, Frosini D, Rossi C, *et al.* Spectrum of addictions in Parkinson's disease: from dopamine dysregulation syndrome to impulse control disorders. *J Neurol*, 2010; **257**(Suppl. 2): S276–83.

52 Cilia R, Siri C, Canesi M, *et al.* Dopamine dysregulation syndrome in Parkinson's disease: from clinical and neuropsychological characterisation to management and long-term outcome. *J Neurol Neurosurg Psychiatry*, 2014; **85**: 311–18.

53 Giovannoni G, O'Sullivan JD, Turner K, *et al.* Hedonistic homeostatic dysregulation in patients with Parkinson's disease on dopamine replacement therapies. *J Neurol Neurosurg Psychiatry*, 2000; **68**: 423–8.

54 Dodd ML, Klos KJ, Bower JH, *et al.* Pathological gambling caused by drugs used to treat Parkinson disease. *Arch Neurol*, 2005; **62**: 1377–81.

55 Weiner WJ. The initial treatment of Parkinson's disease should begin with levodopa. *Mov Disord*, 1999; **14**(5): 716–24.

56 Montastruc JL, Rascal O, Senard J. Treatment of Parkinson's disease should begin with a dopamine agonist. *Mov Disord*, 1999; **14**(5): 725–30.

57 Clarke C, Guttman M. Dopamine agonist monotherapy in Parkinson's disease. *Lancet*, 2002; **360**: 1767–9.

58 Hely MA, Morris JGL, Traficante R, *et al.* The Sydney multicentre study of Parkinson's disease: progression and mortality at 10 years. *J Neurol Neurosurg Psychiatry*, 1999; **67**: 300–7.

59 Lees AJ, Katzenschlager R, Head J, *et al.* Ten-year follow-up of three different initial treatments in de-novo PD: a randomized trial. *Neurology*, 2001; **57**: 1687–94.

60 Lieberman A, Ranhosky A, Korts D. Clinical evaluation of pramipexole in advanced Parkinson's disease: results of a double-blind, placebo-controlled, parallel-group study. *Neurology*, 1997; **49**: 162–8.

61 Lieberman A, Olanow CW, Sethi K, *et al.* A multicenter trial of ropinirole as adjunct treatment for Parkinson's disease. *Neurology*, 1998; **51**: 1057–62.

62 Onalow CW, Fahn S, Muenter M, *et al.* A multicenter double-blind placebo-controlled trial of pergolide as an adjunct to Sinemet in Parkinson's disease. *Mov Disord*, 1994; **9**(1): 40–7.

63 Baldwin CM, Keating GM. Spotlight on rotigotine in Parkinson's disease. *Drugs Aging*, 2008; **25**(2): 175–7.

64 Pietz K, Hagell P, Odin P. Subcutaneous apomorphine in late stage Parkinson's disease: a long term follow up. *J Neurol Neurosurg Psychiatry*, 1998; **65**: 709–16.

65 Colzi A, Turner K, Lees AJ. Continuous subcutaneous waking day apomorphine in the long term treatment of levodopa induced interdose dyskinesias in Parkinson's disease. *J Neurol Neurosurg Psychiatry*, 1998; **64**: 573–6.

66 Dewey RB, Hutton JT, LeWitt PA, *et al.* A randomized, double-blind, placebo-controlled trial of subcutaneously injected apomorphine for parkinsonian off-state events. *Arch Neurol*, 2001; **58**: 1385–92.

67 Richard IH, Kurlan R, Tanner C, *et al.* Serotonin syndrome and the combined use of deprenyl and an antidepressant in Parkinson's disease. *Neurology*, 1997; **48**: 1070–7.

68 Palhagen S, Heinonen EH, Hagglund J, *et al.* Selegiline delays the onset of disability in de novo parkinsonian patients. *Neurology*, 1998; **51**: 520–5.

69 Ives NJ, Stowe RL, Marro J, *et al.* Monoamine oxidase type B inhibitors in early Parkinson's disease: meta-analysis of 17 randomised trials involving 3525 patients. *BMJ*, 2004; **329**: 593–6.

70 Marras C, McDermott MP, Rochon PA, *et al.* Survival in Parkinson disease: thirteen-year follow-up of the DATATOP cohort. *Neurology*, 2005; **64**: 87–93.

71 Ben-Shlomo Y, Churchyard A, Head J *et al.* Investigation by Parkinson's Disease Research Group of United Kingdom into excess mortality seen with combined levodopa and selegiline treatment in patients with early, mild Parkinson's disease: further results of randomised trial and confidential enquiry. *BMJ*, 1998; **316**: 1191–6.

72 Waters CH, Sethi KD, Hauser RA, *et al.* Zydis selegiline reduces off time in Parkinson's disease patients with motor fluctuations: a 3-month randomized, placebo-controlled study. *Mov Disord*, 2004; **19**(4): 426–32.

73 Parkinson Study Group. A controlled trial of rasagiline in early Parkinson disease: the TEMPO study. *Arch Neurol*, 2002; **59**: 1937–43.

74 Hauser RA, Lew MF, Hurtig HI, *et al.* Long-term outcome of early versus delayed rasagiline treatment in early Parkinson's disease. *Mov Disord*, 2009; **24**(4): 564–73.

75 Rascol O, Brooks DJ, Melamed E, *et al.* Rasagiline as an adjunct to levodopa in patients with Parkinson's disease and motor fluctuations (LARGO, lasting effect in adjunct therapy with rasagiline given once daily, study): a randomised, double-blind, parallel-group trial. *Lancet*, 2005; **365**: 947–54.

76 Verhagen Metman L, Del Dotto P, van den Munckhof P, *et al.* Amantadine as treatment for dyskinesias and motor fluctuations in Parkinson's disease. *Neurology*, 1998; **50**: 1323–6.

77 Snow BJ, Macdonald L, Mcauley D, *et al.* The effect of amantadine on levodopa-induced dyskinesias in Parkinson's disease: a double-blind, placebo-controlled study. *Clin Neuropharm*, 2000; **23**(2): 82–5.

78 Verhagen Metman L, Del Dotto P, LePool K, *et al.* Amantadine for levodopa-induced dyskinesias: a 1-year follow-up study. *Arch Neurol*, 1999; **56**: 1383–6.

79 Uitii RJ, Rajput AH, Ahlskog JE, *et al.* Amantadine treatment is an independent predictor of survival in Parkinson's disease. *Neurology*, 1996; **46**: 1551–6.

80 Perry EK, Kilford L, Lees AJ, *et al.* Increased Alzheimer pathology in Parkinson's disease related to antimuscarinic drugs. *Ann Neurol*, 2003; **54**: 235–8.

81 The Deep-Brain Stimulation for Parkinson's Disease Study Group. Deep-Brain, stimulation of the subthalamic nucleus or the pars interna of the globus pallidus in Parkinson's disease. *N Engl J Med*, 2001; **345**(13): 956–63.

82 Deuschl G, Schade-Brittinger C, Krack P, *et al.* A randomised trial of deep-brain stimulation for Parkinson's disease. *N Engl J Med*, 2006; **355**(9): 896–908.

83 Schuepbach WMM, Rau J, Knudsen K, *et al.* Neurostimulation for Parkinson's disease with early motor complications. *N Engl J Med*, 2013; **368**: 610–22.

84 Vingerhoets FJG, Villemure JG, Temperli R, *et al.* Subthalamic DBS replaces levodopa in Parkinson's disease: two-year follow-up. *Neurology*, 2002; **58**: 396–401.

85 Krack P, Batir A, Van Blercom N, *et al.* Five-year follow-up of bilateral stimulation of the subthalamic nucleus in advanced Parkinson's disease. *N Engl J Med*, 2003; **349**(20): 1925–34.

86 Koller W, Pahwa R, Busenbark K, *et al.* High-frequency unilateral thalamic stimulation in the treatment of essential tremor and parkinsonian tremor. *Ann Neurol*, 1997; **42**: 292–9.

87 Russmann H, Ghika J, Villemure JG, *et al.* Subthalamic nucleus deep brain stimulation in Parkinson's disease patients over age 70 years. *Neurology*, 2004; **63**: 1952–4.

88 Okun MS. Deep-brain stimulation for Parkinson's disease. *N Engl J Med*, 2012; **367**: 1529–38.

89 Schuurman PR, Bosch DA, Bossuyt PMM, *et al.* A comparison of continuous thalamic stimulation and thalamotomy for suppression of severe tremor. *N Engl J Med*, 2000; **342**: 461–8.

90 Fine J, Duff J, Chen R, *et al.* Long-term follow-up of unilateral pallidotomy in advanced Parkinson's disease. *N Engl J Med*, 2000; **342**: 1708–14.

91 Alkhani A, Lozano AM. Pallidotomy for Parkinson disease: a review of contemporary literature. *J Neurosurg*, 2001; **94**: 43–9.

92 Ghika J, Ghika-Schmid F, Frankhauser F, *et al.* Bilateral contemporaneous posteroventral pallidotomy for the treatment of Parkinson's disease: neuropsychological and neurological side-effects: report of four cases and review of the literature. *J Neurosurg*, 1999; **91**: 313–21.

93 Dooneief G, Mirabello E, Bell K, *et al.* An estimate of the incidence of depression in idiopathic Parkinson's disease. *Arch Neurol*, 1992; **49**: 305–7.

94 Jansen Steur ENH. Increase of Parkinson disability after fluoxetine medication. *Neurology*, 1993; **43**: 211–13.

95 Fernandez HH, Trieschmann ME, Burke MA, *et al.* Quetiapine for psychosis in Parkinson's disease versus dementia with Lewy bodies. *J Clin Psych*, 2002; **63**: 513–15.

96 Friedman JH, Factor SA. Atypical antipsychotics in the treatment of drug-induced psychosis in Parkinson's disease. *Mov Disord*, 2000; **15**(2): 201–11.

97 Emre M, Aarsland D, Albanese A, *et al.* Rivastigmine for dementia associated with Parkinson's disease. *N Engl J Med*, 2004; **351**: 2509–18.

98 Wood BH, Bilclough JA, Bowron A, *et al.* Incidence and prediction of falls in Parkinson's disease: a prospective multidisciplinary study. *J Neurol Neurosurg Psychiatry*, 2002; **72**(6): 721–5.

99 Medcalf P. Good practice in the assessment and management of nocturnal Parkinson's disease symptoms. *Age Ageing*, 2005; **34**: 435–8.

100 Bhatia KP, Munchau A, Brown P. Botulinum toxin is a useful treatment in excessive drooling of saliva. *J Neurol Neurosurg Psychiatry*, 1999; **67**: 697.

101 Hussain IF, Brady CM, Swinn MJ, *et al.* Treatment of erectile dysfunction with sildenafil citrate (Viagra) in parkinsonism due to Parkinson's disease or multiple system atrophy with observations on orthostatic hypotension. *J Neurol Neurosurg Psychiatry*, 2001; **71**: 371–4.

102 Miller N, Noble E, Jones D, *et al.* Hard to swallow: dysphagia in Parkinson's disease. *Age Ageing*, 2006; **35**: 614–18.

103 Brennan KA, Genever RW. Managing Parkinson's disease during surgery. *BMJ*, 2010; **341**: 990–3.

104 Jarman B, Hurwitz B, Cook A, *et al.* Effects of community based nurses specialising in Parkinson's disease on health outcome and costs: randomised controlled trial. *BMJ*, 2002; **324**: 1072–5.

105 Ramig LO, Countryman S, O'Brien C, *et al.* Intensive speech treatment for patients with Parkinson's disease: short- and long-term comparison of two techniques. *Neurology*, 1996; **47**: 1496–1504.

106 Ramig LO, Sapir S, Fox C, *et al.* Changes in vocal loudness following intensive voice treatment (LSVT) in individuals with Parkinson's disease: a comparison with untreated patients and normal age-matched controls. *Mov Disord*, 2001; **16**(1): 79–83.

107 Comella CL, Stebbins GT, Brown-Toms N, *et al.* Physical therapy and Parkinson's disease: a controlled clinical trial. *Neurology*, 1994; **44**: 376–8.

108 McKeith I, Mintzer J, Aarsland D, *et al.* Dementia with Lewy bodies. *Lancet Neurology*, 2004; **3**(1): 19–28.

109 Litvan I, Campbell G, Mangone CA, *et al.* Which clinical features differentiate progressive supranuclear palsy (Steel-Richardson-Olszewski syndrome) from related disorders? A clinicopathological study. *Brain*, 1997; **120**: 65–74.

110 McKeith IG, Galasko D, Kosaka K, *et al.* Consensus guidelines for the clinical and pathologic diagnosis of dementia with Lewy bodies (DLB): report of the consortium on DLB international workshop. *Neurology*, 1996; **47**: 1113–24.

111 Ferman TJ, Smith GE, Boeve BF, *et al.* DLB fluctuations: specific features that reliably differentiate ALD from AD and normal aging. *Neurology*, 2004; **62**: 181–7.

112 Kraybill ML, Larson EB, Tsuang W, *et al.* Cognitive differences in dementia patients with autopsy-verified AD, Lewy body pathology or both. *Neurology*, 2005; **64**: 2069–73.

113 McKeith IG, Dickson DW, Lowe J, *et al.* Diagnosis and management of dementia with Lewy bodies: third report of the DLB consortium. *Neurology*, 2005; **65**: 1863–72.

114 McKeith I, Fairbairn A, Perry R, *et al.* Neuroleptic sensitivity in patients with senile dementia of Lewy body type. *BMJ*, 1992; **305**: 673–8.

115 Schrag A, Ben-Shlomo Y, Quinn NP. Prevalence of progressive supranuclear palsy and multiple system atrophy: a cross-sectional study. *Lancet*, 1999; **354**: 1771–5.

116 Nath U, Ben-Shlomo Y, Thomson RG, *et al.* The prevalence of progressive supranuclear palsy (Steel–Richardson–Olszewski syndrome) in the UK. *Brain*, 2001; **124**: 1438–49.

117 Litvan I, Mangone CA, McKee A, *et al.* Natural history of progressive supranuclear palsy (Steele–Richardson–Olszewski syndrome) and clinical predictors of survival: a clinicopathological study. *J Neurol Neurosurg Psychiatry*, 1996; **61**: 615–20.

118 Maher ER, Lees AJ. The clinical features and natural history of the Steele–Richardson–Olszewski syndrome (progressive supranuclear palsy). *Neurology*, 1986; **36**: 1005–8.

119 Conrad C, Andreadis A, Trojanowski JQ, *et al.* Genetic evidence for the involvement of tau in progressive supranuclear palsy. *Ann Neurol*, 1997; **41**(2): 277–81.

120 Litvan I, Agid Y, Calne D, *et al.* Clinical research criteria for the diagnosis of progressive supranuclear palsy (Steel–Richardson–Olszewski syndrome): report of the NINDS-SPSP International Workshop. *Neurology*, 1996; **47**: 1–9.

121 Wenning GR, Ebersbach G, Verny M, *et al.* Progression of falls in postmortem-confirmed parkinsonian disorders. *Mov Disord*, 1999; **14**(6): 947–50.

122 Ghika J, Bogousslavsky J. Presymptomatic hypertension is a major feature in the diagnosis of progressive supranuclear palsy. *Arch Neurol*, 1997; **54**: 1104–8.

123 Litvan I, Phipps M, Pharr VL, *et al.* Randomized placebo-controlled trial of donepezil in patients with progressive supranuclear palsy. *Neurology*, 2001; **57**: 467–73.

124 Polo KB, Jabbari B. Botulinum toxin-A improves the rigidity of progressive supranuclear palsy. *Ann Neurol*, 1994; **35**(2): 237–9.

125 Wenning GK, Ben Shlomo Y, Magalhaes M, *et al.* Clinical feature and natural history of multiple system atrophy: an analysis of 100 cases. *Brain*, 1994; **117**: 835–45.

126 Litvan I, Goetz CG, Jankovic J, *et al.* What is the accuracy of clinical diagnosis of multiple system atrophy? A clinicopathologic study. *Arch Neurol*, 1997; **54**: 937–44.

127 Schrag A, Kingsley D, Phatouros C, *et al.* Clinical usefulness of magnetic resonance imaging in multiple system atrophy. *J Neurol Neurosurg Psychiatry*, 1998; **65**: 65–71.

128 Wenning GK, Litvan I, Jankovic J, *et al.* Natural history and survival of 14 patients with corticobasal degeneration confirmed at postmortem examination. *J Neurol Neurosurg Psychiatry*, 1998; **64**: 184–9.

129 Boeve BF, Lang AE, Litvan I. Corticobasal degeneration and its relationship to progressive supranuclear palsy and frontotemporal dementia. *Ann Neurol*, 2003; **54**(Suppl. 5): S15–19.

130 Schneider JA, Watts RL, Gearing M, *et al.* Corticobasal degeneration: neuropathologic and clinical heterogeneity. *Neurology*, 1997; **48**: 959–69.

131 Morgante L, Rocca WA, Di Rossa AE, *et al.* Prevalence of Parkinson's disease and other types of parkinsonism: a door-to-door survey in three Sicilian municipalities. *Neurology*, 1992; **42**: 1901–7.

132 Jeste D, Lacro JP, Bailey A, *et al.* Lower incidence of tardive dyskinesia with risperidone compared with haloperidol in older patients. *J Am Geriatr Soc*, 1999; **47**: 716–19.

133 Jeste DV, Okamoto A, Napolitano J, *et al.* Low incidence of persistent tardive dyskinesia in elderly patients with dementia treated with risperidone. *Am J Psychiatry*, 2000; **157**: 1150–5.

134 Lee PE, Sykora K, Gill SS, *et al.* Antipsychotic medications and drug-induced movement disorders other than parkinsonism: a population-based cohort study in older adults. *J Am Geriatr Soc*, 2005; **53**(8): 1374–9.

135 Rosenberg MR, Green M. Neuroleptic malignant syndrome: review of response to therapy. *Arch Intern Med*, 1989; **149**: 1927–31.

136 Ebadi M, Srinivasan SK. Pathogenesis, prevention, and treatment of neuroleptic-induced movement disorders. *Pharmacological Rev*, 1995; **47**(4): 575–99.

137 Suh H, Bronson B, Martin R. Neuroleptic malignant syndrome and low-dose olanzapine. *Am J Psychiatry*, 2003; **160**(4): 796.

138 Goveas JS, Hermida A. Olanzapine induced 'typical' neuroleptic malignant syndrome. *J Clin Psychopharmacology*, 2003; **23**(1): 101–2.

139 Hasan S, Buckley P. Novel antipsychotics and the neuroleptic malignant syndrome: a review and critique. *Am J Psychiatry*, 1998; **155**(8): 1113–16.

140 Ueda M, Hamamoto M, Nagayama H, *et al.* Susceptibility to neuroleptic malignant syndrome in Parkinson's disease. *Neurology*, 1999; **52**: 777–81.

141 Ohkoshi N, Satoh D, Nishi M, *et al.* Neuroleptic malignant-like syndrome due to donepezil and maprotiline. *Neurology*, 2003; **60**(6): 1050–1.

142 Chandran GJ, Mikler JR, Keegan DL. Neuroleptic malignant syndrome: case report and discussion. *CMAJ*, 2003; **169**(5): 439–42.

143 Rosebush PI, Stewart T, Mazurek MF. The treatment of neuroleptic malignant syndrome: are dantrolene and bromocriptine useful adjuncts to supportive care? *Br J Psychiatry*, 1991; **159**: 709–12.

144 Velamoor VR. Neuroleptic malignant syndrome: recognition, prevention and management. *Drug Safety*, 1998; **19**(1): 73–82.

145 Thanvi B, Lo N, Robinson T. Vascular parkinsonism – an important cause of parkinsonism in older people. *Age Ageing*, 2005; **34**(2): 114–19.

146 Duinkerke A, Williams MA, Rigamonti D, *et al.* Cognitive recovery in idiopathic normal pressure hydrocephalus after shunt. *Cognitive Behav Neurol*, 2004; **17**(3): 179–4.

147 Marmarou A, Young HF, Aygok GA, *et al.* Diagnosis and management of idiopathic normal-pressure hydrocephalus: a prospective study in 151 patients. *J Neurosurg*, 2005; **102**: 987–97.

148 Esmonde T, Cooke S. Shunting for normal pressure hydrocephalus (NPH). *Cochrane Database Syst Rev* 2002, Issue 3. Art. No.: CD003157. DOI: 10.1002/14651858.CD003157.

149 Hebb AO, Cusimano MD. Idiopathic normal pressure hydrocephalus: a systematic review of diagnosis and outcome. *Neurosurgery*, 2001; **49**(5): 1166–86.

150 Iddon JL, Pickard JD, Cross JJL, *et al.* Specific patterns of cognitive impairment in patients with idiopathic normal pressure hydrocephalus and Alzheimer's disease: a pilot study. *J Neurol Neurosurg Psychiatry*, 1999; **67**: 723–32.

151 Elble RJ. Diagnostic criteria for essential tremor and differential diagnosis. *Neurology*, 2000; **54**(Suppl. 4): S2–6.

152 Koller WC, Hristova A, Brin M. Pharmacologic treatment of essential tremor. *Neurology*, 2000; **54**(Suppl. 4): S30–8.

153 Ondo W, Hunter C, Vuong KD, *et al.* Gabapentin for essential tremor: a multiple-dose, double-blind, placebo-controlled trial. *Movt Disord*, 2000; **15**(4): 678–82.

154 Connor GS. A double-blind placebo-controlled trial of topiramate treatment for essential tremor. *Neurology*, 2002; **59**: 132–4.

155 Brin MF, Lyons KE, Doucette J, *et al.* A randomized, double masked, controlled trial of botulinum toxin type A in essential hand tremor. *Neurology*, 2001; **56**: 1523–8.

156 Limousin P, Speelman JD, Gielen F, *et al.* Multicentre European study of thalamic stimulation in parkinsonism and essential tremor. *J Neurol Neurosurg Psychiatry*, 1999; **66**: 289–96.

157 Pahwa R, Lyons KL, Wilkinson SB, *et al.* Bilateral thalamic stimulation for the treatment of essential tremor. *Neurology*, 1999; **53**: 1447–50.

158 Hening W, Allen RP, Tenzer P, *et al.* Restless legs syndrome: demographics, presentation and differential diagnosis. *Geriatrics*, 2007; **62**(9): 26–9.

159 Winkelman JW, Allen RP, Tenzer P, *et al.* Restless legs syndrome: nonpharmacologic and pharmacologic treatments. *Geriatrics*, 2007; **62**(10): 13–16.

CHAPTER 10

Stroke

DEFINITIONS

➤ *Stroke*: a sudden onset of a focal neurological deficit or reduced consciousness that is most likely caused by vascular aetiology and of duration greater than 24 hours (or resulting in death). However, conventionally, subarachnoid haemorrhage is also considered a form of stroke (usually presenting with a sudden onset of headache and meningism).

➤ *Transient ischaemic attack* (TIA): a sudden onset of a focal neurological deficit or monocular dysfunction that is most likely due to a vascular aetiology and of symptom duration less than 24 hours.

EPIDEMIOLOGY

Stroke is the most common acute vascular disorder, accounting for 45% of such events.[1] Its overall incidence is around 200–250 per 100 000 per year.[2] This figure for stroke, but not subarachnoid haemorrhage, increases with age. Eighty per cent of events occur in those over the age of 65 and 54% in those over the age of 75.[1] Currently the mean age of people having a cerebrovascular event in the UK is around 74 years.[1] It is the second commonest cause of death worldwide (after heart disease).[3]

SUBTYPES OF STROKE

Strokes are divided into those caused by a blocked blood vessel and those caused by a bleed (haemorrhagic). The former of these is conventionally termed 'ischaemic', although this is a little imprecise as both types of stroke involve the death of brain cells due to hypoxia. Conventionally, subarachnoid haemorrhage (SAH) is also classified as a form of stroke. Approximately 85% of strokes are ischaemic and 15% are haemorrhagic (10% primary intracerebral haemorrhage and 5% SAH).[4]

Overall, the 30-day mortality rate for stroke has been found to be 19%. However, this varies according to stroke subtype, with better outcomes for those sustaining an ischaemic event (10%) than those with a haemorrhagic one (50%).[4] Prognosis is discussed further within the relevant sections for different stroke subtypes.

ASSESSMENT

The diagnosis of stroke is not always easy, especially to the non-specialist. One study has found that 20% of patients initially classified as having had a stroke by emergency physicians were subsequently shown to have an alternative pathology (e.g. post-ictal states, cerebral tumours, and toxic/metabolic disorders).[5] Common differential diagnoses are discussed on p. 227. The clinical findings, rather than the results of imaging studies, are the key to achieving a successful diagnosis.

History

Onset

The history of a sudden onset of symptoms is crucial to the diagnosis of stroke. This is even more relevant with TIA, where neurological signs will usually have resolved prior to medical assessment. Activities at the time of symptom commencement may give clues to alternative explanations (e.g. postural change causing neurocardiovascular symptoms) (*see* p. 341). The deficits of a stroke are usually maximal at the time of onset and will, characteristically, gradually improve after the event (albeit often over days to weeks), whereas with alternative diagnoses (e.g. tumours) deficits will tend to increase. Occasionally the symptoms of stroke will worsen over the first few days following onset (e.g. if cerebral oedema or haemorrhagic transformation develop). Symptoms of stroke are typically 'negative' – i.e. some function is lost (e.g. weakness or loss of sensation). 'Positive' symptoms (e.g. jerking movements or tingling sensations) suggest an alternative pathology.

The presence of headache is not a good discriminator between ischaemia and haemorrhage, and commonly accompanies both. Severe headache at the onset could indicate SAH, giant cell arteritis (*see* p. 436) or arterial dissection. Vomiting around the time of symptom onset is suggestive of a haemorrhagic aetiology.

Deficit

It is important to clarify the specific symptoms – patients may use vague terms such as 'my arm was dead' to mean either motor or sensory loss (or a combination). When available, a witness history is valuable. This is especially so if unconsciousness is reported or seizures are suspected. Non-medical people's accounts of events may mistake dysphasia for confusion. Patients with significant neglect may be unaware of the degree of their deficit. Associated factors should be directly asked about. These include weakness or sensory disturbance in the face, arm and leg of each side of the body, changes in speech or vision, and the presence of headache. The greater eloquence of left-sided brain tissue in most individuals leads to a greater recognition of strokes on this side compared to those on the right.[6]

Risk factors

Vascular risk factors (e.g. smoking, hypertension, diabetes, other vascular disorders and atrial fibrillation) should be sought. A history of previous strokes is clearly important. The body parts or functions affected by any such prior events should be noted along with any residual deficits. Old impairments may be made more prominent under certain conditions – including during acute medical illnesses. This should be suspected when a very similar deficit to a previous stroke is provoked. A strong family history of stroke at a young age raises the possibility of an inherited vascular disorder (*see* p. 227).

Social

An accurate social history will help to predict difficulties at the time of discharge (e.g. whether the patient lives alone and if there are stairs within the property).

Examination

Clearly, a detailed neurological examination is crucial to assessment in those who have had a stroke. A thorough review of this is beyond the scope of this book but some of the aspects that are particularly relevant to stroke are discussed.

Motor deficit

A downward drift of an outstretched arm while the eyes are closed is suggestive of a subtle motor impairment, but this may also occur with proprioceptive sensory loss. Asking the patient to touch the tip of their nose with each finger in turn while the eyes remain closed can crudely assess this later problem. An evaluation of the functional impact of impairments is more informative than a numerical value (e.g. the MRC scale 0–5). Despite their (predominant) upper motor neuron aetiology, strokes often cause early flaccidity with later development of spasticity. Marked hypertonia at the onset may be due to a stroke affecting the basal ganglia.

Sensory deficit

Sensory inattention is a sign of a parietal lobe lesion. It is tested for by asking the patient to close their eyes with their hands placed in front of them. The patient is told to inform the examiner which hand if they feel one being touched. The hands are then touched individually, followed by both together. A patient with intact sensation but sensory inattention will correctly report the individual hands being touched but will only report the hand of the unaffected side when both are touched together.

Speech

A speech disorder may be identified while taking the patient's history. When testing for speech problems it is important to ensure that the patient has the best chance of responding appropriately, for example their hearing aid is fitted and working. Asking the patient to obey commands tests comprehension of speech (i.e. identify receptive dysphasia). These should initially be one-stage commands (e.g. 'close your eyes'), but then can be more complex sequences (e.g. 'point to the door, the window and then the ceiling'). Expressive dysphasia can be detected by asking the patient to name objects (e.g. pen and watch, then the smaller components of each, such as the nib, hands, etc.). Subtle dysarthria may be detected by asking the patient to repeat difficult phrases, for example 'West Register Street', 'baby hippopotamus' and 'biblical criticism'. Agnosia is a high-level sensory disturbance that leads to a failure to recognise objects despite intact sensory systems. Patients with dysphasia can usually mime how an object is used (e.g. a pen) even if they cannot name it, whereas those with agnosia cannot. Language disorders and the language areas of the brain are discussed on p. 85.

Swallowing

The assessment of swallowing is important in all patients who have sustained a stroke. It is discussed on p. 40.

Visual fields

Some patients may be unaware of a homonymous hemianopia. Formal confrontation technique is not always possible; for example, in patients with reduced conscious levels or those with receptive dysphasia. An absence of a blink response to a threatening stimulus from the side (e.g. the examiner's finger brought rapidly towards the patient's eye) may detect a homonymous hemianopia. Visual inattention is similar to sensory inattention. While standing in front of the patient with his or her arms outstretched, the examiner asks the patient to look directly at their nose and say if a hand is seen to move. The fingers of each outstretched hand are then wiggled in turn, followed by both hands together. The patient with visual inattention will correctly identify the individual movements but when both are moved together they will only report movement in the unaffected field.

Neglect

Neglect can occur in various forms. It can be neglect of own person (e.g. failing to use one side of the body) or of the environment (e.g. not appreciating obstacles on one side). It may be caused by lesions in the parietal lobe on either side of the brain, but is often more severe when it affects the non-dominant hemisphere. Functional impairment may be out of proportion with motor and sensory loss. A variety of techniques have been developed to aid its detection. These include clock-drawing (*see* p. 90) and the star cancellation test.[7]

Gait

When a patient is capable of standing safely, gait should be examined. This may reveal subtle deficits in coordination or motor function not obvious when the patient is lying down.

Level of consciousness

In patients with a reduced conscious level, the Glasgow Coma Scale (GCS) score should be recorded (performed on the unaffected side of the body). Early unconsciousness suggests SAH or a brainstem haemorrhage. A very large cortical infarct may cause a reduced conscious level that worsens over the following few days due to the development of oedema.

Vascular system

The examination of the vascular system is also relevant. Of particular note are the detection of atrial fibrillation (AF) (*see* Chapter 19) and hypertension (*see* Chapter 18). Auscultation over the carotid arteries for the detection of carotid bruits is an unreliable way to detect carotid stenosis.[8] It should not be used in the place of a carotid doppler and therefore has little value in the physical examination of a patient who has suffered a stroke or TIA.

Investigations

Blood tests

Basic blood tests should include a glucose level (to identify diabetes and exclude hypoglycaemia as a cause of symptoms), erythrocyte sedimentation rate (ESR) (to exclude vasculitis), and if the patient is on warfarin or in AF (when anticoagulation is likely to be considered in the near future) an international normalised ratio (INR). A high cholesterol level may identify a vascular risk factor, but in light of the Heart Protection Study (*see* p. 210) patients even with normal levels should be considered for statin therapy.

In younger patients with no clear vascular risk factors, especially those with personal or family histories of thrombosis, a thrombophilia screen (e.g. factor V Leiden, anti-thrombin III, proteins C and S, and antiphospholipid antibodies) may be considered. It is controversial whether thrombophilias that increase the risk of venous thrombosis also increase the risk of arterial stroke. However, even if antiphospholipid syndrome is diagnosed, the current recommended treatment is the same as for those without this diagnosis.[9] Therefore the usefulness of these investigations is questionable.[10]

ECG

An electrocardiogram (ECG) should be performed to accurately identify the cardiac rhythm.

Brain imaging

Clinical criteria alone do not reliably distinguish between ischaemic and haemorrhagic strokes;[11] this is the primary aim of imaging the brain of patients who have sustained an acute stroke. On occasions it will have the additional benefit of detecting an alternative explanation for symptoms – such as a structural lesion. Guidelines recommend that this should be within one hour if thrombolysis is being considered, and always within 12 hours.[9] Some clinical situations make more rapid brain imaging preferable. These are outlined below:

➤ consideration of thrombolysis
➤ current anticoagulant use or known bleeding disorder
➤ reduced level of consciousness (GCS less than 13)
➤ progressive or fluctuating symptoms
➤ severe headache, neck stiffness, papilloedema, or fever
➤ papilloedema, neck stiffness or fever
➤ symptom onset coincides with head trauma.

Computerised tomography (CT) scanning is widely available, quick to perform, and easy for patients to tolerate. However, it often does not show abnormalities immediately following an ischaemic stroke, especially with small infarcts and within the first six hours.[12] Changes may be subtle – such as loss of grey-white matter differentiation, obscuration of the lentiform nucleus, sulcal effacement and loss of insular ribbon.[13] Several days later, hypodense (dark grey or black) areas will develop with breakdown of the dead cells. However, around 50% of infarcts will never become visible on CT scans.[14] They are of most use in detecting bleeding straight after an event as blood appears hyperdense (white) and remains so for approximately 10 days (depending on the size of the bleed). After this time the blood is gradually broken down to intermediary products, which are isodense (grey like brain tissue) and then become hypodense. At this stage CT scanning cannot distinguish whether a haemorrhagic or ischaemic event has occurred.[15] Therefore, CT scans are best performed within one week of an event.

In general terms magnetic resonance imaging (MRI) scans give better definition than CT scans and so acute infarcts are more likely to be detected. In one series MRI scanning detected acute ischaemic changes in 46% of patients compared to just 10% detected by CT.[16] This is particularly true for lesions within the posterior fossa (i.e. brainstem and cerebellum). However, acute haemorrhage is typically less distinct on MRI scans, but it can be made more apparent with the 'gradient echo' technique. A study did not demonstrate any significant difference between CT and gradient echo MRI for detecting acute haemorrhage, and MRI scanning appeared superior in detecting early haemorrhagic transformation of infarcts.[17] MRI is also capable of detecting the breakdown products of blood (haemosiderin), which allows the distinction of haemorrhagic and ischaemic strokes well beyond one week after the event (up to several months). Another possibility is 'diffusion-weighted' MRI, with which acute infarcts appear hyperdense (white) and are therefore more easily detected.[12] The efficacy of this has been demonstrated in a randomised trial setting,[18] although alternative pathologies may have a similar appearance (e.g. demyelination plaques). Lesions are usually seen within minutes of infarction, although a small proportion will never be detected by this method.[14] Approximately 20% of patients are unable to undergo MRI scanning due to either being unable to tolerate the noisy and claustrophobic procedure, or due to metallic implants (e.g. cerebral aneurysm clips or cardiac pacemakers).[12]

At the present time CT scanning all patients with acute stroke to enable early detection of haemorrhage (and exclusion of some other pathology) seems the best option. MRI scanning is reserved for difficult cases where identifying an ischaemic lesion would be clinically helpful or those presenting beyond 10 days to exclude a haemorrhagic event.

Trans-oesophageal echocardiography

Trans-oesophageal echocardiography (TOE) has been reported to detect potential sources of embolism in around 40% of patients with cryptogenic stroke (strokes where there are no apparent causes).[19] However, many of these cases will be due to patent foramen ovale, which has an unclear role in the pathogenesis of stroke (*see* p. 224), or the finding of aortic thrombus (the optimal management of which is unknown). As such it is unlikely to affect the management of many patients. There is a 0.2% risk of serious complications with this procedure (including hypoxia, gastrointestinal bleeding and arrhythmias).[20] It is not a suitable routine test but may have a role in selected patients. Examples would include patients with suspected bacterial endocarditis or atrial myxoma (both of which are rare).

SUBTYPES OF STROKE

The Bamford classification is a clinical method of distinguishing strokes into four subtypes derived from the Oxfordshire Community Stroke Project.[21] The subtype of stroke sustained has prognostic significance (*see* p. 213).

Lacunar stroke syndromes

Lacunar stroke syndromes (LACS) are usually caused by intrinsic thrombus within small penetrating cerebral blood vessels. The major risk factor for their development is hypertension. They are not associated with any cortical signs (e.g. dysphasia, inattention or hemianopia). The lenticulostriate arteries arise from the middle cerebral artery (MCA) and supply blood to the internal capsule. As the motor fibres are tightly packed together in this region, such a lesion will cause a deficit affecting a large body area (*see* Figure 10.1). This will either be the face and arm, arm and leg, or face, arm and leg. A more limited deficit is likely to have arisen from a cortical lesion (i.e. not LACS).

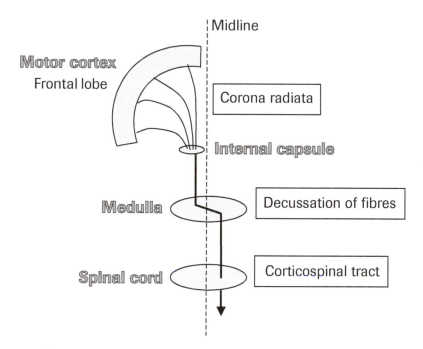

FIGURE 10.1 The motor pathways.

Lacunar events may also disturb the posterior circulation affecting the pons (causing an ataxic hemiparesis by affecting both motor and cerebellar fibres) or thalamus (where they may cause a pure sensory stroke) (*see* Figure 10.2). Mixed sensorimotor impairments have also been described. Many of these events are clinically silent.

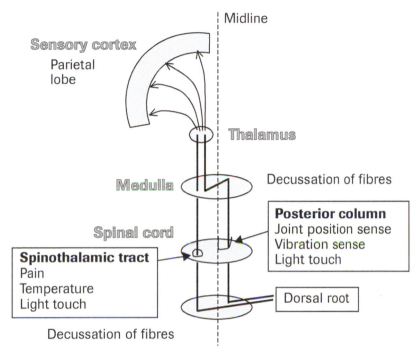

FIGURE 10.2 The sensory pathways.

The accumulation of multiple events can cause a subcortical dementia, small-stepping gait ('marche à petits pas') and/or pseudobulbar palsy. The small size of the lesions makes it common for them to not be seen on CT scanning.

Posterior circulation syndromes

Posterior circulation syndromes (POCS) involve lesions relating the vertebrobasilar system or posterior cerebral arteries. The clinical features of these are discussed on p. 198.

Anterior circulation syndromes

Anterior circulation syndromes are subdivided into partial (PACS) and total (TACS) depending on the extent of the infarct. They are more likely than a lacunar stroke to be due to either a cardiac or large vessel embolus, or haemorrhage.

A TACS involves the combination of hemiplegia, hemianopia and at least one higher cognitive disturbance (e.g. dysphasia or inattention). A TACS is more likely than a PACS when there is an associated reduction in conscious level (indicating an extensive area of infarction).

A PACS causes a lesser combination of the features of a TACS or can cause a localised motor or sensory deficit (due to affecting a small area of either the motor or sensory cortex).

Infarcts

After a CT scan has been performed, if haemorrhage has been excluded, the names of the Bamford subtypes are changed – the 'S' for syndrome is replaced by an 'I' for infarct, for example LACI, POCI, TACI and PACI.

LOCALISATION OF THE EVENT

Cerebral vascular supply

The basic anatomy of the circle of Willis is shown in Figure 10.3. The approximate cortical regions supplied by the major vessels are shown in Figure 10.4. The main functions of the cortical regions are shown in Figure 10.5.

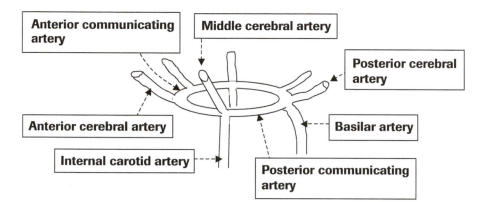

FIGURE 10.3 A three-dimensional representation of the circle of Willis.

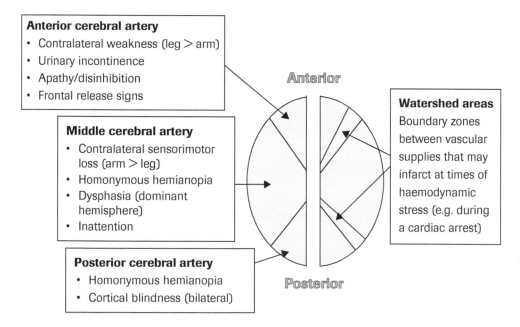

FIGURE 10.4 The approximate cortical areas supplied by the major blood vessels.

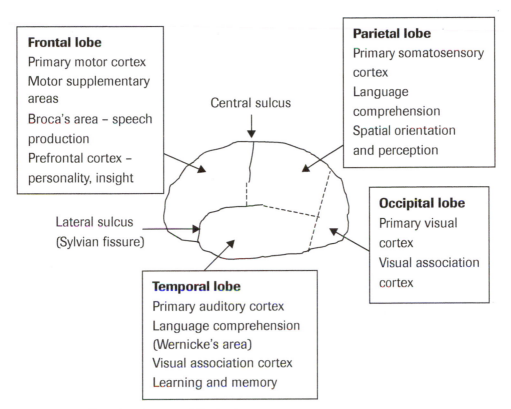

Frontal lobe
Primary motor cortex
Motor supplementary
areas
Broca's area – speech
production
Prefrontal cortex –
personality, insight

Central sulcus

Parietal lobe
Primary somatosensory
cortex
Language
comprehension
Spatial orientation
and perception

Lateral sulcus
(Sylvian fissure)

Occipital lobe
Primary visual
cortex
Visual association
cortex

Temporal lobe
Primary auditory cortex
Language comprehension
(Wernicke's area)
Visual association cortex
Learning and memory

FIGURE 10.5 Functional areas of the brain.

Anterior circulation strokes

Anterior cerebral artery

The anterior cerebral artery (ACA) supplies a large portion of the frontal lobes. Infarction here may cause either apathy or disinhibition. There may also be emotional lability and urinary incontinence (due to loss of inhibitory reflexes and involvement of the nervous supply of the bladder). Examination may show frontal release signs (e.g. the grasp reflex (*see* p. 92)). The medial aspect of the motor cortex is affected, leading to a more marked motor deficit in the leg than that seen in the arm.

Middle cerebral artery

The middle cerebral artery (MCA) supplies the majority of the parietal and temporal lobes. Any motor deficit is usually more severe in the arm than in the leg. Due to the large representation of the hand in the motor cortex, it is possible to have a localised infarct that affects solely hand function. There will usually be associated cortical deficits, such as sensory inattention and dysphasia. Visual function may be affected with either a homonymous hemianopia or an upper or lower quadrantanopia (due to involvement of all or part of the optic radiation).

Posterior circulation strokes

The main components of the posterior circulation are shown in Figure 10.6. Around 24% of ischaemic strokes affect the posterior circulation.[21]

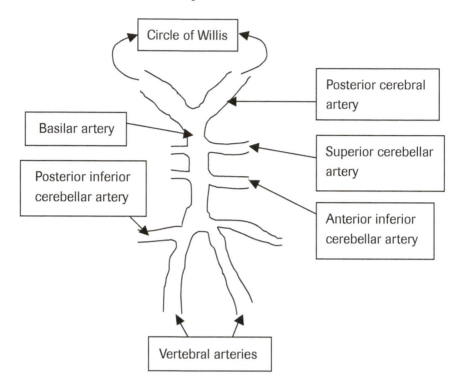

FIGURE 10.6 Simplified diagram of the posterior circulation of the brain.

Posterior cerebral artery

Lesions of the posterior cerebral artery (PCA) usually cause visual disturbances. This may be an isolated homonymous hemianopia (with macular sparing due to collateral supply from the MCA). Bilateral infarcts may lead to cortical blindness. This may be associated with confabulation of vision (Anton syndrome). Strokes within the visual association areas can provoke visual hallucinations. Visuospatial function is more likely to be affected with non-dominant hemisphere lesions.

Vertebrobasilar system

Cerebrovascular lesions of the vertebrobasilar system commonly present with light-headedness or vertigo (*see* Chapter 13), double or lost vision, ataxia, and/or loss of power/sensation affecting one or both sides of the body.[22] However, the compact nature of structures in the region makes the occurrence of one symptom in isolation very unlikely. Signs of cerebellar involvement are listed in Table 10.1.

TABLE 10.1 Signs of cerebellar involvement

Vermis*	Hemispheres (ipsilateral signs)
Truncal ataxia	Nystagmus (fast phase towards affected side; *see* p. 319)
	Dysarthria ('staccato speech')
	Past-pointing
	Intention tremor
	Dysdiadochokinesia
	Rebound phenomena (arms outstretched and eyes closed)
	Pendular reflexes
	Gait: ataxic, broad-based

*The vermis is the central part of the cerebellum; the two hemispheres lie laterally to it.

Brainstem lesions may also cause a disturbance of conjugate eye movements, Horner syndrome, or, rarely, a unilateral internuclear ophthalmoplegia. 'Top-of-the-basilar syndrome' is a term for patients with reduced conscious level, memory disturbance, small pupils and vertical gaze palsy secondary to infarction of the midbrain and thalamus.[22] Basilar artery occlusion may cause bilateral limb signs or even the 'locked in' syndrome (the inability to move any part of the body except the eyes and eyelids in association with retained consciousness) due to bilateral pontine infarction. A diagram representing the anatomical levels of some structures within the brainstem to help localise a lesion is shown in Figure 10.7.

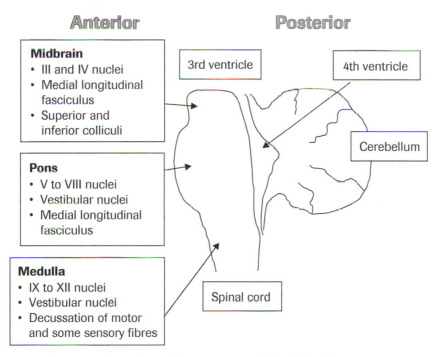

FIGURE 10.7 Anatomical location of key structures within the brainstem.

Various eponymous syndromes have been described relating to infarcts of the many small vessels supplying this region. They often result in ipsilateral cranial nerve palsies with contralateral limb signs (e.g. Weber syndrome – ipsilateral III nerve palsy plus contralateral limb weakness) – this is termed a 'crossed' syndrome. Lateral medullary (or Wallenberg) syndrome is a rare but well-described combination of signs secondary to posterior inferior cerebellar artery territory infarction. The full features are listed in Table 10.2, but variants with only some features are equally likely (compare with Figures 10.1, 10.2 and 10.6 for an anatomical explanation of the make-up of deficits).

TABLE 10.2 The constellation of signs seen with lateral medullary syndrome

Ipsilateral	Contralateral
↓ facial sensation	↓ pain and temperature sensation trunk and limbs
Lower cranial nerve palsies	
Horner syndrome (miosis, ptosis, reduced facial sweating)	
Cerebellar signs	

Thalamic infarction can cause a range of symptoms and signs. These include pure sensory strokes and some neuropsychological deficits. Amnesia can be caused by lesions affecting the limbic system (*see* Figure 6.7), but other neurological deficits would be expected to occur simultaneously. Lesions affecting the basal ganglia may induce movement disorders, such as hemiballismus or focal dystonia.

Bilateral vertebrobasilar atheromatous disease can lead to symptoms due to hypoperfusion of the brainstem provoked by stimuli that further reduce blood flow (*see* p. 322). These include increases in antihypertensive medication or rapid postural change.[23] Typically multiple brief, stereotyped episodes occur and common symptoms include light-headedness, dysarthria, ataxia, blurred vision and diplopia.

ISCHAEMIC STROKES AND TIAS

A blood vessel blockage may occur due to thrombus formation within the blood vessel itself or due to embolised thrombus from elsewhere. This is most commonly from clots formed on the walls of larger vessels (i.e. the carotid arteries or aorta) or within the left atrium of people in AF. Around half of ischaemic strokes are thought to be caused by emboli from large vessels, a quarter due to intracranial vessel disease, a fifth from cardiac emboli (but more common in the elderly due to a higher prevalence of AF – *see* Chapter 19) and a small proportion due to rare causes (*see* Figure 10.8).

Risk factors

Hypertension

The SHEP trial randomised 4736 people over the age of 60 (mean age 72 years) with isolated systolic hypertension (systolic blood pressure (BP) >160 mmHg, diastolic BP<90 mmHg) to receive active treatment (a thiazide (chlorthalidone) plus a beta-blocker (atenolol) if required) or placebo.[24] The systolic BP readings averaged

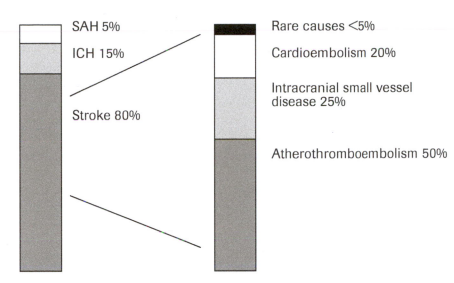

FIGURE 10.8 A breakdown of the causes of ischaemic stroke.

143 mmHg in the treatment arm and 155 mmHg in the placebo group. The five-year stroke incidence rates were 5.2 per 100 people with treatment and 8.2 per 100 with placebo – a relative risk reduction of 36%.

Atrial fibrillation

Between 6% and 20% of people who sustain a stroke are found to be in AF, and these people have around a 15% risk of recurrence within the following year.[25] These patients have a worse prognosis than those in sinus rhythm, probably due to a greater tendency for large, cortical strokes to occur. People in AF who have not previously sustained a stroke have on average a 4.5% risk of thromboembolism per year.[26] But individual risk is highly variable depending on comorbidities (*see* p. 406).

Others

Smoking, diabetes and a history of vascular disease (including stroke) confer an increased risk of stroke. A positive family history is very occasionally relevant as there are some rare familial causes of stroke (*see* p. 227). Obstructive sleep apnoea (OSA) has been found to carry around a doubling of the risk of stroke after correction for other variables.[27] Low physical activity, high alcohol intake, and a diet low in fruit and vegetables may also increase the risk of stroke.[28]

Transient ischaemic attacks

TIAs are defined by their symptom duration of less than 24 hours. However, 24 hours is an arbitrary figure and most TIAs are of duration less than three hours. They are almost always assumed to be caused by vessel blockages, as the symptoms from a haemorrhagic lesion are extremely unlikely to fully resolve within this time period. Symptoms lasting only seconds at a location other than the eye are unlikely to be due to a TIA. It was thought that TIAs represent a period of focal brain ischaemia rather than infarction (analogous to angina compared to a myocardial infarction). However, CT imaging of the brain has been shown to reveal an area of cerebral infarction in 13% of TIA patients,[29] and a much higher proportion when MRI scanning is used.[30] The probability of an infarct being detected on scanning appears to increase linearly with duration of symptoms, being found in 35% of those with symptoms lasting days to weeks, and 49% of those with persistent symptoms following a minor stroke. TIAs share the same risk factors and secondary prevention strategies with ischaemic stroke. The risk of future stroke is similar in people who have had a TIA to those who have sustained a minor stroke (*see* p. 213).

Migraine attacks and syncopal episodes are common causes of TIA misdiagnosis. Non-focal neurological symptoms (e.g. dizziness, confusion or loss of consciousness) occurring in isolation are not due to TIAs. The most frequent symptoms are unilateral weakness or sensory loss, dysarthria, dysphasia and transient visual problems.

Visual disturbances seen with TIAs include monocular vision loss, homonymous hemianopia and diplopia. Patients are often unable to distinguish between the loss of vision in one eye and the loss of one visual field (homonymous hemianopia). They may have tried covering each eye during the episode, which would provide more information, and so this should be asked about.

Transient monocular blindness (also known as 'amaurosis fugax') is a term for the sudden onset of visual loss in one eye. This may feel like a dark curtain coming across the visual field. There is no associated eye pain. Ophthalmoscopy should always be performed to detect abnormalities such as cholesterol emboli (yellow blobs within the retinal arterioles), haemorrhages, optic nerve pallor and papilloedema. In this way a primary ocular disorder that mimics a TIA may be detected. Eye pain, redness and pupillary changes suggest an alternative cause to the visual symptoms. ESR should be measured to exclude a vasculitic process.

Brain imaging is not always necessary in cases of TIA as a haemorrhagic event would not lead to rapid symptom resolution. Imaging should be performed when the diagnosis or vascular territory are uncertain.[9] In these situations a diffusion-weighted MRI scan is the investigation of choice. Following a high risk TIA (ABCD2 score 4 or above (*see* p. 213), atrial fibrillation or multiple events within a week) specialist investigation and treatment should occur within 24 hours, otherwise guidance is to complete these within one week.[9]

ACUTE TREATMENT OF ISCHAEMIC STROKE
Thrombolysis

Intravenous (IV) recombinant tissue plasminogen activator (rt-PA) has been found to be of benefit in some people following acute stroke. It works by converting plasminogen to plasmin, which breaks down the fibrin polymers that form clots – *see* Figure 10.9. Other thrombolytic agents have not been found to be similarly effective.

In one trial, 624 patients were randomised to either rt-PA or placebo within three hours of an acute ischaemic stroke (haemorrhage excluded by CT scanning).[31] A three-month assessment revealed a higher proportion of patients had a favourable outcome

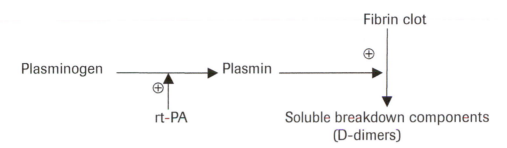

FIGURE 10.9 The mechanism of action of recombinant tissue plasminogen activator (rt-PA).

(absence of death or severe disability) in the rt-PA group than placebo (odds ratio (OR) 1.7; 95% CI 1.2–2.6, p=0.008). There were no significant differences in mortality between the groups. Symptomatic intracranial haemorrhage (SICH) occurred in 20 patients (6.0%) with rt-PA compared to two (0.6%) with placebo.

A report of open-label cases thrombolysed within Canada has demonstrated similar outcomes to the above randomised controlled trial.[32] Over 2.5 years a total of 1135 patients (59% over the age of 70) had been treated, and 37% of these had a favourable outcome. There was a lower rate (4.6%) of SICH but 75% of these patients died while in hospital. Orolingual angio-oedema was seen in 1.3% of patients. The study suggests that the results of the randomised controlled trial may be realistically recreated in standard practice. However, the proportion of stroke patients treated with rt-PA in all of Canada over this period was <2%. A similar analysis from European centres gathered data from 6483 patients (mean age 68 years).[33] They found a lower rate of SICH of 1.7% within 24 hours. Mortality was 11.3% at three months.

A Cochrane systematic review of the available trials demonstrated a large degree of heterogeneity in outcomes, partly due to differing protocols used.[34] Overall, thrombolysis with rt-PA was associated with a significant reduction in the combined end-point of death or dependency (OR 0.80; 95% CI 0.69–0.93), and a non-significant increase in deaths from all causes (OR 1.17; 95% CI 0.95–1.45). The use of thrombolysis significantly increased the risk of fatal intracranial haemorrhage (OR 3.60; 95% CI 2.28–5.68). Some signs seen on CT scanning may be able to detect those patients who are more likely to have haemorrhagic adverse events. There is evidence that it is more likely to occur when there is a marked early appearance of brain oedema, mass effect or a large area of hypodensity.[35]

The ECASS III trial randomised 821 patients (mean age 65 years) and found that thrombolysis appears to effective and safe between 3 and 4.5 hours from stroke onset.[36] A favourable outcome (not dead or severely disabled (modified Rankin score <2 (mRS – *see* Appendix A)) was found in 52.4% of the treatment group compared to 45.2% of the controls (OR 1.34, 95% CI 1.02–1.76).

Initial thrombolysis protocols used an age cut-off limit of 80 years. However, data suggest that thrombolysis is still beneficial in selected older patients.[37–40] Many stroke physicians would consider patients aged over 80 who previously functioned well and who meet other criteria as suitable for thrombolysis. In a review of patients over the age of 90 years (n=22; median age 93, range 90–101) who had received thrombolysis, after 30 days 36% had severe disability and 45% were dead.[33]

Current typical criteria for thrombolysis include age less than 80 years (but this is not absolute), a persisting neurological deficit (i.e. not rapidly resolving), absence of recent surgery or bleeding problem (last three weeks), no recent prior stroke (last three months), the patient being reasonably independent prior to the event, and being responsive to noxious stimuli (i.e. not in a deep coma). High blood pressure (180/105 or above), seizures since symptom onset and a high blood sugar (>22 mmol) are all associated with higher risk of bleeding and so are contraindications to thrombolysis (*see* Table 10.3). Patients taking warfarin may safely be given thrombolysis if their INR is 1.7 or below.[41] Some clinicians consider a visible area of hypodensity in more than a third of the MCA territory also to be a contraindication to thrombolysis, but this is controversial.[14] The National Institutes of Health Stroke Scale (NHISS – *see* Appendix A) is used to rate stroke severity. Typically very severe strokes (scores of 25 or above) are considered inappropriate for thrombolysis due to higher risk of adverse outcome. Also mild strokes (scores <5) are often excluded on the basis that risks may exceed possible functional gains, although an exception might be made for isolated dysphasia (as it would have a large functional impact).

In summary, there is evidence that selected stroke patients benefit through reduced long-term disability following thrombolysis. The treatment can be effective up to 4.5 hours from stroke onset, but chances of benefit are highest when given as soon after the event as possible.[40]

TABLE 10.3 Indications and contraindications to receiving thrombolysis for acute ischaemic stroke

Indication	Contraindication
• Age <80 – but most recent evidence suggests this should not be a barrier • Persisting neurological deficit (i.e. not rapidly resolving)	• Surgery or bleeding problem in last three weeks • Prior stroke in last three months • Unresponsive to noxious stimuli • Functionally dependent (e.g. nursing home resident) • BP > 180/105 despite attempts to lower it (e.g. intravenous labetolol) • Seizure since symptom onset • Blood sugar > 22 mmol • On warfarin with INR >1.7

Physiological parameters

The outcomes of stroke appear to be worse in those with pyrexia at the time of admission and better in those with low body temperature.[42,43] Paracetamol can reduce body temperature but its efficacy in this situation has not been proven. Forty per cent of patients admitted following acute stroke are hyperglycaemic, yet the optimal management of hyperglycaemia after stroke is unknown.[44] Given the benefits following acute MI, there is logic in thinking glucose control may be beneficial, and hyperglycaemia has been associated with worse post-stroke outcomes.[44] However, the GIST-UK trial did not demonstrate a reduction in 90-day mortality rates through the use of insulin infusions to control blood glucose.[45] It makes sense to correct hypoxia when present. However, the routine use of high-flow oxygen in non-hypoxic acute stroke patients has not been shown to convey any advantage.[46] Dehydration at presentation appears to be associated with worse outcomes, but interventional studies showing a benefit of rigorous rehydration have not been performed.[47] Both very high and very low BP recordings at baseline have been associated with less favourable outcomes after stroke.[48]

The optimal management of BP immediately following stroke has been unclear. Approximately 60% of patients have been found to have a systolic BP >160 mmHg following an acute stroke.[49] However, the BP will normalise spontaneously over a seven-day period in most of these people.[50] If a patient is already on BP-lowering medications, it is common practice to continue them (providing the patient can swallow or they can be given nasogastrically). A recent trial randomised 4071 patients to either receive BP lowering medications (to achieve a target of <140/90 mmHg within seven days) or placebo following an acute stroke.[51] No significant difference was found between groups for either death or major disability at 14 days or three months. The Royal College of Physicians (RCP) stroke guidelines recommend that an elevated BP should only be acutely lowered (within the first two weeks or prior to hospital discharge) when hypertensive complications are likely, for example encephalopathy.[9] Another subgroup of patients has a low BP at presentation and whether steps to increase this parameter may be beneficial is unknown.

Other acute treatments

There have been a number of trials testing the use of agents that may limit brain damage following a stroke (i.e. 'neuroprotective'). In theory a reversible area of ischaemic 'penumbra' surrounds the core. It is postulated that drugs could interfere with the neurochemical cascade in this region that ultimately leads to cell death.[3] Unfortunately they have all, so far, been unsuccessful.

Intra-arterial thrombolysis has been tried in acute stroke. A trial that randomised patients (n=180, mean age 64 years) to this treatment plus heparin, or heparin alone, found a reduced rate of disability (mRS of two or less: 40% vs 25%), with similar rates of mortality.[52] The median time from stroke onset to initiation of treatment was 5.3 hours. SICH was more common in the treatment group (10% vs 2%). Over 12 000 patients were screened to randomise just 180. Therefore, this treatment is unlikely to be suitable for many patients, and its role may be limited to those presenting within 4.5 and 6 hours of stroke.

Clot retrieval (thrombectomy) devices are able to be inserted endovascularly into cerebral arteries and physically remove blood clots. The 'Mechanical Embolus Removal in Cerebral Ischaemia' (MERCI) trial had no control group (n=141, mean age 67 years).[53] They recruited patients between three and eight hours of a stroke, or less than three hours if ineligible for rt-PA treatment (27% of the patients). Adjuvant intra-arterial rt-PA was used when thought necessary. Vessel recanalisation was achieved in 48% of patients. Clinically significant complications occurred in 7%, and 30-day mortality was 37%. This latter figure is similar to 30-day mortality for untreated total anterior circulation infarct (TACI) stroke (*see* later). It may be that blood flow is simply being restored to already dead brain tissue. A more recent trial randomised 362 patients (mean age 67 years, median NIHSS score 13) within 4.5 hours of acute ischaemic stroke to receive either endovascular treatment (clot retrieval/disruption and/or intra-arterial thrombolysis) or intravenous rt-PA.[54] No significant differences were found in three-month survival without disability or intracranial haemorrhage rates.

Decompressive surgery has been used for patients with malignant middle cerebral artery syndrome. In this condition there is excessive oedema of a cerebral hemisphere due to extensive infarction in the MCA territory. It mainly affects younger adults (cerebral atrophy presumably protects the elderly). In an analysis of trial data, decompressive surgery was associated with significantly less disability (mRS of 3 or less: 43% vs 21%; 95% CI 5–41%) and greater chance of survival (78% vs 29%; 95% CI 33–67%) than conservative management.[55]

SECONDARY PREVENTION OF ISCHAEMIC STROKE

In general terms, the absolute benefits of secondary prevention are proportional to the baseline risk of recurrence in an individual. Advanced age increases the chance of recurrent events. Yet adults aged over 75 are less likely to be started on anti-platelets, anti-hypertensives and cholesterol-lowering drugs than younger people following stroke.[56] Maximising secondary prevention strategies in combination may lead to as much as an 80% relative risk reduction in recurrent vascular event rates.[57]

Antiplatelet agents

Aspirin

Aspirin is absorbed in the stomach and upper small intestine. It has a half-life of just 20 minutes in the blood but has a much longer duration of action due to its irreversible binding with platelet enzymes.[58] Therefore, its effects last for the lifetime of the platelet (around 10 days). The platelets are replaced at around 10% per day, and so a single dose of aspirin still impairs the action of around 50% of circulating platelets after five days.[58] At low doses its main effect is to inhibit the enzyme cyclo-oxygenase 1 (COX 1). This results in the inability of platelets to produce thromboxane, which promotes platelet aggregation and induces vasoconstriction.[58] After one week of therapy, doses as low as 30 mg per day result in near complete inhibition of platelet thromboxane production.[59]

Low doses have little effect on either BP control or renal function but do increase the risk of gastrointestinal haemorrhage.[59] The risk of haemorrhage while taking aspirin is approximately doubled, resulting in around one to two major bleeding complications per 1000 patient-years. This is dose-dependent and so the lowest effective dose of aspirin should be used (probably 75–100 mg daily); higher doses do not appear to offer any additional vascular protection advantages.[58] The evidence for benefit below 75 mg per day is less clear.[60] There is also an increased risk of haemorrhagic stroke. A meta-analysis of aspirin trials involving over 50 000 patients found that the use of aspirin for three years resulted in 12 more haemorrhagic strokes per 10 000 population than placebo.[61]

In acute settings, where rapid and complete inhibition of platelets is required, a single higher loading dose of aspirin should be used (150–300 mg).[60] Gastric-coated formulations are associated with a reduced risk of gastrointestinal haemorrhage. However, this comes at the cost of a much-reduced bioavailability of the drug.[58] Occasionally, people may have a hypersensitivity reaction to aspirin.

The use of aspirin is associated with around a 25% RRR in the risk of serious vascular events (including a 33% RRR in non-fatal MI, 25% RRR in non-fatal stroke and a 17% RRR in vascular death).[60] The absolute size of the benefit is proportional to the baseline risk within an individual. Primary prevention in those at low baseline risk is unlikely to be effective.

There is evidence that early commencement of aspirin has a beneficial effect. When started within 48 hours of an acute stroke, at a dose of 160 mg per day, it is associated with a 14% RRR in four-week mortality compared to placebo (absolute risk 3.3% vs 3.9%).[62] Another study has confirmed this finding with a 300 mg daily dose of aspirin.[63] Here, recurrent stroke within 14 days was seen in 2.8% of those on aspirin compared to 3.9% in the placebo arm, without a significant increase in bleeding risk. So, in the immediate post-stroke period an aspirin dose of 160–300 mg is of proven value. Current UK guidelines recommend a dose of 300 mg for the first two weeks following a stroke unless aspirin intolerant.[9] In people unable to swallow it can be given rectally (300 mg PR daily) or in solution via a nasogastric (NG) tube.

See p. 411 for the use of aspirin in AF.

Dipyridamole

Dipyridamole acts by blocking the breakdown of cyclic adenosine monophosphate (AMP), which prevents the activation of second messengers in the pathway that leads to platelet aggregation. Clinically, the most significant side-effect is headache, which leads to a number of patients discontinuing therapy.

A large randomised controlled trial (ESPS2) demonstrated a benefit of a modified release formulation of dipyridamole in combination with aspirin for the prevention of stroke.[64] Here 6602 patients who had had a recent stroke or TIA (within three months) were randomised to aspirin 25 mg bd, dipyridamole modified-release (MR) 200 mg bd, both, or placebo, and were followed up for a two-year period. The primary outcome of stroke or death showed a non-significant trend favouring aspirin and dipyridamole over aspirin alone (event rates 17% vs 20%, respectively). For the individual outcome of stroke there was a significant 23% relative risk reduction (p=0.006) for the combination of agents compared to aspirin by itself.

More recently the ESPRIT study has supported a benefit of the combination of aspirin and dipyridamole.[65] Here 2763 patients (mean age 63 years) who had had a minor stroke or TIA within the last six months were randomised to aspirin (mean dose 75 mg) plus dipyridamole 200 mg bd (83% on MR preparation) or aspirin plus placebo over a mean follow-up period of 3.5 years. The primary outcome of vascular death, stroke, MI or major bleeding complication occurred in 16% of the aspirin group compared to 13% of those on combination therapy. The number needed to treat (NNT) for one year is around 100. There was no significant difference in bleeding rates between the groups. However, side-effects were common with combination of medications, especially headache – which resulted in 9% of patients discontinuing therapy. When the results of this trial are added to previous meta-analysis data, a significant benefit is seen in rates of vascular death, stroke and MI (RR 0.82; 95% CI 0.74–0.91). Current guidance recommends a combination of aspirin 75 mg once daily and dipyridamole MR 200 mg twice daily for people unable to tolerate clopidogrel for long term prevention following an ischaemic stroke or TIA.[9]

Clopidogrel

Clopidogrel prevents the aggregation of platelets by blocking the binding of adenosine diphosphate (ADP) to its receptor on their surface. This inhibits the binding of platelets to fibrin strands.

The CAPRIE study compared clopidogrel (75 mg) to aspirin (325 mg) in 19 185 patients (mean age 63 years) with a history of vascular disease (stroke, MI or peripheral vascular disease) over a mean follow-up of 1.9 years.[66] The primary outcome was combined rates of ischaemic stroke, MI or vascular death, for which there was a rate of 5.3% and 5.8% in the clopidogrel and aspirin groups, respectively. This just reached clinical significance (p=0.043) and represents a relative risk reduction of 8.7% (95% CI 0.3–16.5%). Subgroup analysis suggests that this benefit is most marked for those with peripheral vascular disease and the results are not significant for either stroke or MI alone. Withdrawal rates were similar in both groups. Adverse effects seen more commonly with clopidogrel included rash and diarrhoea, those seen with aspirin included upper gastrointestinal (GI) discomfort, and GI and intracranial haemorrhage.

A more recent study has compared aspirin plus clopidogrel vs aspirin plus placebo in 15 603 patients (mean age 64, range 39–95 years) with vascular risk factors over a mean follow-up period of 28 months.[67] For the primary outcome of MI, stroke or vascular death there was no significant difference between the groups (6.8% with clopidogrel vs 7.3% with placebo; relative risk (RR) 0.93; 95% CI 0.83–1.05; p=0.22). There was a higher rate of bleeding adverse events in the combination therapy group. A meta-analysis of studies suggested that clopidogrel may have around an additional 10% RRR compared to aspirin.[60]

Trials that have added clopidogrel to aspirin in the period immediately following unstable angina or myocardial infarction have demonstrated a clear benefit.[68,69] A recent study tested a combination of aspirin plus clopidogrel for 21 days (followed by clopidogrel alone) to aspirin alone for 90 days after a high risk TIA or minor stroke.[70] Stroke occurred in 8.2% of the patients in the combination of aspirin and clopidogrel group compared to 11.7% of those on aspirin alone (HR 0.68, 95% CI 0.57 to 0.81). However, aspirin plus clopidogrel has been found to have no additional benefit in secondary stroke prevention compared to clopidogrel alone and is associated with a significantly increased rate of adverse events, especially in those who had a lacunar stroke.[71,72]

A trial has compared the combination of aspirin and dipyridamole to clopidogrel in 20 332 people (mean age 66 years) with previous stroke.[73] After a mean follow-up period of 2.5 years, there were no significant differences in recurrent stroke rates (9.0% vs 8.8%; HR 1.01, 95% CI 0.92–1.11). However, major haemorrhagic events were more common with aspirin and dipyridamole (4.1% vs 3.6%; HR 1.15, 95% CI 1.00–1.32).

Guidance

Current guidance recommends clopidogrel 75 mg daily for long-term prevention following an ischaemic stroke or TIA for patients in sinus rhythm.[9]

Anticoagulants

Anticoagulation should be considered for people in atrial fibrillation (*see* Chapter 19). Due to the increased risk of bleeding into an area of infarct immediately following an ischaemic stroke, guidelines recommend that anticoagulation is not started (or is withheld if already taking) in the initial two weeks (one week for those with mechanical heart valves) and an antiplatelet agent be used in the interim.[9] Following a TIA, patients with atrial fibrillation should receive anticoagulation as soon as possible, typically with a rapid onset agent such as one of the novel anticoagulant drugs (*see* below).

Warfarin

Warfarin is indicated for the prevention of stroke in those with AF who are at a moderate to high risk of recurrence. Its use has also been proposed in other groups at high risk of recurrent stroke (e.g. those with significant intracranial arterial stenosis[74]) but to date there is no randomised controlled trial evidence of superior efficacy to antiplatelet agents within people in sinus rhythm.[75] Therefore, the elevated risk of bleeding complications with warfarin means that its use cannot be justified outside those with AF unless there is an alternative clinical indication (e.g. a prosthetic heart valve).

Novel anticoagulants

The oral drugs dabigatran (a direct thrombin inhibitor), apixaban and rivaroxaban (both factor Xa inhibitors) have recently been developed as alternatives to warfarin. These drugs have the advantage of being given at a standardised dose that does not need titrating or monitoring. The two potential limitations are the current higher financial cost (but some money is saved by not needing to monitor drug levels) and the inability to rapidly reverse the anticoagulant effect. Broadly speaking they have a similar efficacy as warfarin in preventing stroke in patients with AF but may have fewer bleeding complication rates (*see* p. 410).

Heparin

The use of subcutaneous heparin (various doses) has been compared to aspirin (300 mg) in over 19 000 acute stroke patients.[63] The study found a reduction in recurrent ischaemic events but this was offset by a similar increase in haemorrhagic complications, making heparin ineffective. When low molecular weight heparin has been compared to aspirin in those with atrial fibrillation in the first two weeks from a stroke, no benefit was found.[25,76] Therefore, heparin does not appear to have a significant role in the management of acute stroke.

Cholesterol reduction

A meta-analysis of trials involving over 90 000 patients on either a statin or placebo treatment found five-year RRR of around 20% for major vascular events (including stroke) per 1 mmol/L lowering of low-density lipoprotein (LDL) cholesterol.[77] The absolute benefits clearly are greater in those at higher baseline vascular risk. This appears to be irrespective of baseline cholesterol level or agent used to produce the reduction.

The Heart Protection study randomised 20 536 people with vascular risk factors to receive simvastatin 40 mg daily or placebo over a five-year period.[78] They found a 25% RRR of stroke with active therapy (4.3% vs 5.7% absolute risk). There was also a reduction in those having TIAs or requiring carotid endarterectomy. The difference became significant after two years of therapy. LDL cholesterol was around 1.0 mmol/L lower with the statin therapy. The benefit appears to be present irrespective of starting cholesterol level. The SPARCL study demonstrated a benefit of atorvastatin at a dose of 80 mg per day in reducing vascular events in people with a history of stroke (n=4731; mean age = 63 years) over a five-year period (HR 0.80, 95% CI 0.69–0.92).[79] The risk of haemorrhagic stroke was higher in the treatment arm.

Current guidelines recommend that treatment is started with simvastatin 40 mg at night.[9] However, if a total cholesterol level of <4.0 or an LDL cholesterol of <2.0 is not achieved, this should be intensified to atorvastatin 80 mg daily. Atorvastatin may have an additional advantage over simvastatin in not having an interaction with calcium channel blocking drugs.

Blood pressure control

The control of hypertension is discussed in Chapter 18. The PROGRESS trial is of particular note to post-stroke patients.[80] In this study, 6105 patients who had sustained a previous stroke or TIA (mean age 64 years, median time of eight months since stroke event) were randomised to receive either a placebo or an angiotensin-converting enzyme inhibitor (ACEi) (perindopril) with a thiazide diuretic (indapamide), if required, over a four-year period. The active treatment was associated with a larger average reduction in BP of 9/4 mmHg (mean initial BP 147/86 mmHg), and a lower risk of recurrent stroke than placebo (10% vs 14%; RRR 28%; $p<0.0001$). The combination of therapeutic agents resulted in a greater mean fall in BP and subsequent larger positive effect. The benefit seen was irrespective of patients' starting BP.

Some physicians feel that this study demonstrates a specific benefit of ACEi therapy in this patient subgroup. However, most believe that is it the degree of control of BP, rather than the specific agent(s) used that is of most importance in the prevention of future stroke. Current guidelines recommend a BP target following stroke of better than 130/80 mmHg,[81] although a BP target of below 150/90 mmHg for people aged over 80 years may be more appropriate.

Diabetes

In diabetic patients who have had a stroke tight blood sugar control is usually advised to reduce the risk of further events. However, evidence of a benefit in reducing stroke in those with type 2 diabetes is lacking (*see* p. 446). The early control of abnormal sugar levels is discussed on p. 204.

Smoking cessation

Smoking is a major modifiable risk factor for vascular disease, including stroke. However, even among younger smokers, only 22% have been noted to quit following a cerebrovascular event.[82] Up to half of all smokers die prematurely – on average 10 years earlier than non-smokers.[83] It is estimated that around 20% of all deaths in the developed world can currently be attributed to tobacco.[84] The main causes of death are cardiovascular, malignant and respiratory diseases. The prevalence of smoking is falling but is currently between 20% and 30% of the population in most developed countries. Smokers who manage to quit will see early benefits in respiratory function (possibly after a period of rebound increased mucus production) and later benefits in reduced cardiovascular risk. This increased risk falls to 50% after one year and approximates to the risk in non-smokers after 15 years.[84] The symptoms following quitting include anxiety, irritability, reduced concentration and weight gain.

To promote smoking cessation, doctors should enquire about smoking, advise on the benefits of stopping and offer referral to a specialist service. The mainstays of treatment are counselling and pharmacological treatments. Counselling should be performed by a trained person but this may be provided as a telephone service. Pharmacological treatments include nicotine replacement (available in various preparations including patches and gum) and some atypical antidepressants (e.g. bupropion) that reduce cravings and withdrawal symptoms. They may be used alone or in combination.

Cochrane reviews on the efficacy of both nicotine and bupropion have suggested an approximate doubling of benefit compared to placebo (from around a 10% success rate to 20% with treatment).[85,86] A review of the efficacy of telephone quit lines also suggests a benefit.[87] Given the enormous numbers of smokers and the large detrimental effect on health, even a small positive effect may have profound public health benefits.

Carotid endarterectomy

Carotid atherosclerotic stenosis of at least moderate severity (i.e. 50–99%) is found in 2–8% of people aged over 60 years, but is more prevalent in those with a history of vascular disease (e.g. 25% of people with peripheral vascular disease and 15% with coronary artery disease).[88] It usually causes no symptoms, but emboli from carotid artery plaques are thought to cause 15–20% of ischaemic strokes.[89] Carotid endarterectomy (CE) is a surgical technique that removes the inner layers of the carotid artery and any associated atheroma. The relative benefit of this procedure is proportional to the degree of vessel narrowing attributed to atheroma formation. The amount of internal carotid artery (ICA) stenosis can be estimated with carotid Doppler but is more accurately assessed by standard or magnetic resonance angiography. To complicate matters, there are differing systems for calculating the severity of any stenosis, which yield significantly different estimations. A recent study has found that patients seem to do as well with either local or general anaesthesia.[90]

The NASCET trial randomised 659 patients (mean age 66 years) who had sustained a TIA or non-disabling stroke in the relevant carotid territory within the last 120 days, and had a stenosis of 70–99%, to surgical intervention or usual medical care.[91] After two years the stroke rate was 26% in the medical arm compared to 9% in those who underwent surgery. However, the perioperative stroke or death rate was 5.8% despite using only highly skilled surgeons.

A further component of the NASCET trial randomised 2226 patients with stenoses less than 70% to surgery or control groups.[92] No benefit of surgery was found compared to control subjects with stenoses less than 50% (death or stroke occurred in 15% vs 19%; p=0.16) and only a small benefit in those with stenoses between 50% and 69% (16% vs 22%; p=0.045).

In the ECST trial 3024 patients (mean age 62 years) with carotid territory symptoms within the last six months were randomised to early surgery or a control group and followed up for a period of six years.[93] The participants had a range of degrees of carotid stenosis. Overall there was no benefit of surgery for the primary outcome measure of death or major stroke (37% in both groups). However, the subgroup that had stenosis of 80% or more did benefit (primary outcome reached in 15% of the surgery group compared to 27% of control subjects). There was a 7% risk of death or major stroke within 30 days of undergoing surgery.

In summary, CE is of proven benefit in patients with a stenosis of 70–99% who have sustained a recent stroke or TIA in that vascular territory.[89] It is of borderline benefit in those with stenoses of 50–70%, depending on the surgical complication rate and of no benefit in those with a symptomatic stenosis below 50%. CE for asymptomatic stenosis may have a small benefit for patients with stenoses of 60–99%, an expected survival of more than five years and when operated on by a surgeon, with a perioperative stroke or death rate of less than 3%.

The timing of the surgery is also critical. Analysis of data from the major carotid surgery trials has shown a large benefit for having surgery within 2 weeks of a symptomatic event compared to a delay of over 12 weeks (the NNT to prevent one stroke is 5 with early surgery vs 125 when delayed).[94] Previously in the UK as few as 20% of eligible people received their surgery within 2 weeks with 30% waiting over 12 weeks.[95] With greater awareness of the importance of early surgery these figures are improving. The current aim is to ideally perform surgery within 48 hours of an event, and certainly within one week.[88]

Having a surgeon with a very low complication rate is crucial. As medical therapy for the secondary prevention of stroke improves, the risk versus benefit profile of carotid surgery may change. In the ECST trial less than 10% of participants were on lipid-lowering medications, in the NASCET trial around 15% of participants were initially on lipid-lowering therapy and this rose to around 40% by the end of the trial.[92,93] It is not recommended for patients with a probable cardio-embolic source (e.g. those in AF) – these patients were excluded from the major trials.

The benefit of CE is highest in the elderly. Those over the age of 75 years have an absolute risk reduction over two years of 29%, compared to 15% in those aged 65 to 74, and 10% in those <65 years.[96] The NNT to prevent one stroke over a 5-year period has been calculated as 5 for those aged over 75, compared to 18 for those aged below 65 years.[94] Yet despite carotid stenosis being more common in older individuals, beyond the age of 80, patients are less likely to be referred for carotid imaging.[97]

Studies so far have not distinguished between different subtypes of anterior circulation stroke. Logic would suggest that the benefits of CE would be greatest in those whose stroke's mechanism was most likely due to an embolus from the relevant carotid artery (i.e. not lacunar circulation infarct (LACIs) (*see* p. 194)) and who have significant brain remaining in that territory to protect (i.e. not TACIs). Also, pure sensory strokes are likely to be due to posterior circulation aetiology and, therefore, be uninfluenced by carotid atheroma. This would suggest that partial anterior circulation infarct (PACI) strokes (or following a TIA/transient monocular blindness) are the group most likely to benefit from CE.

Carotid stenting

Arterial stenting is a less invasive revascularisation option for the carotids. However, initial studies found a high rate of emboli formation during the procedure. This has been lessened by the use of emboli-prevention devices. When the technique has been compared to endarterectomy in a randomised controlled trial recruiting patients who were deemed to be at high risk to undergo surgical intervention, the results suggested it was at least as effective for these patients.[98] However, a more recent trial comparing stenting to CE has shown a higher 30-day stroke or death rate with stenting (9.6% vs 3.9%).[99] Its use is currently restricted to specialist centres.[9]

PROGNOSIS OF ISCHAEMIC STROKE

It is difficult to predict individual patients' outcomes after a stroke. Overall, 10% of people who sustain ischaemic strokes are dead after one month, and this figure rises to 23% after one year.[21] A breakdown of the prognosis with specific stroke subtypes is shown in Table 10.4. The risk of recurrence over a five-year period is estimated to be 15–40%.[2] The highest risk of recurrent stroke is seen with those of the PACI subtype.[21] The risk of future stroke in those who have sustained a TIA has been found to be 8% after one week, 12% after one month and 17% after three months.[100] Equivalent figures for those who have sustained a minor stroke are very similar (12%, 15% and 19%, respectively). After 10 years, 54% of those who have had a TIA or minor stroke will have had at least one further vascular event and 60% will be dead.[101]

TABLE 10.4 A comparison of the composition and prognosis of stroke subtypes in the Bamford classification scheme[21]

Stroke subtype	Percentage of all ischaemic strokes	Independent at one year (%)	Dead at 30 days from stroke (%)	Dead at one year from stroke (%)
Lacunar infarct	25	60	2	11
Posterior circulation infarct	24	62	7	19
Partial anterior circulation infarct	34	55	4	16
Total anterior circulation infarct	17	4	39	60

A scoring tool has been developed to try to stratify those patients at highest risk of stroke following a TIA in order to more rapidly assess them and address modifiable risk factors. This is called the 'ABCD²', standing for **A**ge (1 point scored if aged 60 or above), **B**lood pressure (1 point if either systolic >140 mmHg or diastolic >90 mmHg), **C**linical features (2 points if unilateral weakness, 1 point if only speech affected, anything else doesn't score), **D**uration of symptoms (2 points if lasted 60 minutes or longer, 1 point if 10–59 minutes, 0 if <10 minutes) and **D**iabetes (1 point if present). This gives a total score of between 0 and 7. It has been found that the risk of stroke within seven days of a TIA is low (1.2%) in those with an ABCD² score of <4, but 5.9% in those with a score of 4 or 5, and 11.7% in those with a score >5.[102] Around 20% of patients were in the highest risk group (scores >5). This group could be targeted for more rapid assessment when resources are limited, but in an ideal world everyone would receive rapid assessment. One criticism of this scoring system is that the clinical features component will fail to detect posterior circulation symptoms, but such patients would not be candidates for carotid surgery.

A further study found that the risk of stroke within 24 hours of a TIA was 5.1%, representing 42% of all recurrent stroke within 30 days.[103] This highlights the importance of rapid assessment (i.e. within 24 hours). In this study, 20% of recurrent events were in people with an ABCD² score <4. This suggests that all patients should have rapid assessment, irrespective of ABCD² score.

Given the risk of early recurrent stroke it is highly important that patients are assessed and treated rapidly after their first symptoms. In a before and after comparative study, by reducing the median time for assessment (from three days to less than one day) and commencement of treatment (from 20 days to 1 day), the 90-day recurrent stroke risk was reduced from 10.3% to 2.1%.[104]

INTRACEREBRAL HAEMORRHAGE
Epidemiology
Approximately 15% of all strokes are haemorrhagic. They are subdivided into intracerebral haemorrhage (ICH) and subarachnoid haemorrhage (SAH) (*see* later). Around 80% of ICH is related to vascular damage to perforating arteries caused by hypertension or cerebral amyloid angiopathy (CAA).[105] Other events are related to an alternative underlying abnormality, which includes arteriovenous malformations, aneurysms, tumours and coagulopathies. ICH is subdivided according to anatomical location, into deep (at the basal ganglia, brainstem or cerebellum) and lobar (cortical). The incidence of ICH is around 10–20 per 100 000 population per year, but it is more common in the elderly, males and certain ethnic groups (especially Black and Japanese).[105]

Pathophysiology
Hypertension causes damage to the walls of small vessels. In the elderly, lobar bleeds are associated with CAA, whereas deep bleeds are associated with hypertension.[26] CAA is especially likely when two or more bleeds have occurred (together or at separate times).[106] Older bleeds may be detected by gradient-echo MRI scanning. The bleeds associated with CAA are usually at the grey-white matter border, but occasionally they

may affect the cerebellum. The increased bleeding tendency is caused by beta-amyloid deposition in the vessel walls. CAA is implicated in around 10% of ICH, and up to 30% of lobar ICH, in the elderly.[107] It may also increase the risk of bleeding while on warfarin. It is present to some degree in around 60% of those aged over 90 years, but is seen more commonly in the brains of people with neurodegenerative diseases (e.g. Alzheimer's) – probably due to higher accumulated levels of intracerebral amyloid protein.

Arteriovenous malformations are the most common cause of ICH in those aged below 45 years (*see* p. 226). Intracranial aneurysms and cerebral venous thrombosis (*see* p. 229) are infrequent causes of ICH. Anticoagulant (*see* p. 408) and, to a lesser extent, antiplatelet (*see* p. 206) use may also be implicated. There may be genetic factors that play a role in haemorrhage as a positive family history conveys an elevated risk. Lobar haemorrhage is more common with those who possess an apolipoprotein E4 or E2 allele.[108]

Clinical features

Like other strokes types, the presentation may be an abrupt onset of a focal neurological deficit. However, ICH is a more common cause of reduced consciousness due to the haematoma's mass effect causing compression of the brainstem structures (i.e. the reticular activating system).[105] A low GCS score at presentation carries a worse prognosis. Headache and vomiting may be due to either raised intracranial pressure or meningism secondary to leakage of blood into the ventricular system. When seizures are associated, they are most likely in the first 24 hours after onset.

Early clinical deterioration (within 24 hours) due to an increase in the size of the haematoma is seen in around 40% of patients (increase in size of >33%).[109] In the majority of these cases this enlargement occurs in the first hour from onset. It has been shown that worsening within the first 48 hours can also occur secondary to vasogenic oedema.[105] Corticosteroids have not been found to be beneficial in this form of cerebral oedema. Osmotic diuretics such as mannitol may have a role, but randomised controlled trial evidence of benefit is lacking.

Haemorrhagic stroke treatment

Blood pressure control

The control of BP in the acute phase, as with ischaemic stroke (*see* p. 205), is a controversial area and the best management is unclear. A recent trial found that intensive early lowering of systolic BP (within six hours of onset of ICH to <140 mmHg within one hour) do not improve rates of death or severe disability at 90 days.[110] After the acute phase, BP guidance is as for the secondary prevention of ischaemic strokes (*see* p. 210).

Recombinant activated factor VII

Early haematoma enlargement (mainly within the first four hours) is thought to be a significant factor associated with poor outcomes following ICH.[111] A randomised trial has compared the use of various doses of recombinant activated factor VII to placebo in 399 people (median age 66 years) with acute intracerebral haemorrhage (within four hours of onset).[112] It was found that the active therapy was associated with less early haematoma enlargement. This led to a lower 90-day mortality rate with the active treatment compared to placebo (18% vs 29%; *p*=0.02). However, there was a higher rate of serious thromboembolic complications (mainly MI and ischaemic stroke) with active treatment (7% vs 2%). Overall this is a promising result but further studies are required before this can become accepted therapy.

Reversal of anticoagulation

When ICH is associated with oral anticoagulant use (most commonly warfarin), early haematoma expansion may continue for up to 48 hours after the onset.[111] For this reason it is felt that rapid reversal of anticoagulation is of key importance. Studies have found that prothrombin complex concentrate (PCC) is more effective at achieving this than vitamin K and/or fresh frozen plasma (FFP).[113] PCC contains concentrated amounts of the vitamin K-dependent clotting factors II (prothrombin), VII, IX and X. The interaction of these factors with vitamin K and warfarin is shown in Figure 10.10. FFP contains clotting factors but in a non-concentrated format and with variable amounts of each component. It is usually fast acting but short-lived. Vitamin K has the disadvantage of a slow onset of action. Current guidelines recommend the use of PCC (dose calculated by weight) plus vitamin K (usually 5 mg IV).[114] When PCC is unavailable, FFP is an alternative. The most effective way to reverse the effect of novel anticoagulants is currently poorly understood.[115]

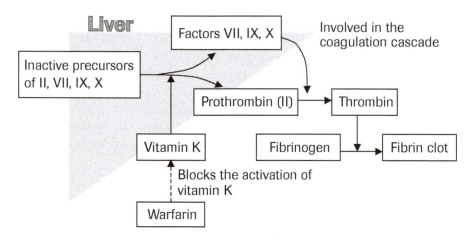

FIGURE 10.10 The roles of vitamin K, warfarin and the vitamin K-dependent clotting factors in thrombus formation.

Anticoagulation or antiplatelets after intracerebral haemorrhage

Generally speaking, people who have survived ICH are at a greater future risk of ICH rather than ischaemic stroke.[116] However, there is a subgroup of patients who have sustained an intracerebral bleed who are at an increased risk of ischaemic stroke (e.g. those who have prosthetic heart valves or are in AF). The question as to whether these patients should receive some form of blood-thinning therapy has not been well answered by current evidence.[117] Extrapolating from available data, it is usual practice that anticoagulant or antiplatelet therapy is avoided in patients in atrial fibrillation alone.[11,26] Overall, patients with prosthetic heart valves have been calculated to have a 4% per year risk of thromboembolism while off warfarin, compared to a 1% annual risk on warfarin (2% per year on antiplatelet agents).[118] It is generally accepted that a one to two-week period off warfarin carries a low (but not zero[119]) risk of embolus while the bleeding source repairs itself. Typically, such patients are then re-anticoagulated. The treatment of deep vein thrombosis (DVT) after ICH is discussed on p. 222.

Surgery

The STICH trial randomised 1033 patients (mean age 62 years) with acute ICH to either early surgery (within 24 hours) or initial conservative management.[120] Eligible patients had a haematoma seen on CT scanning of at least 2 cm diameter and a GCS score of five or more. The responsible neurosurgeon was also to be uncertain about the benefits of either treatment. The surgical technique was left to the choosing of the surgical team. Those in the conservative arm were allowed later surgery if the treating team felt it would be beneficial. This occurred in 26% of these patients at a mean time interval of 31 hours from randomisation. The results did not show a significant benefit of early surgery. A favourable outcome (absence of death or significant disability) was reported in 26% of those with early surgery compared to 24% of the conservative treatment group (OR 0.89; 95% CI 0.66–1.19). Those patients presenting with a GCS score of eight or less almost universally had a poor outcome. So, where surgical uncertainty exists, patients do not appear to benefit from early surgical intervention. Of course, there may be subgroups, such as posterior fossa haematomas or following the development of hydrocephalus, where surgical intervention is beneficial. For this reason, obtaining neurosurgical advice is usually still appropriate for cases of ICH.

Prognosis

ICH carries a high early mortality rate of between 30% and 50% in the first 30 days.[109] Coupled to this, only 20% of those afflicted manage to regain functional independence. Factors associated with worse prognosis include low GCS score at admission, advanced age, large bleed volume and the presence of blood within the ventricular system. When the ICH is associated with oral anticoagulant use, the mortality rate is around 70%.[111] Overall the recurrence rate has been estimated at around 2.4% per year.[116] However, the risk in the elderly is higher[121] and figures of 15% per year for lobar bleeds, but only 2% per year for deep hemispheric bleeds have been detected.[26] The association with CAA may explain why lobar bleeds are more likely to recur. The control of hypertension after the acute phase is associated with a reduction in recurrence rates.[105] If an underlying anatomical abnormality is suspected then a conventional or MR angiogram should be performed.

SUBARACHNOID HAEMORRHAGE

Subarachnoid haemorrhage (SAH) accounts for around 2–5% of all strokes, and ruptured intracranial aneurysms cause around 80% of SAH.[122] It is more common in women than men, and the mean age of onset is 55 years. Risk factors for bleeding include hypertension, smoking, excessive alcohol intake and cocaine use. The occurrence of intracranial aneurysms has a familial component due to the association with some genetic conditions (e.g. polycystic kidney disease and some connective tissue disorders). The aneurysms are most likely to occur at arterial branching sites at, or close to, the circle of Willis (*see* Figure 10.3). Autopsy studies suggest they are present in 1 to 5% of the population, but most are small and never rupture.[123]

SAH should be suspected in patients with a sudden onset of severe headache ('worst ever'), and will be detected in around a quarter of these people.[124] The pain may be diffuse or localised. Additional suggestive features that may be present include neck pain, photophobia, nausea/vomiting and reduced consciousness. Sudden loss of consciousness may be the presenting feature. Focal neurological signs are occasionally present. A third nerve palsy can be caused by compression by an expanding, or bleeding, posterior communicating artery aneurysm.

When SAH is clinically suspected it is recommended that urgent CT scanning is obtained. When performed within 12 hours, this will detect around 95% of SAH. If the CT is negative, a lumbar puncture (LP) should be performed.[9] A period of at least 12 hours should have passed since the symptom onset to the time of the LP and the direct measurement of bilirubin concentration, or spectrophotometry should be used to maximise the chance of detecting xanthochromia (the result of breakdown of blood cells in the cerebrospinal fluid (CSF) to form yellow bilirubin, which cannot be caused by a traumatic tap).

Treatment

Acute BP control following SAH is often recommended in those with markedly elevated blood pressures, but this approach lacks randomised controlled trial evidence of benefit, and a target value has not been defined. Intercollegiate guidelines recommend the use of the anti-vasospastic agent, nimodipine (a calcium channel blocker), in cases of SAH.[9] A Cochrane review suggested evidence of a benefit with 60 mg of nimodipine four-hourly.[125] A neurosurgical opinion should be sought and most patients will be transferred to a neurosurgical unit. When SAH is secondary to the rupture of an intracranial aneurysm, the treatment of the aneurysm can reduce the probability of recurrent bleeding. A recent trial that compared open surgery with vessel clipping to endovascular embolisation with coiling for intracranial aneurysms that were anatomically suitable for either technique found a survival benefit with the less invasive technique of coiling (death or dependency at one year: 24% vs 31%).[126] When there is a strong family history of SAH, or with a history of polycystic kidney disease, screening family members for aneurysms is probably indicated.

Prognosis

Aneurysmal SAH has a poor prognosis with a 50% fatality rate, and around one-third of survivors require long-term care.[122] Non-aneurysmal SAH has a better prognosis. Adverse prognostic indicators include a reduced GCS score at the time of admission, large volume of bleed and older age. Common complications in the first two weeks after SAH, which worsen outcomes, include vasospasm, hydrocephalus and rebleeding.

Vasospasm has a peak incidence between 5 and 14 days after SAH and is usually only seen following aneurysmal bleeds. Hydrocephalus is more likely to develop in patients who have intraventricular extravasation of the bleed.

SUBACUTE TREATMENT OF STROKE

Stroke units

Following an acute stroke, patients should be transferred to a specialist stroke unit as soon as possible. The nature of stroke units varies but the basic components are similar, being based around multidisciplinary rehabilitation delivered by specialist staff in a ward that is geographically discrete from the rest of the hospital. In comparison to usual care, stroke units have been found to be associated with a reduction in one-year mortality (OR 0.83; 95% CI 0.69–0.98; $p<0.05$) and the combined outcome of death and institutionalisation (OR 0.75; 95% CI 0.65–0.87; $p<0.0001$) with no net increase in length of stay.[127] The benefits are still apparent in patients followed up 10 years after their stroke.[128] It is estimated that for every 1000 strokes 50 patients could be prevented from death or disability by stroke unit care, compared to 6 for rt-PA and 4 for aspirin.[3]

Rehabilitation

Stroke is a major cause of disability. Fortunately, almost always some, and occasionally complete, functional recovery is expected. After one year around two-thirds of the survivors of strokes will be functionally independent.[4] Rehabilitation is, clearly, a very important aspect of post-stroke recovery. It is discussed in Chapter 3.

Post-stroke nutrition

Malnutrition is a real concern for any elderly person admitted to hospital for a prolonged period (*see* p. 10). When this is complicated by dysphagia secondary to stroke, the risks are further elevated. The normal swallowing process and treatment methods are discussed on p. 40. The recent publication of the FOOD trials (three separate randomised controlled trials evaluating post-stroke nutrition) has increased our understanding of this area.[129,130] They are discussed below under the relevant subheadings.

Nutritional supplements

In the FOOD trial of patients who were hospitalised following an acute stroke, but able to swallow normally, 4023 patients (mean age 71 years) were randomised to receive either standard hospital meals alone or with additional nutritional supplements.[129] No significant benefit was found in death or poor outcome with this intervention. However, only 8% of patients were deemed to be undernourished at the start of the trial. This suggests that nutritional supplements should not be used routinely, but they may have a role in selected undernourished individuals.

Enteral tube feeding

The two common methods of enteral tube feeding are discussed below, followed by a review of the components of the FOOD trials that recruited dysphagic patients, which may guide clinical practice in this area.

Nasogastric (NG) tubes

NG tubes are usually easily inserted on hospital wards. They can be irritating to the patient's nasopharynx, and are prone to becoming dislodged (accidentally or deliberately). The maintenance of such tubes is more difficult in the significant number of individuals with associated acute confusional states.

Percutaneous endoscopic gastrostomy (PEG) tubes

PEG tubes are feeding tubes that are inserted through the stomach wall under endoscopic guidance (although alternative methods involving either radiologically guided or surgically placed tubes are occasionally used).[131] They have the advantage over NG tubes of not being irritating to the nasopharynx and generally being more comfortable for longer-term usage. The disadvantage is that they are invasive and need a minor surgical procedure to insert them. The most common reason for PEG insertion in the UK is for dysphagia following a stroke.

The insertion procedure itself is usually well tolerated and has a low complication rate (less than 2%).[132] However, in the hospitalised elderly there is a 30-day mortality rate of 24–28%, rising to 63% at one year.[133,134] Studies looking at patients admitted for elective PEG insertion have found lower mortality rates;[135] however, this is not applicable to those who are hospitalised following an acute stroke. Those at highest risk include patients with a history of aspiration pneumonia or an age over 75 years.[136] The presence of dementia is also an adverse predictive factor (*see* p. 115). Complications related to the PEG tube commonly occurring in the year after insertion include obstruction of the tube (11%), infection (9%) and bleeding (7%) at the insertion site, leakage around the tube (4%) and peritonitis (2%).[135]

PEG tubes do not exclude the development of an aspiration pneumonia.[137] Patients continue to be at risk of aspirating oral secretions or regurgitated stomach contents. The best patient position for feeding and the optimal duration and frequency of feeds are unknown. Logic suggests that being upright during feeds may reduce the regurgitation risk compared to being recumbent. If so, feeds at discrete times when sitting upright out of bed may be better than prolonged slow feeds when reclined, especially overnight. Guidelines suggest that patients should be propped up to 30 degrees or more during feeding and for at least 30 minutes afterwards.[138]

The FOOD trials for dysphagic patients

The FOOD trials had two further components that enrolled patients who were dysphagic following an acute stroke.[130] In both arms the patients were allowed to commence oral feeding if their swallow improved during the study period.

The first of these randomised 859 patients (mean age 76 years) to receive enteral tube feeding (PEG or NG) as soon as possible or to avoid enteral feeding for at least seven days (these patients received IV or subcutaneous (SC) fluids alone). Tube feeding was associated with a non-significant trend towards a reduction in absolute mortality of 5.8% (95% CI −0.8 to 12.5; $p=0.09$) with a non-significant reduction in death or poor outcome (severe disability) of 1.2% (95% CI −4.2 to 6.6; $p=0.7$). This suggests that early feeding may have a modest effect on improvement in mortality but is likely to increase the number of patients who survive with severe disability. The authors recommend that early tube feeding should be offered to dysphagic acute stroke patients.

The second FOOD trial in dysphagic acute stroke patients randomised 321 people (mean age 76 years) who were judged appropriate for enteral feeding to receive either a PEG or NG tube within three days of randomisation and continued for as long as practical. They found that PEG tubes were associated with a borderline significant increase in death or poor outcome, compared to NG feeding, of 7.8% (95% CI 0.0–15.8; p=0.05). This suggests that, at least within the first few weeks of an acute stroke, NG feeding is preferable to PEG feeding. Of course, there may be patients in whom PEG insertion is a better option, for example due to intolerance of NG tubes.

Refeeding syndrome

During periods of starvation the usual mechanisms for bodily ion homeostasis are down-regulated to conserve energy.[138] This results in reduced intracellular levels of potassium, magnesium, calcium and phosphate. The recommencement of feeding causes a rapid uptake of these ions into cells. The result can be a rapid fall in extracellular concentrations. This complication is thought to be most likely to occur in the most malnourished. If untreated this can cause arrhythmias, neuromuscular dysfunction, confusion and death. Therefore it is usually recommended that feeding is started at a slow rate and blood tests are initially monitored daily. Supplements of vitamins that may have become depleted are also given.

Complications following stroke

Complicating conditions occurring while in hospital after an acute stroke are common. One study found a rate of 59%,[139] the most common being falls (22%), skin breaks (18%), urinary tract infection (UTI) (16%) and chest infections (12%). Depression and shoulder subluxation tend to occur later in the course of recovery.

Some degree of haemorrhagic transformation may be detected on follow-up brain imaging in around one-third of ischaemic strokes, but a far smaller number are symptomatic. It is thought to be more common after large-sized infarcts than smaller ones.

Thromboembolism

Estimates of the incidence of DVT and pulmonary embolus (PE) after stroke vary widely, perhaps reflecting differing diagnostic criteria. A UK hospital-based study reported a DVT rate of 3% when identified by case note review.[139] PEs may account for up to 20% of early deaths following stroke.[140]

Prophylaxis

When heparin has been given following acute stroke, the increased rate of haemorrhagic complications negated any anti-thrombotic benefits.[63] Routine use of prophylactic anticoagulation is typically not recommended in post-stroke patients.

Compression hosiery has been found to be beneficial in preventing thromboembolic complications after surgical intervention.[141] However, a trial has addressed this issue by comparing thigh length graduated compression stockings to no stockings in

2518 patients (mean age 76 years) who had recently had a stroke.[142] DVT (symptomatic or asymptomatic) was detected by ultrasound in 10.0% of those with stockings and 10.5% of those without (non-significant). Adverse events included skin ulcers, blisters and necrosis, and were more common with stocking use (5% vs 1%). Coupled to the discomfort experience by patients, it can no longer be recommended to routinely use compressing hosiery following stroke.

More recently the CLOTS3 Trial has demonstrated a benefit of intermittent pneumatic compression (IPC) of the lower legs in reducing the risk of DVT following stroke.[143] Here 2876 patients were randomised to IPC or no treatment. DVT was detected within 30 days in 8.5% of the IPC group compared to 12.1% of the no treatment group (absolute risk reduction 3.6%, 95% CI 1.4–5.8%). The 30-day mortality rate was also lower with IPC (11% vs 13%). Rates of adverse events related to the treatment were low.

Treatment of DVT after intracerebral haemorrhage

An alternative approach in the prevention of a PE following a DVT is the use of a caval filter. Here a device is percutaneously inserted into the inferior vena cava to act as a filter preventing emboli travelling from the deep leg veins to the lungs. It is proposed that they may have a role in patients with contraindications to anticoagulation therapy (e.g. ICH). However, randomised controlled trial evidence of benefit is lacking. When they have been assessed in conjunction with heparin for those at high risk of thromboembolic event, an early lower incidence of PE (1% vs 5% after 12 days) was offset by a higher late incidence of DVT (21% vs 12% after two years) compared to those without filters.[144] Thrombus formation on the filter is a recognised complication that may increase the risk of emboli. Some physicians advocate the use of anticoagulation, rather than filters, in those with DVT following ICH when the risk of rebleeding is lowest (i.e. with non-lobar ICH (*see* p. 217)).[145]

Post-stroke depression

Depression after stroke is common. Screening for it may be made difficult by cognitive changes such as dysphasia. Some alternative rating scales have been developed for such patients.[146] The SSRI citalopram has been found to be effective in the management of post-stroke depression.[147] However, a significant number of cases will spontaneously resolve in the first two months. Depression is discussed in more detail in Chapter 8.

Pain

Central post-stroke pain is a form of neuropathic pain occurring in the affected side of the body. It should be treated in the same way as other neuropathic pains (*see* p. 62). Shoulder pain is also seen following stroke. Shoulder–hand syndrome is autonomically medicated (reflex sympathetic dystrophy). Here the pain may be associated with swelling and changes in colour or temperature of the affected arm. An alternative cause is shoulder subluxation related to motor weakness. This can largely be prevented by appropriate patient positioning/support and careful use of handling techniques to avoid strain on the shoulder joint.

Other problems

Falls, incontinence, pressure ulcers, dementia and delirium are all common problems following a stroke. They are discussed in detail within the relevant chapters.

Driving

Currently, in the UK, drivers of standard vehicles are required to stop driving for one month after a stroke. They may resume driving after this time if a satisfactory recovery has been made. They only need to inform the DVLA if there is a persisting deficit beyond one month. An exception to this rule is if recurrent TIAs have occurred within a short time interval, in this instance the DVLA should be informed. Full guidance is available at the DVLA website (www.gov.uk/government/publications/at-a-glance – accessed November 2014). As with any change in health status, the driver should inform his or her insurance company of their diagnosis. Links to driving regulation resources in countries other than the UK are shown in Box 6.2.

LESS COMMON CAUSES OF STROKE

The following text discusses some of the less common causes of stroke. Most are very rare in the elderly but more frequently a cause of stroke in younger people. Approximately 1% of strokes occur in people aged 15–45 years.[82] The term 'cryptogenic stroke' is used to describe stroke where there is no obvious underlying cause. This is a much more common occurrence in younger people (up to 40% of such patients).

A review of the causes of stroke in the young found that the most common definite causes were: carotid or vertebrobasilar artery dissection (19%) or atheroma (8%); cardio-embolic sources (5% – mainly AF or bacterial endocarditis); vascular inflammation (2%); and cerebral autosomal dominant arteriopathy with subcortical infarcts and leukoencephalopathy (CADASIL) (1%, *see below*).[82] These strokes had a mortality rate of 4.5% in the first year. The stroke recurrence rate was around 1% per year.

Arterial dissection

Arterial dissection is, essentially, a tear in the artery wall. It can cause a stroke by two mechanisms. First, blood can accumulate between the arterial layers resulting in stenosis; second, the tear may expose the circulating blood to thrombogenic underlying tissues, resulting in clot formation and/or subsequent embolisation. Usually it is triggered by some form of mild trauma, although the actual incident may not be recalled. This may vary from major accidents to trivial occurrences such as a violent cough or sneeze. Spontaneous events are more likely in those with underlying connective tissue disorders. Dissection may account for around 2% of strokes overall and perhaps 20% of those in younger age groups.[148]

It should be suspected when pain at the side (carotid) or back of the head (vertebrobasilar) is a major feature just before the onset of focal symptoms. Other clues are the history of trauma and the occurrence in younger people without clear vascular risk factors. A partial Horner syndrome (miosis and ptosis only) is a clinical feature of carotid dissection due to the close anatomical association of sympathetic fibres with the internal carotid artery. Dissection here may also result in lower cranial nerve palsies. Presently, diagnosis is most frequently confirmed by MR angiography.

It is believed that embolisation of thrombus is the most common mechanism leading to cerebral ischaemia. For this reason some physicians advocate the use of anticoagulation with an INR of 2–3 for three to six months, although there are no randomised trials demonstrating a benefit with this approach.[148] An alternative option is the use of antiplatelet agents.

Patent foramen ovale

A patent foramen ovale (PFO) occurs in around 27% of the adult population.[149] Essentially, it is a hole between the right and left atria (*see* Figure 10.11) and is a normal component of the fetal circulation that usually closes at the time of birth. It is speculated that a PFO could allow a venous embolism to pass from the right to the left side of the heart and cause a stroke (a paradoxical embolism). This may be more likely to occur at times when right atrial pressure is elevated and the pressure gradient with the left atrium is reversed, for example during straining.[150] The role of PFO in the genesis of stroke remains controversial.

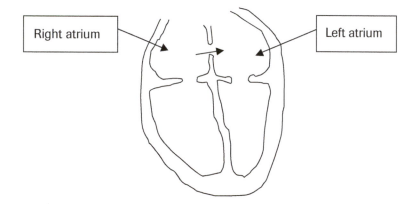

FIGURE 10.11 Patent foramen ovale.

Retrospective reviews of echocardiography results have found an elevated detection of PFO among those under the age of 55 who have sustained a stroke compared to control subjects (40% vs 10%).[151] However, the investigators were not blinded to the patients' past histories and indications for performing the scans varied between groups. Against PFO being a risk factor for stroke is the fact that patients with a cryptogenic stroke are rarely found to have a venous source of embolism. However, this has been seen with confirmed cases of pulmonary embolism.

One meta-analysis of case-control studies supported the idea that the presence of a PFO increases the risk of stroke in patients below the age of 55 but an association was less clear in older subjects.[152] However, a more recent meta-analysis did not find an increased stroke risk associated with PFO status.[153] Some studies have suggested that the combination of a PFO with an atrial septal aneurysm confers a particularly high risk,[154] but other studies have not supported this idea.[155]

Even if a PFO is thought to be causative in stroke, there is little trial evidence to define the best management strategy and so it remains a matter of some debate.[156] The results of studies of the use of aspirin or warfarin are conflicting. Perhaps the best currently available evidence comes from a subgroup of the Warfarin–Aspirin Recurrent Stroke Study (WARSS) who underwent TOE.[155] Patients in this study were randomly allocated to warfarin or aspirin. The subgroup contained 630 patients (mean age 59, range 30–85 years), 34% of whom were found to have a PFO. After two years there was no significant difference in stroke or TIA rates between the group with and those without a PFO. Nor was there any difference in events between those allocated to warfarin or aspirin. A recent meta-analysis of trials also found no difference in efficacy with aspirin or warfarin but increased rates of bleeding complications in those allocated to anticoagulation.[153]

A percutaneous technique of mechanical PFO closure has been developed, but there are no randomised controlled trials demonstrating its efficacy at reducing the risk of stroke.[156] The risk of recurrent stroke or TIA in patients with a PFO treated with warfarin or aspirin has been found to be between 3.4% and 3.8% per year.[157] One series found a similar annual recurrence rate of 3.4% following percutaneous closure.[157] Serious complications occur in around 1.5% of people undergoing the procedure. They include major haemorrhage, cardiac tamponade, pulmonary embolism and death. The recruitment of sufficient patients to perform suitably powered randomised controlled trials in this area is in part hampered by the trend for the open-label insertion of devices.[158]

Until better evidence becomes available, based on the risks of causing harm with the proposed therapies, aspirin seems to be the current safest option. If a paradoxical embolism is suspected, a source should be searched for; clearly, if identified, a course of warfarin may then be appropriate. Risk factors for thromboembolism (e.g. oral contraceptive use and the thrombophilias) should be considered. The role of percutaneous closure will remain unclear until randomised controlled trial evidence becomes available.

Other cardiac sources of emboli

AF is by far the most common cardiac source of emboli. Less common alternatives include thrombus formed on a less mobile ventricle wall following an acute MI, valvular vegetations secondary to infective endocarditis, and thrombus formed on the surface of atrial myxomas.

Vasculitis

The most common vasculitis causing cerebral ischaemia in the UK is giant cell arteritis (GCA) (*see* p. 436). This is seen only in those over the age of 50 years. It is usually associated with non-specific symptoms, such as fatigue, myalgia and weight loss. Less common alternative vasculitides include systemic lupus erythematosus (SLE). When suspected, an ESR and autoantibody studies should be performed. In the case of GCA, a temporal artery biopsy may confirm the diagnosis. Characteristically it responds very rapidly to high-dose steroids.

Arteriovenous malformations

Arteriovenous malformations (AVMs) are congenital abnormalities of blood vessels that result in the formation of an abnormal coil of arteries and veins. The basic anatomy of an AVM is shown in Figure 10.12. There are no capillaries between the larger vessels, resulting in direct shunting of blood from the arterial to the venous system. They are estimated to have a prevalence of less than 0.01% of the total population.[159]

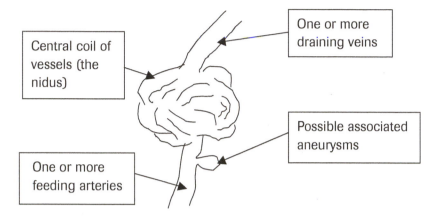

One or more draining veins

Central coil of vessels (the nidus)

Possible associated aneurysms

One or more feeding arteries

FIGURE 10.12 The basic anatomy of an arteriovenous malformation (AVM).

AVMs may be asymptomatic or produce symptoms. Over half present with haemorrhagic stroke, and around a quarter with seizures.[160] Headache and progressive neurological deficit are less common presentations. They appear to be more likely to cause symptoms in the young with a mean age of onset of 31 years.[159] They may account for around 3% of strokes, and around one-third of ICH in people below the age of 45 years.[161]

The annual risk of haemorrhage has been estimated to be around 2–3%.[160] The presence of associated aneurysms and a history of hypertension are thought to increase bleeding risk. The mortality with such events is between 10% and 20%.[159] However, the natural history is poorly understood, in part due to the trend towards early intervention.

Occasionally there are clinical signs of AVMs. These include overlying skin pigmentation (the Sturge–Weber syndrome), a cranial bruit or evidence of associated hereditary haemorrhagic telangiectasia. They may be seen on CT scanning (especially with contrast) but are more readily detected on MRI images. Arteriography may provide more anatomical and functional information.

Intervention is usually undertaken on the premise that it will reduce future bleeding risk. Alternative indications include the treatment of intractable seizures and progressive neurological impairment. Due to the lower cumulative lifetime risk in the elderly, intervention is rarely undertaken. Treatment options include microsurgical techniques, endovascular embolisation and radiosurgery.[159] The larger and deeper the AVM, the higher the complication rate. There are no randomised controlled trials to evaluate the benefits of interventional techniques compared to a conservative approach.

Mitochondrial disorders

Mitochondria were originally symbiotic bacteria that migrated into animal cells with the advantage of being able to perform aerobic metabolism. They posses their own DNA and are inherited by division of the mitochondria contained with the maternal egg cell. Various disorders have been described relating to mutations in the mitochondrial DNA.[162] One of these is 'mitochondrial encephalomyopathy, lactic acidosis and stroke-like episodes' (MELAS).

This disorder is very rare and usually presents in children or young adults with focal neurological deficits, seizures and progressive cognitive impairment. There may be an associated history of exercise intolerance, deafness, diabetes, migraine and/or learning disability. Fasting plasma and CSF lactate levels are elevated. Muscle biopsy may demonstrate ragged red fibres or abnormal mitochondria. There is no treatment for this condition.

CADASIL

Cerebral autosomal dominant arteriopathy with subcortical infarcts and leukoencephalopathy (CADASIL) is a very rare (autosomal-dominantly) inherited disorder. It presents with migraine attacks and cerebrovascular events in early adulthood, and leads to a progressive cognitive impairment. Death usually occurs prior to the age of 60 years. It is caused by mutations in the notch 3 gene located on chromosome 19, which leads to abnormalities in the structure of small blood vessels. Vascular lesions will be seen on brain imaging. Blood vessel abnormalities can sometimes be detected in tissue samples from skin or muscle biopsies.

DIFFERENTIAL DIAGNOSES OF STROKE

Migraine

The classic presentation of migraine (an aura, particularly flashing/zigzag lights, followed by headache) is easily distinguished from stroke. The onset of symptoms is also more gradual, worsening over several minutes. There may be associated nausea and photophobia. Occasionally atypical migraines without headache can occur ('acephalgic migraine'). Rarely a migraine may be followed by prolonged neurological symptoms due to cerebral infarction thought secondary to vascular spasm. Observational studies have suggested an increased risk of stroke in people with a history of migraine (RR 2.16, 95% CI 1.89–2.48).[163] In those with a history of migraine with classic aura, the risk of stroke and ischaemic heart disease are both elevated.[164] The finding of 'infarct-like' lesions on MRI scanning is also more common in people with a history of classic migraine.[165]

Seizures

Seizures may cause symptoms that are mistaken for stroke. Following an ictal episode there may be poor recollection of the event and there may also be an associated transient weakness in the affected limbs (Todd paresis). A further complicating factor is that some strokes will provoke seizures at their onset. In patients with no history of stroke, the onset of seizures after the age of 60 is associated with an increased risk of cerebrovascular disease (*see* p. 429).[166]

Symptoms of seizures tend to be 'positive' – resulting in additional phenomena such as jerking movements or hallucinations, compared to stroke that tends to cause 'negative' symptoms – loss of functions such as sensation or power. An MRI scan should be performed in patients with suspected seizures to exclude a structural lesion that may not be detected on CT scanning.

Brain tumours

Classically, brain tumours cause slowly progressive neurological deficits that can be easily distinguished from strokes by careful history, although it is reported that transient neurological symptoms can occur. Possible explanations for these include partial seizures, vascular 'steal' phenomenon or haemorrhage into the tumour with compression of surrounding tissues. Other presentations include seizures, signs of raised intracranial pressure, or cognitive impairment. The clinical finding of papilloedema makes the diagnosis more likely to be a tumour than a stroke. They are usually detected on CT scanning – especially when contrast is used and peripheral enhancement is seen. MRI scans may provide more information if the diagnosis is in doubt.

In adults the majority of primary tumours (80%) are supratentorial. They rarely metastasise, and there is no lymphatic spread in the CNS (no true lymphatic system). Around half are of glial cell origin. Low-grade gliomas (e.g. astrocytomas and oligodendrogliomas) are uncommon in the elderly. High-grade 'glioblastoma multiforme' (GBM), which has signs of necrosis, haemorrhage and oedema on imaging, is unfortunately common. This tumour has around a 30% one-year survival when untreated. Other possibilities include meningiomas (around 25%; benign and slow-growing; may be vascular (enhance with contrast) or calcified), pituitary adenomas (20%), vascular (e.g. angiomas), and, rarely, lymphoma.

Regarding the management of GBM, surgical resection is non-curative (debulking), technically challenging and possibly only of a small benefit. Steroids can be used to reduced surrounding oedema. The response seen is similar in the elderly as to that of younger individuals. Symptomatic improvement is usually rapid (begins within hours). Dexamethasone crosses the blood–brain barrier well. Divided doses of 12 to 16 mg per day are typical. The dose should be reduced rapidly following symptomatic response (e.g. 2 mg per day after 48 hours) to the lowest effective maintenance dose (typically 2–4 mg per day). Healthy brain tissue is poorly tolerant of radiotherapy and some tumours may be less sensitive in older adults. Early complications of radiotherapy include headache, fever and worsening of focal signs. In a trial comparing radiotherapy and supportive care in 81 people over the age of 70 years (half of whom had prior debulking surgery) with a new diagnosis of GBM, median survival was extended by 12 weeks (from 17 to 29 weeks) without an associated reduction in cognition or quality of life.[167] Chemotherapy is generally difficult for brain tumours due to the protective effect of blood–brain barrier. Recently a chemotherapeutic agent, temozolomide, has been found to be of benefit in GMB. A trial randomised 573 patients (mean age

56 years) to receive radiotherapy and temozolomide or radiotherapy alone.[168] The two-year survival rate was 27% in the temozolomide arm and just 10% in the controls.

The majority of brain tumours detected in the elderly are metastatic deposits of extra-cranial tumours. The commonest primary sites are lung (50–60%), breast (15–20%), melanoma (5–10%), and gastrointestinal tract (4–6%).[169] They tend to be frontoparietal or cerebellar. They are usually well circumscribed and enhance with contrast. Management is typically with palliative radiotherapy and dexamethasone. Occasionally surgical resection is considered if the primary tumour is well controlled and only one or two lesions are present in the brain.

Subdural haematoma

Occasionally, subdural haematomas can cause focal neurological symptoms. They are more common in those who take warfarin, the elderly and alcoholics (probably due to brain shrinkage causing venous stretching). There may be no history of head trauma. The onset is usually subacute. Headache is commonly associated. There may also be impaired consciousness, confusion and/or a fluctuating course. The haemorrhage is usually seen on CT scanning. The difficulty may arise between one and three weeks from the onset when the blood may appear isodense to surrounding brain tissue.

Cerebral venous thrombosis

Venous thrombosis can occur in the intracranial veins or venous sinuses. This can result in venous infarction and associated haemorrhage. The annual incidence has been estimated to be between three and four cases per million, and the majority of cases occur in women of child-bearing age.[170] There is a spectrum of clinical presentations, ranging from a rapidly declining conscious level to slowly progressive lesions that mimic cerebral tumours or abscesses.[171] The majority of patients will have headache and 40% develop seizures.[170] Intracranial hypertension may be present with papilloedema and associated brief visual disturbances. Risk factors include the use of oral contraceptives and pregnancy (especially the third trimester and immediately post-birth). Minor cranial or venous trauma (including central venous cannulation and lumbar punctures) can precipitate events.[170]

Cavernous sinus thrombosis is usually precipitated by infections in the paranasal sinuses or orbit.[170] It is associated with proptosis, chemosis and oculomotor palsies.

Central venous thrombosis should be considered in younger patients with atypical headache or stroke-like symptoms in the absence of vascular risk factors.[170] Lesions may be seen on CT scanning (haemorrhagic infarcts that may be multiple and not confined to arterial territories), but the advent of MRI and MR venography has improved its recognition.[170]

Anticoagulant treatment, initially with heparin and then warfarin (INR 2–3) for at least six months, is usually advised. This is based on data from several small, randomised trials and larger non-randomised series.[170] Over 80% of patients will have a favourable outcome.[170]

Transient global amnesia

Transient global amnesia (TGA) is a condition in which there is a loss of memory lasting less than 24 hours (typically less than two hours). During an episode subjects are able to function normally and have no other evidence of abnormality, but are likely to repeatedly ask the same question and not recall recent events. The mechanism is unknown. The idea that it could be a variant of cerebrovascular disease has been suggested but vascular risk factors are not strongly associated and prognosis is far better than that of individuals who have sustained a TIA.[172] Alternative explanations include a form of migraine or epilepsy. No specific treatment is required.

Functional symptoms

'Functional symptoms' is a term that covers a range of presentations that cannot be explained by a physical disease process and are felt to have a psychiatric/psychological basis (sometimes termed 'conversion reactions'). They may have a presentation mimicking stroke. Clues to the diagnosis include a past psychiatric history, young age at onset, inconsistent history, lack of objective neurological signs and normal brain imaging. Helpful clinical features of functional paralysis include a positive Hoover's sign and a monoplegic 'dragging' gait.[173] Hoover's sign is elicited by asking the patient, while lying on an examination bed, to push down with their heel on to the examiner's hand. The 'weak' leg will not push down strongly. The patient is then asked to raise the opposite leg while the examiner's other hand pushes it downwards. A positive Hoover's sign is elicited when the affected heel pushes down strongly on the examiner's hand during the raising of the opposite leg. The 'dragging' gait is present when the patient pulls their affected leg along behind them (rather than circumducting as seen following stroke).

Other differentials

Metabolic disorders are occasionally mistaken for stroke, for example hypo- or hyperglycaemia, and hyponatraemia. They are likely to have a subacute onset and be associated with cognitive impairment. Cerebral abscesses may cause a focal neurological deficit, but would usually be of subacute onset and associated with delirium and fever.

REFERENCES

1 Rothwell PM, Coull AJ, Fairhead JF, *et al.* Population-based study of event-rate, incidence, case fatality, and mortality for all acute vascular events in all arterial territories (Oxford Vascular Study). *Lancet*, 2005; **366**: 1773–83.
2 Wolfe CDA. The impact of stroke. *Br Med Bulletin*, 2000; **56**(2): 275–86.
3 Donnan GA, Fisher M, Macleod M, *et al.* Stroke. *Lancet*, 2008; **371**: 1612–23.
4 Bamford J, Sandercock P, Dennis M, *et al.* A prospective study of acute cerebrovascular disease in the community: the Oxfordshire Community Stroke Project –1981–86. *J Neurol Neurosurg Psychiatry*, 1990; **53**: 16–22.
5 Libman RB, Wirkowski E, Alvir J, *et al.* Conditions that mimic stroke in the emergency department: implications for acute stroke trials. *Arch Neurol*, 1995; **52**: 1119–22.
6 Foerch C, Misselwitz B, Sitzer M, *et al.* Difference in recognition of right and left hemispheric stroke. *Lancet*, 2005; **366**: 392–3.

7   Halligan PW, Marshall JC, Wade DT. Visuospatial neglect: underlying factors and test sensitivity. *Lancet*, 1989: **2**(8668): 908–11.

8   Hankey GJ, Warlow CP. Symptomatic carotid ischaemic events: safest and most cost effective way of selecting patients for angiography, before carotid endarterectomy. *BMJ*, 1990; **300**: 1485–91.

9   Intercollegiate Stroke Working Party. *National Clinical Guideline for Stroke*, 4th ed. 2012. Available at: www.rcplondon.ac.uk/sites/default/files/national-clinical-guidelines-for-stroke-fourth-edition.pdf (accessed 18 September 2014).

10 Hankey GJ, Eikelboom JW. Routine thrombophilia testing in stroke patients in unjustified. *Stroke*, 2003; **34**: 1826–7.

11 Keir S, Wardlaw JM, Sandercock PAG, *et al.* Antithrombotic therapy for patients with any form of intracranial haemorrhage: a systematic review of the available controlled studies. *Cerebrovasc Dis*, 2002; **14**: 197–206.

12 Wardlaw JM, Farrall AJ. Diagnosis of stroke on neuroimaging: 'scan all immediately' strategy improves outcomes and reduces cost. *BMJ*, 2004; **328**: 655–6.

13 Wardlaw JM, Mielke O. Early signs of brain infarction at CT: observer reliability and outcome after thrombolytic treatment – systematic review. *Radiology*, 2005; **235**(2): 444–53.

14 Warlow C, Sudlow C, Dennis M, *et al.* Stroke. *Lancet*, 2003; **362**: 1211–24.

15 Wardlaw JM, Keir SL, Dennis MS. The impact of delays in computed tomography of the brain on the accuracy of diagnosis and subsequent management in patients with minor stroke. *J Neurol Neurosurg Psychiatry*, 2003; **74**: 77–81.

16 Chalela JA, Kidwell CS, Nentwich LM, *et al.* Magnetic resonance imaging and computed tomography in emergency assessment of patients with suspected acute stroke: a prospective comparison. *Lancet*, 2007; **369**: 293–8.

17 Kidwell CS, Chalela JA, Saver JL, *et al.* Comparison of MRI and CT for detection of acute intracerebral haemorrhage. *JAMA*, 2004; **292**(15): 1823–30.

18 Fiebach JB, Schellinger PD, Jansen O, *et al.* CT and diffusion-weighted MR imaging in randomized order: diffusion-weighted imaging results in higher accuracy and lower interrater variability in the diagnosis of hyperacute ischemic stroke. *Stroke*, 2002; **33**: 2206–10.

19 Harloff A, Handke M, Reinhard M, *et al.* Therapeutic strategies after examination by transesophageal echocardiography in 503 patients with ischaemic stroke. *Stroke*, 2006; **37**: 859–64.

20 Daniel WG, Erbel R, Kasper W, *et al.* Safety of transesophageal echocardiography: a multicenter survey of 10,419 examinations. *Circulation*, 1991; **83**: 817–21.

21 Bamford J, Sandercock P, Dennis M, *et al.* Classification and natural history of clinically identifiable subtypes of cerebral infarction. *Lancet*, 1991; **337**: 1521–6.

22 Savitz SI, Caplan LR. Vertebrobasilar disease. *N Engl J Med*, 2005; **352**(25): 2618–26.

23 Shin H, Yoo K, Chang HM, *et al.* Bilateral intracranial vertebral artery disease in the New England Medical Center Posterior Circulation Registry. *Arch Neurol*, 1999; **56**: 1353–8.

24 SHEP Cooperative Research Group. Prevention of stroke by antihypertensive drug treatment in older persons with isolated systolic hypertension. *JAMA*, 1991; **265**(24): 3255–64.

25 Saxena R, Lewis S, Berge E, *et al.* Risk of early death and recurrent stroke and effect of heparin in 3169 patients with acute ischemic stroke and atrial fibrillation in the international stroke trial. *Stroke*, 2001; **32**: 2333–7.

26 Eckman MH, Rosand J, Knudsen KA, *et al.* Can patients be anticoagulated after intracerebral haemorrhage? A decision analysis. *Stroke*, 2003; **34**: 1710–16.

27 Yaggi HK, Concato J, Kernan WN, *et al.* Obstructive sleep apnea as a risk factor for stroke and death. *N Engl J Med*, 2005; **353**(19): 2034–41.

28 Myint PK, Luben RN, Wareham NJ, *et al.* Combined effect of health behaviours and risk of first ever stroke in 20,040 men and women over 11 years' follow-up in Norfolk cohort of European

Prospective Investigation of Cancer (EPIC Norfolk): prospective population study. *BMJ*, 2009; **338**: 639–42.

29 Koudstaal PJ, van Gijn J, Frenken CWGM, *et al*. TIA, RIND, minor stroke: a continuum, or different subgroups? *J Neurol Neurosurg Psychiatry*, 1992; **55**: 95–7.

30 Awad I, Modic M, Little JR *et al*. Focal parenchymal lesions in transient ischemic attacks: correlation of computed tomography and magnetic resonance imaging. *Stroke*, 1986; **17**(3): 399–403.

31 National Institute of Neurological Disorders; Stroke rt-PA Stroke Study Group. Tissue plasminogen activator for acute ischaemic stroke. *N Engl J Med*, 1995; **333**(24): 1581–7.

32 Hill MD, Buchan AM. Thrombolysis for acute ischaemic stroke: results of the Canadian Alteplase for Stroke Effectiveness Study. *Canadian Med Assoc J*, 2005; **172**(10): 1307–12.

33 Mateen FJ, Nasser M, Spencer BR, *et al*. Outcomes of intravenous tissue plasminogen activator for acute ischemic stroke in patients aged 90 or over. *Mayo Clin Proc*, 2009; **84**(4): 334–8.

34 Wardlaw JM, del Zoppo G, Yamaguchi T, *et al*. Thrombolysis for acute ischaemic stroke. *Cochrane Database Syst Rev* 2003, Issue 3. Art. No.: CD000213. DOI: 10.1002/14651858.CD000213.

35 Albers GW, Amarenco P, Easton JD, *et al*. Antithrombotic and thrombolytic therapy for ischemic stroke: the Seventh ACCP Conference on Antithrombotic and Thrombolytic Therapy. *Chest*, 2004; **126**(Suppl.): S483–512.

36 Hacke W, Kaste M, Bluhmki E, *et al*. Thrombolysis with alteplase 3 to 4.5 hours after acute ischaemic stroke. *N Engl J Med*, 2008; **359**(13): 1317–29.

37 Engelter ST, Bonati LH, Lyrer PA. Intravenous thrombolysis in stroke patients of >80 versus <80 years of age – a systematic review across cohort studies. *Age Ageing*, 2006; **35**: 572–80.

38 Ford GA, Ahmed N, Azevedo E, *et al*. Intravenous alteplase for stroke in those older than 80 years old. *Stroke*, 2010; **41**: 2568–74.

39 Mishra N, Ahmed A, Anderson G, *et al*. Thrombolysis in very elderly people: controlled comparison of SITS International Stroke Thrombolysis Registry and Virtual International Stroke Trials Archive. *BMJ*, 2010; **341**: c6046.

40 Wardlaw JM, Murray V, Berge E, *et al*. Recombinant tissue plasminogen activator for acute ischaemic stroke: an updated systematic review and meta-analysis. *Lancet*, 2012; **379**: 2364–72.

41 Xian Y, Liang L, Smith EE, *et al*. Risks of intracranial hemorrhage among patients with acute ischemic stroke receiving warfarin and treated with intravenous tissue plasminogen activator. *JAMA*, 2012; **307**: 2600–8.

42 Wang Y, Lim LL, Levi C, *et al*. Influence of admission body temperature on stroke mortality. *Stroke*, 2000; **31**(2): 404–9.

43 Kammersgaard LP, Jorgensen HS, Rungby JA, *et al*. Admission body temperature predicts long-term mortality after acute stroke: the Copenhagen Stroke Study. *Stroke*, 2002; **33**(7): 1759–62.

44 Williams LS, Rotich J, Qi R, *et al*. Effects of admission hyperglycemia on mortality and costs in acute ischemic stroke. *Neurology*, 2002; **59**: 67–71.

45 Gray CS, Hildreth AJ, Sandercock PA, *et al*. Glucose-potassium-insulin infusions in the management of post-stroke hyperglycaemia: the UK Glucose Insulin in Stroke Trial (GIST-UK). *Lancet Neurol*, 2007; **6**(5): 397–406.

46 Ronning OM, Guldvog B. Should stroke victims routinely receive supplemental oxygen? A quasi-randomized controlled trial. *Stroke*, 1999; **30**(10): 2033–7.

47 Bhalla A, Sankaralingam S, Dundas R, *et al*. Influence of raised plasma osmolality on clinical outcome after acute stroke. *Stroke*, 2000; **31**(9): 2043–8.

48 Leonardi-Bee J, Bath P, Phillips SJ, *et al*. Blood pressure and clinical outcomes in the International Stroke Trial. *Stroke*, 2002; **33**(5): 1315–20.

49 Robinson TG, Potter JF. Blood pressure in acute stroke. *Age Ageing*, 2004; **33**(1): 6–12.

50 Morfis L, Schwartz RS, Poulos R, *et al.* Blood pressure changes in acute cerebral infarction and hemorrhage. *Stroke*, 1997; **28**(7): 1401–5.

51 He J, Zhang Y, Xu T, *et al.* Effects of immediate blood pressure reduction on death and major disability in patients with acute ischemic stroke: the CATIS randomized clinical trial. *JAMA*, 2014; **311**(5): 479–89.

52 Furlan A, Higashida R, Wechsler L, *et al.* Intra-arterial prourokinase for acute ischemic stroke: the PROACT II study: a randomized controlled trial. *JAMA*, 1999; **282**(21): 2003–11.

53 Smith WS, Sung G, Starkman S, *et al.* Safety and efficacy of mechanical embolectomy in acute ischemic stroke: results of the MERCI trial. *Stroke*, 2005; **36**: 1432–40.

54 Ciccone A, Valvassori L, Nichelatti M, *et al.* Endovascular treatment for acute ischaemic stroke. *N Engl J Med*, 2013; **368**: 904–13.

55 Vahedi K, Hofmeijer J, Juettler E, *et al.* Early decompressive surgery in malignant infarction of the middle cerebral artery: a pooled analysis of three randomised controlled trials. *Lancet Neurol*, 2007; **6**(3): 215–22.

56 Rudd AG, Lowe D, Hoffman A, *et al.* Secondary prevention for stroke in the United Kingdom: results from the National Sentinel Audit of Stroke. *Age Ageing*, 2004; **33**(3): 280–6.

57 Hackam DG, Spence JD. Combining multiple approaches for the secondary prevention of vascular events after stroke: a quantitative modeling study. *Stroke*, 2007; **38**(6): 1881–5.

58 Patrono C, Coller B, Fitzgerald GA, *et al.* Platelet-active drugs: the relationships among dose, effectiveness, and side-effects. *Chest*, 2004; **126**(Suppl.): S234–64.

59 Patrono C, Garcia Rodriguez LA, Landolfi R, *et al.* Low-dose aspirin for the prevention of atherothrombosis. *N Engl J Med*, 2005; **353**(22): 2373–83.

60 Antithrombotic Trialists' Collaboration. Collaborative meta-analysis of randomised trials of antiplatelet therapy for prevention of death, myocardial infarction, and stroke in high risk patients. *BMJ*, 2002; **324**: 71–86.

61 He J, Whelton PK, Vu B, *et al.* Aspirin and risk of hemorrhagic stroke: a meta-analysis of randomized controlled trials. *JAMA*, 1998; **280**(22): 1930–35.

62 CAST (Chinese Acute Stroke Trial) Collaborative Group. CAST: randomised placebo-controlled trial of early aspirin use in 20,000 patients with acute ischaemic stroke. *Lancet*, 1997; **349**: 1641–9.

63 International Stroke Trial Collaborative Group. The International Stroke Trial (IST): a randomised trial of aspirin, subcutaneous heparin, both, or neither among 19,435 patients with acute ischaemic stroke. *Lancet*, 1997; **349**: 1569–81.

64 Diener H, Cunha L, Forbes C, *et al.* European Stroke Prevention Study 2. Dipyridamole and acetylsalicylic acid in the secondary prevention of stroke. *J Neurological Sciences*, 1996; **143**: 1–13.

65 The ESPRIT Study Group. Aspirin plus dipyridamole versus aspirin alone after cerebral ischaemia of arterial origin (ESPRIT): randomised controlled trial. *Lancet*, 2006; **367**(9523): 1665–73.

66 CAPRIE Steering Committee. A randomised, blinded, trial of clopidogrel versus aspirin in patients at risk of ischaemic events (CAPRIE). *Lancet*, 1996; **348**: 1329–39.

67 Bhatt DL, Fox KAA, Hacke W, *et al.* Clopidogrel and aspirin versus aspirin alone for prevention of atherothrombotic events. *N Engl J Med*, 2006; **354**(16): 1706–17.

68 The Clopidogrel in Unstable Angina to Prevent Recurrent Events Trial Investigators. Effects of clopidogrel in addition to aspirin in patients with acute coronary syndromes without ST-segment elevation. *N Engl J Med*, 2001; **345**(7): 494–502.

69 COMMIT (ClOpidogrel and Metoprolol in Myocardial Infarction Trial) collaborative group. Addition of clopidogrel to aspirin in 45,852 patients with acute myocardial infarction: randomised placebo-controlled trial. *Lancet*, 2005; **366**: 1607–21.

70 Wang Y, Wang Y, Zhao X, *et al.* Clopidogrel with aspirin in acute minor stroke or transient ischemic attack. *NEJM*, 2013; **369**: 11–19.

71 Diener H, Bogousslavsky J, Brass LM, *et al.* Aspirin and clopidogrel compared with clopi-dogrel alone after recent ischaemic stroke or transient ischaemic attack in high-risk patients (MATCH): randomised, double-blind, placebo-controlled trial. *Lancet*, 2004; **364**: 331–7.

72 SPS3 Investigators. Effects of clopidogrel added to aspirin in patients with recent lacunar stroke. *N Engl J Med*, 2012; **367**: 817–25.

73 Sacco RL, Diener H, Yusuf S, *et al.* Aspirin and extended-release dipyridamole versus clopi-dogrel for recurrent stroke. *N Engl J Med*, 2008; **359**(12): 1238–51.

74 Chimowitz MI, Lynn MJ, Howlett-Smith H, *et al.* Comparison of warfarin and aspirin for symptomatic intracranial arterial stenosis. *N Engl J Med*, 2005; **352**(13): 1305–16.

75 Mohr JP, Thompson JLP, Lazar RM, *et al.* A comparison of warfarin and aspirin for the preven-tion of recurrent ischemic stroke. *N Engl J Med*, 2001; **345**(20): 1444–51.

76 Berge E, Abdelnoor M, Nakstad PH, *et al.* Low molecular weight heparin versus aspirin in patients with acute ischaemic stroke and atrial fibrillation: a double-blind randomised study. *Lancet*, 2000; **355**: 1205–10.

77 Cholesterol Treatment Trialists' (CTT) Collaborators. Efficacy and safety of cholesterol-lowering treatment: prospective meta-analysis of data from 90,056 participants in 14 randomised trials of statins. *Lancet*, 2005; **366**: 1267–78.

78 Heart Protection Study Collaborative Group. Effects of cholesterol-lowering with simvastatin on stroke and other major vascular events in 20,536 people with cerebrovascular disease or other high-risk conditions. *Lancet*, 2004; **363**: 757–67.

79 Amarenco P, Bogousslavsky J, Callahan A, *et al.* High-dose atorvastatin after stroke or transient ischemic attack. *N Engl J Med*, 2006; **355**(6): 549–59.

80 PROGRESS Collaborative Group. Randomised trial of a perindopril-based blood-pressure-lowering regimen among 6105 individuals with previous stroke or transient ischaemic attack. *Lancet*, 2001; **358**: 1033–41.

81 National Institute of Health and Care Excellence. *Hypertension: clinical management of primary hypertension in adults.* CG127, 2011. Available at: www.nice.org.uk/guidance/cg127 (accessed 8 October 2014).

82 Leys D, Bandu L, Henon H, *et al.* Clinical outcome in 287 consecutive young adults (15 to 45 years) with ischemic stroke. *Neurology*, 2002; **59**: 26–33.

83 Schroeder SA. What to do with a patient who smokes. *JAMA*, 2005; **294**(4): 482–7.

84 Peto R, Boreham J, Lopez AD, *et al.* Mortality from tobacco in developed countries: indirect estimation from national vital statistics. *Lancet*, 1992; **339**: 1268–78.

85 Hughes JR, Stead LF and Lancaster T. Antidepressants for smoking cessation. *Cochrane Database Syst Rev* 2004, Issue 4. Art. No.: CD000031. DOI: 10.1002/14651858.CD000031.pub2.

86 Silagy C, Lancaster T, Stead L *et al.* Nicotine replacement therapy for smoking cessation. *Cochrane Database Syst Rev* 2004, Issue 3. Art. No.: CD000146. DOI: 10.1002/14651858. CD000146.pub2.

87 Stead LF, Lancaster T, Perera R. Telephone counselling for smoking cessation. *Cochrane Database Syst Rev* 2003, Issue 1. Art. No.: CD002850. DOI: 10.1002/14651858.CD002850.

88 Thapar A, Jenkins IH, Mehta A, *et al.* Diagnosis and management of carotid atherosclerosis. *BMJ*, 2013; **346**: 29–33.

89 Chaturvedi S, Bruno A, Feasby T *et al.* Carotid endarterectomy – an evidence-based review: report of the Therapeutics and Technology Assessment Subcommittee of the American Academy of Neurology. *Neurology*, 2005; **65**: 794–801.

90 GALA Trial Collaborative Group. General anaesthesia versus local anaesthesia for carotid surgery (GALA): a multicentre, randomised controlled trial. *Lancet*, 2008; **372**: 2132–41.

91 North American Symptomatic Carotid Endarterectomy Trial Collaborators. Beneficial effect of carotid endarterectomy in symptomatic patients with high-grade carotid stenosis. *N Engl J Med*, 1991; **325**(7): 445–53.

92 Barnett HJM, Taylor DW, Eliasziw M, *et al.* Benefit of carotid endarterectomy in patients with symptomatic moderate or severe stenosis. *N Engl J Med*, 1998; **339**(20): 1415–25.

93 European Carotid Surgery Trialists' Collaborative Group. Randomised trial of endarterectomy for recently symptomatic carotid stenosis: final results of the MRC European Carotid Surgery Trial (ECST). *Lancet*, 1998; **351**: 1379–87.

94 Rothwell PM, Eliaszew M, Gutnikov SA, *et al.* Endarterectomy for symptomatic carotid stenosis in relation to clinical subgroups and timing of surgery. *Lancet*, 2004; **363**: 915–24.

95 Halliday AW, Lees T, Kamugasha D, *et al.* Waiting times for carotid endarterectomy in UK: observational study. *BMJ*, 2009; **338**: 1423–5.

96 Alamowitch S, Eliasziw M, Algra A, *et al.* Risk, causes, and prevention of ischaemic stroke in elderly patients with symptomatic internal carotid artery stenosis. *Lancet*, 2001; **357**: 1154–60.

97 Fairhead JF, Rothwell PM. Underinvestigation and undertreatment of carotid disease in elderly patients with transient ischaemic attack and stroke: comparative population based study. *BMJ*, 2006; **333**: 525–7.

98 Yadav JS, Wholey MH, Kuntz RE, *et al.* Protected carotid-artery stenting versus endarterectomy in high-risk patients. *N Engl J Med*, 2004; **351**(15): 1493–501.

99 Mas J, Chatellier G, Beyssen B, *et al.* Endarterectomy versus stenting in patients with symptomatic severe carotid artery stenosis. *N Engl J Med*, 2006; **355**(16): 1660–71.

100 Coull AJ, Lovett JK, Rothwell PM. Population based study of early risk of stroke after transient ischaemic attack or minor stroke: implications for public education and organisation of services. *BMJ*, 2004; **328**: 326.

101 van Wijk I, Kapple LJ, van Gijn J, *et al.* Long-term survival and vascular event risk after transient ischaemic attack or minor ischaemic stroke: a cohort study. *Lancet*, 2005; **365**: 2098–104.

102 Johnston SC, Rothwell PM, Nguyen-Huynh MN, *et al.* Validation and refinement of scores to predict very early stroke risk after transient ischaemic attack. *Lancet*, 2007; **369**: 283–92.

103 Chandratheva A, Mehta Z, Geraghty OC, *et al.* Population-based study of risk and predictors of stroke in the first few hours after TIA. *Neurology*, 2009; **72**: 1941–7.

104 Rothwell PM, Giles MF, Chandratheva A, *et al.* Effect of urgent treatment of transient ischaemic attack and minor stroke on early recurrent stroke (EXPRESS study): a prospective population-based sequential comparison. *Lancet*, 2007; **370**: 1432–42.

105 Qureshi AI, Tuhrim S, Broderick JP, *et al.* Spontaneous intracerebral hemorrhage. *N Engl J Med*, 2001; **344**(19): 1450–60.

106 Knudsen KA, Rosand J, Karluk D, *et al.* Clinical diagnosis of cerebral amyloid angiopathy: validation of the Boston criteria. *Neurology*, 2001; **56**: 537–9.

107 Thanvi B, Robinson T. Sporadic cerebral amyloid angiopathy – an important cause of cerebral haemorrhage in older people. *Age Ageing*, 2006; **35**: 565–71.

108 Woo D, Sauerbeck LR, Kissela BM, *et al.* Genetic and environmental risk factors for intracerebral hemorrhage: preliminary results of a population-based study. *Stroke*, 2002; **33**(5): 1190–6.

109 Brott T, Broderick J, Kothari R, *et al.* Early hemorrhage growth in patients with intracerebral hemorrhage. *Stroke*, 1997; **28**: 1–5.

110 Anderson CS, Heeley E, Huang Y, *et al.* Rapid blood-pressure lowering in patients with acute intracerebral hemorrhage. *NEJM*, 2013; **368**: 2355–65.

111 Steiner T, Rosand J, Diringer M. Intracerebral hemorrhage associated with oral anticoagulant therapy: current practices and unresolved questions. *Stroke*, 2006; **37**(1): 256–62.

112 Mayer SA, Brun NC, Bergtrup K *et al.* Recombinant activated factor VII for acute intracerebral hemorrhage. *N Engl J Med*, 2005; **352**(8): 777–85.

113 Cartmill M, Dolan G, Byrne JL, *et al.* Prothrombin complex concentrate for oral anticoagulant reversal in neurosurgical emergencies. *Br J Neurosurg*, 2000; **14**(5): 458–61.

114 Hankey JP. Warfarin reversal. *J Clin Pathology*, 2004; **57**: 1132–9.

115 Siegal DM, Cuker A. Reversal of novel oral anticoagulants in patients with major bleeding. *J Thromb Thrombolysis*, 2013; **35**(3): 391–8.

116 Bailey RD, Hart RG, Benavente O, *et al.* Recurrent brain hemorrhage is more frequent than ischemic stroke after intracranial hemorrhage. *Neurology*, 2001; **56**: 773–7.

117 Wani M, Nga E, Navaratnasingham R. Should a patient with primary intracerebral haemorrhage receive antiplatelets or anticoagulant therapy? *BMJ*, 2005; **331**: 439–42.

118 Ananthasubramaniam K, Beattie JN, Rosman HS, *et al.* How safely and for how long can warfarin therapy be withheld in prosthetic valve patients hospitalized with a major hemorrhage? *Chest*, 2001; **119**(2): 478–84.

119 Shah N, Dawson SL. Intracerebral haemorrhage, prosthetic heart valve and anticoagulation. *J R Soc Med*, 2004; **97**(3): 129–30.

120 Mendelow AD, Gregson BA, Fernandes HM, *et al.* Early surgery versus initial conservative treatment in patients with spontaneous supratentorial intracerebral haematomas in the International Surgical Trial in Intracerebral Haemorrhage (STICH): a randomised trial. *Lancet*, 2005; **365**: 387–97.

121 Vermeer SE, Algra A, Franke CL, *et al.* Long-term prognosis after recovery from primary intracerebral hemorrhage. *Neurology*, 2002; **59**: 205–9.

122 Suarez JI, Tarr RW, Selman WR. Aneurysmal subarachnoid haemorrhage. *N Engl J Med*, 2006; **354**: 387–96.

123 Brisman JL, Song JK, Newell DW. Cerebral aneurysms. *N Engl J Med*, 2006; **355**(9): 928–39.

124 Al-Shahi R, White PM, Davenport RJ, *et al.* Subarachnoid haemorrhage. *BMJ*, 2006; **333**: 235–40.

125 Rinkel GJE, Feigin VL, Algra A, *et al.* Calcium antagonists for aneurysmal subarachnoid haemorrhage. *Cochrane Database Syst Rev* 2005, Issue 1. Art. No.: CD000277. DOI: 10.1002/14651858.CD000277.pub2.

126 Molyneux AJ, Kerr RSC, Yu L, *et al.* International subarachnoid aneurysm trial (ISAT) of neurosurgical clipping versus endovascular coiling of 2143 patients with ruptured intracranial aneurysm: a randomised comparison of effects on survival, dependency, seizures, rebleeding, subgroups, and aneurysm occlusion. *Lancet*, 2005; **366**: 807–19.

127 Stroke Trialists' Collaboration. Collaborative systematic review of the randomised trials of organised inpatient (stroke unit) care after stroke. *BMJ*, 1997; **314**: 1151–9.

128 Drummond AER, Pearson B, Lincoln NB, *et al.* Ten year follow-up of a randomised controlled trial of care in a stroke rehabilitation unit. *BMJ*, 2005; **331**: 491–2.

129 The FOOD Trial Collaboration. Routine oral nutritional supplementation for stroke patients in hospital (FOOD): a multicentre randomised controlled trial. *Lancet*, 2005; **365**: 755–63.

130 The FOOD Trial Collaboration. Effect of timing and method of enteral tube feeding for dysphagic stroke patients (FOOD): a multicentre randomised controlled trial. *Lancet*, 2005; **365**: 764–72.

131 Pennington C. To PEG or not to PEG. *Clin Med*, 2002; **2**(3): 250–5.

132 Dharmarajan TS, Unnikrishnan D, Pitchumoni CS. Percutaneous endoscopic gastrostomy and outcome in dementia. *Am J Gatroent*, 2001; **96**(9): 2256–63.

133 Sanders DS, Carter MJ, D'Silva J, *et al.* Survival analysis in percutaneous endoscopic gastrostomy: a worse outcome in patients with dementia. *Am J Gatroent*, 2000; **95**: 1472–5.

134 Grant MD, Rudberg MA, Brody JA. Gastrostomy placement and mortality among hospitalized Medicare beneficiaries. *JAMA*, 1998; **279**(24): 1973–6.

135 Callaghan CM, Haag KM, Weinberger M, *et al.* Outcomes of percutaneous endoscopic gastrostomy among older adults in a community setting. *J Am Geriatr Soc*, 2000; **48**(9): 1048–54.

136 Light VL, Slezak FA, Porter JA, *et al.* Predictive factors for early mortality after percutaneous endoscopic gastrostomy. *Gastroint Endosc*, 1995; **42**(4): 330–5.

137 Finucane TE, Bynum JPW. Use of tube feeding to prevent aspiration pneumonia. *Lancet*, 1996; **348**: 1421–4.

138 Stroud M, Duncan H, Nightingale J. Guidelines for enteral feeding in adult hospital patients. *Gut*, 2003; **52**(Suppl. vii): vii1–vii12.

139 Davenport RJ, Dennis MS, Wellwood I, *et al*. Complications after acute stroke. *Stroke*, 1996; **27**(3): 415–20.

140 Kelly J, Rudd A, Lewis R, *et al*. Venous thromboembolism after acute stroke. *Stroke*, 2001; **32**: 262–7.

141 Wells PS, Lensing AWA, Hirsh J. Graduated compression stockings in the prevention of post-operative venous thromboembolism: a meta-analysis. *Arch Int Med*, 1994; **154**: 67–72.

142 The CLOTS Trials Collaboration. Effectiveness of thigh-length graduated compression stockings to reduce the risk of deep vein thrombosis after stroke (CLOTS trial 1): a multicentre, randomised controlled trial. *Lancet*, 2009; **373**: 1958–65.

143 CLOTS (Clots in Legs Or sTockings after Stroke) Trials Collaboration. Effectiveness of intermittent pneumatic compression in reduction of risk of deep vein thrombosis in patients who have had a stroke (CLOTS 3): a multicentre randomised controlled trial. *Lancet*, 2013; **382**: 516–24.

144 Decousus H, Leizorovicz A, Parent F, *et al*. A clinical trial of vena caval filters in the prevention of pulmonary embolism in patients with proximal deep-vein thrombosis. *N Engl J Med*, 1998; **338**(7): 409–15.

145 Barton AL, Dudley NJ. Caval filter placement for pulmonary embolism in a patient with a deep vein thrombosis and primary intracerebral haemorrhage. *Age Ageing*, 2002; **31**: 144–6.

146 Turner-Stokes L, MacWalter R. Use of antidepressant medication following acquired brain injury: concise guidance. *Clinical Med*, 2005; **5**: 268–74.

147 Anderson G, Vestergaard K, Lauritzen L. Effective treatment of poststroke depression with the selective serotonin reuptake inhibitor citalopram. *Stroke*, 1994; **25**: 1099–1104.

148 Schievink WI. Spontaneous dissection of the carotid and vertebral arteries. *N Engl J Med*, 2001; **344**(12): 898–906.

149 Hagen PT, Scholz DG, Edwards WD. Incidence and size of patent foramen ovale during the first 10 decades of life: an autopsy study of 965 normal hearts. *Mayo Clin Proc*, 1984; **59**: 17–20.

150 Falk RH. PFO or UFO? The role of a patent foramen ovale in cyptogenic stroke. *Am Heart J*, 1991; **121**(4): 1264–6.

151 Lechat P, Mas JL, Lascault G, *et al*. Prevalence of patent foramen ovale in patients with stroke. *N Engl J Med*, 1988; **318**(18): 1148–52.

152 Overell JR, Bone I, Lees KR. Interatrial septal abnormalities and stroke: a meta-analysis of case-control studies. *Neurology*, 2000; **55**: 1172–9.

153 Messe SR, Silverman IE, Kizer JR, *et al*. Practice parameter: recurrent stroke with patent foramen ovale and atrial septal aneurysm: report of the Quality Standards Subcommittee of the American Academy of Neurology. *Neurology*, 2004; **62**: 1042–50.

154 Mas J, Arquizan C, Lamy C, *et al*. Recurrent cerebrovascular events associated with patent foramen ovale, atrial septal aneurysm, or both. *N Engl J Med*, 2001; **345**(24): 1740–6.

155 Homma S, Sacco RL, Di Tullio MR, *et al*. Effect of medical treatment in stroke patients with patent foramen ovale: patent foramen ovale in cryptogenic stroke study. *Circulation*, 2002; **105**: 2625–31.

156 Kizer JR, Devereux RB. Patent foramen ovale in young adults with unexplained stroke. *N Engl J Med*, 2005; **353**(22): 2361–72.

157 Windecker S, Wahl A, Chatterjee T, *et al*. Percutaneous closure of patent foramen ovale in patients with paradoxical embolism: long-term risk of recurrent thromboembolic events. *Circulation*, 2000; **101**: 893–8.

158 Maisel WH, Laskey WK. Patent foramen ovale closure devices: moving beyond equipoise. *JAMA*, 2005; **294**(3): 366–9.

159 Fleetwood IG, Steinberg GK. Arteriovenous malformations. *Lancet*, 2002; **359**: 863–73.

160 Ogilvy CS, Stieg PE, Awad I, *et al.* Recommendations for the management of intracranial arteriovenous malformations: a statement for healthcare professionals from a special writing group of the Stroke Council, American Stroke Association. *Circulation*, 2001; **103**: 2644–57.

161 Al-Shahi R, Warlow C. A systematic review of the frequency and prognosis of arteriovenous malformations of the brain in adults. *Brain*, 2001; **124**: 1900–26.

162 DiMauro S, Schon EA. Mechanisms of disease: mitochondrial respiratory-chain diseases. *N Engl J Med*, 2003; **348**(26): 2656–68.

163 Etminan M, Takkouche B, Isorna FC, *et al.* Risk of ischaemic stroke in people with migraine: systematic review and meta-analysis of observational studies. *BMJ*, 2005; **330**: 63–6.

164 Kurth T, Gaziano JM, Cook NR, *et al.* Migraine and risk of cardiovascular disease in women. *JAMA*, 2006; **296**(3): 283–91.

165 Scher AI, Gudmundsson LS, Sigurdsson S, *et al.* Migraine headache in middle age and late-life brain infarcts. *JAMA*, 2009; **301**(24): 2563–70.

166 Cleary P, Shorvon S, Tallis R. Late-onset seizures as a predictor of subsequent stroke. *Lancet*, 2004; **363**: 1184–6.

167 Keime-Guibert F, Chinot O, Taillandier L, *et al.* Radiotherapy for glioblastoma in the elderly. *N Engl J Med*, 2007; **356**(15): 1527–35.

168 Stupp R, Mason WP, van den Bent MJ, *et al.* Radiotherapy plus concomitant and adjuvant temozolomide for glioblastoma. *N Engl J Med*, 2005; **352**(10): 987–96.

169 Nathoo N, Chahlavi A, Barnett GH, *et al.* Pathobiology of brain metastases. *J Clin Pathol*, 2005; **58**: 237–42.

170 Stam J. Thrombosis of the cerebral veins and sinuses. *N Engl J Med*, 2005; **352**(17): 1791–8.

171 van den Bergh WM, van der Schaaf I, van Gijn J. The spectrum of presentations of venous infarction caused by deep cerebral vein thrombosis. *Neurology*, 2005; **65**: 192–6.

172 Lewis SL. Aetiology of transient global amnesia. *Lancet*, 1998; **352**: 397–9.

173 Stone J, Carson A, Sharpe M. Functional symptoms in neurology: diagnosis and management. *ACNR*, 2005; **4**: 8–11.

QUESTIONS FOR PART B

1   Which of the following cognitive tests is *least* likely to detect executive functional impairment?
   A. Addenbrooke's Cognitive Examination
   B. Clock drawing test
   C. Wisconsin Card Sort test
   D. Mini Mental State Examination
   E. Trail making test

2   A 76-year-old man is admitted with a history of stepwise cognitive decline and multiple strokes. His CT scan shows high attenuation lesions in three different cortical regions. What is the most likely underlying cause?
   A. Multiple berry aneurysms
   B. Hypertension
   C. Cerebral amyloid angiopathy
   D. Venous thrombosis
   E. Alcoholism

3   An elderly gentleman presents with Parkinsonism, falls and cognitive impairment. Normal uptake is seen in his substantia nigra on SPECT scanning. Which is the most likely diagnosis?
   A. Normal pressure hydrocephalus
   B. Corticobasal degeneration
   C. Idiopathic Parkinson's disease
   D. Multiple system atrophy
   E. Progressive supranuclear palsy

4   A 78-year-old lady presents with a history of a sudden onset of a right-sided weakness and dysphasia 60 minutes ago. A CT scan of the head excludes haemorrhage. In which of the following situations would it be most appropriate to administer thrombolysis?
   A. Her brain CT shows a large area of low attenuation in the left middle cerebral artery territory
   B. Her blood sugar is 24 mmol/L
   C. She had an intracranial haemorrhage 12 years ago
   D. Her blood pressure is 175/100 mmHg on repeated readings
   E. She had a brief seizure at the time of symptom onset

5   Which of the following statements is most correct regarding intracerebral neoplasms in older adults?
   A. Metastatic deposits of non-cerebral tumours account for around a third of cases
   B. In women, after lung cancer, the second commonest source of metastases is breast tissue
   C. Most primary tumours are of meningeal origin
   D. Tumours are usually highly radio-sensitive
   E. Steroids are less effective at reducing associated oedema in older than younger adults

6 Which of the following features is more likely to be present in older patients presenting with schizophrenia compared to younger patients?
   A. Male gender
   B. Thought disorder
   C. Family history of schizophrenia
   D. Paranoid delusions
   E. Flat affect

7 Mental capacity to decide on place of residence is most likely to be present in which of the following situations?
   A. Patient cannot recall the relevant information
   B. Patient says they live with their parents
   C. Patient does not believe the information
   D. Patient has aphasia
   E. Patient accepts the risks but still wishes to return home

8 A 71-year-old man presents with an unsteady gait and confusion. He has a past history of tuberculosis as a child, partial gastrectomy for a benign gastric ulcer 11 years ago, and a myocardial infarction three years ago. He takes aspirin, omeprazole and atenolol. Rhomberg's test is positive. He scores 19/30 on the MMSE. No other abnormalities are detected on examination. His initial blood tests are as below:

Sodium	137	(133–146 mmol/L)
Potassium	4.5	(3.5–5.3 mmol/L)
Urea	5.3	(2.5–7.8 mmol/L)
Creatinine	82	(64–104 umol/L)
Bilirubin	9	(0–22 umol/L)
Alkaline phosphatase (ALP)	103	(40–117 u/L)
Alanine aminotransferase (ALT)	40	(14–64 u/L)
Gamma-glutamyltransferase (GGT)	54	(18–70 u/L)
Haemoglobin	12.1	(13–18 g/dL)
White cell count	6.2	(4–11 $\times 10^9$/L)
Platelets	353	(150–450 $\times 10^9$/L)
Mean cell volume	104	(80–99 fl)

What is the most likely diagnosis?
   A. Diabetes
   B. Folate deficiency
   C. B_{12} deficiency
   D. Hypothyroidism
   E. Alcohol excess

9 Which of the following non-pharmacological interventions is most likely to be appropriate in the management of an 84-year-old woman with advanced dementia?
A. Turning off all lights at bedtime to limit the tendency to wander
B. Aromatherapy oils to reduce aggression
C. Challenging false beliefs
D. Alcohol to reduce nocturnal agitation
E. Hiding outdoor clothing to reduce the desire to wander outside

10 A 69-year-old lady presents with a four-month history of increasing confusion. Examination reveals myoclonic jerks but no focal neurological deficit. She scores 14/30 on the MMSE. Her brain CT scan shows mild atrophy and small vessel ischaemic changes. Which test should be done next?
A. Brain biopsy
B. Cerebrospinal fluid examination for oligoclonal bands
C. CT with contrast
D. EEG
E. SPECT scan

11 A 90-year-old woman is referred to hospital. She has become unsteady on her feet, increasingly confused and has developed urinary incontinence. On examination her gait has a 'feet stuck to floor' appearance. Which brain scan finding is *unlikely*?
A. Effacement of sulci on MR
B. Widened anterior horns on CT
C. Slit-like lateral ventricles on CT
D. Poorly defined Sylvian fissure on MR
E. Enlarged 3rd ventricle on CT

12 A 73-year-old man presents with a 10-month history of progressive cognitive decline. Which of the following findings on examination would be most suggestive of a diagnosis of Alzheimer's disease?
A. Utilisation behaviour
B. Paraphrasia
C. A positive grasp reflex
D. A score of 28 out of 30 on the Geriatric Depression Scale
E. A score of 28 out of 30 on the Mini-Mental State Examination

13 A 76-year-old woman presents with a four-week history of visual hallucinations. She describes seeing cats and dogs within her home, more commonly in the evenings. She does not appear to be particularly distressed by this. Her past history is of hypertension and glaucoma. Her current medication is aspirin, bendroflumethiazide and latanoprost eye drops. Physical examination reveals poor visual acuity only. She scores 27/30 on the MMSE. Her initial blood tests are normal.

Which of the following diagnoses is most likely?
A. Dementia with Lewy bodies
B. Schizophrenia
C. Delirium
D. Psychotic depression
E. Charles Bonnet syndrome

14 An 82-year-old lady presents with a right hemiparesis and a left 3rd nerve palsy. Which vascular territory is most likely to be involved?
A. Anterior cerebral
B. Middle cerebral
C. Posterior cerebral
D. Vertebral
E. Posterior communicating

15 Which of the following statements is most correct regarding the Mini Mental State Examination (MMSE)?
A. Results are unaffected by baseline education levels
B. It does not have a significant ceiling effect
C. It is useful for distinguishing between Alzheimer's disease and depressive pseudo-dementia
D. It does not test language ability
E. It takes approximately eight minutes to perform in older adults

16 An 81-year-old man presents with a two-day history of diarrhoea and a tremor. One week previously he had developed a cough and had been commenced on erythromycin by his GP for a suspected chest infection. At presentation he has become acutely confused. His past history includes OA, gout, depression and COPD. His usual medications are paracetamol, tramadol, allopurinol, sertraline, and salbutamol and tiotropium inhalers. Examination reveals a pyrexia 38.7°C, BP 195/97, pulse 118 regular, he is generally hyperreflexic and hypertonic, his pupils are 5 mm bilaterally and slowly reactive to light. Initial blood tests are normal with the exception of a raised white cell count 14.1×10^9/L (normal range 4–11) and creatine kinase 1316 u/L (normal range 20–192).

What is the most likely diagnosis?
A. Guillain-Barré syndrome
B. Malignant hyperthermia
C. Neuroleptic malignant syndrome
D. Serotonin syndrome
E. Intracerebral abscess

17 A 74-year-old man presents with a three-month history of a resting tremor and a slow, shuffling gait. He has also fallen several times immediately following rising from a chair and has developed urinary incontinence. An MMSE was performed by his GP, in which he scored 29/30.

Which is the most likely diagnosis?
A. Progressive supranuclear palsy
B. Multiple system atrophy
C. Parkinson's disease
D. Corticobasal degeneration
E. Normal pressure hydrocephalus

18 A 72-year-old woman complains of being unable to keep her legs still at night. This problem has gradually worsened over the last two months.
Her GP has recently done some blood tests:

Sodium	134	(133–146 mmol/L)
Potassium	4.2	(3.5–5.3 mmol/L)
Urea	6.5	(2.5–7.8 mmol/L)
Creatinine	74	(49–90 umol/L)
Bilirubin	8	(0–22 umol/L)
ALP	69	(40–117 u/L)
ALT	24	(14–64 u/L)
GGT	32	(18–70 u/L)
Thyroid stimulating hormone (TSH)	3.2	(0.3–4.5 mu/L)
Glucose	6.3	(2.5–10 mmol/L)
Haemoglobin	9.6	(11.5–16.5/dL)
White cell count	8.1	(4–11 ×10⁹/L)
Platelets	225	(150–450 ×10⁹/L)
Mean cell volume	76	(80–99 fl)

What is the likely cause of her presenting symptoms?
A. Parkinson's disease
B. Iron deficient anaemia
C. Idiopathic restless legs syndrome
D. Nocturnal leg cramps
E. Anxiety disorder

19 A 73-year-old lady presents with partial epilepsy and essential tremor. Which of the following medications is likely to be most beneficial?
A. Gabapentin
B. Sodium valproate
C. Carbamazepine
D. Phenytoin
E. Lamotrigine

20 A 77-year-old man with dementia with Lewy bodies develops disturbing visual hallucinations. He is on the following medications: quinine at night, aspirin, bendroflumethiazide. Which initial action is most appropriate?
   A. Add quetiapine
   B. Add haloperidol
   C. Stop all medication
   D. Stop quinine
   E. Add ropinirole

21 A 78-year-old man has developed stiffness and a shuffling gait. Which feature is most suggestive of a diagnosis of vascular Parkinsonism?
   A. Asymmetric onset
   B. Levodopa responsive
   C. Legs predominantly affected
   D. Pill-rolling tremor
   E. Cognition unaffected

22 An older man presents with Parkinsonism. Which of the following features makes idiopathic Parkinson's disease *least* likely?
   A. Reduced up gaze
   B. No family history of tremor
   C. Asymmetric onset
   D. Loss of arm swing when walking
   E. Tremor more prominent at rest

23 An 83-year-old lady presents to hospital with an acute onset of slurred speech, poor balance and difficulty swallowing. A CT scan at that time shows a cerebellar bleed. The next day she deteriorates and is hard to rouse. Her blood glucose is checked but is in the normal range. What is the most important thing to exclude next?
   A. Epilepsy
   B. Rebleeding
   C. Fourth ventricle compression
   D. Ischaemic stroke
   E. Cardiac arrhythmia

24 Which of the following statements regarding drugs used in the treatment of Parkinson's disease is most correct?
   A. Selegiline is a dopamine receptor agonist
   B. Amantadine is a catecholamine-o-methyl transferase (COMT) inhibitor
   C. Ropinirole increases the synaptic bioavailability of dopamine
   D. Entacapone reduces the conversion of levodopa to inactive metabolites within the central nervous system
   E. Carbidopa inhibits the conversion of levodopa to dopamine

25 An 84-year-old man was diagnosed with Parkinson's disease four years ago. It initially started as a tremor in his right hand but now affects his right leg also. He does not have any symptoms in his left side. He remains mobile independently and has not had any falls. He continues to live alone. Postural instability is demonstrated on examination. According to the Hoehn and Yahr rating scale, which disease stage is he in?
   A. I
   B. II
   C. III
   D. IV
   E. V

26 A 77-year-old man presents with a three-month history of worsening memory problems. He developed an akinetic rigid syndrome 18 months ago, for which he has been on co-careldopa 125 mg three times a day to treat suspected Parkinson's disease, with significant symptomatic benefit. He scores 22 out of 30 on the MMSE. Which of the following diagnoses is most likely?
   A. Dementia with Lewy bodies
   B. Delirium secondary to co-careldopa
   C. Parkinson's disease dementia
   D. Vascular Parkinsonism plus dementia
   E. Progressive supranuclear palsy

27 Which of the following clinical features would favour a diagnosis of Alzheimer's disease over a diagnosis of vascular dementia?
   A. Dysarthric speech
   B. Impaired planning ability
   C. Reduced verbal fluency
   D. Getting lost in familiar environments
   E. Change in food preference

28 Which of the following clinical features would favour a diagnosis of dementia over a diagnosis of depression?
   A. Psychomotor retardation
   B. Reduced appetite
   C. Preserved insight
   D. Less marked deficit later in the day
   E. Reduced visuospatial skills

29 Which of the following statements is most accurate regarding delirium in people aged over 75 years, who are acutely admitted to hospital?
   A. Benzodiazepines should be discontinued at the time of admission
   B. It is associated with higher rates of discharge to care home settings, but not higher mortality rates
   C. Cognitive impairment is typically worse at night
   D. Alcohol withdrawal is a rare problem
   E. Visual impairment does not increase the risk of confusion

30 Which of the following statements regarding the treatment of depression in the elderly is most likely to be correct?
A. Mirtazapine does not cause hyponatraemia
B. Duloxetine is better tolerated than sertraline
C. Beneficial effects from medications are unlikely to be seen within four weeks of commencement
D. Serotonin specific reuptake inhibitors (SSRIs) are associated with an increased risk of gastrointestinal haemorrhage
E. The occurrence of pain limits the use of electroconvulsive therapy

31 A 65-year-old woman presents with a five-month history of progressive confusion. She is no longer able to feed herself and just sits in the chair with no speech. Some twitching of her arm has been noticed. An MRI scan of the brain is reported as normal. A lumbar puncture is performed. Which test should be performed on the fluid obtained?
A. Electrophoresis
B. Prion-related protein
C. Viral serology
D. 14-3-3 protein
E. Syphilis serology

32 Which of the following is part of the Abbreviated Mental Test Score?
A. Name two objects
B. Patient's address
C. Patient's date of birth
D. Copy interlocking pentagons
E. Count backwards from 100 in steps of 7

33 A woman with dementia is admitted from a nursing home. Members of the care staff at the home think she may be in pain. Which of the following is a pain-rating scale for people with advanced dementia?
A. Abbey scale
B. Visual analogue scale
C. Picture pain scale
D. Wong-Baker FACES scale
E. Cornell scale

34 A person presents with disinhibition and you suspect a diagnosis of frontotemporal dementia. What might you see on an MRI brain scan that would support this diagnosis?
A. Pulvinar sign
B. Dilated ventricles
C. Anterior temporal lobe atrophy
D. Caudate nucleus hyperintensities
E. Empty delta sign

35 Which of the following neurodegenerative disorders has a pathogenesis that is thought to primarily involve defective tau protein metabolism?
   A. Parkinson's disease
   B. Dementia with Lewy bodies
   C. Multiple system atrophy
   D. Alzheimer's disease
   E. Progressive supranuclear palsy

36 What is the approximate prevalence of Parkinson's disease per 100 000 people in the developed world?
   A. 20
   B. 50
   C. 85
   D. 150
   E. 260

37 What is the most accurate average survival time for a person aged 75 when first diagnosed with dementia?
   A. 2 years
   B. 4 years
   C. 7 years
   D. 10 years
   E. 15 years

38 Which of the following clinical features is most likely to be seen with bilateral anterior temporal lobe dysfunction (Klüver-Bucy syndrome)?
   A. Emotional blunting
   B. Expressive dysphasia
   C. Alien limb phenomena
   D. Auditory hallucinations
   E. Semantic memory loss

39 A 68-year-old man has had Parkinson's disease for over 12 years. He has been on the same combination of medications for over a year. He presents to the medical admissions unit in an acutely confused state with associated visual hallucinations. He is diagnosed with delirium although the underlying precipitant is unclear. It is felt that his medications are playing a contributory role to his cognitive state. Which medication would you reduce (or discontinue) first?
   A. Levodopa controlled release
   B. Levodopa standard release
   C. Ropinirole
   D. Selegiline
   E. Amantadine

40 A man with a history of Parkinson's disease, for which he is on dopamine agonist therapy, keeps going into the garden to dig it up. He has missed his dinner on a number of occasions and becomes irritable when his family question his activity. How would you describe his behaviour?
A. Obsessive compulsive disorder
B. Punding
C. Depression
D. Mania
E. Parkinson's disease dementia

41 A 76-year-old man presents to the stroke clinic following a TIA. He lost power in his left arm for 15 minutes. His BP is 162/86 mmHg. He has had a normal echocardiogram but a carotid Doppler study shows a 75% occlusion of his right carotid artery. He has no history of previous stroke or TIA, heart disease or diabetes.

What is his ABCD2 score?
A. 1
B. 2
C. 3
D. 4
E. 5

42 Which of the following combinations is most likely to be seen in the refeeding syndrome?
A. Low phosphate, high calcium, normal glucose
B. High phosphate, low calcium, low glucose
C. Low phosphate, low calcium, normal glucose
D. High phosphate, high calcium, high glucose
E. Low phosphate, high calcium, high glucose

43 You wish to prescribe an antidepressant medication to an older depressed patient with multiple comorbidities. Which drug is least likely to result in side-effects and drug interactions?
A. Duloxetine
B. Paroxetine
C. Fluoxetine
D. Venlafaxine
E. Sertraline

44 A 77-year-old man presents with a three-month history of worsening memory problems. He developed an akinetic rigid syndrome 18 months ago, for which he has been on co-careldopa 125 mg three times a day to treat suspected Parkinson's disease, with significant symptomatic benefit. He scores 22 out of 30 on the MMSE. Which of the following diagnoses is most likely?
A. Dementia with Lewy bodies
B. Delirium secondary to co-careldopa
C. Parkinson's disease dementia
D. Vascular Parkinsonism plus dementia
E. Progressive supranuclear palsy

45 Which of the following is most likely to be true of people with mild cognitive impairment?
   A. 5–10% conversion rate to Alzheimer's dementia per year
   B. Functional ability is impaired
   C. Normal scores on ACE-III testing
   D. Only language ability is affected
   E. No increased risk of developing dementia

46 In which clinical situation would it be most appropriate to prescribe memantine?
   A. Mild Alzheimer's dementia
   B. Moderate vascular dementia
   C. Severe Alzheimer's dementia
   D. In combination with a cholinesterase inhibitor
   E. Moderate dementia with Lewy bodies

47 You wish to start a depressed elderly patient on an antidepressant drug. Their past history suggests that they are at an increased risk of ventricular arrhythmias. Which of the following drugs is most likely to cause prolongation of the QT interval on ECG recordings?
   A. Citalopram
   B. Mirtazapine
   C. Sertraline
   D. Venlafaxine
   E. Fluoxetine

48 A 73-year-old man presents following a sudden onset of a two-hour episode of right arm weakness and being unable to find the right words to say the day previously. His deficit has fully resolved and neurological examination is now normal. His blood pressure is 127/76 mmHg. An ECG shows sinus rhythm. He does not currently take any medication. Which of the following would be most appropriate to reduce his long-term risk of future stroke?
   A. Aspirin 75 mg daily
   B. Aspirin 75 mg plus clopidogrel 75 mg daily
   C. Aspirin 75 mg daily plus dipyridamole MR 200 mg twice daily
   D. Clopidogrel 75 mg daily
   E. Warfarin aiming for INR in range 2.0 to 3.0

49 Following an ischaemic total anterior circulation stroke, approximately which percentage of people will be dead at 30 days?
   A. 10%
   B. 15%
   C. 25%
   D. 40%
   E. 50%

50 Which of the following statements regarding cerebral autosomal dominant arterio-pathy with subcortical infarcts and leukoencephalopathy (CADASIL) is most likely to be correct?
A. It is associated with migraine attacks
B. It is primarily a mitochondrial disorder
C. It is associated with mutations in the notch 3 gene located on chromosome 11
D. It is implicated in 10% of strokes in people below the age of 45 years
E. Brain imaging is typically normal prior to a presenting with a stroke

51 A 68-year-old woman is referred to a neurovascular clinic. Her husband reports that three days previously she had an unusual episode that lasted for an hour. During this time she continually asked where she was and couldn't remember her birthday night out that had taken place two days before. Despite this she was able to do her usual activities around the house. She now has only a vague recollection of what went on but otherwise feels well. She has no significant past medical history and takes no medica-tion. Her neurological examination is normal and she scores 30 out of 30 on the MMSE. Her ECG shows sinus rhythm. What action should be taken?
A. Reassurance only
B. CT scan of brain
C. MRI scan of the brain
D. Carotid Dopplers
E. Start clopidogrel 75 mg daily

52 An 80-year-old man with Parkinson's disease has been admitted to the surgical ward for an elective bowel operation. His Parkinson's disease is usually well controlled on co-careldopa 25/100 (carbidopa 25 mg, levodopa 100 mg) four times daily, entacapone 200 mg four times daily and co-careldopa modified release 50/200 (carbidopa 50 mg, levodopa 200 mg) at night. The surgical team plan to give his medication in dispersible form via a nasogastric tube perioperatively. What is the equivalent dose of dispersible levodopa that should be given over a 24-hour period?
A. 420 mg
B. 600 mg
C. 660 mg
D. 780 mg
E. 910 mg

53 What is the approximate prevalence of major depression in people aged over 75 years living in the community?
A. 0.5%
B. 1%
C. 3%
D. 7%
E. 12%

54 Which of the following statements is more likely to be true of selective serotonin reuptake inhibitors compared to other classes of antidepressant medication?
  A. They are associated with a higher incidence of anticholinergic side-effects
  B. They are less well tolerated
  C. They are associated with a lower risk of gastrointestinal bleeding
  D. They are associated with a lower risk of insomnia
  E. They are associated with a higher risk of hyponatraemia

55 Delirium most frequently results in impairment of which of the following cognitive functions?
  A. Attention
  B. Orientation
  C. Short-term memory
  D. Visuospatial skills
  E. Executive function

56 Which of the following methods is most likely to be beneficial in preventing the development of deep vein thrombosis following an ischaemic stroke?
  A. Aspirin 300 mg daily
  B. Subcutaneous low molecular weight heparin
  C. Thigh length compression hosiery
  D. Vena caval filter
  E. Intermittent pneumatic compression of the lower legs

57 Which of the following statements regarding tolcapone use in Parkinson's disease is most likely to be correct?
  A. It does not cross the blood–brain barrier
  B. Its use is limited by the risk of developing pulmonary fibrosis
  C. Its use is limited to people who do not respond to entacapone
  D. Renal function should be monitored every two weeks
  E. It can be used as mono-therapy in early Parkinson's disease

PART C

Bladder and bowel

CHAPTER 11

Urinary tract disorders

URINARY TRACT INFECTION

The overall incidence of urinary tract infection (UTI) rises with increasing age. Factors involved include incomplete bladder emptying, and the increased use of antibiotics and catheters.[1] The frail elderly may also be more prone to infections caused by less virulent organisms than younger people (*see* p. 12). It is associated with faecal incontinence, probably secondary to perineal soiling.[1] UTI is 40 times more common in young women than young men.[2] A key factor in this difference is thought to be the shorter length of the urethra and the closer proximity of its meatus to the anus. Half of all women have a least one UTI in their lifetime.[2] However, this gender gap becomes narrowed in later life and is reported to be almost as common in men as in women over the age of 75.[3] This is thought to be due to the development of benign prostatic hyperplasia (BPH) in men, in some cases causing bladder outflow tract obstruction and urinary retention.[4] The insertion of urinary catheters is another strong risk factor for the development of UTI, and occurs more commonly in older adults (*see* later).

So, there are many reasons why physicians may suspect UTI in the frail elderly. However, there is concern that it is an overused label.[5] A retrospective review of 265 hospital admissions of patients aged over 75 years (mean age 85) with a discharge diagnosis of UTI, found a misdiagnosis rate of over 40% when compared to prespecified criteria.[6]

Asymptomatic bacteriuria

Asymptomatic bacteriuria (ASB) is defined as the presence of bacteria within the urinary tract in the absence of associated symptoms. ASB occurs in around 1–5% of healthy pre-menopausal women,[7] but is rare in young men (0.1%).[4] After the age of 75 years it is found in around 7–10% of men and 17–20% of women.[1,8] Among institutionalised, non-catheterised, elderly people, 25–50% of women and 15–40% of men have ASB.[9] It appears to be most commonly found in the most frail patients, especially those with dementia, incontinence or immobility. All chronic catheter users have bacteriuria. ASB typically triggers a local host inflammatory response, and is associated with white blood cells in the urine (pyuria) in over 90% of cases and systemic antibody detection is also common.[9,10] There is a high rate of turnover with patients developing and becoming negative for ASB over time, often with differing organisms.[1] Its treatment does not improve mortality or morbidity but does increase the risk of antibiotic-related side-effects and the development of infection with resistant organisms.[11-13] A number needed to harm of three has been calculated.[8] In patients with chronic urinary incontinence and ASB, eradication does not result in symptomatic improvement.[14] Additionally, the eradication of ASB is associated with high rates or reinfection over the following weeks.[15] In summary, it is not recommended to treated ASB in the elderly.

Subtypes of infection

➤ **Lower UTI** – an infection of the urine affecting the bladder (cystitis) and below. This typically causes any of dysuria, frequency, urgency, haematuria and suprapubic pain.
➤ **Upper UTI** – an infection of the urine also involving the kidneys (pyelonephritis). Typically this causes fever and flank pain, occasionally with nausea and vomiting.
➤ **Complicated UTI** – an infection occurring in a patient with functional or structural abnormalities of the urinary tract or a metabolic disorder (e.g. diabetes). This definition includes UTIs in catheterised patients. Infections in men are usually considered complicated due to the strong association with bladder tract obstruction secondary to BPH.
➤ **Bacteraemic UTI** – organisms originating from the urinary tract are detected within the bloodstream (i.e. blood and urine cultures are positive for the same organism concurrently). This subtype of UTI carries the worst prognosis with mortality rates of 15 to 33% in those aged over 75 years (compared to overall UTI related mortality rates of around 6% in the hospitalised elderly).[3,6,16,17] UTI accounts for around 30% of bacteraemia in people over the age of 65.[3,18,19]

Organisms

Escherichia coli (*E. coli*) accounts for 80% of UTI in young women.[20] It is also the most common organism causing UTI in older people but accounts for a smaller proportion of cases (around 70% of all UTI in people over 65 years old).[19] It appears to be an even less common cause in older men and those with catheters.[3] Alternative organisms implicated include other Gram negative rods (e.g. *Klebsiella*, *Proteus*, *Enterobacter* and *Pseudomonas aeruginosa*), some Gram positive cocci (e.g. staphylococci, beta haemolytic streptococci and enterococci), and occasionally fungi such as candida. Gram positive organisms account for 10–20% of UTI in the elderly and there are also higher rates of more resistant organisms (e.g. pseudomonas) partly related to higher catheterisation and antibiotic prescription rates.[21] Catheterised patients have higher rates of *Proteus mirabilis*, pseudomonas and Gram-positive organism infection,[16,22] plus they more commonly harbour resistant strains of pathogens.[23] Pseudomonas and Gram-positive organisms more commonly cause UTI in men.[4] Generally speaking, the more frail the patient, the less likely that a coliform (Gram negative bacilli that colonise the intestine, e.g. *E. coli*, *Klebsiella*, *Proteus* and *Enterobacter*) will be the cause (*see* Figure 11.1).

Pathogenic *E. coli* generally have short hairs on their surface called pili (or fimbriae) that aid adhesion to the urinary tract surface and help the colonisation process.

They usually originate from the colonic flora. *Proteus*, *Klebsiella* and *Staphylococcus saprophyticus* produce urease that causes hydrolysis of urea resulting in ammonia production. This elevates urinary pH, making the formation of bladder and kidney stones more likely.

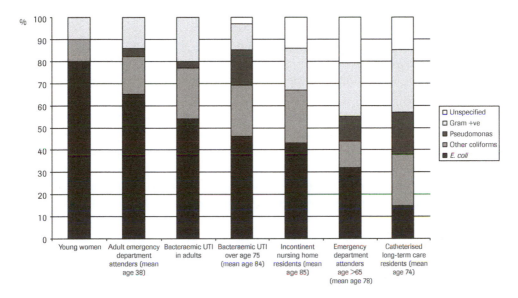

FIGURE 11.1 Proportion of organisms causing UTI in differing populations.[3,16,17,20,22,23,40]

Diagnosis

Symptoms

In young women the presence of any of dysuria, frequency, haematuria, back pain or renal angle tenderness increases the chance of UTI, and the probability is reduced if a vaginal discharge is present.[24] But elderly patients are more prone to atypical presentations of disease (*see* p. 8). In a series of 104 uncatheterised patients with bacteraemic UTI, comparing patients over the age of 70 to patients aged 50 to 70 years, it was found that a presentation with urinary symptoms (except incontinence) was less likely, and a presentation with non-focal (e.g. falls or delirium) or false localising symptoms (e.g. respiratory tract) was more common.[25] In other series of cases of bacteraemic UTI, urinary tract symptoms have been found in only 18–51% of elderly patients.[26,27] So, many older adults with genuine UTIs do not have urinary tract symptoms.

A study has compared community-dwelling patients over the age of 65 years presenting to an emergency department without urinary tract symptoms.[28] The patients were divided into an asymptomatic (100 afebrile patients over the age of 65 (mean age 78) with non-infectious, non-systemic symptoms) and a symptomatic group (100 patients (mean age 79) without urinary tract symptoms but with a least one of acute confusion, weakness or fever). Urine cultures were positive for growth in 14% and 19% of the groups respectively. All of the asymptomatic group would be classified as ASB, and only half of the later group were ultimately diagnosed as having a UTI by the treating medical team. This data suggests that non-specific symptoms are infrequently due to UTI in the elderly.

Chronic symptoms, for example urinary incontinence, increased frequency, urgency, and nocturia are common in older adults and may be confused for signs of acute disease. Studies have suggested that chronic urinary symptoms are prevalent in around 25–40% of men and women over the age of 70 years.[29,30] In a study of older people, the presence of bacteriuria was found to not correlate with the urinary tract symptoms of incontinence, frequency, urgency, suprapubic pain, flank pain or fever (patients with dysuria were excluded).[31]

Subgroups of older adults not reporting typical symptoms despite having a UTI could include those with an indwelling catheter (where the tube is likely to prevent patients experiencing dysuria, frequency and urgency) and those with cognitive impairment (including dementia, delirium and severe dysphasia following a stroke). Such patients may develop an unexplained functional or cognitive decline. In this situation the clinician may have to rely on the presence of one or more signs of a septic illness (e.g. pyrexia, a raised serum white blood cell count or inflammatory marker) in the absence of a better explanation as the basis for diagnosing a UTI.

Signs

Recognised clinical signs of sepsis include a temperature above 38°C (or below 36°C), a pulse rate over 90 beats per minute or a respiratory rate over 20 breaths per minute.[32] Frail elderly patients may be apyrexial when presenting with serious infections. Studies have found that 8–24% of elderly people with bacteraemia had a presenting temperature below 37°C.[27,33,34] In a group of patients aged 75 and over with a diagnosis of bacteraemic UTI, 27% did not have temperature over 38°C.[27] In this group 38% had suprapubic tenderness, 8% had costovertebral angle tenderness and 27% had delirium.

Urine sampling

Urine samples may be tested with urinary dipsticks or by microscopy and culture. Sometimes urine appearance is also used to distinguish those with a UTI. One study found urinary turbidity had a sensitivity of 90% and specificity of 66% for the presence of bacteriuria in the elderly.[35] But alternative explanations do exist, such as the presence of amorphous phosphates in the urine. In older adults there may be difficulty in obtaining urine for sampling, particularly those with incontinence managed with pads or in those with cognitive impairment. Contamination of samples may also be an issue. This is typically considered present when more than one organism is detected in high numbers within the urine. Studies have reported contamination rates between 5 and 31%.[6,35,36] These problems coupled with the high prevalence of ASB limit the usefulness of urine testing and recent guidelines have suggested urine dipsticks should not be used in the diagnosis of UTI in elderly people.[37]

Urine dipsticks

Commonly used urinary dipsticks can test for various parameters suggesting UTI. The most studied are urinary leucocytes and nitrites, both alone and in combination.

Leucocytes   Leukocyte esterase (LE) is an enzyme found in white blood cells and its detection in the urine is a marker of their presence (pyuria). Unfortunately pyuria has been found to be present in 32% of elderly (mean age 86 years), ambulant women without bacteriuria (possible alternative explanations include vaginitis), and in over 90% of patients with ASB in this population.[10]

Nitrites   Coliform organisms can reduce urinary nitrates to nitrites if there is sufficient nitrate in diet and the urine has been in the bladder for several hours. Therefore, a urinalysis positive for nitrites is a marker for the presence of bacteria in the urine. Again, this test is unable to distinguish UTI from ASB. In addition, a false negative result will be obtained when non-coliform organisms are causing the UTI (e.g. Gram-positives and pseudomonas). For both of these reasons it is a less useful test in the elderly.

Leucocytes or nitrites   A urine dipstick positive for either LE or nitrites has been suggested as a way of detecting UTI. Unfortunately this has been found to have both a high false positive and false negative rate. In a study of 200 elderly patients presenting to an emergency department without urinary tract symptoms, only 61% patients with either nitrites or LE on dipsticks had a positive urine culture.[28] Young women with urinary symptoms but a urine dipstick negative for both leukocyte esterase and nitrates have still been found to have a 23% chance of having a UTI.[24]

The higher rate of non-coliform infections in older adults is likely to result in more false negative tests for nitrites, and the high prevalence of ASB will also cause many false positives. In a meta-analysis of studies performing urine dipsticks on elderly patients between 1990 and 1999, the sensitivity and specificity were calculated as 82% and 71% for either nitrites or LE positivity.[38]

A urine dipstick negative for both LE and nitrites has been suggested as a useful way to exclude UTI. In a study of 176 nursing home (NH) residents with episodes of suspected UTI this criteria was found to have a negative predictive value (NPV) of 100%.[39] However, given the high rate of positive tests, UTI could be excluded in only 12 of the 176 episodes (7%) by this method. Additionally, in a different study of incontinent NH residents a negative urine dipstick was found to have an NPV of 80–86% for the detection of bacteriuria, i.e. 14 to 20% of cases may be missed by this criteria.[40] These studies suggest that a negative urine dipstick is an uncommon and unreliable way to exclude UTI in frail older adults.

Urine cultures

Given the high rate of ASB, urine culture is also an unreliable way to diagnose UTI in older adults. But a negative urine culture if taken prior to receiving antibiotics is a useful way to exclude UTI.[9] Additionally, they may be helpful for obtaining sensitivities of organisms to guide treatment in patients diagnosed by other criteria as having a UTI, especially in older adults where atypical organisms are common. Empiric therapy can then be commenced pending culture results. In patients with an indwelling catheter, a change of catheter prior to treatment has been found to result in more rapid symptom resolution and lower rates of treatment failure.[41] This is also an opportunity to obtain a sample of urine from within the bladder, which may be a more reliable guide than a catheter bag specimen, to determine antibiotic sensitivities.

Blood cultures

A blood culture positive for a common uropathogen makes UTI likely,[9] especially if the same organism is also found in the urine (bacteraemic UTI). In a retrospective review of 150 patients over the age of 75 (mean age 85 years) admitted to hospital with a diagnosis of UTI, 69 (46%) had blood cultures sent, of whom 20 (29%) grew a uropathogen.[6] This suggests that the overall incidence of bacteraemic UTI is between 13% (no missed cases of bacteraemia) and 29% in this population. A different study found that around a third of older patients with bacteraemic UTI did not have a pyrexia at the time of admission.[25] Therefore, blood cultures may be a useful additional tool to aid diagnosis in patients who are sufficiently unwell to require hospital admission even if apyrexial.

Other blood tests

Among elderly patients with bacteraemia, 24–26% have been found to have a normal serum white cell count (WCC).[34,42] In a group of people aged over 75 with bacteraemic UTI, 27% did not have a serum WCC above $11.0 \times 10^9/L$ but all had a least a small rise in the inflammatory marker C-reactive protein (above 9 mg/L).[27]

Summary

The diagnosis of UTI in older adults is far more problematic than in younger people. To try to improve diagnosis, consensus criteria have been developed for nursing home populations.[43–45] However, when compared to the presence of bacteriuria and pyuria in a group of patients clinically suspected of having a UTI the sensitivities and specificities were poor (sensitivity 19–30%, specificity 79–89%).[46] In the absence of a gold-standard diagnostic test the diagnosis rests on a combination of clinical features. A suggested simple flow diagram for the evaluation of suspected UTI in unwell older adults is shown in Figure 11.2. If we can improve accuracy of diagnosis, it may be possible to improve access to appropriate treatment, with benefit to patient outcomes, and reduce unnecessary adverse events including hospital-acquired infections.

Treatment

Antibiotics are associated with significant harms in the elderly, including MRSA and *C. difficile* infections (*see* pp. 434 and 296). In addition, around 6% of patients receiving antibiotics within the care homes suffer related adverse reactions (mostly nausea, rashes, diarrhoea and yeast infections), co-amoxiclav (amoxicillin-clavulanate) appears to be most common offending agent.[47] One of the key issues with UTI is avoiding unnecessary treatment of ASB. Urine cultures are often performed in response to non-specific symptoms such as subtle cognitive or functional decline in the elderly.[46,48] Studies have found that 33–36% of systemic antibiotic prescriptions in care homes are for UTI, and 25–30% of these are for ASB.[47,49] The presence of new or increased urinary incontinence was the most common reason for diagnosing UTI. It has been shown that antibiotic prescriptions can be reduced by using protocols and education within nursing homes.[45] In a series of older hospitalised patients 40% of diagnoses of UTI did not meet simple diagnostic criteria, and 46% of these patients had no clinical evidence of a septic illness.[6]

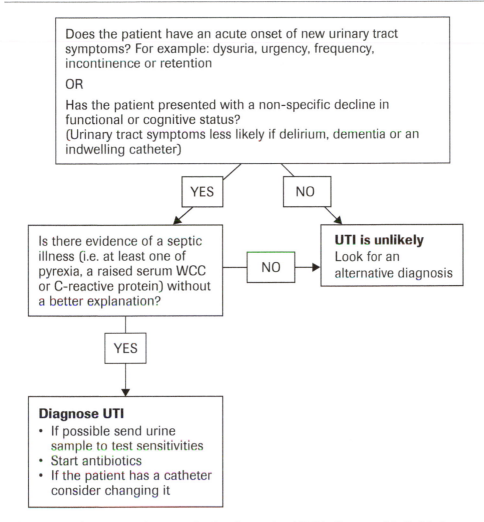

FIGURE 11.2 A suggested system for the diagnosis of UTI in the unwell frail elderly.

The quality of review articles and evidence-based guidelines on the treatment of UTI in the elderly is generally poor and infrequently based on randomised controlled trial data from studies recruiting older people.[50] In addition, doctors' adherence to antibiotic guidelines is poor, resulting in much variability in drug usage.[6,51] The antibiotic chosen should attain a high urinary concentration, i.e. be primarily excreted via the kidneys. This may be more difficult to achieve in older patients with a higher prevalence of renal impairment.

Organism resistance to commonly used antibiotics is rising, especially to penicillins and trimethoprim.[52] In a study of 435 patients (mean age 38 years) attending ED with a symptomatic UTI, risk factors for multidrug-resistant organism infection included advanced age, male gender, residing in a long-term care facility, catheter use and recent antibiotic prescription.[23] The prevalence of multidrug resistance was found to be 10–15% in people beneath the age of 50 without catheters and not living in long-term care. This rose to 45% of those over the age of 65, 56% of those with catheters, and 61% of long-term care residents. Resistance rates vary in differing regions and so local antibiotic guidelines should be followed. Uncomplicated UTIs are less likely to be caused by resistant organisms and so narrow spectrum antibiotics (e.g. trimethoprim) are usually effective and less likely to cause harm. Broader-spectrum antibiotics are usually recommended for complicated UTI (e.g. co-amoxiclav). If urine cultures are sent prior to treatment, antibiotic usage can be adjusted once sensitivities are known – aiming to use the agent with the narrowest spectrum of activity whenever possible.

Generally a three-day course of antibiotics is considered appropriate for uncomplicated UTI even in elderly women. Trials comparing three-day to seven-day courses found similar efficacy and lower rates of side-effects.[53,54] Courses of seven days or longer are usually advocated for complicated UTI.[8] For those with indwelling catheters, a change of catheter prior to treatment should be considered. Evidence for the optimal duration of antibiotic treatment for men is lacking. Some authors propose long durations (>4 weeks) due to possible bacterial prostatitis. However, one study has shown that two weeks of treatment appears to be equally effective as a four-week duration, even in men with suspected prostatic involvement.[55]

Recurrent UTI

The diagnosis of recurrent UTI should not be used lightly. For the reasons stated above, the diagnosis of UTI is often inaccurate. Once someone has been wrongly labelled as having one UTI then further episodes of non-specific symptoms may be inadequately assessed and treated. The person may simply be labelled as 'prone to UTIs' – perhaps reinforced by the finding of ASB on urine culture. Chronic urinary symptoms may also be wrongly diagnosed.

Topical oestrogen therapy has been suggested as a useful therapy to reduce the incidence of recurrent UTI. It is postulated that it may work by altering vaginal pH (to a lower value) and flora. Two small, randomised controlled trials have suggested a benefit of vaginal oestriol cream or an oestradiol-releasing vaginal ring. One trial randomised 93 women (mean age 65 years) with a history of recurrent UTIs to intravaginal oestriol cream or placebo for a eight-month period.[56] The incidence of UTIs was lower in the oestriol arm (0.5 vs 5.9 per patient-year, p<0.001), but the drop-out rate was high (35%). A second trial randomised 108 women (mean age 67 years) to receive an oestradiol-releasing vaginal ring or no treatment over a 36-week period.[57] The chance of having a recurrent UTI over the duration of the trial was 55% in the oestradiol group and 80% in the placebo arm (*p*=0.008). Reported side-effects with topical oestrogens include breast tenderness and vaginal bleeding, burning and itching. Curiously, however, a similar effect has not been observed with systemic oestrogens.[58] Given the current concerns regarding oestrogen use and increased risk of cardiovascular disease, thromboembolism, some forms of cancer, urinary incontinence (*see* p. 273) and dementia (*see* p. 105), they are only recommended for short-term use and so are unlikely to be useful for the long-term prevention of infections. Patient adherence may be an additional problem with some topical therapies.

Continual use of low-dose antibiotics (e.g. trimethoprim) has been tried to reduce recurrent UTI. A Cochrane review found a significant benefit of 6 to 12 months treatment compared to placebo in younger women with uncomplicated UTI, but side-effects were more common.[59] The concerns of using this strategy in older adults would be that infections would simply be of more resistant organisms, and of antibiotic-related side-effects, including *C. difficile* diarrhoea.

Finally, cranberry juice has also been proposed to prevent UTI. A trial compared cranberry juice to trimethoprim in 137 women (mean age 63 years) who had had two or more antibiotic-treated UTIs in the last 12 months, over a six-month period.[60] Trimethoprim was associated with less recurrent UTIs (14 versus 25), although this did not reach statistical significance (RR 1.62, 95% CI 0.93–2.79). But side-effects leading to withdrawal were more common with trimethoprim. A recent analysis of available data did not support the use of cranberry products to prevent UTI.[61] None of the therapeutic options have been shown to be beneficial in the frail elderly.

Urinary catheters

Limiting the use of urinary catheters is an important step in reducing UTI incidence. Catheter insertion results in the development of a 'biofilm' of organic material on both the internal and external surface that acts as a protective medium in which the bacteria can multiply – protected from the host immune response and subject to poor antimicrobial therapy penetration. The inflated balloon within the bladder also prevents complete emptying, leaving a pool of bacteria behind.[62] External 'condom' catheters are also associated with an increased incidence of UTI.[63] Similar to other UTI, catheter-associated UTI (CAUTI) should not be treated with antibiotics if asymptomatic (*see* earlier).

Acceptable reasons for catheter insertion would typically include urinary retention and the need for accurate fluid balance monitoring. Sometimes they are necessary to aid healing of sacral pressure ulcers. They may be used perioperatively or in palliative care settings. Generally they should not be used to manage urinary incontinence (especially if coexisting faecal incontinence) or simply in patients who are unwell.

Despite being strongly implicated in the pathogenesis of UTI, they are often inserted unnecessarily. In a study looking at catheter use within an emergency department, half of all catheters were deemed to have been inserted into inappropriate patients.[64] Another study found that around a quarter of catheters placed in hospitalised patients over the age of 70 years and a third of those in patients aged over 85 years were unnecessary.[65] With catheter insertion being most likely in the most frail patients. Inappropriate urinary catheter insertion in hospitalised elderly people is associated with longer lengths of stay and increased rates of death.[66]

Programmes that have increased awareness of unnecessary catheterisation have been shown to reduce duration of catheterisation and reduce the number of CAUTI.[67,68] Catheters impregnated with either silver alloy or microbial compounds have been developed to try to reduce CAUTI. However, a Cochrane review was unable to identify sufficient evidence to favour any type of catheter.[69] In conclusion, catheters should only be inserted when absolutely essential and should be removed as soon as possible.

URINARY INCONTINENCE

Urinary incontinence (UI) is a major cause of morbidity and frequently a factor in residential care placement. Estimations of its prevalence vary according to the definition used. In a study of post-menopausal women aged over 50 years, 64% had had symptoms of UI within the last year.[70] A study of 6506 community-dwelling adults over the age of 70 years (mean age 77) found that around 18.5% of women and 8.5% of men had had an episode of UI in the preceding month.[71] Seventeen per cent of men aged over 60 report having suffered UI, with 4% reporting daily episodes.[72] UI is common after stroke and has been found in 53% of patients at presentation, falling to 32% at one year.[73] The prevalence of UI in general nursing homes has been found to be 70%.[74] UI is associated with dementia, and it afflicts around 84% of institutionalised demented people.[75] The presence of UI is linked with an increased risk of functional decline, death, hospitalisation and nursing home placement.[71,76] But this may be due to its high prevalence in those who are frail. The cause of incontinence is usually multifactorial in older people and a multidirectional approach rather than a single curative procedure is frequently required. With appropriate, often simple, interventions improvement or cure is commonly possible.

Causes of urinary incontinence

The appropriate passage of urine is dependent not only on adequate bladder and sphincter function, but also on cognitive, mobility, dexterity and environmental factors. The normal control of bladder action requires frontal cortical input in the control of external sphincter contraction/relaxation and also learned behavioural factors that can be affected by frontal lobe pathology (e.g. inappropriate passage of urine due to disinhibition). There is also a need for an intact motor cortex for both mobility and bladder motor control. The bladder motor neurons lie inferomedially and may be affected by

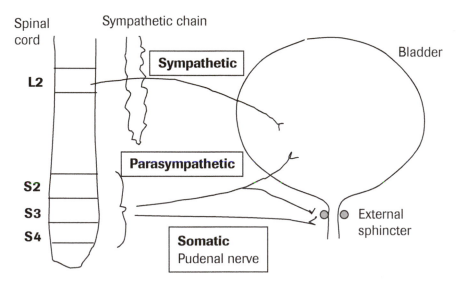

FIGURE 11.3 The nervous supply of the bladder.

such lesions as anterior cerebral artery infraction (*see* p. 197) or normal pressure hydro-cephalus (*see* p. 176). Other cortical processes are also necessary; for example, a patient with a parietal lobe lesion may have difficulty finding the toilet due to geographical apraxia. Lesions affecting the spinal cord or peripheral nerves can impair bladder and sphincter action. A review of the nervous supply to the bladder is shown in Figure 11.3.

Getting to the toilet requires adequate mobility, which is dependent on many different sensory and motor elements (*see* p. 325). A certain amount of dexterity is then necessary to remove clothing. All of these processes may be affected by intercurrent illness, including UTI, and medications. There may be additional environmental obstructions to overcome, such as a flight of stairs between the patient and the toilet.

Factors relating to both quality and quantity of urine may also predispose to UI. This may be excessive urine production due to associated medical conditions (diabetes or hypercalcaemia) or diuretic therapy (ageing itself may also lead to reduced urine

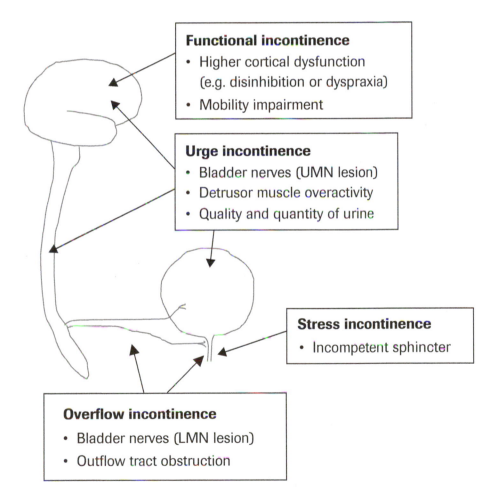

FIGURE 11.4 Factors that are associated with urinary incontinence.
UMN = upper motor neuron; LMN = lower motor neuron.

concentrating ability – *see* p. 7). Or it may be related to the irritant nature of highly concentrated or infected urine on the bladder. The role of the volume of daily fluid drunk in the aetiology of UI is unclear. A study comparing intake to number of micturitions per day in incontinent women did not demonstrate a clear relationship.[77]

On top of all of the above, a number of conditions can affect the bladder and sphincter directly and indirectly (such as a loaded rectum). Bladder activity may be overactive (detrusor instability) or underactive (neurogenic bladder). The bladder sphincter or outlet may be incompetent (stress incontinence) or blocked (e.g. BPH) (*see* Figure 11.4).

Further, ageing alone may make things more difficult. Bladder functional capacity appears to decrease while residual capacity increases. This may be due to increased collagen deposition in the bladder wall. Also, healthy older adults produce a larger proportion of their urine at night than younger people.[78] The nocturnal production of urine may be further increased in the presence of peripheral oedema that can re-enter the circulation while supine at night, which may be caused by heart failure, dependent oedema, or medications (e.g. calcium channel blockers).

Specific subtypes

Urge

Urge UI is also referred to as detrusor instability, overactivity or hyper-reflexia. It is caused by intermittent inappropriate strong contractions of the bladder. It tends to produce symptoms of a sudden sensation of bladder fullness and the need to pass urine, causing the patient to rush to the toilet. When incontinence occurs it is characteristically an infrequent, large-volume loss. It is the most common cause of UI in the institutionalised elderly.[79] 'Overactive bladder' is a term for the occurrence of urgency with or without UI, which is usually associated with frequency and nocturia.[80]

It is caused either by an upper motor neuron (UMN) lesion affecting the bladder nerves or a detrusor muscle disorder. In the elderly, it is often precipitated by cerebrovascular or neurodegenerative disease. It is associated with cerebral white matter lesions (*see* p. 15). In a study of 639 older women (mean age 74 years), a larger volume of white matter lesions was associated with worsened severity of urinary urgency.[81] This may explain some of the association of urge incontinence with cognitive impairment, which may have a quite different pathological basis in older compared to younger people (i.e. primarily a central nervous system disorder rather than a detrusor muscle problem). So, in the frail elderly it may be more a case of 'under-active brain' than 'over-active bladder'.

Stress

Stress UI is due to an inadequate sphincter. This is almost exclusively seen in women and is associated with parity, obesity and previous hysterectomy. Rarely, it occurs in males, for example after prostatic surgery. Characteristically a small amount of urine is leaked following increased intra-abdominal pressure, such as after coughing, sneezing or exercising. It may also be provoked by alpha-adrenergic blocking medications (e.g. prazosin or doxazosin) that affect the sympathetic innervation of the bladder neck and urethral smooth muscle.[82]

Overflow

Overflow UI is usually due to an under-active bladder or a blocked bladder outlet. This can occur with a lesion affecting the spinal cord (e.g. multiple sclerosis) or peripheral nerves (e.g. diabetic neuropathy). It is a common cause of incontinence in older men due to blockage secondary to BPH. It may also be induced by constipation. The incontinence tends to be a continuous loss of small amounts of urine.

Functional

Functional UI is a rather loose term to group together factors outside the bladder and sphincter that lead to incontinence. It includes mobility, cognitive and environmental contributors.

Mixed

Mixed UI is when more than one cause of incontinence is present. This is typically the case in frail older people.

Assessment

History

The history, although imprecise, may give clues to the type of incontinence. It should be remembered that several different mechanisms might coexist. The duration of symptoms may give clues as to the likelihood of an acute causation, such as a UTI or the relative timing to the commencement of medications. Symptoms of duration longer than a week are unlikely to be related to UTI (*see* p. 256). Questions should try to look for specific UI subtypes, for example:

➤ Do you get a sudden desire to pass water and have to rush to the toilet?
➤ Do you ever leak urine when you cough or sneeze?
➤ What's the flow of your urine like?

The frequency and amount of urine lost should be established as well as the distress caused and current coping strategy. The use of a bladder diary to record the timing, frequency and approximate amounts of urine lost may be beneficial. Easily reversible causes should be sought:

➤ UTI (e.g. acute onset and associated with dysuria)
➤ medication-related
➤ constipation.

Nocturia (getting up at night to pass urine) is a distressing symptom and may be associated. It is important to establish if the patient needs to get up and pass water or if they simply were awake and decided to get up (i.e. insomnia). It may be related to other comorbidities (e.g. polyuria due to diabetes or the reabsorption of peripheral oedema while lying flat). But it may simply be a symptom of overactive bladder.

Medications that may induce incontinence include those with anticholinergic properties (e.g. tricyclic antidepressants (TCAs)) that may result in bladder underactivity, and those that may cause increased urine formation (i.e. diuretics). Alpha-adrenergic blockers can cause urethral sphincter relaxation and lead to stress incontinence. Cholinesterase inhibitors may induce urge incontinence.[83] Any sedating medication may reduce either the awareness of the need to pass water or the ability to safely access the toilet. Constipating medications (e.g. calcium channel blockers or opiates) may induce urinary retention.

Past medical history may indicate contributory conditions. A social and functional history may identify likely environmental barriers. Enquire about the amount and type of fluids taken, especially caffeine and alcohol.

Examination

Palpation of the abdomen may reveal a distended bladder or faecally loaded colon. Rectal examination may detect faecal impaction and give an (inaccurate) impression of prostatic size. Neurological examination is necessary to identify any of the many potential contributory factors discussed previously. Mobility should be assessed (*see* p. 327). A formal cognitive assessment including tests for dyspraxia may be indicated (*see* p. 89).

Investigations

The assessment and diagnosis of UTI is discussed on p. 257. Urinalysis may detect microscopic haematuria, when UTI is not suspected this should raise the suspicion of either bladder calculi or malignancy. Baseline blood tests should exclude diabetes and hypercalcaemia. A post-voiding bladder scan can identify incomplete bladder emptying. A residual urine volume of more than 100 mL is abnormal in a younger person. In older people the residual volume of the bladder becomes increased and a value of up to 200 mL may not indicate urinary retention.

Urodynamic studies are sometimes useful in determining the cause of UI. They usually involve the insertion of tubes into the bladder and rectum. The patient requires reasonable cognitive capacity to comply with the tests. Their value is not well defined in the elderly. They are probably most helpful when surgical intervention is being planned, but even then may not always be necessary.[84] A number of different tests come under the heading of urodynamics. The most frequently performed are cystometry and uroflowmetry. Other tests include those that utilise ultrasound or X-ray imaging (with the aid of radio-opaque fluids) and provide more structural information. These investigations are discussed more thoroughly elsewhere.[85]

Cystometry

Cystometry is performed with a pressure-sensing probe in the rectum and a catheter in the bladder that can be used to instil fluid and also measure bladder pressure. Fluid is slowly run into the bladder (up to 100 mL/min). Bladder pressure should only rise slowly with filling. In normal people the first desire to pass urine should not occur until after 200 mL have been put into the bladder and a strong desire should only occur after at least 300 mL. This information gives an idea of bladder capacity. The rectal (abdominal) pressure reading is subtracted from the bladder reading to give an estimate of the pressure being generated by the detrusor muscle. In this way, abnormal detrusor contractions (overactivity) can be detected. During the process the patient is also asked to cough and perform the Valsalva manoeuvre. Leakage of urine in the absence of an increase in detrusor pressure indicates stress incontinence (*see* Figure 11.5).

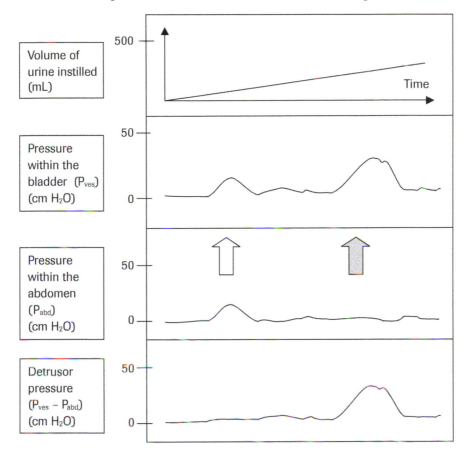

FIGURE 11.5 A representation of data obtained during a urodynamic study.

The light arrow represents the patient coughing – the rise in intra-abdominal pressure is seen in both Pves and Pabd, but the subtracted values (Pves–Pabd) show that there is no increase in detrusor muscular tone. The shaded arrow represents an abnormal strong bladder contraction (triggered by increasing fluid volume within the bladder), which was associated with leakage of urine, indicating an overactive bladder.

Uroflowmetry

Uroflowmetry is the measurement of rate and volume of urine passed during micturition. This is achieved by passing urine into a specialised measurement device. It may be performed following cystometry with the bladder and rectal pressure transducers still in place. In this way the bladder pressure generated can be matched with urine flow. An underactive bladder or a high pressure required to overcome outflow tract obstruction may be observed (*see* Figure 11.6).

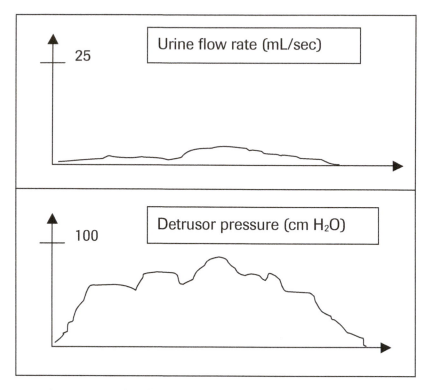

FIGURE 11.6 An example of uroflowmetry: obstructed outflow. Low urine volumes are passed despite high detrusor pressures (Pves–Pabd).

Treatment

In this section general management issues are discussed followed by specific interventions for subtypes of incontinence, and finally the use of catheters and pads. A flow diagram to show an overview of the assessment and management of UI is shown in Figure 11.7.

General management strategies

UI is not always curable, but there is almost always at least some improvement that can be made to the life of the individual. Given the multifactorial nature of most incontinence in elderly people, it is often best managed by a multifaceted approach incorporating different members of a multidisciplinary team. While in hospital this can be helped by goal-setting, careful bladder charting and regular review. In care settings a culture that promotes continence should be adopted. People should be given every opportunity to access toilet facilities rather than accepting incontinence on the basis that it is easier to clean up afterwards.

Clinics led by nurse continence advisers are becoming increasingly common. They are able to combine lifestyle advice with education and treatment strategies tailored for individuals. A study randomised 421 cognitively unimpaired people (approximately half of whom were aged over 65 years) with UI to either four-weekly clinic visits or a

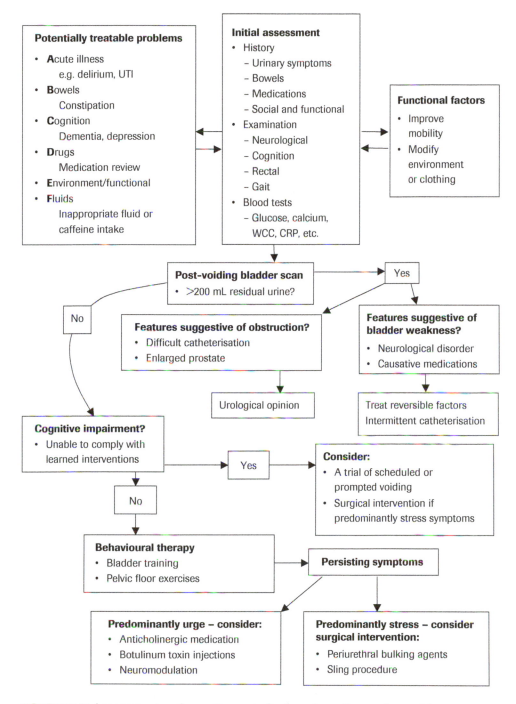

FIGURE 11.7 Assessment and management of urinary incontinence in an older person.

control group for a 25-week period.[86] The most often-used interventions were advice on fluid and caffeine intake, pelvic muscle exercises and bladder training. The results showed an improvement in daily incontinent episodes from a mean of 2.1 to 1.0 in the intervention arm compared with 2.4 to 2.2 in the control subjects ($p=0.001$). A limitation of this study is the absence of a sham intervention for the control group.

A trial randomised 338 overweight women (mean BMI 36, mean age 53 years) with UI (stress and/or urge types) to a weight reduction programme (diet, exercise and behavioural change) or education.[87] They found weight reduction (mean 8 kg) was associated with a 47% reduction in incontinent episodes (28% reduction in the education group).

In patients with urinary incontinence of mixed aetiology, it appears that treating the individual components is an effective strategy. For example, anticholinergic agents can be effective in reducing urge incontinent episodes even in women with mixed urge–stress UI.[88]

Environmental modifications

Sometimes, environmental modifications that reduce the time to access toileting facilities are sufficient to prevent UI. Possible solutions include bedside commodes, anti-spill bottles (that contain a one-way valve for those with reduced manual dexterity) and elasticated or Velcro clothing fasteners to enable rapid removal.

Pelvic floor exercises

Pelvic floor muscle training may be used for stress, urge or mixed stress–urge incontinence. It tends to show promising early results but these do not appear to be maintained. A study found significant initial success rates with an intensive exercise regime compared to a home exercise programme but this benefit had disappeared at a 15-year follow-up.[89]

A group of 204 women (mean age 61 years) with stress, urge or mixed incontinence, were randomised to either bladder training, pelvic muscle exercises or a combined treatment group.[90] The results showed that bladder training and pelvic muscle exercises had similar outcomes irrespective of the urodynamic diagnosis. There was a small initial additional benefit with a combination of both of these therapies but this was not apparent after three months.

Bladder training

Bladder training is a technique whereby individuals are taught to control their bladder activity and then gradually increase the time interval between micturitions. Depending on initial frequency, intervals are commenced at 30–60-minute gaps and then extended by 30 minutes each week. The aim is to be able to have three-hour gaps between toilet visits without the occurrence of UI.

A study compared a six-week bladder training programme to a control group in 123 community-dwelling women (mean age 68, range 55–90 years) who had either stress or urge UI without marked cognitive impairment (Mini Mental State Examination (MMSE) score >23).[91] The treatment group had a significant reduction in the number of incontinent episodes per week compared to the controls (mean 21 pre-treatment falling to nine post-treatment (a 57% reduction), vs 22 falling to 19 episodes (a 14% reduction), respectively, $p=0.0001$). The benefits appeared to be maintained at a six-month follow up assessment.

Urge incontinence
Behavioural treatment

The term 'behavioural treatment' (BT) incorporates several different techniques that share common features. They require patient education on the physiology and anatomy of the urogenital tract. They use patient bladder diaries for initial assessment and subsequent monitoring. There is also some form of intervention that enables the patient to improve control. This may incorporate biofeedback assistance, which helps teach patients how to control their bladder and sphincter muscle tone.

BOX 11.1 Hormone replacement therapy

Hormone replacement therapy (HRT) has previously been advocated as a treatment for female UI. The logic behind this practice is that HRT could reverse the age-related changes in the female urinary tract, for example atrophic vaginitis. Oestrogen receptors have been found within genitourinary tissues, including the bladder wall. Trial results had been mixed, but some small studies had suggested a possible benefit.[92] Recently, a subgroup analysis of the Women's Health Initiative study looked at the effect of HRT on urinary symptoms in 23 296 post-menopausal women over a one-year period.[70] They found that UI was more likely to develop in women on HRT who were continent at baseline than with placebo. Also, those with incontinence at baseline were more likely to become worse following HRT treatment compared to placebo. Therefore, the best available evidence shows that HRT may cause or worsen incontinence and so it has no role in its treatment.

A study that recruited 197 cognitively unimpaired women (mean age 68, range 55–92 years) with urge UI, compared a biofeedback-assisted behavioural strategy to daily anticholinergic medication or a placebo group over an eight-week period.[93] They found an 81% reduction in the incidence of incontinent episodes in the behavioural intervention group compared to 69% and 39% in the drug and placebo arms, respectively ($p=0.04$ and $p<0.001$ for comparison to drug and placebo). There was also a small additional benefit in a subgroup of patients from this study who subsequently combined treatments.[94] However, a number of subjects within this study also had stress UI symptoms that may have responded better to behavioural therapy, biasing the study in its favour.[95] Another study found that behavioural therapy added to tolterodine was more effective than tolterodine alone (n=307, mean age 57 years).[96] But improvements were not maintained at eight-month follow-up.

BT with biofeedback has been compared to BT without feedback or self-administered BT (self-help booklet) in 222 cognitively unimpaired women with urge UI (mean age 65, range 55–92 years) over an eight-week period.[97] No significant differences in efficacy were demonstrated between the groups. This finding suggests that the use of biofeedback is not necessary for a beneficial effect with BT.

Prompted voiding

In those patients who do not have the cognitive capacity to comply with behavioural therapies, prompted voiding is an alternative. This technique involves asking the patient (up to three times) if they would like to go to the toilet at regular intervals, for example two-hourly. When this has been tried with nursing home residents (mean age 85, mean MMSE score 13), around 40% of incontinent individuals had a significant improvement in continence (defined as being wet on less than 20% of checks).[98] The same study proposed that a three-day trial of intervention may adequately identify all of those individuals who would benefit.

In a trial of 133 incontinent women (mean age 85 years, mean MMSE score 13/30) who resided in nursing home care, women randomised to a 13-week programme of prompted voiding demonstrated a reduction in UI frequency compared to baseline and a control group.[99] This was seen as a fall in incontinence episodes from an average of 2.2 to 1.7 per day, compared to a reduction from 2.1 to 1.9 in the control group, that is, a reduction of 26% vs 8%. The actual clinical relevance of this reduction is unclear. Presumably the residents in the treatment group continued to use pads after the intervention period. Also, this was achieved by the use of additional staff within the nursing homes and the practicality of such a scheme outside a clinical trial is unknown. When a prompted-voiding strategy has been attempted to prevent nocturnal incontinence, no significant benefit was demonstrated.[100]

Scheduled toileting

In scheduled toileting, a pattern of toileting is developed with regular, pre-specified timing, for example at two-hour intervals or planned to coincide with an individual's toileting habit. Small trials have suggested a mild benefit but the associated increased workload often leads to poor staff compliance.[75,101]

Anticholinergic medication

Anticholinergic drugs used in the treatment of UI act at muscarinic receptors. Five subtypes of muscarinic receptor have been identified (M1 to M5).[102] The main subtypes found on smooth muscle are M2 and M3, whereas the other subtypes are more commonly found in brain tissue. Available agents include oxybutynin, tolterodine, trospium, solifenacin and darifenacin.

Anticholinergic medications have many potential adverse effects in the elderly (*see* Table 2.2). They have been associated with cognitive deterioration and delirium in elderly patients, particularly those with neurodegenerative disorders.[103–107] They may actually predispose to the development of Alzheimer-type pathology within these patients,[108] and oxybutynin has also been shown to adversely affect cognition in normal individuals.[109] They should only be used with caution in older people and avoided all together in those with baseline cognitive impairment (also, there is little to suggest efficacy within this group[75]). Other common side-effects include dry mouth, constipation, blurred vision, orthostatic hypotension, drowsiness and urinary retention. These often result in discontinuation of the drug.

Extended release (ER) preparations (taken once daily) are available for oxybutynin and tolterodine. They appear to be similarly effective as standard formulations but may have a lower incidence of dry mouth.[110] This finding is probably due to less marked fluctuation in drug levels. Tolterodine ER appears to have similar effects in older and younger cohorts with an incidence of dry mouth of 24% in those over the age of 65 (compared to 7% in the placebo arm).[111]

There has been speculation that newer drugs may cause less cognitive side-effects in older adults than oxybutynin. In animal models, tolterodine appears to have a more marked affect on bladder contraction than salivary gland inhibition. It is less lipophilic and so it is postulated that it may not cross the blood–brain barrier as much as oxybutynin and so it may cause fewer central nervous system (CNS) adverse effects.[112] However, clinical trials have not detected such a difference.[113] Initial studies comparing these two agents have found a similar efficacy with a reduced incidence of dry mouth in the tolterodine group.[101,114,115] A drug company sponsored trial of short duration (three weeks) suggested less impairment on selected cognitive tests in healthy older adults (mean age 67 years) with darifenacin compared to oxybutynin ER.[116] However, the methodological quality was poor and frail elderly or those with baseline cognitive impairment were not included. Until robust trial evidence is available to demonstrate an absence of cognitive side-effects, in at-risk individuals, it is safest to assume that this is a class effect.

The majority of trials have enrolled younger individuals. However, tolterodine has been compared to placebo in 177 ambulant, cognitively unimpaired elderly people (mean age 75, range 62–92 years) with urge UI.[117] Over a four-week period there was a small reduction in frequency of incontinent episodes with 2 mg bd of tolterodine compared to placebo (by a mean of 0.7 episodes per day from a baseline mean of 2.8 episodes per day vs no reduction from 5.1 episodes per day in the control group, $p=0.007$, compared to placebo). It is unclear whether such a change is of clinical significance. A 1 mg bd dose did not significantly reduce incontinent episodes. It should be noted that there were significant differences between the groups at baseline. The main adverse event reported was dry mouth; however, there was only a short study period and detailed cognitive evaluation was not undertaken. A recent drug company sponsored trial randomised 50 cognitively impaired women (mean age 89 years, mean MMSE 15/30) to receive oxybutynin ER 5 mg per day or placebo over a four-week period.[118] No significant differences were detected in Confusion Assessment Method (see Appendix A) scores over this period. The trial did report efficacy in reducing UI episodes. Clearly a trial with so few participants, of such a short duration, and using the lowest drug dose is insufficient to allay concerns of harmful effects.

Several trials have compared oxybutynin and tolterodine. A study of 332 men and women (mean age 58, range 21–87 years) without significant comorbidities, were randomised to either oxybutynin ER 10 mg daily or tolterodine 2 mg bd for a 12-week period.[119] There was a significantly bigger reduction in weekly UI events in the oxybutynin group compared to tolterodine (28.6 at baseline falling to 7.1 vs 27.0 falling to 9.3, respectively, $p=0.02$). There were no significant differences in the incidence of adverse events. The most common side-effect was dry mouth, occurring in approximately 30% of participants in both groups.

A study of 790 women with overactive bladder (mean age 60, range 18–92 years) compared the ER preparations of oxybutynin (10 mg) and tolterodine (4 mg) over a 12-week period.[120] The baseline mean UI episodes per week was 37 in both groups and this fell to 11 episodes per week after 12 weeks of treatment in both groups (a 70% reduction). The only significant difference in adverse events was the incidence of dry mouth, which was 30% in the oxybutynin group and 22% in the tolterodine group.

A transdermal preparation of oxybutynin has also been compared to tolterodine ER.[121] Both drugs appeared to have similar efficacy with less dry mouth in the transdermal oxybutynin group at the cost of application-site pruritis (14% of recipients).

Trospium chloride is another antimuscarinic agent. It has been shown to be more effective than placebo at reducing urge incontinence in 523 men and women (mean age 62) with the most common adverse event being dry mouth.[122] It has no obvious advantage over other available agents.

Meta-analyses of studies using anticholinergic drugs for overactive bladder have found that symptoms were, statistically, significantly improved compared to placebo.[123,124] However, the effect size was small (mean reduction of 0.5 incontinent episodes per day) and of questionable clinical significance. Frail elderly people are likely to have to continue using containment aids, such as pads, but with the additional burden of side-effects from the drugs.

So, it seems that anticholinergic medications may be beneficial in some individuals who have urge UI without cognitive impairment. Unfortunately, urge UI is often associated with cognitive impairment in the elderly. Currently there is insufficient data to demonstrate either efficacy or safety in the frail elderly.[125,126] They appear to be less effective than behavioural strategies in selected patients,[93] and carry significant side-effects. For these reasons they should be reserved for patients at low risk of harm who fail to respond to non-pharmacological measures. ER or transdermal formulations are more expensive but could be tried in those who have significant dry mouth with standard preparations.

Mirabegron

Mirabegron is a beta-3-adrenoceptor agonist that has been used in people with overactive bladder. Preliminary trial data suggest it has a similar efficacy to anticholinergic medications.[127] The incidence of dry mouth was lower but other side-effects, including hypertension (6%) did occur. It has been recommended as a second-line drug for people who do not respond to, or are intolerant of, anticholinergic drugs.[128] However, trials have not been performed in frail older people and the side-effect profile in this population is unknown.

Intravesical therapy

Botulinum toxin has been used to treat urge incontinence. It is injected directly into the detrusor muscle under cystoscopic guidance. In a study recruiting 59 patients (mean age 41, range 20–72 years) with neurogenic urge UI (due to a spinal cord lesion or multiple sclerosis) who currently used intermittent catheterisation, a single botulinum toxin injection was compared to placebo over a 24-week period.[129] There was a significant reduction in incontinent episodes (around 50%) in the treatment group compared to the placebo. Around 25% of the subjects developed a UTI during the study period. Injection site pain was reported by a small number of people. There were no significant differences in adverse effects noted between the two groups.

A non-randomised series of 30 patients found an improvement in symptoms in 73% of subjects.[130] The effects lasted an average of five months. Side-effects included transient urinary dysfunction, difficulty initiating micturition, and an increased residual urine volume.

A more recent study randomised 249 women (mean age 58 years) to receive a single intravesical injection of botulinum toxin (plus placebo tablets) or daily oral anticholinergic (solifenacin 5 mg plus a placebo intravesical injection of saline).[131] Over six months the number of daily episodes of UI fell from an average of 5.0 to 3.3 in the botulinum toxin group and 3.4 in the anticholinergic tablet group. Complete resolution was more common with botulinum toxin (27% vs 13%), but this group was more likely to need a catheter (5% vs 0%) or develop a UTI (33% vs 13%), although less likely to report dry mouth (31% vs 46%).

There have also been studies using this treatment in non-neurogenic urge incontinence. Results suggest that it may be effective and have only a small incidence of inducing urinary retention.[132] It seems likely that botulinum toxin will be used more frequently in the management of UI in the future but whether similar benefits will be seen in the frail elderly is currently unclear.

Neuromodulation

Neuromodulation, or sacral nerve stimulation, involves the use of an implantable electrical stimulation device that acts on the sacral nerve roots to inhibit bladder contractility. It has been trialed in the treatment of refractory urge UI in younger patients (mean age 47, range 20–79) with some success.[133] Disadvantages include cost, the need for an invasive procedure and associated complications (including pain, lead migration and the need for surgical revision).

Acupuncture

A study compared weekly acupuncture sessions to a placebo acupuncture technique in 74 women (median age 51, range 22–82 years) with overactive bladder over a four-week period.[134] They found a 59% reduction in incontinent episodes in the acupuncture group compared to a 40% reduction in the placebo arm but this did not achieve statistical significance. The role of acupuncture in UI, if any, is not yet defined.

Stress incontinence
Pelvic muscle exercises

The theory with pelvic muscle exercises is that pubococcygeus muscle's action can be increased, resulting in an increased closing force on the urethra.[135] They are suitable for cognitively unimpaired, highly motivated women. Exercises need to be repeated 30–200 times per day. They appear to be more effective than no treatment or a placebo treatment but their actual effect size is hard to judge on available evidence.[136] Such exercises must be continued indefinitely. When an exercise programme was compared to a biofeedback technique, there were no significant differences in outcome between the groups (but both did better than a control group).[137]

Vaginal cones

Vaginal cones are a series of objects of varying weight that the incontinent woman holds within the vaginal cavity for around 20 minutes a day. The weight is gradually increased with the aim of strengthening the pelvic floor. When compared to pelvic floor exercises, vaginal cones were less effective.[138] They are occasionally associated with vaginitis or bleeding and patient concordance is poor. Their use can no longer be recommended.

Electrical stimulation

External electrical stimulators have been used to try to improve pelvic floor musculature. This technique appears to be less effective than standard pelvic muscle exercises and is associated with some discomfort and motivational problems.[138] When it has been combined with a behavioural training programme, there was no additional benefit compared to BT alone.[139] Its use can no longer be recommended.

Drugs

An alpha agonist agent (phenylpropanolamine hydrochloride) has been found to be as effective as pelvic floor muscle exercises for stress UI in 157 women (mean age 68, range 55–90 years) over a six-month period.[135] Side-effects limit the clinical use of such agents, the most important being hypertension. A Cochrane review concluded that there was 'weak evidence' of efficacy of a variety of adrenergic compounds in women with stress UI but a number of associated side-effects.[140]

More recently, a combined serotonin and norepinephrine reuptake inhibitor (duloxetine) has been proposed for stress incontinence. The theory is that serotonergic neurons may suppress bladder parasympathetic actions. A trial recruited 494 women (mean age 51, range 24–83 years) with predominant stress UI and randomised to duloxetine or placebo over a 12-week period.[141] There was a reduction in the median frequency of UI (50% vs 29% for placebo, $p=0.002$). However, there was no associated improvement in quality of life scores and there were significant adverse events reported: 22% of the duloxetine group discontinued treatment due to adverse events, compared to 5% of the placebo group ($p<0.001$). Adverse events seen significantly more often were nausea, dry mouth, constipation, fatigue, insomnia, dizziness, increased sweating, vomiting, somnolence and tremor. It may well be that the positive effects of this medication were mediated either by alpha-agonist properties or by an anticholinergic effect in those with mixed incontinence given the high incidence of anticholinergic type side-effects. It seems hard to justify the use of duloxetine on the current evidence of such a small beneficial effect, particularly in the elderly who are more likely to have adverse reactions.

Surgery

A variety of surgical procedures have been developed for the treatment of stress incontinence. Early reports suggest high rates of improvement or cure. Trials of open retropubic colposuspension have found a 69–88% cure rate.[142] However, the longer-term results may be less impressive. In a survey of community-dwelling women, 73% who had previously undergone surgery had had at least one incontinent episode in the last month and 53% were currently using absorbent pads.[143] Colposuspension aims to elevate the tissues that surround the lower bladder and upper urethra. Laparoscopic colposuspension has the advantage of quicker recovery times due to the absence of a major abdominal incision but possibly at the expense of poorer long-term outcomes.[144] Anterior vaginal repair uses an approach through the vaginal wall. Bladder neck needle suspension employs sutures to attach the vaginal to the abdominal wall. Available evidence suggests that both of these methods are less successful than open abdominal retropubic colposuspension.[145,146]

More recent work has focused on less invasive surgical procedures, leading to the pubovaginal sling becoming more popular. Even less invasive methods of this procedure include tension-free vaginal tape. The tape supports the mid-urethra and it is thought that this prevents incontinence by inducing some urethral kinking.[147] A follow-up study of 692 women who had undergone a tension free tape procedure between two and eight years previously showed that those with pure stress incontinence had an 85% chance of cure even after four to eight years, whereas those with mixed incontinence had only a 30% chance of cure after this amount of time.[148]

Periurethral bulking agents

Injectable periurethral bulking agents have become increasingly popular as a minimally invasive treatment for female stress UI. The initial substance injected was collagen; however, there are now various alternative agents.[149] It may be performed under local anaesthesia and endoscopic guidance. The injectable material is placed submucosally, adjacent to the proximal urethra. This appears to increase urethral closing pressure and prevent urine leakage. Early results from small series are mixed, showing improvement in 11–85% and cure in 7–95%.[149] A Cochrane review was unable to find robust evidence of efficacy.[150]

Catheters

Indwelling catheters

In some circumstances catheters will be the most appropriate intervention for the patient. However, they are associated with a number of problems, including blockage, infection (*see* p. 263) and interference with sexual activity. They have also been associated with chronic pyelonephritis and renal inflammation.[151] Recurrent blockage of catheters can be minimised by using silicon-coated devices and maintaining a high fluid intake. Bypassing of catheters can be reduced by using a catheter with a smaller lumen (larger bore tubes can hamper the efficacy of sphincter closure around them) and, if this fails, the concomitant use of bladder-relaxing medication.[152] Mobile patients will use a 300 mL portable leg bag. They, or their carers, need to be educated on the appropriate use of this.

Intermittent catheterisation

Intermittently passing a catheter to drain a full bladder is an alternative to a permanent indwelling catheter. This can either be self-administered or performed by a carer. It may be associated with a lower infection rate than indwelling devices and has other advantages such as preservation of sexual function. Evidence suggests that it is well-tolerated by the elderly.[153]

External catheters

Condom-like external catheters are sometimes appropriate. Their main disadvantage is difficulty retaining them. They are also prone to increased infection rates and skin breakdown.

Pads

There is a variety of pads available for use in incontinent individuals. They can be divided into body-worn pads and flat bed pads. The body-worn pads can be either disposable or machine washable. Flat bed pads are a form of absorbent sheet that can be placed beneath a patient in bed. The body-worn pads are almost always preferable as they are able to absorb more fluid, may have a gel lining that keeps urine away from the skin, do not affect the pressure distribution properties of specialised mattresses and do not become wrinkled under the patient, causing increased pressure damage.[154] The is some evidence that disposable pads are associated with less skin adverse events than their washable equivalents.[155]

PROSTATE DISORDERS
Benign prostatic hyperplasia

An increase in prostate cell number (benign prostatic hyperplasia (BPH)) is very common in older men (80%), with a higher risk associated with obesity and diabetes. This may lead to prostate enlargement, which is seen in around 50% of older men, and 50% of these men will have lower urinary tract symptoms. Bladder outlet obstruction may lead to overflow incontinence.

Alpha-blockers (e.g. tamsulosin or doxazosin) reduce smooth muscle contractility within the bladder neck. They are usually considered the first-line treatment and lead to symptomatic improvement in those who respond (around 70% of men) within 48 hours.[156] All such drugs appear to have a similar efficacy, improving maximal urine flow rate by around 15–30%.[156] The most troublesome side-effect in the elderly is their tendency to cause postural hypotension.

5-alpha reductase inhibitors (e.g. finasteride or dutasteride) block the production of dihydrotestosterone (*see* Figure 16.2). They cause a slow reduction in prostatic size (of about 25–30% of volume). It may take over six months for significant symptomatic benefits to be noted.[156] Side-effects include reduced libido, erectile dysfunction and gynaecomastia. They do not increase the risk of hip fracture in older men.[157] Serum prostate specific antigen (PSA) levels are reduced by around 50% while on these drugs. This may need to be taken into account in those with a history of prostate cancer.

A study of 3047 men (mean age 63 years) with BPH allocated participants to either placebo, doxazosin, finasteride, or a combination of these latter two drugs.[158] The follow-up period was 4.5 years. Compared to placebo all three drug regimens reduced urinary tract symptoms, but the reduction was greatest with combination therapy. Finasteride, alone or in combination, reduced the risk of urinary retention, but doxazosin alone did not. Adverse events seen with doxazosin included postural hypotension. Finasteride was associated with an increased risk of erectile dysfunction and reduced libido.

Surgical procedures (usually transurethral resection) lead to symptomatic benefit in 80–90% of patients. It is especially recommended if urinary retention, hydronephrosis or renal impairment are present. It may also be considered in those who have not had symptomatic relief on medical therapy.

Prostate cancer

Prostate cancer has a median age of presentation of around 70 years. It is the commonest cancer in older men.[159] There is an increased risk in those with a family history of this condition. It is usually asymptomatic. Urinary symptoms are rare as tumours tend to arise in posterior prostate. Occasionally it may present as bone pain secondary to metastatic disease.

Prostate specific antigen is a marker of prostate cancer. There has been controversy as to its efficacy as a screening test for this condition. A recent trial randomised 162 243 men aged 55 to 69 to undergo PSA screening, or not.[160] They found that screening was associated with a significantly lower rate of death from prostate cancer (RR 0.80, 95% CI 0.65–0.98), but did cause considerable over-estimation of diagnosis. However, another study of 76 693 men failed to find a significant difference in either incidence of prostate cancer or mortality rates over a 7 to 10 year period.[161] Definitive diagnosis is usually made by ultrasound-guided transrectal biopsy.

Patients with distant metastases have a poor prognosis, with mean survival times of between 24 and 48 months.[159] Anti-androgen treatment (e.g. bilateral orchidectomy or gonadorelin analogues) is indicated. Around 75% of men will have some symptomatic relief from this treatment (e.g. reduced bone pain).[159] Side-effects of anti-androgen treatments include fatigue, depression, erectile dysfunction and hot flushes. They are also associated with an increased risk of osteoporosis. Other side-effects with long-term treatment may include an increased risk of vascular disease and diabetes.[162] Surgery (radical prostatectomy) and radiotherapy may be appropriate in some patients with high-grade tumours.

In a review of over 200 000 cases of men diagnosed with prostate cancer between the ages of 65 and 84, overall approximately 8% died of prostate cancer.[163] Around 60%

of the men had low to moderate grade tumours. Of these men just 2% died of prostate cancer. Cardiovascular disease and other cancers were more common causes of death. This questions the role of anti-androgens in such men. Patients with localised prostate cancer and a life expectancy of less than 10 years are recommended to initially simply have their disease monitored.[159]

REFERENCES

1 Baldassarre JS, Kaye D. Special problems of urinary tract infection in the elderly. *Med Clin N Am*, 1991; **75**(2): 375–90.

2 McLaughlin SP, Carson CC. Urinary tract infections in women. *Med Clin N Am*, 2004; **88**: 417–29.

3 Tal S, Guller V, Levi S, *et al.* Profile and prognosis of febrile elderly patients with bacteremic urinary tract infection. *J Infection*, 2005; **50**: 296–305.

4 Lipsky BA. Urinary tract infections in men: epidemiology, pathophysiology, diagnosis, and treatment. *Ann Intern Med*, 1989; **110**(2): 138–50.

5 McMurdo MET, Gillespie ND. Urinary tract infection in old age: over-diagnosed and over-treated. *Age Ageing*, 2000; **29**: 297–8.

6 Woodford HJ, George J. Diagnosis and management of urinary tract infection in hospitalized older people. *J Am Geriatr Soc*, 2009; **57**(1): 107–14.

7 Colgan R, Nicolle LE, McGlone A, *et al.* Asymptomatic bacteriuria in adults. *Am Fam Phys*, 2006; **74**(6): 985–90.

8 Scottish Intercollegiate Network (SIGN). *Management of Suspected Bacterial Urinary Tract Infection in Adults No. 88.* 2012 (updated). www.sign.ac.uk/pdf/sign88.pdf (accessed 3 November 2014).

9 Nicolle LE. Urinary infections in the elderly: symptomatic or asymptomatic? *Int J Antimicrob Agents*, 1999; **11**: 265–8.

10 Boscia JA, Abrutyn E, Levison ME, *et al.* Pyuria and asymptomatic bacteriuria in elderly ambulatory women. *Ann Intern Med*, 1989; **110**(5): 404–5.

11 Nicolle LE, Mayhew WJ, Bryan L. Prospective randomised comparison of therapy and no therapy for asymptomatic bacteriuria in institutionalized elderly women. *Am J Med*, 1987; **83**: 27–33.

12 Abrutyn E, Berlin J, Mossey J, *et al.* Does treatment of asymptomatic bacteriuria in older ambulatory women reduce subsequent symptoms of urinary tract infection? *J Am Geriatr Soc*, 1994; **44**(3): 293–5.

13 Abrutyn E, Mossey J, Berlin JA, *et al.* Does asymptomatic bacteriuria predict mortality and does antimicrobial treatment reduce mortality in elderly ambulatory women? *Ann Intern Med*, 1994; **120**(10): 827–33.

14 Ouslander JG, Schapira M, Schnelle JF, *et al.* Does eradicating bacteriuria affect the severity of chronic urinary incontinence in nursing home residents? *Ann Intern Med*, 1995; **122**(10): 749–54.

15 Nicolle LE. Urinary tract infections in long-term-care facilities. *Infect Control Hosp Edipdemiol*, 2001; **22**: 167–75.

16 Ackermann RJ, Monroe PW. Bacteremic urinary tract infection in older people. *J Am Geriatr Soc*, 1996; **44**(8): 927–33.

17 Ginde AA, Rhee SH, Katz ED. Predictors of outcome in geriatric patients with urinary tract infections. *J Emerg Med*, 2004; **27**(2): 101–8.

18 Whitelaw DA, Rayner BL, Willcox PA. Community-acquired bacteremia in the elderly: a prospective study of 121 cases. *J Am Geriatr Soc*, 1992; **40**(10): 996–1000.

19 Eykyn SJ. Urinary tract infections in the elderly. *Br J Urol*, 1998; **82**(Suppl. 1): 79–84.

20 Stamm WE, Hooton TM. Mangement of urinary tract infections in adults. *N Engl J Med*, 1993; **329**(18): 1328–34.

21 Ronald A. The etiology of urinary tract infection: traditional and emerging pathogens. *Am J Med*, 2002; **113**(Suppl. 1A): S14–19.

22 Smith PW, Selp CW, Schaefer SC, *et al.* Microbiologic survey of long-term care facilities. *Am J Infect Control*, 2000; **28**(1): 8–13.

23 Wright SW, Wrenn KD, Haynes M, *et al.* Prevalence and risk factors for multidrug resistant uropathogens in ED patients. *Am J Emerg Med*, 2000; **18**(2): 143–6.

24 Bent S, Nallamothu BK, Simel DL, *et al.* Does this woman have an acute uncomplicated urinary tract infection? *JAMA*, 2002; **287**(20): 2701–10.

25 Barkham TMS, Martin FC, Eykyn SJ. Delay in the diagnosis of bacteraemic urinary tract infection in elderly patients. *Age Ageing*, 1996; **25**: 130–2.

26 Esposito AL, Gleckman RA, Cram S, *et al.* Community-acquired bacteraemia in the elderly: analysis of one hundred consecutive episodes. *J Am Geriatr Soc*, 1980; **28**: 315–19.

27 Woodford HJ, Graham C, Meda M, *et al.* Bacteremic urinary tract infection in hospitalized older patients: are any currently available diagnostic criteria sensitive enough? *J Am Geriatr Soc*, 2011; **59**: 567–8.

28 Ducharme J, Neilson S, Ginn JL. Can urine cultures and reagent test strips be used to diagnose urinary tract infection in elderly emergency department patients without focal urinary symptoms? *CJEM*, 2007; **9**(2): 87–92.

29 Boyle P, Robertson C, Mazzetta C, *et al.* The prevalence of lower urinary tract symptoms in men and women in four centres. The UrEpik study. *BJU Int*, 2003; **92**: 409–14.

30 Kupelian V, Wei JT, O'Leary MP, *et al.* Prevalence of lower urinary tract symptoms and effect on quality of life in a racially and ethnically diverse random sample: the Boston Area Community Health (BACH) survey. *Arch Intern Med*, 2006; **166**: 2381–7.

31 Boscia JA, Kobasa WD, Abrutyn E, *et al.* Lack of association between bacteriuria and symptoms in the elderly. *Am J Med*, 1986; **81**: 979–82.

32 Bone RC, Balk RA, Cerra FB, *et al.* Definitions for sepsis and organ failure and guidelines for the use of innovative therapies in sepsis. ACCP/SCCM Consensus Conference Committee. *Chest*, 1992; **101**: 1644–55.

33 Whitelaw DA, Rayner BL, Willcox PA. Community-acquired bacteremia in the elderly: a prospective study of 121 cases. *J Am Geriatr Soc*, 1992; **40**: 996–1000.

34 Fontanarosa PB, Kaeberlein FJ, Gerson LW, *et al.* Difficulty in predicting bacteremia in elderly emergency patients. *Ann Emerg Med*, 1992; **21**: 842–8.

35 Flanagan PG, Rooney PG, Davies EA, *et al.* Evaluation of four screening tests for bacteriuria in elderly people. *Lancet*, 1989: 1117–19.

36 Lifshitz E, Kramer L. Outpatient urine culture: does collection technique matter? *Arch Intern Med*, 2000; **160**(16): 2537–40.

37 Scottish Intercollegiate Network (SIGN). *Diagnosis and Management of Suspected UTI in Older People. No. 88.* 2014. Available at: www.sign.ac.uk/pdf/sign88_algorithm_older.pdf (accessed 3 November 2014).

38 Deville WLJM, Yzermans JC, van Duijn NP, *et al.* The urine dipstick test useful to rule out infections: a meta-analysis of the accuracy. *BMC Urology*, 2004; **4**: 4.

39 Juthani-Mehta M, Tinetti M, Perrelli E, *et al.* Role of dipstick testing in the evaluation of urinary tract infection in nursing home residents. *Infect Control Hosp Epidemiol*, 2007; **28**: 889–91.

40 Ouslander JG, Schapira M, Fingold S, *et al.* Accuracy of rapid urine screening tests among incontinent nursing home residents with asymptomatic bacteriuria. *J Am Geriatr Soc*, 1995; **43**(7): 772–5.

41 Raz R, Schiller D, Nicolle LE. Chronic indwelling catheter replacement before antimicrobial therapy for symptomatic urinary tract infection. *J Urol*, 2000; **164**(4): 1254–8.

42 Chassagne P, Perol M, Doucet J, *et al.* Is presentation of bacteremia in the elderly the same as in younger patients? *Am J Med*, 1996; **100**: 65–70.

43 McGeer A, Campbell B, Emori TG. Definitions of infection for surveillance in long-term care facilities. *Am J Infect Control*, 1991; **19**: 1–7.

44 Loeb M, Bentley DW, Bradley S. Development of minimum criteria for the initiation of antibiotics in residents of long-term care facilities: results of a consensus conference. *Infect Control Hosp Epidemiol*, 2001; **22**: 120–4.

45 Loeb M, Brazil K, Lohfeld L, *et al.* Effect of a multifaceted intervention on number of antimicrobial prescriptions for suspected urinary tract infections in residents of nursing homes: cluster randomised controlled trial. *BMJ*, 2005; **331**: 669–73.

46 Juthani-Mehta M, Tinetti M, Perrelli E, *et al.* Diagnostic accuracy of criteria for urinary tract infection in a cohort of nursing home residents. *J Am Geriatr Soc*, 2007; **55**: 1072–7.

47 Loeb M, Simor AE, Landry L, *et al.* Antibiotic use in Ontario facilities that provide chronic care. *J Gen Intern Med*, 2001; **16**: 376–83.

48 Walker S, McGreer A, Simor AE, *et al.* Why are antibiotics prescribed for asymptomatic bacteriuria in institutionalized elderly people? A qualitative study of physicians' and nurses' perceptions. *CMAJ*, 2000; **163**(3): 273–7.

49 Warren JW, Palumbo FB, Fitterman L, *et al.* Incidence and characteristics of antibiotic use in aged nursing home patients. *J Am Geriatr Soc*, 1991; **39**(10): 963–72.

50 Lutters M, Vogt N. What's the basis for treating infections your way? Quality assessment of review articles on the treatment of urinary and respiratory tract infections in older people. *J Am Geriatr Soc*, 2000; **48**(11): 1454–61.

51 Martinez MA, Inglada L, Ochoa C, *et al.* Assessment of antibiotic prescription in acute urinary tract infections in adults. *J Infect*, 2007; **54**: 235–44.

52 Gupta K. Addressing antibiotic resistance. *Am J Med*, 2002; 113(Suppl. 1A): S29–34.

53 Lutters M, Vogt-Ferrier NB. Antibiotic duration for treating uncomplicated, symptomatic lower urinary tract infections in elderly women. *Cochrane Database Syst Rev* 2002, issue 3.

54 Vogel T, Verreault R, Gourdeau M, *et al.* Optimal duration of antibiotic therapy for uncomplicated urinary tract infection in older women: a double blind randomized controlled trial. *CMAJ*, 2004; **170**(4): 469–73.

55 Ulleryd P. Sandberg T. Ciprofloxacin for 2 or 4 weeks in the treatment of febrile urinary tract infection in men: a randomized trial with a 1 year follow-up. *Scand J Infect Dis*, 2003; **35**(1): 34–9.

56 Raz R, Stamm WE. A controlled trial of intravaginal estriol in postmenopausal women with recurrent urinary tract infections. *N Engl J Med*, 1993; **329**(11): 753–6.

57 Eriksen B. A randomized, open, parallel-group study on the preventive effect of an estradiol-releasing vaginal ring (Estring) on recurrent urinary tract infections in postmenopausal women. *Am J Obst Gynaecol*, 1999; **180**(5): 1072–9.

58 Perrotta C, Aznar M, Mejia R, *et al.* Oestrogens for preventing recurrent urinary tract infection in postmenopausal women. *Cochrane Database Syst Rev* 2008, Issue 2. Art. No.: CD005131. DOI: 10.1002/14651858.CD005131.pub2.

59 Albert X, Huertas I, Pereiro I, *et al.* Antibiotics for preventing recurrent urinary tract infection in non-pregnant women. *Cochrane Database Syst Rev* 2004, Issue 3. Art. No.: CD001209. DOI: 10.1002/14651858.CD001209.pub2.

60 Allan GM, Nicolle L. Cranberry for preventing urinary tract infection. *Can Fam Phys*, 2013; **59**: 367.

61 McMurdo MET, Argo I, Phillips G, *et al.* Cranberry or trimethoprim for the prevention of recurrent urinary tract infections? A randomized controlled trial in older women. *J Antimicrob Chemother*, 2009; **63**: 389–95.

62 Nicolle LE. Catheter-related urinary tract infection. *Drugs Aging*, 2005; **22**(8): 627–39.

63 Ouslander JG, Greengold B, Chen S. External catheter use and urinary tract infections among incontinent male nursing home patients. *J Am Geriatr Soc*, 1987; **35**(12): 1063–70.

64 Hazlett SE, Tsai M, Gareri M, *et al.* The association between indwelling urinary catheter use in the elderly and urinary tract infection in acute care. *BMC Geriatrics*, 2006; **6**: 15.

65 Holroyd-Leduc JM, Sands LP, Counsell SR, *et al.* Risk factors for indwelling urinary catheterization among older hospitalized patients without a specific medical indication for catheterization. *J Patient Safety*, 2005; **1**: 201–7.

66 Holroyd-Leduc JM, Sen S, Bertenthal D, *et al.* The relationship of indwelling urinary catheters to death, length of hospital stay, functional decline, and nursing home admission in hospitalized older medical patients. *J Am Geriatr Soc*, 2007; **55**(2): 227–33.

67 Robinson S, Allen L, Barnes MR, *et al.* Development of an evidence-based protocol for reduction of indwelling urinary catheter usage. *MedSurg Nursing*, 2007; **16**(3): 157–61.

68 Gotelli JM, Merryman P, Carr C, *et al.* A quality improvement project to reduce the complications associated with indwelling urinary catheters. *Urol Nurs*, 2008; **28**(6): 465–73.

69 Jahn P, Preuss M, Kernig A, *et al.* Types of indwelling urinary catheters for long-term bladder drainage in adults. *Cochrane Database Syst Rev* 2007, Issue 3. Art. No.: 004997. DOI: 10.1002/14651858.CD004997.pub2.

70 Hendrix SL, Cochrane BB, Nygaard IE, *et al.* Effects of estrogen with and without progestin on urinary incontinence. *JAMA*, 2005; **293**(8): 935–48.

71 Holroyd-Leduc JM, Mehta KM, Covinsky KE. Urinary incontinence and its association with death, nursing home admission, and functional decline. *J Am Geriatr Soc*, 2004; **52**(5): 712–18.

72 Stothers L, Thom D, Calhoun E. Urologic diseases in America project: urinary incontinence in males – demographics and economic burden. *J Urology*, 2005; **173**(4): 1302–8.

73 Kolominsky-Rabas PL, Hilz M, Neundoerfer B, *et al.* Impact of urinary incontinence after stroke: results from a prospective population-based stroke register. *Neurourol Urodyn*, 2003; **22**: 322–7.

74 Chiang L, Ouslander J, Schnelle J, *et al.* Dually incontinent nursing home residents: clinical characteristics and treatment differences. *J Am Geriatr Soc*, 2000; **48**(6): 673–6.

75 Skelly J, Flint AJ. Urinary incontinence associated with dementia. *J Am Geriatr Soc*, 1995; **43**(3): 286–94.

76 Thom DH, Haan MN, Van Den Eeden SK. Medically recognized urinary incontinence and risks of hospitalization, nursing home admission and mortality. *Age Ageing*, 1997; **26**: 367–74.

77 Wyman JF, Elswick RK, Wilson MS, *et al.* Relationship of fluid intake to voluntary micturitions and urinary incontinence in women. *Neurourol Urodyn*, 1991; **10**: 463–73.

78 Kirkland JL, Lye M, Levy DW, *et al.* Patterns of urine flow and electrolyte excretion in healthy elderly people. *BMJ*, 1983; **287**: 1665–7.

79 Resnick NM, Yalla SV, Laurino E. The pathophysiology of urinary incontinence among institutionalized elderly persons. *N Engl J Med*, 1989; **320**(1): 1–7.

80 Tubaro A. Defining overactive bladder: epidemiology and burden of disease. *Urology*, 2004; **64**(Suppl. 6A): S2–6.

81 Poggesi A, Pracucci G, Chabriat H, *et al.* Urinary complaints in nondisabled elderly people with age-related white matter changes: the Leukoaraiosis And DISability (LADIS) Study. *J Am Geriatr Soc*, 2008; **56**(9): 1638–43.

82 Mathew TH, McEwen J, Rohan A. Urinary incontinence secondary to prazosin. *Med J Aust*, 1988; **148**: 305–6.

83 Hashimoto M, Imamura T, Tanimukai S, *et al.* Urinary incontinence: an unrecognised adverse effect with donepezil. *Lancet*, 2000; **356**: 568.

84 Nager CW, Brubaker L, Litman HJ, *et al.* A randomized trial of urodynamic testing before stress-incontinence surgery. *N Engl J Med*, 2012; **366**: 1987–97.

85 Stanton S, Morgan AK. *Clinical Urogynaecology*, 2nd ed. London: Churchill Livingston, 2000.

86 Borrie MJ, Bawden M, Speechley M, *et al.* Interventions led by nurse continence advisers in the management of urinary incontinence: a randomized controlled trial. *CMAJ*, 2002; **166**(10): 1267–73.

87 Subak LL, Wing R, West DS, *et al.* Weight loss to treat urinary incontinence in overweight and obese women. *N Engl J Med*, 2009; **360**(5): 481–90.

88 Khullar V, Hill S, Laval K, *et al.* Treatment of urge-predominant mixed urinary incontinence with tolterodine extended release: a randomized, placebo-controlled trial. *Urology*, 2004; **64**(2): 269–75.

89 Bo K, Kvarstein B, Nygaard I. Lower urinary tract symptoms and pelvic floor muscle exercise adherence after 15 years. *Obst Gyn*, 2005; **105**(5): 999–1005.

90 Wyman JF, Fantl JA, McClish DK, *et al.* Comparative efficacy of behavioral interventions in the management of female urinary incontinence. *Am J Obstet Gynecol*, 1998; **179**(4): 999–1007.

91 Fantl JA, Wyman JF, McClish DK, *et al.* Efficacy of bladder training in older women with urinary incontinence. *JAMA*, 1991; **265**(5): 609–13.

92 Moehrer B, Hextall A, Jackson S. Oestrogens for urinary incontinence in women. *Cochrane Database of Syst Rev* 2003; issue 2.

93 Burgio KL, Locher JL, Goode PS, *et al.* Behavioral vs drug treatment for urge urinary incontinence in older women: a randomized controlled trial. *JAMA*, 1998; 280(23): 1995–2000.

94 Burgio KL, Locher JL, Goode PS. Combined behavioural and drug therapy for urge incontinence in older women. *J Am Geriatr Soc*, 2000; **48**: 370–74.

95 Payne CK. Behavioral therapy for overactive bladder. *Urology*, 2000; **55**(Suppl. 5A): 3–6.

96 Burgio KL, Kraus SR, Menefee S, *et al.* Behavioral therapy to enable women with urge incontinence to discontinue drug treatment: a randomized trial. *Ann Intern Med*, 2008; **149**(3): 161–9.

97 Burgio KL, Goode PS, Locher JL, *et al.* Behavioral training with and without biofeedback in the treatment of urge incontinence in older women: a randomized controlled trial. *JAMA*, 2002; **288**(18): 2293–9.

98 Ouslander JG, Schnelle JF, Uman G, *et al.* Predictors of successful prompted voiding among incontinent nursing home residents. *JAMA*, 1995; **273**(17): 1366–70.

99 Hu T, Igou JF, Kaltreider L, *et al.* A clinical trial of a behavioural therapy to reduce urinary incontinence in nursing homes: outcome and implications. *JAMA*, 1989; **261**(18): 2656–62.

100 Ouslander JG, Al-Samarrai N, Schnelle JF. Prompted voiding for night-time incontinence in nursing homes: is it effective? *J Am Geriatr Soc*, 2001; **49**(6): 706–9.

101 Ostaszkiewicz J, Johnston L, Roe B. Habit retraining for the management of urinary incontinence in adults. *Cochrane Database Syst Rev* 2004, Issue 2. Art. No.: CD002801. DOI: 10.1002/14651858.CD002801.pub2.

102 Chapple CR. Muscarinic receptor antagonists in the treatment of overactive bladder. *Urology*, 2000; **55**(Suppl. 5A): 33–46.

103 Donnellan CA, Fook L, McDonald P, *et al.* Oxybutynin and cognitive dysfunction. *BMJ*, 1997; **315**: 1363–4.

104 Edwards KR, O'Connor JT. Risk of delirium with concomitant use of tolterodine and acetylcholinesterase inhibitors. *J Am Geriatr Soc*, 2002; **50**(6): 1165–6.

105 Williams SG, Staudenmeier J. Hallucinations with tolterodine. *Psych Services*, 2004; **55**(11): 1318–19.

106 Tsao JW, Heilman KM. Transient memory impairment and hallucinations associated with tolterodine use. *N Engl J Med*, 2003; **349**(23): 2274–5.

107 Ancelin ML, Artero S, Portet F, *et al.* Non-degenerative mild cognitive impairment in elderly people and use of anticholinergic drugs: longitudinal cohort study. *BMJ*, 2006; **332**: 445–9.

108 Perry EK, Kilford L, Lees AJ, *et al.* Increased Alzheimer pathology in Parkinson's disease related to antimuscarinic drugs. *Ann Neurol*, 2003; **54**: 235–8.

109 Katz IR, Sands LP, Bilker W, *et al.* Identification of medications that cause cognitive impairment in older people: the case of oxybutynin chloride. *J Am Geriatr Soc*, 1998; **46**(1): 8–13.

110 Van Kerrebroeck P, Kreder K, Jonas U, *et al.* Tolterodine once–daily: superior efficacy and tolerability in the treatment of the overactive bladder. *Urology*, 2001; **57**(3): 414–21.

111 Zinner NR, Mattiasson A, Stanton SL. Efficacy, safety, and tolerability of extended-release once-daily tolterodine treatment for overactive bladder in older versus younger patients. *J Am Geriatr Soc*, 2002; **50**: 799–802.

112 Scheife R, Takeda M. Central nervous system safety of anticholinergic drugs for the treatment of overactive bladder in the elderly. *Clin Therap*, 2005; **27**(2): 144–53.

113 Chu FM, Dmochowski RR, Lama DJ, *et al.* Extended-release formulations of oxybutynin and tolterodine exhibit similar central nervous system tolerability profiles: a subanalysis of data from the OPERA trial. *Am J O&G*, 2005; **192**(6): 1849–54.

114 Abrams RF, Anderstrom C, Mattiasson A. Tolterodine, a new antimuscarinic agent: as effective but better tolerated than oxybutynin in patients with an overactive bladder. *Br J Urol*, 1998; **81**: 801–10.

115 Appell RA. Clinical efficacy and safety of tolterodine in the treatment of overactive bladder: a pooled analysis. *Urology*, 1997; **50**(Suppl. 6A): 90–6.

116 Kay G, Crook T, Rekeda L, *et al.* Differential effects of the antimuscarinic agents darifenacin and oxybutynin ER on memory in older subjects. *European Urol*, 2006; **50**: 317–26.

117 Malone-Lee JG, Walsh JB, Maugourd M *et al.* Tolterodine: a safe and effective treatment for older patients with overactive bladder. *J Am Geriatr Soc*, 2001; **49**(6): 700–5.

118 Lackner TE, Wyman JF, McCarthy TC, *et al.* Randomised, placebo-controlled trial of the cognitive effect, safety, and tolerability of oral extended-release oxybutynin in cognitively impaired nursing home residents with urge urinary incontinence. *J Am Geriatr Soc*, 2008; **56**(5): 862–70.

119 Appell RA, Sand P, Dmochowski R, *et al.* Prospective randomized controlled trial of extended-release oxybutynin chloride and tolterodine tartrate in the treatment of overactive bladder: results of the OBJECT study. *Mayo Clin Proc*, 2001; **76**: 358–63.

120 Diokno AC, Appell RA, Sand PK. Prospective, randomized, double-blind study of the efficacy and tolerability of the extended-release formulations of oxybutynin and tolterodine for overactive bladder: results of the OPERA trial. *Mayo Clin Proc*, 2003; **78**: 687–95.

121 Dmochowski RR, Sand PK, Zinner NR, *et al.* Comparative efficacy and safety of transdermal oxybutynin and oral tolterodine versus placebo in previously treated patients with urge and mixed urinary incontinence. *Urology*, 2003; **62**(2): 237–42.

122 Zinner N, Gittelman M, Harris R, *et al.* Trospium chloride improves overactive bladder symptoms: a multicenter phase III trial. *J Urology*, 2004; **171**: 2311–15.

123 Herbison P, Hay-Smith J, Ellis G, *et al.* Effectiveness of anticholinergic drugs compared with placebo in the treatment of overactive bladder: systematic review. *BMJ*, 2003; **326**: 841–4.

124 Nabi G, Cody JD, EllisG, *et al.* Anticholinergic drugs versus placebo for overactive bladder syndrome in adults. *Cochrane Database Syst Rev* 2006, Issue 4. Art. No.: CD003781. DOI: 10.1002/14651858.CD003781.pub2.

125 Paquette A, Gou P, Tannenbaum C. Systematic review and meta-analysis: do clinical trials testing antimuscarinic agents for overactive bladder adequately measure central nervous system adverse events? *J Am Geriatr Soc*, 2011; **59**: 1332–9.

126 Lackner TE, Wyman JF, McCarthy TC, *et al.* Efficacy of oral extended-release oxybutynin in cognitively impaired older nursing home residents with urge urinary incontinence: a randomized placebo-controlled trial. *J Am Med Dir Assoc*, 2011; **12**: 639–47.

127 Caremel R, Loutochin O, Corcos J. What do we know and not know about mirabegron, a novel β3 agonist, in the treatment of overactive bladder? *Int Urogynecol J*, 2014; **25**: 165–70.

128 National Institute for Health and Care Excellence. *Mirabegron for Treating Symptoms of Overactive Bladder*. NICE technology appraisal guidance 290, 2013. Available at: www.nice.org.uk/guidance/ta290 (accessed: 5 November 2014).

129 Schurch B, de Sèze M, Denys P *et al.* Botulinum toxin type a is a safe and effective treatment for neurogenic urinary incontinence: results of a single treatment, randomized, placebo controlled 6-month study. *J Urology*, 2005; **174**(1): 196–200.

130 Kuo H. Urodynamic evidence of effectiveness of botulinium A toxin injection in treatment of detrusor overactivity refractory to anticholinergic agents. *Urology*, 2004; **63**(5): 868–72.

131 Visco AG, Brubaker L, Richter HE, *et al.* Anticholinergic therapy vs. onabotulinum toxinA for urgency urinary incontinence. *N Engl J Med*, 2012; **367**(19): 1803–13.

132 Cruz F, Silva C. Botulinum toxin in the management of lower urinary tract dysfunction: contemporary update. *Curr Opin Urol*, 2004; **14**(6): 329–34.

133 Schmidt RA, Jonas U, Oleson KA, *et al.* Sacral nerve stimulation for treatment of refractory urinary urge incontinence. *J Urology*, 1999; **162**(2): 352–7.

134 Emmons SL, Otto L. Acupuncture for overactive bladder: a randomized controlled trial. *Obst Gyn*, 2005; **106**(1): 138–43.

135 Wells TJ, Brink CA, Diokno AC, *et al.* Pelvic muscle exercise for stress urinary incontinence in elderly women. *J Am Geriatr Soc*, 1991; **39**(8): 785–91.

136 Hay-Smith EJC, Bo K, Berghmans LCM, *et al.* Pelvic floor muscle training for urinary incontinence in women. *Cochrane Database Syst Rev* 2001, Issue 1. Art. No.: CD001407. DOI: 10.1002/14651858.CD001407.

136 Burns PA, Pranikoff K, Nochajski TH, *et al.* A comparison of effectiveness of biofeedback and pelvic muscle exercise treatment of stress incontinence in older community-dwelling women. *J Gerontol* 1993; **48**(4): M167–74.

138 Bo K, Talseth T, Holme I. Single blind, randomised controlled trial of pelvic floor exercises, electrical stimulation, vaginal cones and no treatment in management of genuine stress incontinence in women. *BMJ*, 1999; **318**: 487–93.

139 Goode PS, Burgio KL, Locher JL, *et al.* Effect of behavioural training with or without pelvic floor electrical stimulation on stress incontinence in women: a randomized controlled trial. *JAMA*, 2003; **290**(3): 345–52.

140 Alhasso A, Glazener CMA, Pickard R, *et al.* Adrenergic drugs for urinary incontinence in adults. *Cochrane Database Syst Rev* 2005, Issue 3. Art. No.: CD001842. DOI: 10.1002/14651858.CD001842.pub2.

141 Van Kerrebroeck P, Abrams P, Lange R, *et al.* Duloxetine versus placebo in the treatment of European and Canadian women with stress urinary incontinence. *BJOG*, 2004; **111**: 249–57.

142 Lapitan MC, Cody DJ, Grant AM. Open retropubic colposuspension for urinary incontinence in women. *Cochrane Database Syst Rev* 2005, Issue 3. Art. No.: CD002912. DOI: 10.1002/14651858.CD002912.pub2.

143 Diokno AC, Burgio K, Fultz NH, *et al.* Prevalence and outcomes of continence surgery in community dwelling women. *J Urol*, 2003; **170**: 507–11.

144 Moehrer B, Ellis G, Carey M, *et al.* Laparoscopic colposuspension for urinary incontinence in women. *Cochrane Database Syst Rev* 2000, Issue 3. Art. No.: CD002239. DOI: 10.1002/14651858.CD002239.

145 Glazener CMA, Cooper K. Anterior vaginal repair for urinary incontinence in women. *Cochrane Database Syst Rev* 2001, Issue 1. Art. No.: CD001755. DOI: 10.1002/14651858.CD001755.

146 Glazener CMA, Cooper K. Bladder neck needle suspension for urinary incontinence in women. *Cochrane Database Syst Rev* 2004, Issue 2. Art. No.: CD003636. DOI: 10.1002/14651858.CD003636.pub2.

147 Atherton MJ, Stanton SL. The tension-free vaginal tape reviewed: an evidence-based review from inception to current status. *BJOG*, 2005; **112**: 534–46.

148 Holmgren C, Nilsson S, Lanner L, *et al.* Long-term results with tension-free vaginal tape on mixed and stress urinary incontinence. *O&G*, 2005; **106**(1): 38–43.

149 Kershen RT, Dmochowski RR, Appell RA. Beyond collagen: injectable therapies for the treatment of female stress urinary incontinence in the new millennium. *Urol Clin N Am*, 2002; **29**: 559–74.

150 Keegan PE, Atiemo K, Cody JD, *et al.* Periurethral injection therapy for urinary incontinence in women. *Cochrane Database Systc Rev* 2007, Issue 3. Art. No.: CD003881. DOI: 10.1002/14651858.CD003881.pub2.

151 Warren JW, Muncie HL, Hebel JR, *et al.* Long-term urethral catheterization increases risk of chronic pyelonephritis and renal inflammation. *J Am Geriatr Soc*, 1994; **42**(12): 1286–90.

152 Resnick NM. Geriatric incontinence. *Urol Clin N Am*, 1996; **23**(1): 55–74.

153 Pilloni S, Krhut J, Mair D, *et al.* Intermittent catheterisation in older people: a valuable alternative to the indwelling catheter? *Age Ageing*, 2005; **34**: 57–60.

154 Hampton S. Importance of the appropriate selection and use of continence pads. *Br J Nursing*, 2005; **14**(5): 265–9.

155 Brazzelli M, Shirran E, Vale L. Absorbent products for containing urinary and/or faecal incontinence in adults. *Cochrane Database Syst Rev* 1999, Issue 3. Art. No.: CD001406. DOI: 10.1002/14651858.CD001406.

156 Patel AK, Chapple CR. Benign prostatic hyperplasia: treatment in primary care. *BMJ*, 2006; **333**: 535–9.

157 Jacobsen SJ, Cheetham TC, Haque R, *et al.* Association between 5-alpha reductase inhibition and risk of hip fracture. *JAMA*, 2008; **300**(14): 1660–4.

158 McConnell JD, Roehrbom CG, Bautista OM, *et al.* The long-term effect of doxazosin, finasteride, and combination therapy on the clinical progression of benign prostatic hyperplasia. *N Engl J Med*, 2003; **349**: 2387–98.

159 Damber J, Aus G. Prostate cancer. *Lancet*, 2008; **371**: 1710–21.

160 Schroder FH, Hugosson J, Roobol MJ, *et al.* Screening and prostate-cancer mortality in a randomized european study. *N Engl J Med*, 2009; **360**: 1320–8.

161 Andriole GL, Crawford ED, Grubb RL, *et al.* Mortality results from a randomized prostate-cancer screening trial. *N Engl J Med*, 2009; **360**(13): 1310–19.

162 Saylor PJ, Smith MR. Metabolic complications of androgen deprivation therapy for prostate cancer. *J Urol*, 2009, **181**(5): 1998–2006.

163 Ketchandji M, Kuo YF, Shahinian VB, *et al.* Cause of death in older men after the diagnosis of prostate cancer. *J Am Geriatr Soc*, 2009; **57**(1): 24–30.

CHAPTER 12

Bowel disorders

CONSTIPATION

Constipation is classically defined as passing stools less often than once every three days. It may alternatively be described as difficulty passing stools (dyschezia) due to their hard or pebble-like nature, or difficulty in initiating evacuation despite regular bowel motions.[1] A distinction of subtypes of constipation into either slow transit time or difficult stool expulsion has been proposed but some overlap does exist.[2] Constipation is more common in older than younger people, but its incidence and prevalence are hard to establish accurately as people's perception of constipation often differs from the clinical definition. A survey of older people found that around 30% reported constipation but only 3% actually opened their bowels less than three times per week.[3] A study of the community-dwelling elderly (aged 65–93 years) found a prevalence of chronic constipation of 24% (defined as straining at stool or less than three motions per week more than 25% of the time).[4] Changes in the bowel associated with ageing that may increase the likelihood of developing constipation include reduced neuronal function and anal sphincter fibrosis.

A number of factors are necessary to maintain normal bowel function (*see* Figure 12.1). These include adequate hydration, dietary fibre and mobility. The colon usually removes 90% of water from its contents. Despite this, the normal composition of faeces is approximately three-quarters water with the rest being mainly fibre, bacteria and inorganic matter (e.g. calcium and phosphate). The percentage of absorbed water is increased in the presence of dehydration or a prolonged bowel transit time. Dietary fibre helps retain stool water by assisting peristalsis due to its bulk and by an osmotic effect. Moving around appears to have an additive effect to bowel peristalsis in reducing the transit time. The gastrocolic reflex is a normal hormonally mediated physiological occurrence whereby colonic contraction is stimulated 20–30 minutes after gastric distension. Hence, bowel evacuation is more likely after eating. Defecation is also more likely to occur first thing in the morning.[5]

Parasympathetic activity and the effects of various hormone agents are important in maintaining bowel propulsion.[6] The surrounding striated muscle structures of the diaphragm, abdominal wall and pelvic floor are important in the normal defecation process.

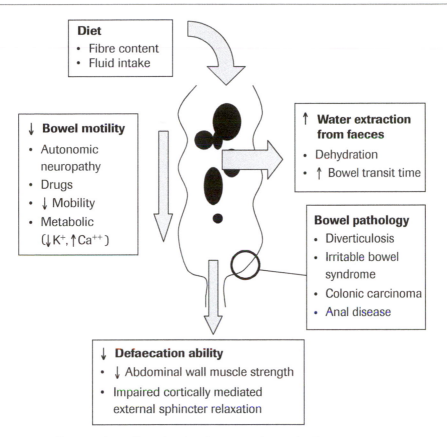

FIGURE 12.1 Factors that affect the development of constipation.

Pathological conditions of the bowel, including diverticulosis, irritable bowel syndrome, colonic carcinoma and painful anal disorders (e.g. fissures), are additional factors in constipation in some individuals. The normal process is often disturbed by illness due to immobility, dehydration, change in dietary intake and medications that reduce bowel motility (*see* Table 12.1). Some comorbidities predispose to constipation,

TABLE 12.1 Medications that commonly cause constipation in the elderly

Opiates
Metallic ions (e.g. iron and calcium)
Calcium channel blockers (especially verapamil)
Antispasmodics (e.g. hyoscine)
Anticholinergics (e.g. tricyclic antidepressants (TCAs), oxybutynin and tolterodine) – a two to three times increased risk of constipation is noted with the use of these agents in nursing home residents[7]
Dopamine agonists
Diuretics (via dehydration)
Memantine

for example autonomic neuropathy (e.g. Parkinson's disease and diabetes) and hypothyroidism. Metabolic disturbances, including hypercalcaemia and hypokalaemia, can cause constipation. Defecation requires abdominal muscle contraction, which can be disturbed by conditions such as herniation of the abdominal wall. Raised toilet seats that help immobile patients to access toilets may be counterproductive as they can disrupt the normal abdominal wall actions during defecation.[6]

If untreated constipation can cause urinary retention, overflow diarrhoea, bowel obstruction and, rarely, perforation. Faecal impaction is discussed on p. 301.

Assessment

History

A history of recent change in bowel habit should always raise the concern that there may be an underlying bowel malignancy. Red flags include weight loss and rectal bleeding. It is important to qualify what the patient actually means by constipation; this may be aided by the use of a stool diary. For patients in hospital, a stool chart can be utilised. The accuracy of stool description may be increased by use of the Bristol Stool Scale.[8] This is a seven-point descriptive scale ranging from hard lumps of stool (1) to watery motions (7) that correlates with bowel transit time. The timing of symptom onset may coincide with potential precipitants, such as the commencement of medications.

Examination

Abdominal examination may demonstrate faecal loading in the colon. Rectal examination can detect faecal loading, assess stool consistency and detect contributory lesions such as a rectal carcinoma, anal fissure or thrombosed haemorrhoid.

Investigations

Blood tests should exclude hypothyroidism, hypokalaemia and hypercalcaemia. A full blood count (FBC) showing a microcytic anaemia, or a low serum ferritin level, increases the likelihood of a gastrointestinal malignancy. Abdominal X-ray can detect bowel obstruction or high faecal impaction if clinically suspected. Colonoscopy is useful for detecting colonic neoplasia when indicated. Barium enemas are usually less well tolerated than colonoscopy and may provide less information, including the inability to take biopsies of suspicious lesions. In studies looking at colonoscopy in the over seventy-fives, there is around a 10% pick-up rate for colonic neoplasia (*see* p. 424).[9,10] These patients may go on to have surgical treatment or, possibly, endoscopic palliative stenting. Serious complications are rare (<1%) but there are high rates of incompletion (around 40%) due either to poor bowel preparation or procedural intolerance. Further testing, including transit studies, manometry and defecography, may be considered in specialist clinics for resistant, unexplained constipation.

Treatment

If an underlying cause can be identified, this should be addressed. Contributory factors such as dehydration and immobility should be improved when possible. If the patient's diet is believed to contain insufficient fibre, dietary advice is appropriate (aiming for

20–40 g of fibre per day[11]). When constipation is opiate-induced, there is some evidence from studies in younger people that inhibitors of opiate receptors may be beneficial.[12]

Laxatives

In general there is very little evidence for the treatment of constipation.[13] When considering the subgroup that is elderly people, the evidence is even more scarce. Trials tend to be small and of low quality.[14] A systematic review of the efficacy of various constipation treatments found a pooled effect of bulk laxatives of an increase of 1.4 bowel movements per week (95% CI 0.6–2.2) compared to 1.5 for all other laxative agents combined (95% CI 1.1–1.8).[15] There was insufficient data to adequately compare individual agents. The main available agents are discussed below. As there is little to choose between the agents in terms of evidence of efficacy, their use is usually driven by potential adverse effects and financial cost.

Bulking agents

➤ *Natural fibres*: bran, psyllium (the ground husk of the psyllium seed), ispaghula.
➤ *Synthetic agents*: e.g. methylcellulose, polycarbophil.

Bulking agents cause an increased stool mass due to unabsorbed fibre and increased stool water retention attributed to an associated osmotic effect; this leads to a reduced bowel transit time by peristalsis assistance and softer stools.

Bacterial metabolism of these substances within the gut can lead to abdominal bloating and excessive flatus production. Major problems in the elderly include cases of intestinal obstruction both of the lower bowel and oesophagus.[16] In the most extreme case bowel perforation has been reported.[17] Problems may be related to excessive dietary fibre or insufficient water intake. Oesophageal problems may be more likely in association with an impaired swallowing reflex or reduced oesophageal motility. Therefore, these agents should be avoided in individuals who cannot drink adequate amounts of fluid. They play an important role in the treatment of diverticular disease and irritable bowel syndrome – both of which may cause constipation.

Osmotic laxatives

Osmotic laxatives increase stool water content by preventing water absorption by the bowel endothelium and thus make them easier to pass. The disadvantage of this is the potential to cause dehydration, especially in the elderly.

Poorly absorbed ions, such as magnesium and phosphate, may cause hypermagnesaemia, hyperphosphataemia and subsequent hypercalcaemia. The risk of side-effects is increased in the elderly, those with renal impairment and with prolonged exposure of the large bowel to the ions, for example when there is faecal impaction.[16]

Lactulose (a disaccharide) and sorbitol (a sugar alcohol) are partially metabolised by bacteria in the large bowel, which may cause flatulence and abdominal pain due to CO_2 production. When these two agents have been compared in a clinical trial, no significant difference in efficacy was detected.[18] Lactulose has been compared to a senna-fibre (ispaghula) combination in 77 older people (mean age 83 years) in long-stay hospital wards or nursing homes in a crossover design study.[19] There was a significantly higher mean daily stool frequency with the senna-fibre combination (0.8 stools per day vs 0.6; p=0.001). No significant side-effect differences were reported.

Polyethylene glycol (PG) is a mixture of polymers that increase stool water content due to an osmotic effect. Molecules with a molecular weight of 3350 or above are used as they cannot be absorbed by the gut.[11] PG has been shown to be effective in the treatment of faecal impaction (*see* p. 301). It comes as a sachet that is added to sufficient water so as to remove the risk of dehydration. It is not metabolised by bowel bacteria and is not absorbed.

In a study of 70 patients with constipation (mean age 42 years), PG was compared to placebo over a six-month period.[20] A significantly higher rate of remission was seen in the treatment group (77% vs 22% in the placebo arm; p<0.01). There were no significant differences in adverse event rates between the two groups. It has been compared to lactulose in 115 patients (mean age 55 years but 37% between the ages of 65 and 89) with chronic constipation over a four-week period.[21] There was a small but significant increase in mean daily stool frequency with PG compared to lactulose (1.3 vs 0.9; p=0.005). Adverse event rates were similar for both groups; there was an increased incidence of diarrhoea in the PG group early in the treatment regimen but it appeared to be associated with less flatus production.

PG appears to be a safe and effective agent for use in the elderly. Its higher cost than other agents means that it should be reserved for those who are unresponsive to initial, cheaper therapies.

Stimulant laxatives

Senna is derived from plants of the genus *Cassia*, and it passes to the large bowel where it is converted by bacteria to its active compound.[11] It may have a toxic effect on the colonic mucosa, leading to melanosis coli (pigment deposition in bowel epithelial macrophage cells). This was previously thought to be associated with colonic neoplasia following long-term usage but a recent study challenges this association.[22] Its effects commence when it arrives in the colon which, depending on transit time, usually takes around six to eight hours. Therefore, if taken at bedtime its effects should coincide with the post-breakfast gastrocolic reflex. Bisacodyl has similar actions and speed of onset to senna.[11] Danthron is associated with carcinoma formation in animal studies.

Stool softeners

Docusate sodium is a synthetic detergent that is thought to allow greater penetration of water and fat into the faeces and thereby soften them. It may also have a mild stimulatory effect. It has been compared to psyllium in 170 people (mean age 37, range 20–74 years) with chronic constipation over a two-week period.[23] The make-up of this study group was heterogeneous with 73% of participants having a definition of constipation based on passing less than three stools per week and 27% being included on the basis of passing hard, small volume stools. After two weeks, the stool frequency of the psyllium group had increased from 3.1 motions per week to 3.5, compared to a fall in the docusate group from 3.4 at baseline to 2.9 per week (p=0.02). There was an associated, non-significant difference in stool weights. The psyllium group increased from 261 g/week to 354 g/week compared to a rise from 282 g/week to 312 g/week in the docusate arm after two weeks. This study suggests that psyllium may be more effective than docusate. However, given the young and heterogeneous nature of the study population, it is hard to know whether these results are applicable to older people with constipation. There is no evidence of a benefit of stool softeners in preventing constipation in the chronically ill or immobile elderly.[11,24]

Newer drugs

Prucalopride is a pro-kinetic agent acting at gut 5-HT$_4$ receptors. Lubiprostone activates chloride channels in the intestinal wall to increase fluid and electrolyte secretion into the bowel. Linactolide is a guanylate cyclise-C receptor agonist that promotes intestinal fluid secretion. Currently there is very little data to support either efficacy or safety of these drugs in frail older people.[25,26]

Enemas

Phosphate enemas

Phosphate enemas contain sodium acid phosphate and sodium phosphate, which have an osmotic effect resulting in increased stool water. They usually induce defecation within 10 minutes of administration, but there is no robust evidence of efficacy in the treatment of constipation.[27] They have, rarely, been associated with significant side-effects. These include hyperphosphataemia and hypernatraemia, which appear to be more likely in patients with either renal impairment or significant dehydration. Adverse events are also more common in the elderly.[28] They have been associated with rectal bleeding and perforation and should be avoided in people with rectal or anal disease. People who are subsequently incontinent are at risk of skin lesions from the solution. Given the lack of evidence of efficacy and the potential harms, they should only be used with caution in the frail elderly.

Other enemas

Simple water or osmotically active agents (such as sorbitol) have been used as enemas in people with constipation. They are associated with fewer adverse effects than phosphate enemas.

Suppositories

Glycerin and bisacodyl suppositories are available. Bisacodyl has a local stimulatory effect on bowel contractions. The suppositories have an effect in around 10–15 minutes.[11] Glycerin has an osmotic action, drawing water into the stools.

Therapeutic recommendations

A suggested protocol for the management of constipation is shown in Figure 12.2. In constipated elderly people who are otherwise well and ambulant, a wide range of oral agents could be tried. These include bulking agents, osmotic agents (lactulose, sorbitol and PG), stimulants (bisacodyl and senna) and docusate. All of these agents have few side-effects and there is little evidence of variance in efficacy. The choice of agent tried first should be based on cost. Suppositories and enemas are an alternative but evidence of benefit is lacking and patient acceptance is likely to be lower.

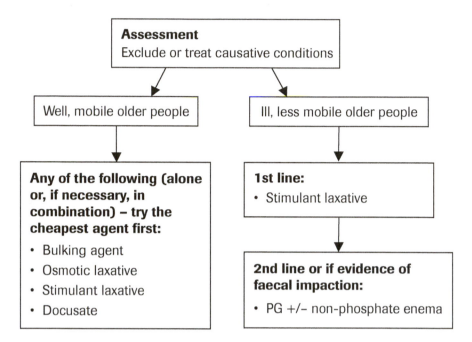

FIGURE 12.2 A suggested protocol for the management of constipation.

In the constipated elderly who are unwell, hospitalised and less mobile, there are fewer appropriate treatments. Osmotic agents that may lead to dehydration should be avoided in those with reduced fluid intake. Bulking agents should also be avoided in this group and those with impaired swallowing due to a risk of bowel obstruction. Docusate has little evidence of efficacy in this situation. So, a stimulant laxative may be appropriate as a first-line agent. If this fails or if there is evidence of faecal impaction, PG should be tried. Enemas may also be useful in cases of faecal impaction. If pharmacotherapy fails to resolve faecal impaction, manual evacuation may be necessary (*see* p. 302).

CLOSTRIDIUM DIFFICILE DIARRHOEA

Clostridium difficile is a spore-forming anaerobic Gram-positive rod bacterium that is sometimes present as a normal commensal organism in the gut (2–3% of healthy, non-hospitalised adults). It is more commonly found in older, hospitalised patients who have an asymptomatic carriage rate of about 20%.[29] It is the major cause of antibiotic-associated diarrhoea, and in the frail elderly it is a significant disease with a mortality rate of up to 25%.[29] Although traditionally associated with hospitalised patients, the community prevalence is rising.[30] A number of community cases are not associated with either antibiotic exposure or recent hospitalisation, suggesting other, yet unknown, factors may also be involved.[31]

Characteristically, clinical features start between four and nine days after antibiotic exposure. The most frequently causative antibiotics are third-generation cephalosporins and clindamycin, but other agents, including penicillins (especially amoxicillin-clavulanate combinations) and fluoroquinolones, have also been implicated.[32] The risk of developing diarrhoea increases with age, which may be due to both an increased colonisation prior to antibiotics and an increased susceptibility to developing disease. Transmission is by the faecal–oral route. Hospital environments harbour the organism and its spores (which can survive for months or years). Around three-quarters of patients with *C. difficile* isolated have contracted it while in hospital – usually through the ingestion of spores. Sites from which the organism has been isolated, not surprisingly, include toilets and bedpans, but also hospital floors and the hands of medical staff. Bedpan washers may not kill the spores and therefore bedpans of infected patients should be autoclaved. The spores are also resistant to some disinfectant agents.

Factors other than advanced age and antibiotic use that increase the risk of *C. difficile* infection include the use of proton pump inhibitors (PPI), nasogastric (NG) tube insertion, shared toilet facilities and long duration of hospitalisation.[29] PPIs could reduce a gastric acid-mediated natural protection from the organism.[30] Although this idea is controversial.[33] Gastric acid is probably ineffective at killing the bacterial spores that typically spread the disease. Other implicated drugs include H_2 blockers (presumably for a similar reason) and NSAIDs, although the mechanism of the latter class is unknown.[34]

C. difficile can produce two toxins (named 'A' and 'B'). The toxins may be produced in varying amounts by different strains of bacteria and both probably cause a disruption in the mucosal layer leading to fluid and protein loss with or without frank haemorrhage. At least one form that produces toxin B, but not toxin A, has been isolated, which has implications when testing for the organism. More recently a highly pathogenic ribotype 027 strain has been identified. This is associated with much higher levels of toxin production, lower response rates to treatment and worse patient outcomes.[35,36]

Clinical features

In the elderly the most common presentation is watery diarrhoea that may have a characteristic greenish appearance. Vomiting, abdominal pain and fever are sometimes associated. It is a recognised cause of delirium. A form of disease without diarrhoea also exists. It should be considered in the differential diagnosis of a non-specifically unwell, hospitalised, elderly patient with a very high white cell count (WCC) ($20 – 30 \times 10^9$/L). It may present as a severe colitis or an acute abdomen and lead to toxic megacolon.[37] Pseudomembranous colitis (PMC) is a severe form of the disease, resulting in an endoscopic appearance of the bowel resembling thin membranes overlying the bowel wall. Due to protein loss, oedema may be detected. Extremely severe disease has been known to cause colonic perforation. Life-threatening disease may cause hypotension and an ileus or toxic megacolon. The presence of any of the following features is typically considered a marker of severe disease:[36]

➤ serum white blood cell count > 15×10^9/L
➤ acute rise in serum creatinine (>50% from baseline value)

➤ temperature >38.5°C

➤ signs of severe colitis (on abdominal examination or radiology).

Stool frequency is an unreliable marker of severity as it may be hard to record in those with faecal incontinence or reduced in those who have developed an ileus. A serum lactate of 5.0 mmol/L or more is a very poor prognostic sign.

Diagnosis

The mnemonic 'SIGHT' has been recommended to aid the diagnosis and reduce the spread of spores.[36]

S	Suspect infection as a cause of diarrhoea when unexplained
I	Isolate in a side room and speak to infection control while awaiting stool test results
G	Gloves and aprons should be used
H	Hand washing with soap and water between all contacts
T	Test the stool for toxin as soon as possible

Immunoassays to detect toxins A or B are the most commonly used diagnostic tests. They can be performed in less than two hours. Sensitivities and specificities are around 80–95% depending on the test used. Many test only for the presence of toxin A and so toxin A-negative, B-positive strains may go undetected. Culture of the organism is difficult (and hence its name) and is more expensive and takes longer (up to three days). Sigmoidoscopy may detect the pseudomembranes of PMC but the disease sometimes only affects more proximal large bowel. Therefore, a colonoscopy would be required to adequately exclude all such changes. Given the frailty of this population and the increased risk of colonic perforation in the presence of inflammation, this procedure can rarely be justified. A plain abdominal X-ray should be performed if megacolon is suspected.

Repeat stool testing to look for clearance of toxins following symptom resolution is not appropriate as it may remain positive for several weeks even when the infection has resolved.

Treatment

The causative antibiotic(s) should be discontinued if possible. Careful attention needs to be given to the frail elderly regarding electrolyte balance, hydration status, nutrition and complications such as pressure ulcers.[36] Antiperistaltic drugs should be avoided as they may reduce the clearance of toxins and increase the risk of toxic megacolon. Consideration should be given to withholding or discontinuing any PPI medication. Stool type and frequency should be monitored using the Bristol Stool Scale.

Either oral metronidazole or vancomycin for 10 days are usually effective (as metronidazole is cheaper than vancomycin it is first-line therapy in mild to moderate disease).[36,38] Oral vancomycin is probably more effective and is typically preferred for severe disease (there is some evidence of emerging resistance to metronidazole).[36] If unable to take oral medication, either intravenous (IV) metronidazole (not vancomycin) or oral medication via an NG tube may be tried. In some situations it may be reasonable to try rectal vancomycin delivered via a urinary catheter. Fidaxomicin is an oral macrocyclic antibacterial agent that is poorly absorbed from the gut. It has a higher financial cost but may be considered for patients with severe disease at high risk of recurrence, such as the frail elderly.[36] Patients with severe disease that does not respond to initial treatment may be considered for oral rifampicin or intravenous immunoglobulin, but evidence of benefit is lacking.[36]

Probiotics are live microorganisms (e.g. *Saccharomyces boulardii* and *Lactobacillus* species) that may improve the colonic flora. Their role is not well established.[39] A Cochrane review was unable to find sufficient evidence of benefit of probiotics, in conjunction with standard antibiotic therapy, in the treatment of *C. difficile* diarrhoea.[40] They may have a benefit in reducing the chance of recurrent disease[29] or prevention (*see* below).

Surgery is occasionally indicated for fulminant colitic forms of the disease. This usually involves subtotal colectomy with end ileostomy. In this setting it is associated with high mortality rates of around 50%.[37,41] Colectomy may be considered when colonic dilatation is >10 cm and blood lactate is raised (but less than 5 mmol/L as above this level survival becomes unlikely). Surgery appears to be most successful in patients aged over 65, without immunocompromise, with a white cell count >20 × 10^9/L, and a lactate level between 2.2 and 4.9 mmol/L.[41]

Some patients can have continuing diarrhoea despite effective treatment of the *C. difficile* diarrhoea, possibly due to post-infective irritable bowel syndrome. In stable patients with persisting diarrhoea despite 20 days of treatment, plus a reduction in stool frequency, a normal serum white blood cell count and no signs of abdominal pain or distension, an anti-motility agent (e.g. loperamide) may be considered.[36]

Relapse

Around 20% of patients will relapse several days after completion of their eradication therapy.[36] This is most often due to reinfection by uncleared spores. A further 10-day course of antibiotics should be tried (typically with vancomycin). Fidaxomicin is associated with a lower recurrence rate than vancomycin but is more expensive.[42] Sometimes a prolonged period of tapered dose or pulsed administration of antibiotics is necessary (to ensure clearance of spores).[36] Rarely, a colectomy is considered for unresponsive, progressive colonic disease. The technique of faecal transplantation has also been tested.[43] Here a suspension of donors' faeces are instilled into the bowel of patients with recurrent disease (via an enema or nasoduodenal tube) with apparent success. A recent small study (n=43, mean age 70 years) found that this technique resulted in cure of recurrent *C. difficile* diarrhoea in 94% of cases, compared to 31% with vancomycin alone.[44]

Prevention

Antibiotic policies that reduce the exposure of susceptible individuals (e.g. the elderly) to the most common causative agents should be implemented. Antibiotics should only be prescribed when the clinical indication is well established and the shortest possible duration of treatment should be used. Antibiotics with narrow spectrums of action should be selected wherever possible. When a broad-spectrum agent is required, there is evidence that use of the piperacillin-tazobactam combination is less likely to result in *C. difficile* infection compared to cefotaxime use.[45]

Hand washing between patients, isolation of cases and adequate ward cleaning to remove spores are all extremely important. Alcohol hand gel is thought to be ineffective at removing spores, so is not recommended. Decontamination of the ward environment from spores, which may survive outside the body for several months, may also play a preventative role.

Probiotics have been tried in the prevention of *C. difficile* diarrhoea, and meta-analyses of data have suggested some benefit.[46,47] A trial randomised 135 hospitalised patients (mean age 74 years), who were taking antibiotics, to receive either a drink containing *Lactobacillus* or placebo.[48] Fewer people developed diarrhoea in the treatment arm (12% vs 34%, $p=0.007$). However, less than 10% of patients initially screened were entered into the trial, mainly due to strict inclusion criteria. This raises questions about the generalisability of the findings. Current guidance does not recommend their routine use.[36]

FAECAL INCONTINENCE

Faecal incontinence (FI) is an embarrassing and debilitating problem that often goes undetected by healthcare professionals. It should be specifically asked about when other bowel symptoms are reported. It ranges in severity from occasional leakage of gas to regular loss of solid stools. The prevalence depends on the population studied and the definition employed. In community-dwelling people, when defined as losing control of 'bowels or gas' in the preceding year, a 2.2% prevalence has been detected.[49] When community-dwelling people over the age of 65 have been studied, 3% report difficulty controlling their bowels.[50] In a similar population, using a definition of stool leakage at least once a week or the requirement to wear a pad, a 7% prevalence was found.[51] When defined as losing control of the bowels within the last year sufficient to cause stained underwear or worse, it has been reported to have a prevalence of 12% in a community-based population with a mean age of 75 years.[52] The prevalence is increased in residential and nursing home settings, being 62% in one nursing home population.[53] Further, it represents a common reason for nursing home admission.

It is often associated with urinary incontinence (UI) in the elderly. When a population of 413 nursing home residents (mean age 84 years) was studied, there were prevalences for continence, UI and dual incontinence (DI) of 28%, 70% and 60%, respectively, with only 2% having FI alone.[53] The same study found that 90% of those with DI had cognitive impairment and 94% had transfer and mobility problems – values that were significantly higher than those in either the continent or UI-alone groups.

Faecal impaction or diarrhoea are both frequent precipitants within the nursing home population. In a community-based sample of people (aged 65–93 years) around 60% of those with FI had either an associated chronic diarrhoea or constipation.[51] Other risk factors include the presence of neurological disease, reduced mobility, cognitive decline, and advanced age.[54]

In the elderly it may be induced by diarrhoea or laxatives that cause stool liquefaction. Chronic diarrhoea has been found to be strongly correlated with FI.[52] It may occur with overflow diarrhoea secondary to faecal impaction (*see* below). Autonomic neuropathy in diabetes may induce diarrhoea and FI. It commonly develops in advanced dementia where, similar to urinary problems, there may be reduced mobility, decreased awareness of the need to defecate or disinhibited behaviour. It frequently occurs in the early post-stroke period when both cognition and mobility may be affected. It may also be precipitated by neurological conditions affecting sphincter function. FI in older people is associated with a reduced anal resting pressure and reduced anal sensation.[55] It appears that internal anal sphincter dysfunction is an important factor. Rectal prolapse and subsequent disruption of the innervation can cause FI. It is more common in post-partum women, around half of whom will be incontinent of faeces.[56]

Faecal impaction

'Faecal impaction' is a term for a mass of hard faeces within the rectum that cannot be easily passed. The mechanism that provokes FI appears to be a reduced rectal sensation capacity secondary to the faecal mass rather than the faecal mass affecting internal anal sphincter function.[57] The causes are those of constipation (*see* p. 291) but the frail elderly are particularly susceptible. It should be suspected when such a patient has an unexplained clinical deterioration, especially when bowel habit alters.[58] Specific presenting symptoms include nausea, vomiting, abdominal pain, paradoxical diarrhoea and subsequent FI, but non-specific presentations such as delirium are well recognised in the elderly. The faecal bulk may precipitate urinary retention or incontinence (*see* p. 266). Rarely, pressure on the intestinal wall may provoke ulceration, bleeding or perforation. It is usually managed with a combination of laxatives and enemas. Infrequently, failed medical therapy necessitates manual evacuation. A regimen of high-dose polyethylene glycol/electrolyte solution for up to three days has been shown to be effective in resolving impaction with minimal adverse effects.[59]

Assessment

History

The consistency and frequency of the stools should be established. A stool diary may help to quantify the problem. The patient may be aware of the need to pass stool but unable to reach the toilet in time (urgency), which may be compounded by mobility or environmental factors. Therefore, it is important to distinguish this from unrecognised, passive leakage of stools. When loose stools are reported, medical conditions or drugs that may be causative should be enquired about (*see* Table 12.2). Chronic diarrhoea has a prevalence of around 14% in the community-dwelling elderly.[51] When infrequent or difficult-to-pass stools precede the onset of FI, causes of constipation should be pursued (*see* p. 291). The occurrence of rectal prolapse should be sought.

TABLE 12.2 Conditions and drugs that more commonly cause diarrhoea in the elderly

Conditions	Drugs
Irritable bowel syndrome (IBS)	Laxatives
Inflammatory bowel disease	Antibiotics (erythromycin)
Lactose intolerance	*C. difficile* (as a consequence of antibiotic therapy)
Radiation enteritis	Proton pump inhibitors
Coeliac disease	Cholinesterase inhibitors
Small bowel bacterial overgrowth	Entacapone

Examination

Rectal examination should be performed to exclude faecal impaction. A neurological examination and cognitive assessment are often helpful.

Investigations

A stool sample should be obtained when diarrhoea is reported to exclude an infective cause. A change in bowel habit should raise concern that there is an underlying malignant lesion. Colonoscopy should be considered especially if there is associated weight loss or rectal bleeding. More detailed studies of anal structure and function, such as anal ultrasound and manometry or defecating proctograms, are usually unnecessary unless surgical intervention is being planned.

Treatment

A simple algorithm to guide the initial assessment and management of FI in the elderly is presented in Figure 12.3. When an underlying bowel condition has been identified, treatment should be undertaken to try to improve this. When FI is associated with faecal impaction, the use of laxatives and enemas to promote complete rectal emptying is associated with a reduction in the frequency of incontinent episodes.[60] Polyethylene glycol (PG) has been shown to be useful in the treatment of faecal impaction in a small, uncontrolled study (n = 30, age range 17–87 years).[61] If pharmacological disimpaction fails, manual evacuation (possibly under anaesthesia) may be required. When FI is associated with chronic diarrhoea, antimotility agents (e.g. loperamide or codeine) may be beneficial.

A regular toileting pattern can sometimes be produced by the alternating use of constipating drugs followed by enemas, for example on a thrice-weekly basis. Alternatively regular toileting at times when the passage of stools is more likely (e.g. following meals) can sometimes establish an effective regimen.[62] When prompted-voiding (identical to that used for UI – *see* p. 274) has been tried in nursing home residents, no beneficial effect has been demonstrated.[63] If the patient is aware of the need to pass stools but unable to access the toilet, simple environmental modifications should be tried, such as a bedside commode.

Occasionally, biofeedback or surgical intervention will be appropriate in older patients. These therapies are discussed below. Despite careful assessment and attempts at treatment, FI cannot always be improved. In this situation pads are often the most

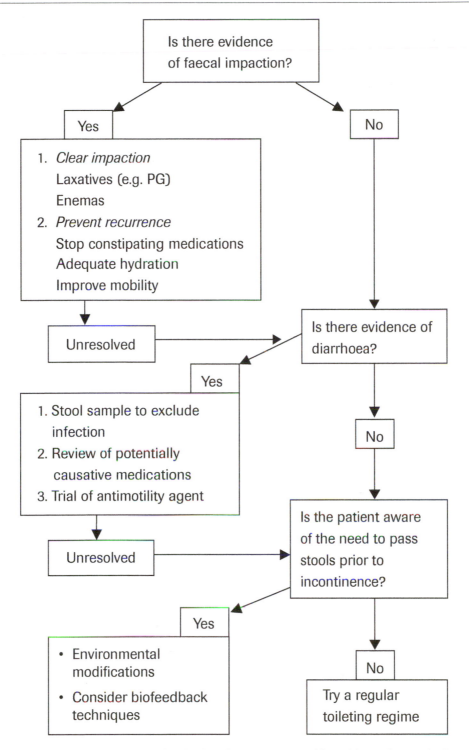

FIGURE 12.3 A simple scheme for the initial management of faecal incontinence in the elderly.

practical solution. Rarely, anal plugs are employed to prevent faecal leakage. These are often poorly tolerated by patients but may have a minor beneficial role in carefully selected people.[64]

Biofeedback training

Biofeedback techniques have been used to improve sphincter control in patients who are cognitively able to comply with such a programme. For a successful outcome there also needs to be some preserved rectal sensation and voluntary sphincter contraction. It aims to teach a method of increasing external anal sphincter closure in response to rectal filling. There have been reports of benefit in around 70% of well-selected groups of patients and no associated adverse effects have been noted.[62,65] However, a Cochrane review was unable to find sufficient high-quality evidence to endorse this approach.[66] Given the frequent association of dementia with FI in the elderly, it is unlikely to be a useful strategy in most older patients.

Surgical intervention

If there is an associated rectal prolapse with FI, this should be repaired. Around two-thirds of such patients will regain continence.[56] In cases where FI is due to sphincteric damage, for example after childbirth or a surgical procedure, an overlapping sphincter repair (sphincteroplasty) is often performed. There have been no randomised controlled trials of this therapy but data suggests that around two-thirds of such patients may benefit.[67] However, longer-term results may be less favourable as there is a tendency for this repair to break down.

An alternative technique is to transpose a muscle (usually the gracilis) so that it loops around the anus to form a new sphincter. This being a skeletal muscle, there are problems maintaining the prolonged contraction necessary to retain the bowel contents. Using an implantable stimulator can circumvent this problem. This combination is termed 'dynamic graciloplasty'. Unfortunately there is a high complication rate with this procedure, most commonly due to infection.[67]

Artificial anal sphincters have also been developed. These use an inflated balloon that can be deflated on demand by a switch positioned in the scrotum or labia. So far there is limited data available on outcomes with this technique, mainly coming from very small studies.[68] Sacral nerve stimulation, as used in UI, has also been used in FI.[69] The mechanism of action is unknown and, to date, there is only limited efficacy data. Injectable bulking agents, similar to those used in UI, have also been proposed but to date there is no randomised controlled trial data.[70]

If all else fails and it is deemed appropriate, colostomy has occasionally been performed for FI. The role of all of these surgical techniques in the management of FI in older people without anal sphincter traumatic injury is unclear. It seems likely that the vast majority of patients will not be suitable for such intervention.

COELIAC DISEASE

Coeliac disease typically presents with diarrhoea and weight loss. It may present with symptoms consequent to absorption problems, i.e. iron deficient anaemia, osteomalacia (increasing the risk of osteoporotic fractures) or folate deficiency (e.g. macrocytic anaemia). B_{12} is absorbed in the terminal ileum and so its absorption is unaffected (*see* Table 12.3). Coeliac disease may present with fatigue. Weight may be normal or even increased. The rash of dermatitis herpetiformis is occasionally associated. The disorder is caused by intolerance to gluten (found in wheat, rye and barley). It is associated with autoimmune disease. Untreated there is an increased risk of small bowel lymphoma and hyposplenism.

It is thought to have a prevalence of 0.5–1% in the general population in the West.[71] An Italian study found that around 4% of cases were diagnosed in people over the age of 65 years.[72] The most common presenting features were diarrhoea (77%), weight loss (60%) and anaemia (58%). Only 3% were asymptomatic at the time of diagnosis. Studies in the UK and USA have suggested the proportion diagnosed over age 65 may be as high as 15–19%.[73,74] There are often long delays in reaching the correct diagnosis, with many patients labelled as having irritable bowel syndrome.

Diagnosis is by duodenal biopsy. Alternatively the transglutaminase antibody test can be used. It has a sensitivity of around 95% and a specificity of nearly 100%.[75] This test has superseded the endomysial antibody test. Treatment is by the avoidance of gluten in the diet. When this is achieved, improvements are seen in weight and nutrient absorption.

SMALL BOWEL BACTERIAL OVERGROWTH

Small bowel bacterial overgrowth causes symptoms secondary to a proliferation of bacteria in the small bowel. It may cause diarrhoea, weight loss and abdominal pain, or symptoms secondary to nutrient deficiencies. It may be detected in 50–70% of elderly people with symptoms suggestive of malabsorption.[76] Its higher prevalence in the elderly may be due to reduced gastric acid secretion (atrophic gastritis or acid-suppressing medication use), impaired small intestinal motility, and more frequent small bowel diverticulae.

Bacteria consume carbohydrate, producing hydrogen and carbon dioxide. They may metabolise bile salts, which reduces the absorption of fats and fat-soluble vitamins (A, D, E and K). Subsequent osteomalacia may result in an increased risk of osteoporotic fractures. Vitamin B_{12} is also metabolised by the bacteria, leading to its deficiency. They may produce folate, leading to normal or even increased levels of this vitamin (*see* Table 12.3).

Diagnosis is either by culture of small bowel aspirates or, more commonly, by a hydrogen breath test. In this latter test the patient is administered glucose or lactulose and breath hydrogen and methane are measured. These gases can only originate from abnormal metabolism by bacteria in the small bowel. The condition can be improved with antibiotics. Repeated cycles may be necessary to prevent recurrence.

TABLE 12.3 Folate, ferritin and vitamin B$_{12}$ changes in coeliac disease and bacterial overgrowth.

	Folate	Ferritin	B$_{12}$
Coeliac disease	↓	↓	−
Bowel overgrowth	− or ↑	−	↓

REFERENCES

1 Schiller LR. Constipation and fecal incontinence in the elderly. *Gastroent Clin N Am*, 2001; **30**(2): 497–515.
2 Rao SSC. Constipation: evaluation and treatment. *Gastroent Clin N Am*, 2003; **32**: 659–83.
3 Whitehead WE, Drinkwater D, Cheskin LJ *et al.* Constipation in the elderly living at home: definition, prevalence, and relationship to lifestyle and health status. *J Am Geriatr Soc*, 1989; **37**: 423–9.
4 Talley NJ, O'Keefe EA, Zinsmeister AR, *et al.* Prevalence of gastrointestinal symptoms in the elderly: a population-based study. *Gastroenterol*, 1992; **102**: 895–901.
5 Heaton KW, Radvan J, Mountford RA, *et al.* Defecation frequency and timing, and stool form in the general population: a prospective study. *Gut*, 1992; **33**: 818–24.
6 Wrenn K. Fecal impaction. *N Engl J Med*, 1989; **321**(10): 658–62.
7 Monane M, Avorn J, Beers MH, *et al.* Anticholinergic drug use and bowel function in nursing home patients. *Arch Int Med*, 1993; **153**: 633–8.
8 O'Donnell LJ, Virjee J, Heaton KW. Detection of pseudodiarrhoea by simple clinical assessment of intestinal transit rate. *BMJ*, 1990; **300**: 439–40.
9 Syn W, Tandon U, Ahmed MM. Colonoscopy in the very elderly is safe and worthwhile. *Age Ageing*, 2005; **34**: 510–13.
10 Cardin F, Barbato B, Terranova O. Outcomes of safe, simple colonoscopy in older adults. *Age Ageing*, 2005; **34**: 513–15.
11 Schiller LR. The therapy of constipation. *Aliment Pharmacol Ther*, 2001; **15**: 749–63.
12 Yuan C, Foss JF, O'Connor M, *et al.* Methylnaltrexone for reversal of constipation due to chronic methadone use: a randomized controlled trial. *JAMA*, 2000; **283**(3): 367–72.
13 Ram Kumar D, Rao SSC. Efficacy and safety of traditional medical therapies for chronic constipation: systematic review. *Am J Gastroent*, 2005; **100**(4): 936–71.
14 Petticrew M, Watt I, Brand M. What's the 'best buy' for treatment of constipation? Results from a systematic review of the efficacy and comparative efficacy of laxatives in the elderly. *Br J Gen Practice*, 1999; **49**: 387–93.
15 Tramonte SM, Brand MB, Mulrow CD, *et al.* The treatment of chronic constipation in adults: a systematic review. *J Gen Intern Med*, 1997: **12**: 15–24.
16 Xing JH, Soffer EE. Adverse effects of laxatives. *Dis Colon Rectum*, 2001; **44**(8): 1201–9.
17 Elliot D, Glover GR. Large bowel perforation due to excessive bran ingestion. *Br J Clin Prac*, 1983; **37**: 32–3.
18 Lederle FA, Busch DL, Mattox KM, *et al.* Cost-effective treatment of constipation in the elderly: a randomized double-blind comparison of sorbitol and lactulose. *Am J Med*, 1990; **89**: 597–601.
19 Passmore AP, Wilson-Davies K, Stoker C, *et al.* Chronic constipation in long-stay elderly patients: a comparison of lactulose and a senna-fibre combination. *BMJ*, 1993; **307**: 769–71.
20 Corazziari E, Badiali D, Bazzocchi G, *et al.* Long term efficacy, safety, and tolerability of low daily doses of isosmotic polyethylene glycol electrolyte balanced solution (PMF-100) in the treatment of functional chronic constipation. *Gut*, 2000; **46**: 522–6.
21 Attar A, Lemann M, Ferguson A, *et al.* Comparison of a low dose polyethylene glycol electrolyte solution with lactulose for treatment of chronic constipation. *Gut*, 1999; **44**(2): 226–30.

22 Nusko G, Schneider B, Schneider I, *et al.* Anthranoid laxative use is not a risk factor for colo-rectal neoplasia: results of a prospective case controlled study. *Gut*, 2000; **46**: 651–5.

23 McRorie JW, Daggy BP, Morel JG, *et al.* Psyllium is superior to docusate sodium for treatment of chronic constipation. *Aliment Pharmacol Ther*, 1998; **12**(5): 491–7.

24 Hurdon V, Viola R, Schroder C. How useful is docusate in patients at risk for constipation? A systematic review of the evidence in the chronically ill. *J Pain Symptom Management*, 2000; **19**(2): 130–6.

25 Gandell D, Straus SE, Bundookwala M, *et al.* Treatment of constipation in older people. *CMAJ*, 2013; **185**: 633–70.

26 Gras-Miralles B, Cremonini F. A critical appraisal of lubiprostone in the treatment of chronic constipation in the elderly. *Clin Interventions Aging*, 2013; **8**: 191–200.

27 Davies C. The use of phosphate enemas in the treatment of constipation. *Nursing Times*, 2004; **100**(18): 32–5.

28 Mendoza J, Legido J, Rubio S, *et al.* Systematic review: the adverse effects of sodium phosphate enema. *Alimentary Pharmacol Therapeutics*, 2007; **26**(1): 9–20.

29 Starr J. *Clostridium difficile* associated diarrhoea: diagnosis and treatment. *BMJ*, 2005; **334**: 498–501.

30 Dial S, Delaney JAC, Barkun AN, *et al.* Use of gastric acid-suppressive agents and the risk of community-acquired *Clostridium difficile*-associated disease. *JAMA*, 2005; **294**(23): 2989–95.

31 Wilcox MH, Mooney L, Bendall R, *et al.* A case-control study of community associated *Clostridium difficile* infection. *J Antimicrob Chemother*, 2008; **62**(2): 388–96.

32 Yip C, Loeb M, Salama S, *et al.* Quinolone use as a risk factor for nosocomial *Clostridium difficile*-associated diarrhoea. *Infect Control Hosp Epidemiol*, 2001; **22**: 572–5.

33 Lowe DO, Mamdani MM, Kopp A, *et al.* Proton pump inhibitors and hospitalization for *Clostridium difficile*-associated disease: a population-based study. *Clin Infect Dis*, 2006; **43**(10): 1272–6.

34 Cunningham R, Dale B, Undy B, *et al.* Proton pump inhibitors as a risk factor for *Clostridium difficile* diarrhoea. *J Hosp Infect*, 2003; **54**: 243–5.

35 Warny M, Pepin J, Fang A, *et al.* Toxin production by an emerging starin of *Clostridium difficile* associated with outbreaks of severe disease in North America and Europe. *Lancet*, 2005; **366**: 1079–84.

36 Public Health England. *Updated Guidance on the Management and Treatment of* Clostridium difficile *Infection*, 2013. Availabe at: www.gov.uk/government/uploads/system/uploads/attach ment_data/file/321891/Clostridium_difficile_management_and_treatment.pdf (accessed 11 November 2014).

37 Longo WE, Mazuski JE, Virgo KS *et al.* Outcome after colectomy for *Clostridium difficile* colitis. *Dis Col Rec*, 2004; **47**(10): 1620–6.

38 McFarland LV. Alternative treatments for *Clostridium difficile* disease: what really works? *J Med Micro*, 2005; **54**: 101–11.

39 Anonymous. Probiotics for gastrointestinal disorders. *Drugs and Therapeutics Bulletin*, 2004; **42**(11): 85–8.

40 Pillai A, Nelson RL. Probiotics for treatment of Clostridium difficile-associated colitis in adults. *Cochrane Database Systc Rev* 2008, Issue 1. Art. No.: CD004611. DOI: 10.1002/14651858. CD004611.pub2.

41 Lamontagne F, Labbe A, Haeck O, *et al.* Impact of emergency colectomy on survival of patients with fulminant *Clostridium difficile* colitis during an epidemic caused by a hypervirulent strain. *Ann Surg*, 2007; **245**(2): 267–72.

42 Aas J, Gessert CE, Bakken JS. Recurrent *Clostridium difficle* colitis: case series involving 18 patients treated with donor stool administered via a nasogastric tube. *Clin Infect Dis*, 2003; **36**: 580–5.

43 Drekonja DM, Butler M, McDonald R, *et al.* Comparative effectiveness of *Clostridium difficile* treatments: a systematic review. *Ann Intern Med*, 2011; **155**: 839–47.

44 Wilcox MH, Freeman J, Fawley W, *et al.* Long-term surveillance of cefotaxime and piperacillin-tazobactam prescribing and incidence of *Clostridium difficile* diarrhoea. *J Antimicrob Chemother*, 2004; **54**(1): 168–72.

45 van Nood E, Vrieze A, Nieuwdorp M, *et al.* Duodenal infusion of donor feces for recurrent *Clostridium difficile*. *N Engl J Med*, 2013; **368**: 407–15.

46 McFarland LV. Meta-analysis of probiotics for the prevention of antibiotic associated diarrhea and the treatment of *Clostridium difficile* disease. *Am J Gastroenterol*, 2006; **101**(4); 812–22.

47 Johnston BC, Ma SSY, Goldenberg JZ, *et al.* Probiotics for the prevention of *Clostridium difficile*-associated diarrhea: a systematic review and meta-analysis. *Ann Intern Med*, 2012; **157**(12): 878–8.

48 Hickson M, D'Souza AL, Muthu N, *et al.* Use of probiotic Lactobacillus preparation to prevent diarrhoea associated with antibiotics: randomised double blind placebo controlled trial. *BMJ*, 2007; **335**: 80–4.

49 Nelson R, Norton N, Cautley E, *et al.* Community-based prevalence of anal incontinence. *JAMA*, 1995; **274**(7): 559–561.

50 Edwards NI, Jones D. The prevalence of faecal incontinence in older people living at home. *Age Ageing*, 2001; **30**: 503–7.

51 Talley NJ, O'Keefe EA, Zinsmeister AR, *et al.* Prevalence of gastrointestinal symptoms in the elderly: a population-based study. *Gastroenterol*, 1992; **102**: 895–901.

52 Goode PS, Burgio KL, Halli AD, *et al.* Prevalence and correlates of fecal incontinence in community-dwelling older adults. *J Am Geriatr Soc*, 2005; **53**: 629–35.

53 Chiang L, Ouslander J, Schnelle J, *et al.* Dually incontinent nursing home residents: clinical characteristics and treatment differences. *J Am Geriatr Soc*, 2000; **48**(6): 673–6.

54 Chassagne P, Landrin I, Neveu C, *et al.* Fecal incontinence in the institutionalized elderly: incidence risk factors, and prognosis. *Am J Med*, 1999; **106**: 185–90.

55 Barrett JA, Brocklehurst JC, Kiff ES, *et al.* Anal function in geriatric patients with faecal incontinence. *Gut*, 1989; **30**: 1244–51.

56 Madoff RD, Williams JG, Caushaj PF. Fecal incontinence. *N Engl J Med*, 1992; **326**(15): 1002–7.

57 Read NW, Abouzekry L. Why do patients with faecal impaction have faecal incontinence? *Gut*, 1986; **27**: 283–7.

58 Wrenn K. Fecal impaction. *N Engl J Med*, 1989; **321**(10): 658–62.

59 Culbert P, Gillet H, Ferguson A. Highly effective new oral therapy for faecal impaction. *Br J Gen Pract*, 1998; **48**: 1599–1600.

60 Chassagne P, Jego A, Gloc P, *et al.* Does treatment of constipation improve faecal incontinence in institutionalized elderly patients? *Age Ageing*, 2000; **29**: 159–64.

61 Culbert P, Gillett H, Ferguson A. Highly effective oral therapy (polyethylene glycol/electrolyte solution) for faecal impaction and severe constipation. *Clin Drug Invest*, 1998; **16**(5): 355–60.

62 Hinninghofen H, Enck P. Fecal incontinence: evaluation and treatment. *Gastr Clin N Am*, 2003; **32**: 685–706.

63 Ouslander JG, Simmons S, Schnelle J, *et al.* Effects of prompted voiding on fecal incontinence among nursing home residents. *J Am Geriatr Soc*, 1996; **44**(4): 424–8.

64 Deutekom M, Dobben A. Plugs for containing faecal incontinence. *Cochrane Database Syst Rev* 2005, Issue 3. Art. No.: CD005086. DOI: 10.1002/14651858.CD005086.pub2.

65 Schiller L. Constipation and fecal incontinence in the elderly. *Gastroent Clin North Am*, 2001; **30**(2): 497–515.

66 Norton C, Hosker G, Brazzelli M. Biofeedback and/or sphincter exercises for the treatment of faecal incontinence in adults. *Cochrane Database Syst Rev* 2000, Issue 2. Art. No.: CD002111. DOI: 10.1002/14651858.CD002111.

67 Madoff RD. Surgical treatment options for fecal incontinence. *Gastroent*, 2004; **126**(1 Suppl.): S48–54.

68 O'Brien PE, Dixon JB, Skinner S, *et al.* A prospective, randomized, controlled clinical trial of placement of artificial bowel sphincter (action neosphincter) for the control of fecal incontinence. *Dis Colon Rectum*, 2004; **47**(11): 1852–60.

69 Ganio E, Luc AR, Clerico G, *et al.* Sacral nerve stimulation for treatment of fecal incontinence. *Dis Colon Rectum*, 2001; **44**(5): 619–31.

70 Vaizey CJ, Kamm MA. Injectable bulking agents for treatment of faecal incontinence. *Br J Surg*, 2005; **92**: 521–7.

71 Sanders DS, Hurlstone DP, McAlindon ME, *et al.* Antibody negative coeliac disease presenting in elderly people: an easily missed diagnosis. *BMJ*, 2005; **330**: 775–6.

72 Gasbarrini G, Coccicioppo R, De Vitis I, *et al.* Coeliac disease in the elderly: a mulitcentre Italian study. *Gerontology*, 2001; **47**: 306–10.

73 Hankey GL, Holmes GKT. Coeliac disease in the elderly. *Gut*, 1994; **35**: 65–7.

74 Patel D, Kalkat P, Baisch D, *et al.* Celiac disease in the elderly. *Gerontology*, 2005; **51**: 213–14.

75 Jones R, Sleet S. Coeliac disease. *BMJ*, 2009; **338**: 539–40.

76 Elphick HL, Elphick DA, Sanders DS. Small bowel bacterial overgrowth: an underrecognized cause of malnutrition in older adults. *Geriatrics*, 2006; **61**(9): 21–6.

QUESTIONS FOR PART C

1 A 92-year-old lady with cognitive impairment is on the rehabilitation ward following surgery for a hip fracture. The nurses report flooding with urinary incontinence every time she is stood up. This is not being adequately managed by pad and pants and has not improved following a toileting regime. Which action is most likely to be helpful?
   A. Indwelling catheter insertion
   B. Amitriptyline
   C. Tolterodine
   D. Pelvic floor exercises
   E. Urodynamic investigations

2 A 75-year-old lady with a 20-year history of diabetes with autonomic neuropathy has developed dribbling urinary incontinence. Which treatment is most likely to be appropriate?
   A. Tolterodine
   B. Duloxetine
   C. Amitriptyline
   D. Intermittent self-catheterisation
   E. Pelvic floor exercises

3 An 84-year-old lady is referred for further assessment of her urinary incontinence. Which of the following findings on urodynamic testing would be most consistent with a diagnosis of detrusor overactivity?
   A. A high detrusor pressure with a low urine flow rate during uroflowmetry
   B. A strong desire to pass urine after 350 mL of water has been instilled into the bladder during cystometry
   C. Leakage of urine associated with a rise in both intra-abdominal and bladder pressure during cystometry
   D. High urine flow rate in association with high detrusor pressure during uroflowmetry
   E. A rise in bladder pressure in the absence of a rise in intra-abdominal pressure during cystometry

4 Regarding urinary tract infection in older adults, which of the following statements is most likely to be correct?
   A. It is under-diagnosed
   B. A three-day course of antibiotics is appropriate for all women
   C. Bacteria in the urine commonly cause no symptoms
   D. Coliform bacteria are likely to give false negative results to dipstick testing for urinary nitrites
   E. Nitrofurantoin is usually an effective antibiotic

5 Which of the following statements is most correct regarding the treatment of benign prostatic hyperplasia in older men?
   A. Tamsulosin blocks the enzyme 5-alpha reductase
   B. Finasteride is associated with an increased risk of osteoporosis
   C. Tamsulosin and finasteride should not be used in combination
   D. Finasteride typically needs to be taken for several months for a significant symptomatic benefit
   E. Tamsulosin use is not associated with postural hypotension

6 A 77-year-old lady presents with a five-day history of diarrhoea. She had a course of co-amoxiclav (amoxicillin-clavulanate) several weeks ago for a pneumonia episode. She takes no regular medications. Blood tests are as below:

Sodium	141	(133–146 mmol/L)
Potassium	4.3	(3.5–5.3 mmol/L)
Urea	6.2	(2.5–7.8 mmol/L)
Creatinine	63	(49–90 umol/L)
Liver enzymes normal		
TSH	3.2	(0.3–4.5 mu/L)
Glucose	5.1	(2.5–10 mmol/L)
Haemoglobin	11.9	(11.5–16.5 g/dL)
White cell count	4.5	(4–11 $\times 10^9$/L)
Platelets	301	(150–450 $\times 10^9$/L)
Mean cell volume	87	(80–99 fl)
Vitamin B_{12}	253	(200–900 ng/L)
Folate	1.6	(3–13 ug/L)
Ferritin	10	(17–322 ug/L)

What is the most likely cause?
   A. Coeliac disease
   B. Bowel overgrowth
   C. *Clostridium difficile* infection
   D. Bowel cancer
   E. Diverticulitis

7 Which of the following statements regarding faecal incontinence in older adults is most correct?
   A. It is frequently associated with chronic diarrhoea or faecal impaction in community-dwelling populations
   B. A trial of biofeedback techniques is an appropriate option for most patients
   C. Prompted voiding has been found to be beneficial in nursing home populations
   D. In nursing homes it is associated with cognitive impairment in 70% of cases
   E. Regular toileting regimes are most effective when performed prior to meal times

8 Which of the following statements is most correct regarding *Clostridium difficile*?
   A. It is a spore-forming Gram-negative rod bacterium
   B. It is found in the faecal flora in around of 10% of well non-hospitalised adults
   C. Hands should be cleaned with alcohol gel between patients to prevent the spread of spores
   D. Following treatment a repeat stool sample should be tested to confirm cure
   E. Intravenous vancomycin is ineffective for treating diarrhoea

9 Which of the following medications is *least* likely to cause constipation in older adults?
   A. Diltiazem
   B. Donepezil
   C. Tolterodine
   D. Ropinirole
   E. Bendroflumethiazide

10 Which of the following statements is most correct regarding the use of anticholinergic medications for the treatment of urge urinary incontinence in the frail elderly?
   A. Selective M2 muscarinic receptor-blocking drugs do not cause cognitive impairment
   B. Constipation is the commonest side-effect
   C. They typically prevent the recurrence of incontinent episodes in around half of patients
   D. Tolterodine is significantly more effective than oxybutynin
   E. There is little data regarding long-term safety in those with cognitive impairment

11 Regarding prostate cancer, which statement is most likely to be correct?
   A. It is the commonest cause of cancer death in men aged over 70 years
   B. Anti-androgen treatments are associated with an increased risk of vascular disease
   C. Diagnosis is usually confirmed by transurethral biopsy
   D. It usually presents with lower urinary tract symptoms
   E. Radiotherapy is an appropriate and effective treatment for the majority of men

12 An 81-year-old woman has had a course of metronidazole for *C. difficile* diarrhoea, but then relapsed and needed vancomycin, followed by a further relapse and needed both drugs. Three weeks later she returns with diarrhoea again and a dilated oedematous colon (>10 cm) on abdominal X-ray. Blood test results: sodium 138, potassium 4.1, urea 7.5, creatinine 92, albumin 36, lactate 3.2, Hb 116, WCC 16.3. Which treatment is now most appropriate?
   A. Metronidazole orally 400 mg tds
   B. Vancomycin intravenous 250 mg qds
   C. Faecal transplant
   D. Colectomy
   E. Intravenous immunoglobulin

13 A 75-year-old man with dementia, hypertension and osteoarthritis develops diarrhoea. Which of the following drugs is most likely to be responsible?
   A. Codeine phosphate
   B. Ibuprofen
   C. Amlodipine
   D. Rivastigmine
   E. Calcium and vitamin D tablets

14 An elderly lady is admitted from a nursing home with a grade 4 pressure ulcer on her sacrum. The plastic surgery team have advised that this could be effectively treated with a skin graft if her faecal incontinence could be controlled. What intervention would be most appropriate?
   A. Formation of a defunctioning stoma
   B. Alternate day enemas with loperamide at other times
   C. Prompted voiding regime
   D. Sacral nerve stimulation
   E. Anal sphincter biofeedback

15 A 68-year-old lady presents with leakage of urine which is worse when coughing. What is the first-line treatment for stress incontinence?
   A. Pelvic floor exercises
   B. Oxybutynin
   C. Duloxetine
   D. Transvaginal tape
   E. Injection of a urethral bulking agent

16 Which of the following clinical features is considered a marker of severe disease when detected in someone with *Clostridium difficile* diarrhoea?
   A. Acute rise in serum creatinine (>50% from baseline value)
   B. Serum white blood cell count >11 $\times10^9$/L
   C. High-pitched bowel sounds
   D. Stool frequency more than three times per day
   E. Temperature above 37.5°C

17 Which of the following is not part of the 'SIGHT' scheme for the initial management of patients with suspected *Clostridium difficile* diarrhoea?
   A. Stop antibiotics as soon as possible
   B. Isolate in a side room and speak to infection control while awaiting stool test results
   C. Gloves and aprons should be used
   D. Hand washing with soap and water between all contacts
   E. Test the stool for toxin as soon as possible

18 An 87-year-old lady has developed urinary incontinence while on the rehabilitation ward. Two weeks previously she had surgery following fall and hip fracture. She describes continually leaking small volumes of urine. She has several comorbidities and takes a large number of medications. A post-void bladder scan shows 435 mL of residual urine. She scored 27/30 on the MMSE. Which of the following medications is most likely to be contributing to her incontinence?

A. Doxazosin
B. Codeine
C. Furosemide
D. Diltiazem
E. Lorazepam

PART D

Falls and related topics

INTRODUCTION

The first part of this section concerns dizziness (divided into light-headedness and vertigo), falls, drop attacks and syncope. In this the following definitions will be used:

➤ *Fall*: unintentionally coming to rest on the ground or a lower level without apparent loss of consciousness.
➤ *Drop attack*: suddenly falling without warning, apparent cause or loss of consciousness.
➤ *Syncope*: an episode of loss of consciousness due to a transient global reduction in cerebral blood flow.
➤ *Light-headedness*: an imbalance or pre-syncopal sensation often described by patients as felling 'swimmy', 'woozy', 'giddy' or 'as though I was drunk'.
➤ *Vertigo*: a sensation of movement, usually the room spinning.

In elderly people a large overlap between light-headedness, falls, drop attacks and syncope has been demonstrated.[1] Given this overlap, many components of assessment are common for all of these conditions. Single pathologies, such as carotid sinus syndrome, have been shown to be able to produce all of these presentations. Older people appear to be prone to such symptoms after minor insults (e.g. mild reductions in cerebral blood flow), which are insufficient to cause problems in younger individuals.[2] Their distinction is made more difficult due to a 30% occurrence of amnesia for unconsciousness in people experiencing syncope.[3] An assessment scheme that considers all of these diagnoses is shown later on (Figure 15.6).

The latter of Part D covers osteoporosis. As falls are the most common cause of fractures in the elderly, these subjects are clearly related. The National Institute for Health and Care Excellence (NICE) guidelines recommend that the assessment and treatment of osteoporosis be incorporated into a comprehensive falls service.[4]

REFERENCES

1 Shaw FE, Kenny RA. The overlap between syncope and falls in the elderly. *Postgrad Med J*, 1997; **73**: 635–9.

2 Kenny RA, Richardson DA, Steen N, *et al.* Carotid sinus syndrome: a modifiable risk factor for nonaccidental falls in older adults (SAFE PACE). *J Am Coll Cardiol*, 2001; **38**(5): 1491–6.

3 Kenny RA, Traynor G. Carotid sinus syndrome – clinical characteristics in elderly patients. *Age Ageing*, 1991; **20**: 449–54.

4 NICE guideline. *Falls: assessment and prevention of falls in older people.* CG161, 2013. Available at: www.nice.org.uk/guidance/cg161 (accessed 14 November 2014).

CHAPTER 13

Dizziness

Dizziness appears to have a very high prevalence among the elderly. In response to a postal questionnaire, a study found that 30% of people aged over 65 reported having experienced dizziness.[1] In another community-based study of older people, any form of dizziness was reported by 33% of patients aged 70, rising to 51% of patients aged 90 years.[2] Symptoms occurring on a daily frequency were reported by 5% of those aged 70, and 25% of those aged 90 years.

'Dizziness' is a very vague term that is used to describe the symptoms of a wide range of conditions. For simplicity, here it will be divided into 'vertigo' and 'light-headedness', as these can usually be distinguished by a careful history. Vertigo is a clear sensation of movement, usually the room spinning. Light-headedness is a sensation of pre-syncope that is often described as a giddiness, wooziness or drunkenness sensation. Sometimes patients describe disequilibrium – a sense of reduced balance and unsteadiness while walking. This is typically due to a combination of gait and balance disorders, sensory loss and possibly medication effects. It can be viewed as a precursor to falls and should be evaluated in a similar way (*see* Chapter 14). Vertigo, light-headedness and disequilibrium may coexist within a patient and all may be caused by some conditions, for example brainstem vascular disease. In a study of elderly patients in primary care who reported dizziness for at least two weeks, pre-syncope was judged to be the commonest type of dizziness affecting 69% of patients, but 44% had more than one subtype.[3] Vertigo was present in 41%, disequilibrium in 40% and a small number of cases were deemed unclassifiable.

The incidence of the pathologies causing dizziness varies according to the subgroup studied. For example, a peripheral vestibular disorder is most likely to be diagnosed in older patients presenting to an ear, nose and throat (ENT) service.[4] In a study recruiting unselected dizzy older patients, light-headedness or unsteadiness has been reported in around two-thirds of patients with only one-third describing vertigo.[1] Also, when patients describing dizziness were subjected to both ENT and neurocardiovascular assessment, 28% were diagnosed with a cardiovascular condition compared to 18% receiving a diagnosis of a peripheral vestibular disorder.[5] In contrast, a study looking at a wide range of ages found the most common diagnoses made were vestibular and psychiatric disorders,[6] suggesting that these are more important causes of dizziness in younger people.

VERTIGO

Vertigo can be caused by lesions affecting the inner ear, eighth nerve or vestibular nuclei in the brainstem. A simplified version of the vestibular system and its main connections is shown in Figure 13.1. More common potential causes are discussed below.

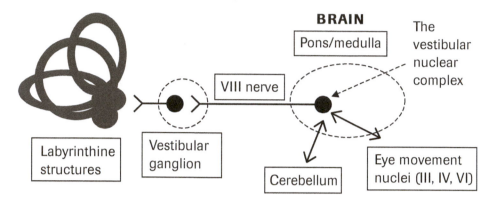

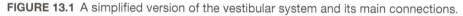

FIGURE 13.1 A simplified version of the vestibular system and its main connections.

Specific conditions

Benign paroxysmal positional vertigo

The labyrinthine structures form a key part of the peripheral vestibular system. They include three semicircular canals that contain sensory structures and fluid (*see* Figure 13.2). They are able to detect rotational movement. Benign paroxysmal positional vertigo (BPPV) is caused by free-floating debris within these semicircular canals that causes inappropriate activation of the sensory structures. It presents as acute episodes of short-lived vertigo (seconds to minutes) often induced by specific movements such as rolling over in bed or looking up to hang out washing. There may be associated nausea and vomiting. It may be diagnosed by the Hallpike test – *see* p. 320. It is best treated by the Epley manoeuvre – a series of movements that transfer the debris within the semicircular canal into the utricle where it no longer causes any symptoms.[7]

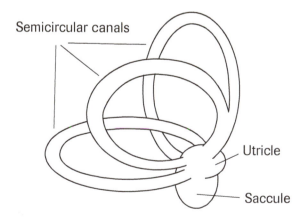

FIGURE 13.2 The peripheral vestibular system.

Vestibular neuritis

Vestibular neuritis is poorly understood condition causing acute vertigo sometimes associated with nausea, vomiting and ataxia. It spontaneously resolves over several days. It is thought to be due to a viral infection of the vestibular pathway.

Vestibular migraine

Vestibular migraine causes vertigo that gradually worsens over a five-minute period and resolves within an hour. Typically it is followed by the characteristic severe throbbing headache of migraine but may present atypically in older people.

Ménière's disease

Ménière's disease is a condition that causes intermittent attacks of vertigo (lasting between 20 minutes and 24 hours) with associated tinnitus (usually unilateral at onset) and hearing deficit.[8] Sufferers often complain of a sense of 'fullness' of the affected ear. The exact cause is unknown and treatment is often ineffective. The vertigo remits after several years in the majority of patients but the hearing deficit usually persists.

Brainstem vascular disease

Lesions affecting the central vestibular nuclei can cause vertigo, for example lateral medullary syndrome (*see* p. 200). There will be associated neurological signs dependent on the vascular territory involved, for example dysarthria, diplopia, hemianopia and sensory/motor signs. Vertigo in isolation is unlikely to be due to a stroke. A study found that 10% of cerebellar strokes (confirmed by MRI findings) presented with vertigo in isolation.[9]

Drug-induced

Ototoxic agents may cause vertigo. Some of the more common causative agents are listed below:
➤ furosemide
➤ gentamicin
➤ non-steroidal anti-inflammatory drugs (NSAIDs)
➤ quinine.

Cerebellopontine angle tumour

Cerebellopontine angle tumours (e.g. acoustic neuroma) usually present with unilateral sensorineural hearing loss due to compression of the eighth nerve. The trigeminal nerve may also be affected, causing facial numbness and loss of the corneal reflex. When vertigo occurs it is usually a late feature.

Assessment

Clinical

History and examination will reveal clinical features leading to a diagnosis in most cases. Nystagmus is a physical sign often associated with vertigo. It is described by the direction of the fast (corrective) phase rather than the slow (pathological) phase. When it is caused by peripheral (labyrinthine) lesions it is usually horizontal in nature and the fast phase is in a direction away from the affected side. It is characteristically diminished on visual fixation of an object. In contrast, nystagmus associated with a central (cerebellar) lesion usually has vertical and rotatory components and tends to be unaffected by visual fixation. The fast phase of the horizontal component is in a direction towards the affected side. There may also be other cerebellar signs, including reduced balance. The 'head thrust test' (also called the 'head impulse test') can be used to help differentiate peripheral from central causes. In this test the patient's head is turned quickly to one side while they attempt to maintain their gaze on a fixed object. The test is positive when the patient's eyes are observed to make a corrective saccade and this suggests a peripheral causation. Sensitivity is around 63% and specificity around 93%.[10] The value and safety of this test in frail older people is unknown and so its routine use in this group is not recommended. The Hallpike test is useful in the diagnosis of BPPV (*see* Figure 13.3).

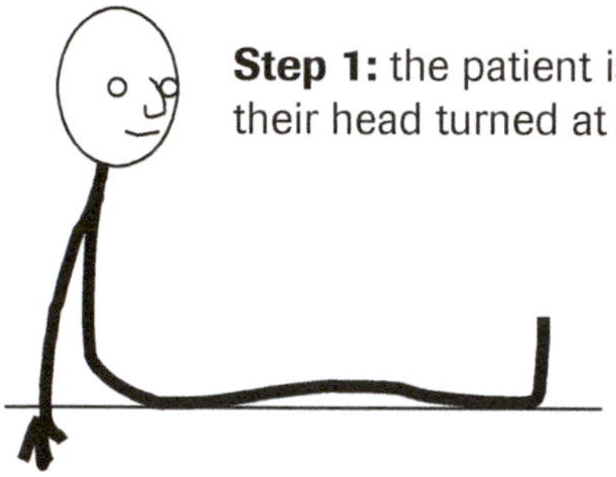

Step 1: the patient is seated on an examination bed with their head turned at 45 degrees to the right.

Step 2: they are laid backwards so their head hangs over the end of the bed, still facing to the right with their eyes open.

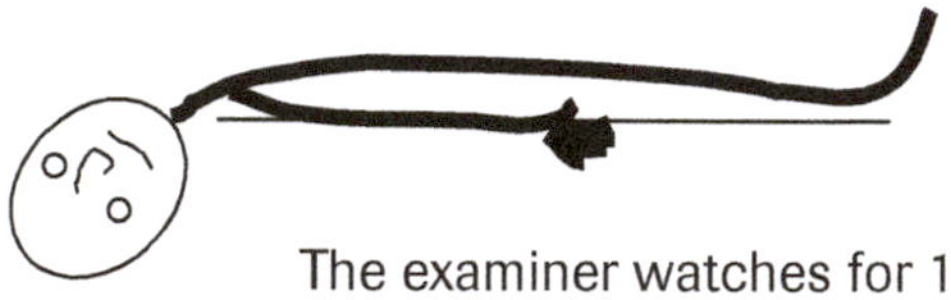

The examiner watches for 1 minute for the occurrence of nystagmus and enquires about symptoms. The process is then repeated, after a minute's rest, with the patient facing to the left.

A positive test is one in which the patient's symptoms are reproduced and nystagmus is provoked.

FIGURE 13.3 The Hallpike test for benign paroxysmal positional vertigo (BPPV).

Investigations

Specialised vestibular testing including electronystagmography and detailed brain imaging with magnetic resonance imaging (MRI) have not proved to be good discriminators of causes of vertigo within an elderly population.[11] Brain imaging is required when clinical features are suggestive of a cerebellopontine angle tumour or a brainstem stroke.

Treatment

If possible any underlying cause should be treated, for example discontinuation of causative medications or performing the Epley manoeuvre for BPPV.

Drugs

A wide range of medications has been tried in the management of vertigo with varying success.[12] The most commonly used are histamine receptor antagonists (e.g. cyclizine (H_1) and betahistine (H_3)). They may have a role in the short-term management of vertigo but prolonged use should be avoided as they may paradoxically worsen symptoms. Some of these drugs also have anticholinergic effects. Reported side-effects include sedation, confusion and dizziness. Newer antihistamine agents that are used in the management of allergies, such as loratadine, have fewer anticholinergic effects but do not cross the blood–brain barrier and so are not useful in the management of vertigo.

Vestibular rehabilitation

Vestibular rehabilitation is a form of exercise programme involving movements that induce the vertigo. These movements are taught by a nurse but then self-administered at home. The theory is that this invokes neurological adaptation that lessens the symptom impact. In a study looking at 170 patients with chronic movement-provoked symptoms believed to be of inner ear origin, 67% of participants reported an improvement compared to 38% in the control group after three months.[13] However, there was no sham treatment in the control group and participants included had a number of different diagnoses and symptoms as well as many undiagnosed patients (42%).

LIGHT-HEADEDNESS

In the elderly, light-headedness appears to be a more common reason for complaining of dizziness than vertigo.[1] The most common cause of this symptom is transient cerebral hypoperfusion in relation to neurocardiovascular disorders (e.g. orthostatic hypotension, vasovagal syndrome and carotid sinus hypersensitivity). The presence of posterior cerebral circulation atheromatous disease may make this symptom more likely to occur. Light-headedness unrelated to postural change may be caused by brainstem cerebrovascular disease, drugs or, occasionally, by paroxysmal cardiac arrhythmias or psychological disorders. An overall scheme for the assessment of light-headedness is discussed later in Chapter 15 (*see* Figure 15.6).

Specific conditions

Neurocardiovascular disorders

Neurocardiovascular disorders are discussed on p. 341. Orthostatic hypotension typically causes light-headedness on standing from sitting or lying. Vasovagal syndrome typically causes symptoms following prolonged standing. Carotid sinus hypersensitivity classically presents following head turning but often no particular movement is noted prior to events. A reduction in blood pressure following meals (post-prandial hypotension)[14] has been noted in elderly subjects and this may be a factor in the aetiology of symptoms.

Brainstem vascular disease

Bilateral vertebrobasilar atherosclerotic disease may cause multiple similar transient ischaemic attack (TIA)-like episodes.[15] These can be triggered by any event further reducing blood flow, such as orthostatic hypotension on standing. They may also be provoked at rest by posterior circulation emboli or by cardiac dysrhythmias. The most common complaints caused are light-headedness, blurred vision, and ataxia which is usually short-lived.[16] Patients presenting with these symptoms who have risk factors for vascular disease should be considered for secondary prevention measures, that is, antiplatelet and statin therapy (*see* p. 206). A number of patients who have sustained a brainstem stroke develop a chronic sensation of light-headedness that is unaffected by postural change (sometimes termed 'central dizziness'). No effective treatment exists for this condition.

Subclavian steal syndrome is a potential, although rare, cause of similar symptoms. In some cases it may result in syncope.[17] It is caused by an occlusion of the proximal subclavian artery which results in retrograde blood flow in the ipsilateral vertebral artery ('steal' of the blood flow to the brainstem). In the vast majority of cases this is secondary to atheromatous disease. Characteristically, symptoms are provoked by vigorous exercise of the affected arm. Physical signs include absent pulses, a difference in blood pressure of >20 mmHg between the arms and a supraclavicular bruit. Diagnosis is made by demonstrating retrograde flow in the vertebral artery with Doppler studies and then proceeding to angiography. Treatment involves addressing vascular risk factors and considering revascularisation procedures such as percutaneous angioplasty.

Drugs

Many drugs are potentially causative. Some of the more common agents are listed below.

➤ *Antihypertensives* and *antidepressants*: as a cause of orthostatic hypotension (*see* p. 344).
➤ *Antiarrhythmics* and *anticonvulsants*: causing paradoxical arrhythmias.

Cardiac arrhythmias

An arrhythmia that is fast or slow enough to cause reduced cerebral perfusion may provoke light-headedness. Bradyarrhythmias may occur secondary to a neurocardio-vascular mechanism. When 24-hour electrocardiograph (ECG) monitoring was used in the assessment of dizzy patients, two of 50 patients had a tachyarrhythmia coinciding with symptoms (one fast atrial fibrillation (AF), one ventricular tachycardia (VT)).[5] A primary cardiac cause is more likely when the symptoms are intermittent and unrelated to postural change. Also, there is a greater chance with a previous history of cardiac disease and pallor is often noted during these attacks.

Psychological disorders

Anxiety and depression are often cited as causes of dizziness. It is hard to know whether these are a cause or effect of the symptom. A light-headedness that is constant in nature and unchanged by movement is most often reported. It would seem reasonable to screen such patients presenting with an unexplained light-headedness for a psychiatric disorder and trying a course of therapy where indicated.

Assessment

Taking a careful history is vital. The events surrounding the symptoms give a clue to the diagnosis. A witness report is very useful when available. Light-headedness caused by neurocardiovascular or cardiac mechanisms may be associated with facial pallor during the episodes. Investigation should be targeted to diagnose or exclude potential causes (*see* Figure 15.6).

Treatment

Treatment is dependent on the underlying cause. The management of neurocardiovascular disorders is discussed on p. 345. Cardiac arrhythmias may be controlled with rate limiting medications ± cardiac pacemakers. Electrophysiology studies and implantable defibrillators may be indicated in cases of VT. If brainstem ischaemia is suspected, secondary stroke prevention measures should be instituted (*see* p. 206). Causative medications should be reassessed for clinical need and alternative agents considered. If anxiety or depression is thought to be playing a significant role a trial of therapy should be considered (*see* Chapter 8).

REFERENCES

1 Colledge NR, Wilson JA, MacIntyre CCA, *et al.* The prevalence and characteristics of dizziness in an elderly community. *Age Ageing*, 1994; **23**: 117–20.

2 Jonsson R, Sixt E, Landahl S, *et al.* Prevalence of dizziness and vertigo in an urban elderly population. *J Vest Res*, 2004; **14**: 47–52.

3 Maarsingh OR, Dros J, Schellevis SG, *et al.* Causes of persistent dizziness in elderly patients in primary care. *Ann Fam Med*, 2010; **8**: 196–205.

4 Katsarkas A. Dizziness in aging: a retrospective study of 1194 cases. *Otolaryn Head Neck Surg*, 1994; **110**(3): 296–301.

5 Lawson J, Fitzgerald J, Birchall J, *et al.* Diagnosis of geriatric patients with severe dizziness. *J Am Geriatr Soc*, 1999; **47**: 12–17.

6 Kroenke K, Lucas CA, Rosenberg ML, *et al.* Causes of persistent dizziness: a prospective study of 100 patients in ambulatory care. *Ann Intern Med*, 1992; **117**(11): 898–904.

7 Epley JM. The canalith repositioning procedure: for treatment of benign paroxysmal positional vertigo. *Otolaryn Head Neck Surg*, 1992; **107**(3): 399–404.

8 Harcourt J, Barraclough K, Bronstein A. Ménière's disease. *BMJ*, 2014; **349**: g6544.

9 Lee H, Sohn S, Cho Y, *et al.* Cerebellar infarction presenting isolated vertigo: frequency and vascular topographical patterns. *Stroke*, 2006; **67**: 1178–83.

10 Dros J, Maarsingh OR, van der Horst HE, *et al.* Tests used to evaluate dizziness in primary care. *CMAJ*, 2010; **182**: E621–31.

11 Colledge NR, Barr-Hamilton RM, Lewis SJ, *et al.* Evaluation of investigations to diagnose the cause of dizziness in elderly people: a community based controlled study. *BMJ*, 1996; **313**: 788–92.

12 Darlington CL, Smith PF. Drug treatment for vertigo and dizziness. *NZ Med J*, 1998; **111**: 332–4.

13 Yardley L, Donovan-Hall M, Smith HE, *et al.* Effectiveness of primary care-based vestibular rehabilitation for chronic dizziness. *Ann Intern Med*, 2004; **141**(8): 598–605.

14 Lipsitz LA, Nyquist RP, Wei JY, *et al.* Postprandial reduction in blood pressure in the elderly. *N Engl J Med*, 1983; **309**(2): 81–3.

15 Shin H, Yoo K, Chang HM, *et al.* Bilateral intracranial vertebral artery disease in the New England Medical Center Posterior Circulation Registry. *Arch Neurol*, 1999; **56**: 1353–8.

16 Caplan LR, Wityk RJ, Glass TA, *et al.* New England Medical Center Posterior Circulation Registry. *Ann Neurol*, 2004; **56**: 389–98.

17 Chan-Tack KM. Subclavian steal syndrome: a rare but important cause of syncope. *Southern Med J*, 2001; **94**(4): 445–7.

CHAPTER 14

Falls

BACKGROUND

It has been shown that around 30% of people over the age of 65 will fall in any given year and that this figure increases to 40% of those aged over 80 years.[1,2] People in nursing homes seem at particular risk, an estimate has been made of 1.5 falls per bed per year.[3] Also, those recently discharged from hospital appear to have a higher chance of falling.[4] Even in the absence of injury, 47% of people over the age of 72 will be unable to get up after a fall at home.[5] Falls have been found to account for 39% of emergency department attendances in those aged over the age of 50 years.[6] A large proportion of falls in the elderly result in hospital admission and on discharge a significant number will be placed in residential facilities.[7]

The process of remaining upright depends on the interaction of multiple systems, including balance (visual, proprioceptive, vestibular and cerebellar components), coordination and limb power. There are also external factors that make falls more likely to occur, such as obstacles and uneven flooring. On top of this there are specific medical conditions that make falls more likely, for example orthostatic hypotension (OH). Therefore, it is unsurprising that many falls are multifactorial in nature and almost any acute illness can increase their likelihood. A comprehensive assessment tries to identify all of the factors that increase their probability. This is best performed by a multidisciplinary team involving medical, nursing, physiotherapy and occupational therapy components.

A wide range of risk factors for falling has been identified. These include gait and balance disorders, visual impairment, arthritis, depression, cognitive impairment and old age itself. Older people more often sustain injuries after a fall than younger people. This difference is partly attributed to blunted reaction times for protective reflexes, and a higher prevalence of osteoporosis. Serious complications of falling include hip fracture. Following a fall there is also a high incidence of 'fear of falling' that can lead to reduced mobility and social isolation. A negative spiral can develop where older people mobilise less due to this fear, and thereby become deconditioned. Then, on the occasions that they do walk, they are less steady on their feet and more likely to fall, further worsening the fear.

ASSESSMENT

The causes of falls in elderly people can be divided into four key groups (*see* below). As with many problems in the frail elderly, frequently the cause is multifactorial with a number of seemingly minor problems combining with dramatic effect.

1. Acute medical illness – almost anything
2. Chronic conditions – e.g. gait and balance abnormalities, sensory and cognitive impairment
3. Drugs – especially psychotropics, cardiovascular drugs and the overall burden of polypharmacy
4. Environmental hazards – e.g. trip hazards, poor lighting and insufficient hand rails.

'Mechanical fall' is an unhelpful term and does not represent a diagnosis – look for the underlying causes so that you may reduce the risk of future harm.

History

It is recommended that all elderly people coming into contact with a healthcare professional should be asked whether they have fallen in the past year.[8] The number of falls in the last year gives an idea of the scale of the problem.

➤ Onset of the symptoms – do any other factors coincide, for example medication changes or illnesses?

Try to get as much information about each fall as possible.

➤ *Activity at the time of falling*: syncope is occasionally provoked by actions such as coughing or micturition (situational syncope). Occurrence following prolonged standing suggests vasovagal syncope. Sudden head turning may trigger carotid sinus hypersensitivity (CSH). OH usually occurs after postural change (lying or sitting to standing). Ask the patient if they feel light-headed or 'woozy' when they stand up. A drop in blood pressure can occur following a meal (post-prandial hypotension). Proximal myopathy or foot drop may cause tripping on going up stairs or when stepping over kerbstones. Falls at times when vision is reduced (e.g. while washing hair in the shower or under poor lighting at night) may suggest a proprioceptive problem.

➤ *Pattern of the falls*: is there a particular time of the day associated with falling? Visual and proprioceptive problems become worse in dim lighting, OH is characteristically worse in the mornings.

➤ *Preceding symptoms*: such as light-headedness (suggestive of OH or syncope).

➤ *Loss of consciousness*: this may or may not be recalled. Ask the patient if they remember the act of falling. If available, a witness account is extremely useful, ask about colour change (neurocardiovascular causes often result in pallor, generalised seizures may cause cyanosis), the presence of seizure activity, duration of unconsciousness and the time taken to return to the normal self following arousal.

➤ *Consequence of the falls*: were any injuries sustained? Was the patient able to get up by him or herself? Have they resulted in a loss of confidence and subsequent social withdrawal?

➤ *Associated depression*: either as a contributory factor or a result of falling (*see* Chapter 8).

A full list of medications is particularly important, as many substances are likely to cause falls, in particular all psychotropic drugs[9] and all hypertension treatments (especially vasodilators and diuretics). Despite this, psychotropic agents are commonly prescribed in the elderly. A study of nursing home residents found that 36% were on an antidepressant, 24% on sedatives/hypnotics and 17% on antipsychotics.[10] There is no apparent benefit of atypical compared to typical neuroleptic agents in terms of fall risk. Fall hazard ratios (HR) have been found to be increased for typical antipsychotic agents (HR 1.35, 95% CI 0.87–2.09), risperidone (HR 1.32, 95% CI 0.57–3.06) and olanzapine (HR 1.74, 95% CI 1.04–2.90).[11] Tricyclic antidepressants and selective serotonin reuptake inhibitors have been associated with similarly increased risks of hip fracture.[12] A systemic enquiry should look for factors associated with falls, such as urinary frequency or incontinence, cognitive decline and visual impairment. People with cognitive impairment may forget to use their mobility aids, fail to recognise risks or move too quickly for someone with their degree of functional impairment. A simple guide to visual ability can be gained by asking the patient if they can still read books and watch the television. A past medical history may identify potentially causative illnesses.

A detailed social and functional history will help guide further assessments such as a home visit by an occupational therapist. In a study looking at community-dwelling people over the age of 70, 39% were found to have five or more safety hazards within their home with the bathroom being most often implicated.[13] Alcohol excess may also be a factor. Where syncope is suspected, establish if the patient is a current driver.

EXAMINATION
The following elements should be emphasised:
➤ *Cardiovascular*: pulse rate and rhythm, presence of murmurs (particularly that of aortic stenosis), blood pressure (lying and standing ideally done as part of an active stand test – *see* p. 328), peripheral oedema and carotid bruits (if carotid sinus massage is being considered).
➤ *Neurological*: cerebellar signs, joint position sense, proximal or focal weakness, foot drop, spatial neglect and Parkinsonism.
➤ *Cognition*: *see* p. 89.
➤ *Locomotor system*: reduced range of motion, pain/tenderness and deformity of joints.
➤ *Gait and balance*: observe the patient walking, note stride width, length and height, path deviation, posture, arm swing and smoothness/steadiness of turning. Heel-toe walking may detect a subtle balance disorder. A 'timed get up and go' test is a useful screening tool for gait abnormality[14] – *see* Figure 14.1. A normal, elderly individual would perform this in less than 20 seconds. It may also be used to measure response to interventions.
➤ *Vision*: using a Snellen chart, with and without glasses (where applicable). Visual impairment is associated with approximately a two-fold increase in falls risk.[15]

Bifocal glasses may cause particular problems when negotiating stairs – they may need to be changed to a more appropriate type.

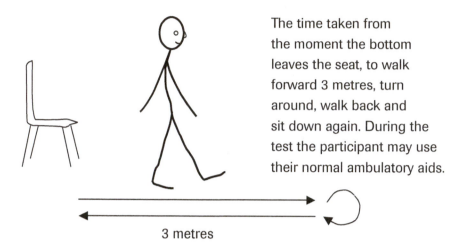

The time taken from the moment the bottom leaves the seat, to walk forward 3 metres, turn around, walk back and sit down again. During the test the participant may use their normal ambulatory aids.

3 metres

FIGURE 14.1 The 'timed get up and go' test.

INVESTIGATIONS

Baseline investigation should include the following:

➤ *Blood tests*: to exclude common contributory conditions such as anaemia, dehydration, hypoglycaemia, hypothyroidism and vitamin B_{12} deficiency.

➤ *Electrocardiogram* (ECG): to ensure sinus rhythm and a normal QT interval. An ECG suggesting previous cardiac disease may raise the suspicion of a cardiogenic aetiology (*see* Chapter 15). Potentially important abnormalities include any degree of heart block, left or right bundle branch block, a short or prolonged QT interval or any ST segment or T wave abnormalities.[16]

➤ *Active stand*: the patient is connected to a beat-to-beat blood pressure monitor (digital plethysmography) and rested flat on a bed for at least five minutes. They are then asked to stand up and remain standing for at least three minutes. The blood pressure is recorded when resting, on initial standing and then at 30-second intervals. The lowest recording is also noted (the nadir). Any symptoms experienced by the patient are recorded. Genuine OH is identified as a drop in blood pressure of more than 20 mmHg systolic and 10 mmHg diastolic that develops shortly after standing, remains present after a minute and is associated with symptoms such as light-headedness. Very transient drops without associated symptoms are of doubtful clinical significance.

Further investigations should be guided by the findings from assessment so far. If loss of consciousness is detected or suspected, neurocardiovascular (head-up tilt (HUT) and carotid sinus massage (CSM)) or cardiological investigation (ambulatory ECG monitoring and electrophysiological studies (EPS)) may be performed. These are discussed on p. 338.

TREATMENT

The treatment of falls is primarily aimed at identifying and, where possible, improving all possible contributory mechanisms. Given the relationship between falls and syncope in the elderly, neurocardiovascular assessment is also often necessary. An algorithm integrating these approaches is shown in Figure 15.6.

Multifactorial intervention programmes

Given the multifactorial nature of falls in the elderly, it is not surprising that a multifactorial treatment strategy has been found to be most effective in meta-analyses.[17,18] An effect size of around a 25% reduction in the incidence of falls is characteristically seen. Most of this data comes from community-based studies, which employed a number of different interventions tested together. Frequent components of these schemes include withdrawal of psychotropic medications, exercise ± gait and balance training, home environment adaptation, visual acuity assessment and information given to both patients and carers.

Further, a guideline has been devised by the National Institute for Health and Care Excellence (NICE).[8] It is recommended that the following components be included in an intervention strategy: strength and balance training; home hazard assessment and modification; visual assessment and correction; and medication review and withdrawal, where appropriate. Also, information should be available in both written and oral forms for patients, their carers and healthcare staff. Topics covered should include strategies to avoid falls and ways to cope if a fall occurs. It is also recommended that an assessment of osteoporosis be incorporated into a falls programme. Osteoporosis is discussed in Chapter 16.

A study recruiting 981 nursing home residents with a mean age of 85 investigated the use of a multifactorial intervention.[19] The intervention consisted of educational sessions for residents and staff, a review of environmental hazards, an exercise programme and the use of hip protectors (to which there was only a 28% adherence). They found a significant reduction in falls in the treatment arm (RR 0.55, 95% CI 0.41–0.73). Therefore, it seems logical that such multifactorial schemes should be implemented to both community-dwelling individuals and those in residential care.

A multi-component intervention has also been tested in a group of visually impaired people (acuity 6/24 or worse) aged 75 or over (mean age 84 years).[20] A combination of a home safety assessment and/or home exercise programme plus vitamin D supplementation or social visits only was implemented. The home safety element was effective at reducing falls (incidence rate ratio 0.59, 95% CI 0.42–0.83), but the other components were not.

It appears that multifactorial intervention programmes, at present, are effective in reducing the incidence of falls by about a third. However, they are probably not effective for all people. In two community-based studies that included cognitively impaired patients, multifactorial intervention programmes have been found to be ineffective (definitions of cognitive impairment were MMSE scores of less than 19 and 24, respectively).[21,22] This probably reflects the difficulty of this subgroup complying with interventions such as gait and balance training. So the selection of patients who are most likely to benefit is important. Some of the frequently incorporated components are discussed in more detail below.

Medication review

A wide range of medications can potentially contribute to falls. It is important to assess the risks versus benefits of all agents in a particular individual. For example, blood pressure-reducing medication may reduce the risk of a stroke but may also increase the risk of a fractured neck of femur, both of which may be fatal. Sedating medications such as benzodiazepines and neuroleptics are particularly harmful and their dose should be reduced and then discontinued whenever possible. A trial of 93 elderly patients (mean age 75 years) compared psychotropic drug withdrawal by gradual substitution with a placebo to a control group of usual care.[23] After a 44-week follow-up period a significant reduction in falls was demonstrated (relative hazard 0.34, 95% CI 0.16–0.74).

Visual intervention

Some 70–79% of visual problems in the elderly are said to be correctable.[15] These are usually caused by cataracts and inadequate glasses. Bifocal and varifocal glasses are associated with increased falls risk.[24] The other common causes are age-related macular degeneration, glaucoma and diabetic retinopathy. Treatment of these conditions is aimed at preventing deterioration in vision. Logic would suggest that improvements in vision would reduce the risk of falling. However, a trial that randomised 616 patients over the age of 70 (mean age 81 years) who lived in the community to either visual assessment (plus, when appropriate, new glasses or referral to an ophthalmologist (generally cataract or glaucoma treatment)) or usual care over a 12-month period failed to show a benefit.[25] In fact falls were significantly more common in the intervention group (65% fell vs 50%, rate ratio 1.57, 95% CI 1.20–2.05) and fractures were also increased (31 vs 18, RR 1.74, 95% CI 0.97–3.11). The reasons for these findings are unclear. A different study has found a lower risk of fracture following cataract surgery (hip fracture adjusted odds ratio 0.84, 95% CI 0.81–0.87),[26] which suggests that falls risk was reduced.

Strength and balance training

Strength and balance training regimens are common components of effective intervention programmes. The exact nature of the most effective format is unknown. One study failed to show a benefit of specific balance training over standard physiotherapy sessions in 198 individuals with a mean age of 83 years.[27] It could be that any form of neuromuscular improvement is beneficial. There is some evidence that a once-weekly exercise regimen may be sufficient to provide this.[28] A more recent meta-analysis has suggested a 17% reduction in falls (rate ratio 0.83, 95% CI 0.75–0.91) in people undergoing exercise programmes compared to controls.[29] In this analysis, higher total doses of exercise training and programmes including challenging balance exercises were most effective. Physiotherapy input should also include guidance on how to get up off the floor after a fall.

T'ai-chi has been suggested as a suitable form of exercise to increase strength and balance and therefore prevent falls. Early trial results have been mixed. A study randomised 269 patients (mean age 77 years) to two hours of t'ai-chi per week for 13 weeks, or standard care.[30] After one year no significant reduction in falls was seen.

Home environment assessment

A home visit performed by an occupational therapist may identify and subsequently improve environmental hazards. The types of simple interventions that have been found to be effective include removing rugs or poorly fitted carpets, installing bilateral stair rails and providing a raised toilet seat, a rubber shower mat, an emergency call alarm and nightlights for the bedroom and bathroom. A recent study recruited 360 community-dwelling people with a mean age of 82 years and a high risk of falling, and randomised them to either home environmental modifications or to a control group.[31] It demonstrated a significant reduction in fall incidence in the intervention arm (RR 0.69, 95% CI 0.51–0.97).

Vitamin D

Deficiency in vitamin D is common among the elderly (*see* p. 360). It has been associated with both proximal myopathy and falls.[32] A trial that compared vitamin D supplementation to placebo (both groups received calcium) in people in residential care (mean age 83 years), over a two-year period, found a reduction in falls in the treatment arm.[33] The participants recruited all had vitamin D levels in the low normal range (25–90 nmol/l). However, this was not associated with a significant reduction in fracture rates.

PREVENTING FALLS IN HOSPITALS

While there is a large body of evidence supporting the efficacy of community-based falls prevention schemes, there is less knowledge about practice within the hospital setting. A systematic review from the year 2000 identified two randomised controlled trials, one prospective study with a parallel control group and a further seven prospective studies with historical controls.[34] The randomised controlled trials investigated the single interventions of bed alarms and identification bracelets.[35,36] Neither demonstrated a significant reduction in falls. The remainder of the studies used a multifaceted strategy including some or all of education programmes, environmental and equipment adjustment, high-risk identification signs/wrist bands, physical restraints and individualised care plans. The meta-analysis of all trials suggested a pooled effect rate ratio of 0.79 (95% CI 0.69–0.89). However, the majority of the positive studies used historical control groups for comparison. On further analysis, none of the interventions showed significant benefit when looked at in isolation. A later randomised controlled trial investigated the use of additional exercise training and an altered type of flooring without significant benefit.[37]

A more recent randomised controlled trial demonstrated a trend to reduction in number of falls (RR 0.78, 95% CI 0.56–1.06) with a combination of a risk-alert card, information for patients, education sessions for staff, an exercise programme and hip protectors.[38] The difference between the groups was not apparent until after six weeks of intervention. There was no difference in fracture rates between groups, although the overall rate was low.

Another trial tested the introduction of a care plan consisting of a risk factor screening tool and appropriate interventions on alternate geriatric wards within a district general hospital with the other geriatric wards acting as a control group.[39] The mean age of patients was 81 years, the mean length of stay was 18 days on the control group wards and 21 days for the intervention group. Patients with a history of falls or those deemed to have either fallen or had a 'near miss' during their admission were targeted. The assessments included an eyesight screen, a review of medications, a lying and standing blood pressure measurement, a urine dip test, a mobility screen, an environment check (including bed rails, bed height and position on ward) and a footwear assessment. Appropriate interventions were then triggered according to the care plan. Comparing a preceding six-month evaluation period to a six-month period of intervention or control on both of the groups of wards, a significant reduction in the incidence of falls was seen in the intervention arm (RR 0.71, 95% CI 0.55–0.90; p=0.006). A systematic review from 2007 has supported a modest benefit from multifactorial intervention programmes (rate ratio 0.82, 95% CI 0.68–0.997),[40] as has a review from 2010 (rate ratio 0.69, 95% CI 0.49–0.96).[41]

Guidelines recommend assessing ward environments to ensure appropriate flooring, lighting, furniture and hand rails are utilised.[8] Four basic steps have been suggested: ask all patients if they have had a recent fall, avoid psychotropic medications, ensure the patients have suitable footwear, and place call bells within easy sight and reach.[42]

Although broader policies, such as ward environment and prescribing practice adjustments, may affect all inpatients, it seems likely that specific interventions will only succeed if targeted at the highest risk patients. A review of falls risk-assessment tools found the following factors best predictors of falls: lower limb weakness; gait instability; agitated confusion; urinary incontinence, increased frequency or the need for assisted toileting; a history of previous falls; and the use of sedative medications.[43] However, no risk assessment tool is currently considered effective and all elderly people in hospital should be considered at risk.[8]

Bed rails

The use of bed rails (also called 'cot sides') is commonplace within hospitals. One UK survey found that overall they were deployed on 32% of hospital beds, a figure that rose to 76% in acute geriatric wards.[44] Despite this, there is no randomised controlled trial evidence of efficacy in reducing falls and non-randomised studies have failed to demonstrate a benefit.[45] Where a policy of reducing their use has been implemented, there has been no apparent increase in fall or injury rates.[46] Also, they are not without the potential to cause harm, which may be that of falling from a greater height to the floor after scaling the rail, but also a number of fatal complications have been reported.[47] Given the absence of evidence of benefit and the fact that they represent a form of patient restraint, their use may be construed as unethical.[48]

In patients with a high risk of falling out of bed, an alternative strategy such as placing the mattress directly on the floor or the use of beds that can be lowered to ground level would appear more appropriate.

Restraints

Physical restraints, such as tying a patient down, have not been shown to reduce the incidence of falls,[49,50] act as a barrier to rehabilitation and are unethical. Their use should be strongly discouraged.

Prevention strategies

The following may be beneficial in reducing the incidence of falls in hospitalised patients.

➤ A screening proforma utilised to identify higher risk patients at the time of admission. The following information is likely to be a useful guide: falls history, a delirium screening test, urinary incontinence/frequency, gait assessment (e.g. timed get up and go) and potential culprit medication checklist.

➤ Patients in the high risk group should then undergo the following interventions:
  — a risk identifier worn on their wrist or above their bed (a symbol rather than written information to try to help preserve patient confidentiality)
  — education in oral and written form on falls risk
  — preferential placement nearer the nursing station
  — a review of medications likely to increase falls risk, and a visual acuity assessment.

➤ Delirium and incontinence should be accurately diagnosed and treated (*see* Chapters 7 and 11).

➤ Education sessions for staff.

➤ Periodic review with ward team members of falls that have occurred.

➤ Exercise and balance training as deemed appropriate by the physiotherapist involved.

➤ Consideration of the falls risk when planning discharge, for example home assessment visits.

DROP ATTACKS

The term 'drop attack' refers to an event whereby the patient suddenly collapses to the ground without any preceding warning symptoms, and without apparent loss of consciousness. Unless an injury is sustained with the fall, there are no lasting effects and the patient quickly returns to normal. Such episodes probably account for around 20% of elderly patients presenting to a falls service.[51,52]

A wide range of conditions has been proposed as causative for these events, including otological disorders and forms of epilepsy.[53,54] It is likely that, along with other falls, they are often multifactorial in nature. When older individuals with drop attacks have been systematically evaluated for neurocardiovascular disorders, 40% have been found to suffer from carotid sinus syndrome and smaller numbers found to have OH and vasovagal syncope.[55] Therefore, in the elderly, drop attacks further blur the distinction between falls and syncope. Their assessment should be a combination of measures used in falls and syncopal events (*see* Figure 15.6). Treatment should be directed towards the underlying causative factors that are identified. Despite intensive investigation, around a third will go undiagnosed (sometimes termed 'cryptogenic drop attacks'), suggesting that we do not fully understand the aetiology of all such events.

REFERENCES

1 Prudham D, Grimley Evans J. Factors associated with falls in the elderly: a community study. *Age Ageing*, 1981; **10**: 141–6.

2 Campbell AJ, Reinken J, Allan BC, *et al.* Falls in old age: a study of frequency and related clinical factors. *Age Ageing*, 1981; **10**: 264–70.

3 Rubenstein LZ, Josephson KR, Robbins AS. Falls in the nursing home. *Ann Intern Med*, 1994; **121**: 442–51.

4 Mahoney J, Sager M, Dunham NC, *et al.* Risk of falls after hospital discharge. *J Am Geriatr Soc*, 1994; **42**: 269–74.

5 Tinetti ME, Liu W, Claus EB. Predictors and prognosis of inability to get up after falls among elderly persons. *JAMA*, 1993; **269**(1): 65–70.

6 Richardson DA, Bexton RS, Shaw FE, *et al.* Prevalence of cardioinhibitory carotid sinus hypersensitivity in patients 50 years or over presenting to the accident and emergency department with 'unexplained' or 'recurrent' falls. *Pace*, 1997; **20** (Part II): 820–3.

7 Sattin RW, Lambert Huber DA, DeVito CA, *et al.* The incidence of fall injury events among the elderly in a defined population. *Am J Epidem*, 1990; **131**(6): 1028–37.

8 NICE guideline. *Falls: assessment and prevention of falls in older people.* CG161, 2013. Available at: www.nice.org.uk/guidance/cg161 (accessed 14 November 2014).

9 Leipzig RM, Cummings RG, Tinetti ME. Drugs and falls in older people: a systematic review and meta-analysis: I. Psychotropic drugs. *J Am Geriatr Soc*, 1999; **47**(1): 30–9.

10 Gurwitz JH, Field TS, Avorn J, *et al.* Incidence and preventability of adverse drug events in nursing homes. *Am J Med*, 2000; **109**: 87–94.

11 Hien LTT, Cummings RG, Cameron ID, *et al.* Atypical antipsychotic medications and risk of falls in residents of aged care facilities. *J Am Geriatr Soc*, 2005; **53**(8): 1290–5.

12 Liu B, Anderson G, Mittmann N, *et al.* Use of selective serotonin-reuptake inhibitors or tricyclic antidepressants and risk of hip fractures in elderly people. *Lancet*, 1998; **351**: 1303–7.

13 Carter SE, Campbell EM, Sanson-Fisher RW, *et al.* Environmental hazards in the homes of older people. *Age Ageing*, 1997; **26**: 195–202.

14 Podsiadlo D, Richardson S. The timed 'up and go': a test of basic functional mobility for frail elderly persons. *J Am Geriatr Soc*, 1991; **39**(2): 142–8.

15 Harwood RH. Visual problems and falls. *Age Ageing*, 2001; **30**(Suppl. 4): S13–18.

16 National Institute of Health and Care Excellence. *Transient Loss of Consciousness ('Blackouts') Management in Adults and Young People.* CG109, 2010. Available at: www.nice.org.uk/guidance/cg109 (accessed 3 December 2014).

17 Gillespie LD, Robertson MC, Gillespie WJ, *et al.* Interventions for preventing falls in older people living in the community. *Cochrane Database Syst Rev*, 2012, Issue 9. Art. No.: CD007146. DOI: 10.1002/14651858.CD007146.pub3.

18 Chang JT, Morton SC, Rubenstein LZ, *et al.* Interventions for the prevention of falls in older adults: systematic review and meta-analysis of randomised clinical trials. *BMJ*, 2004; **328**: 680–3.

19 Becker C, Kron M, Lindemann U, *et al.* Effectiveness of a multifaceted intervention on falls in nursing home residents. *J Am Geriatr Soc*, 2003; **51**: 306–13.

20 Campbell AJ, Robertson MC, La Grow SJ, *et al.* Randomised controlled trial of prevention of falls in people aged > 75 with severe visual impairment: the VIP trial. *BMJ*, 2005; **331**: 817–20.

21 Jensen J, Nyberg L, Gustafson Y, *et al.* Fall and injury prevention in residential care – effects in residents with higher and lower levels of cognition. *J Am Geriatr Soc*, 2003; **51**: 627–35.

22 Shaw FE, Bond J, Richardson DA, *et al.* Multifactorial intervention after a fall in older people with cognitive impairment and dementia presenting to the accident and emergency department: randomised controlled trial. *BMJ*, 2003; **326**: 73–5.

23 Campbell AJ, Robertson MC, Gardner MM, *et al.* Psychotropic medication withdrawal and a home-based exercise program to prevent falls: a randomized, controlled trial. *J Am Geriatr Soc*, 1999; **47**(7): 850–3.

24 Lord SR, Dayhew J, Howland A. Multifocal glasses impair edge-contrast sensitivity and depth perception and increase the risk of falls in older people. *J Am Geriatr Soc*, 2002; **50**(11): 1760–6.

25 Cummings RG, Ivers R, Clemson L, *et al.* Improving vision to prevent falls in frail older people: a randomized trial. *J Am Geriatr Soc*, 2007; **55**(2): 175–81.

26 Tseng VL, Yu F, Lum F, *et al.* Risk of fractures following cataract surgery in Medicare beneficiaries. *JAMA*, 2012; **308**: 493–501.

27 Steadman J, Donaldson N, Kalra L. A randomized controlled trial of an enhanced balance training program to improve mobility and reduce falls in elderly patients. *J Am Geriatr Soc*, 2003; **51**: 847–52.

28 Taaffe DR, Duret C, Wheeler S, *et al.* Once-weekly exercise improves muscle strength and neuromuscular performance in older adults. *J Am Geriatr Soc*, 1999; **47**(10): 1208–14.

29 Sherrington C, Whitney JC, Lord SR, *et al.* Effective exercise for the prevention of falls: a systematic review and meta-analysis. *J Am Geriatr Soc*, 2008; **56**: 2234–43.

30 Logghe IH, Zeeuwe PE, Verhagen AP, *et al.* Lack of effect of Tai Chi Chuan in preventing falls in elderly people living at home: a randomized clinical trial. *J Am Geriatr Soc*, 2009; **57**(1): 70–5.

31 Nikolaus T, Bach M. Preventing falls in community-dwelling frail older people using a home intervention team (HIT): results from the randomized falls-HIT trial. *J Am Geriatr Soc*, 2003; **51**: 300–5.

32 Venning G. Recent developments in vitamin D deficiency and muscle weakness among elderly people. *BMJ*, 2005; **330**: 524–6.

33 Flicker L, MacInnis RJ, Stein MS, *et al.* Should older people in residential care receive vitamin D to prevent falls? Results of a randomized trial. *J Am Geriatr Soc*, 2005; **53**: 1881–8.

34 Oliver D, Hooper A, Seed P. Do hospital fall prevention programs work? A systematic review. *J Am Geriatr Soc*, 2000; **48**: 1679–89.

35 Tideiksaar R, Feiner CF, Maby J. Falls prevention: the efficacy of a bed alarm system in an acute care setting. *Mt Sinai J Med*, 1993; **60**: 522–7.

36 Mayo NE, Gloutney L, Levy AR. A randomised trial of identification bracelets to prevent falls among patients in a rehabilitation hospital. *Arch Phys Med Rehab*, 1994; **75**: 1302–8.

37 Donald I, Shuttleworth H. Preventing falls on an elderly care rehabilitation ward. *Clin Rehab*, 2000; **14**: 178–5.

38 Haines TP, Bennell KL, Osborne RH, *et al.* Effectiveness of targeted falls prevention programme in subacute hospital setting: randomised controlled trial. *BMJ*, 2004; **328**: 676–9.

39 Healey F, Monro A, Cockram A, *et al.* Using targeted risk factor reduction to prevent falls in older in-patients: a randomised controlled trial. *Age Ageing*, 2004; **33**: 390–5.

40 Oliver D, Connelly JB, Victor CR, *et al.* Strategies to prevent falls and fractures in hospitals and care homes and effect of cognitive impairment: systematic review and meta-analyses. *BMJ*, 2007; **334**: 82–7.

41 Cameron ID, Murray GR, Gillespie LD, *et al.* Interventions for preventing falls in older people in nursing care facilities and hospitals. *Cochrane Database Syst Rev*, 2010, Issue 1. Art. No.: CD005465. DOI: 10.1002/14651858.CD005465.pub2.

42 Patient Safety First Campaign. The 'How to' Guide for Reducing Harm from Falls, 2009. Available at: www.patientsafetyfirst.nhs.uk (accessed 14 November 2014).

43 Oliver D, Daly F, Martin FC, *et al.* Risk factors and risk assessment tools for falls in hospital in-patients: a systematic review. *Age Ageing*, 2004; **33**: 122–30.

44 Mildner R, Snell A, Arora A, *et al.* The prevalence of bedrail use in British hospitals. *Age Ageing*, 2002; **31**: 555–6.

45 Capezuti E, Maislin G, Strumpf N, *et al.* Side rail use and bed-related fall outcomes among nursing home residents. *J Am Geriatr Soc*, 2002; **50**(1): 90–6.

46 Hanger HC, Ball MC, Wood LA. An analysis of falls in the hospital: can we do without bedrails? *J Am Geriatr Soc*, 1999; **47**(5): 529–31.

47 Parker K, Miles SH. Deaths caused by bedrails. *JAGS*, 1997; **45**: 797–802.

48 Oliver D. Bed falls and bedrails – what should we do? *Age Ageing*, 2002; **31**: 415–18.

49 Tinetti ME, Liu W, Ginter SF. Mechanical restraint use and fall-related injuries among residents of skilled nursing facilities. *Ann Intern Med*, 1992; **116**: 369–74.

50 Ejaz FK, Jones JA, Rose MS. Falls among nursing home residents: an examination of incident reports before and after restraint reduction programs. *J Am Geriatr Soc*, 1994; **42**: 960–4.

51 Sheldon JH. On the natural history of falls in old age. *BMJ*, 1960; **2**: 1685–90.

52 O'Mahony D, Foote C. Prospective evaluation of unexplained syncope, dizziness, and falls among community-dwelling elderly adults. *J Gerontology Med Sci*, 1998; **53A**(6): M435–40.

53 Ishiyama G, Ishiyama A, Jacobson K, *et al.* Drop attacks in older patients secondary to an otologic cause. *Neurology*, 2001; **57**: 1103–6.

54 Gambardella A, Reutens DC, Andermann F, *et al.* Late-onset drop attacks in temporal lobe epilepsy: a re-evaluation of the concept of temporal lobe syncope. *Neurology*, 1994; **44**: 1074–8.

55 Parry SW, Kenny RA. Drop attacks in older adults: systematic assessment has a high diagnostic yield. *J Am Geriatr Soc*, 2005; **53**: 74–8.

CHAPTER 15

Syncope

Syncope is defined as an episode of loss of consciousness due to a transient global reduction in cerebral blood flow. In elderly, institutionalised individuals (mean age 87 years) it has been found to occur in around 6% of people per year.[1] Its community prevalence is hard to establish because of the frequent amnesia for unconsciousness in people who present with simple falls. In elderly individuals it is typically multifactorial in aetiology. Physiological changes making it more likely include alterations in cerebral blood flow autoregulation and reduced baroreceptor sensitivity. Comorbidities such as heart failure may also affect cerebral blood flow.

One of the differential diagnoses is epilepsy. The distinction can be made more difficult by the presence of associated seizure-like movements with the onset of syncope (usually myoclonic jerks). In situations where the hypoxia is prolonged, for example if the subject is propped up rather than being laid flat following the onset, seizure activity is more likely. Clinical features that are more suggestive of syncope than epilepsy include preceding symptoms of nausea or light-headedness, a pallid appearance, a brief ictal phase without rhythmic clonic movements, and a rapid recovery phase without significant confusion or disorientation (*see* Table 15.1). Epileptic seizures may be associated with a preceding aura (e.g. a peculiar smell), a cyanotic appearance and tongue biting (especially deep bites to the lateral aspects of the tongue) (*see* p. 429). Incontinence of urine, and occasionally faeces, may be associated with either syncope or seizures. When patients with a questionable diagnosis of epilepsy (due to poor response to treatment or atypical clinical features) have been evaluated for syncopal conditions,

TABLE 15.1 A comparison between typical features of syncope and epilepsy

	Syncope	Epilepsy
Preceding symptoms	Light-headedness, nausea, sweating	Possible aura (e.g. taste or smell)
Fitting	Brief jerks	Prolonged and rhythmical
Colour	Pale or grey	Cyanosed
Incontinence	Occasionally	Not always
Tongue biting	Sometimes to the tip of the tongue	May have deep bites to lateral tongue
Following event	Rapidly back to normal	Post ictal (drowsy, confused)

around 40% were assigned an alternative diagnosis.[2] A suggested assessment algorithm is shown in Figure 15.6.

Subclavian steal syndrome is a rare cause of syncope (*see* p. 322). Occasionally, metabolic disorders such as hypoglycaemia can present as syncope. Clinical features and baseline investigations should exclude such conditions. Rarely, psychiatric conditions present with similar symptoms to syncope. This group of patients tends to be younger. Conditions implicated include conversion reactions and somatisation disorders related to anxiety and depression.[3] In a systematic evaluation of 231 older patients (mean age 79 years, range 65–98) presenting with syncope, none was found to have a psychiatric cause for their symptoms.[4] Despite extensive investigation, a number of patients presenting with syncope will remain undiagnosed.

Syncope can impair an individual's ability to drive safely. Guidelines on what is approved within the UK are available at the DVLA website (www.gov.uk/government/publications/at-a-glance – accessed November 2014). Essentially, the guidance reflects the risk of recurrence while seated behind the wheel of a vehicle. Patients who drive should be made aware of the guidelines that apply to them. Web resources for driving regulations in countries outside the UK are shown in Box 6.2.

ASSESSMENT

The assessment of patients with suspected syncope begins with a clinical evaluation the same as for those presenting with falls (*see* Chapter 14). Additional investigations that are useful in determining the cause of suspected syncope are discussed below.

Head-up tilt

The head-up tilt (HUT) test is used to diagnose vasovagal syncope. After a five-minute period of lying flat, the patient is placed at angle of 70 degrees from the horizontal on a specialised table (Figure 15.1). The blood pressure (BP) and heart rate (HR) are carefully monitored. This position is maintained for around 40 minutes.[5] Provocation substances

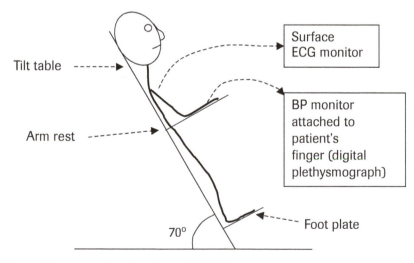

FIGURE 15.1 The set-up for a head-up tilt (HUT) test.

such as glycerol trinitrate (GTN) spray or isoprenaline infusions may be used to increase the sensitivity (a 'provoked HUT'). However, these may reduce the specificity of the test – it is critical that the reproduction of symptoms, rather than haemodynamic consequences alone, is sought. A positive test shows a gradually declining BP, with or without a change in heart rate, which ultimately produces unconsciousness with the reproduction of the same symptoms previously experienced by the patient. These changes have been found to occur at a mean time of 24 minutes into the investigation.[6] On production of a positive result, the bed is rapidly lowered and the patient's legs are raised until the symptoms pass (Figure 15.2). A variant of this test in which the patient receives GTN provocation after 20 minutes of unprovoked tilting has been described.[7] Alternatively, the GTN may be given at the start of the test with the patient then stood for just 20 minutes. This technique appears to increase the sensitivity of the test, but at the expense of more false positive results.[8]

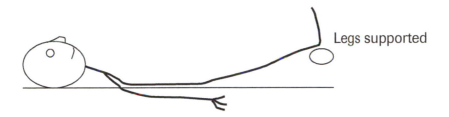

Legs supported

FIGURE 15.2 Recovery position following a positive head-up tilt test.

Carotid sinus massage

Carotid sinus massage (CSM) is a test used to diagnose carotid sinus syndrome (CSS). It is recommended that it should not be performed in people who have sustained a stroke, transient ischaemic attack or myocardial infarction within the last three months or in people with a history of ventricular dysrhythmias.[5] There is a reported 1% risk of inducing transient neurological symptoms with a 0.1% risk of stroke, which the patient needs to be made aware of during the consent process.[9] For this reason it is suggested that the neck be auscultated for carotid bruits and if present a carotid Doppler scan is recommended prior to proceeding in order to assess patient risk and advise on safety (in the absence of definitive evidence this is considered best practice).[5] The patient's neck is then palpated to identify the point of maximal carotid pulsation. This approximates to the location of the carotid sinus and is usually at the level of the cricoid cartilage, medial to the sternocleidomastoid muscle (Figure 15.3). While continuously monitoring the BP and HR, the point of maximal pulsation is rubbed (firm, longitudinal pressure is recommended) for five seconds on the right side, lying flat on a bed. The right side is assessed first as this has been found to be more sensitive than the left.[10] If a positive result is not produced, the process is repeated at an interval of more than one minute on the left, and subsequently on the right and then left while tilted at 70 degrees on a specialised table. A 31% additional benefit of detecting CSS by performing the test at 70 degrees has been demonstrated.[11] A positive result is a pause in HR of more than three seconds or a drop in systolic BP of more than 50 mmHg. If a positive result occurs, steps as for the HUT should be commenced. Atropine and equipment for external cardiac pacing should be available for the unlikely event of a prolonged cardiac pause.

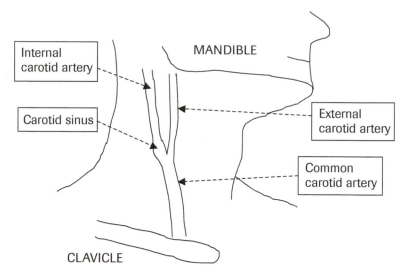

FIGURE 15.3 The position of the carotid sinus.

Ambulatory ECG

Ambulatory electrocardiograph (ECG) recording may be useful if a paroxysmal cardiac arrhythmia is suspected. But the diagnostic yield for cause of syncope is low (<10%), especially in those without structural heart disease.[12] The standard 24-hour ECG (Holter monitor) will only be reliable if symptoms occur on a daily basis. If symptoms are occurring several times a week, then a 48-hour ECG monitor may be appropriate.[13] The less frequent the symptoms, the less likely that the abnormal rhythm will be captured. Continuation of the recording over a seven-day period may be more helpful. An alternative method, also using adhesive surface electrodes, is an external event recorder. The patient wears this device for periods of up to several weeks. On the occurrence of a symptomatic episode, the patient activates the device and the heart beat over the preceding 10 minutes is stored in its memory for later analysis. This type of investigation is useful when symptoms occur at least every two weeks.[13]

Implantable loop recorder

An implantable loop recorder is useful when symptoms are infrequent (intervals of greater than every two weeks), and a longer recording period is necessary. This device is placed under the skin much like a pacemaker. Similar to surface event recorders, it can be activated following a symptomatic episode. The advantage of the device is that it can be used reliably for periods of up to two years. The obvious disadvantages are the requirement for a minor surgical procedure and the financial cost involved. In a series of 95 consecutive cases (mean age 64 years) of unexplained syncope (despite extensive investigations), after a mean follow-up of 10 months, 43 patients (45%) had further syncope, and of these patients 27 (63%) had a detected causative arrhythmia.[14]

Electrophysiological studies

Electrophysiological studies (EPS) are techniques for identifying abnormal cardiac rhythms (e.g. ventricular tachycardia) that have not been detected by less invasive methods. They involve the percutaneous placement of a catheter that is fed through the femoral vein to the right atrium and ventricle. Electric stimulation or intravenous medications can then be used to try to stimulate abnormal heart rhythms. A positive test is one causing the reproduction of symptoms at the same time as a significant arrhythmia. Yield is highest in patients with either a history of cardiac disease or an abnormal baseline ECG.[15]

Ambulatory blood pressure recording

Ambulatory BP recording is unlikely to help with the diagnosis of the aetiology of falls or syncope. Its main use is to guide BP treatment in cases of orthostatic hypotension. It is discussed in more detail on p. 396.

NEUROCARDIOVASCULAR SYNCOPE

There is a great deal of overlap among the neurocardiovascular disorders, suggesting similarities in causative mechanisms. In a group of patients with CSS, a 27% prevalence of orthostatic hypotension (OH) and a 20% prevalence of vasovagal syndrome (VVS) was also detected.[16] These conditions also appear to be more common in people with neurodegenerative dementias, possibly suggesting a common neurotransmitter deficit in their aetiology.[17] This association may explain the feature of loss of consciousness in patients with dementia with Lewy bodies (*see* p. 169). A neurocardiovascular cause is found in around two-thirds of older adults presenting with syncope.[4]

Vasovagal syncope

VVS is produced by an autonomic reflex that leads to hypotension and bradycardia, resulting in a temporary reduction in cerebral perfusion. The precise mechanism is incompletely understood. When normal individuals are standing, there is a gradual gravity-driven accumulation of interstitial fluid in the legs. This is usually compensated for by peripheral vasoconstriction. This is mainly driven by baroreceptor activation and increased vagally mediated parasympathetic actions (*see* Figure 15.4). In susceptible individuals, this corrective reflex malfunctions, leading to VVS.

VVS is classically triggered by periods of prolonged standing. There are several variants of this condition. It is proposed that young individuals may have a *hyper*-sensitive autonomic reflex which, when triggered, causes a rapid drop in BP. This pattern is associated with a history of fainting since childhood. Older individuals who develop symptoms may have a *hypo*-sensitive reflex that causes a gradual reduction in BP on prolonged standing.[3] Alternative triggers may be situations that cause increased abdominal pressure (*see* p. 345) and painful or anxiety-causing stimuli (e.g. cannulation or the sight of blood). It is commonly associated with preceding symptoms of sweating and nausea and a pallid facial appearance.

The diagnostic test is the HUT. If a standard HUT is negative, provocation substances such as GTN may be used to try to reproduce symptoms. The test has not been

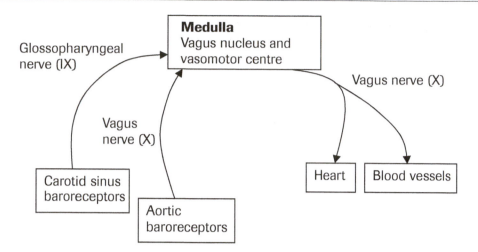

FIGURE 15.4 Vagally mediated blood pressure homeostasis.

associated with significant complications apart from rare reports of arrhythmias on provocation with isoprenaline. The reproducibility of the HUT test is significantly less than 100%.

Differential diagnoses that have been identified during head-up tilt, attributed to an absence of associated BP change, include psychogenic and hyperventilation syncope.[15,18] The latter appears to be mediated by cerebral vasoconstriction in response to a reduced pCO_2. Both of these conditions are more common in younger age groups.

Treatment

The first stage of management is education and reassurance. A number of lifestyle adjustments have been found to reduce the occurrence of symptoms. They are discussed, along with other treatment options, on p. 345.

Carotid sinus syndrome

The carotid sinus is an area of dilatation of the internal carotid artery just distal to the carotid bifurcation (Figure 15.3). It contains a number of nerve receptors that sense change in pressure within the vessel wall (baroreceptors). Signals from these travel in a branch of the glossopharyngeal nerve (IX) to the medulla. From here a vagally mediated response can be triggered (Figure 15.4). As a response to increased pressure within the vessel wall the resultant effect is peripheral vasodilatation and a reduction in HR, leading to a drop in BP. In normal individuals this important mechanism maintains homeostasis of BP during changing physical activities.

CSS (also known as 'carotid sinus hypersensitivity') is a condition of abnormal activation of this structure, which causes symptoms due to changes in HR and BP that lead to cerebral hypoperfusion. It appears to be increasingly common with advancing years, probably due to a combination of increased baroreceptor sensitivity and reduced cerebral autoregulatory mechanisms. The resultant presentations include light-headedness, falls, drop attacks and syncope. A study that systematically evaluated elderly patients (mean age 78, range 67–89 years) with these complaints found that around 25% had CSS.[10] When patients presenting to an emergency department with unexplained or recurrent falls were evaluated, 23% were found to have the cardio-inhibitory (*see* below) variant of CSS.[19] This may have significant consequences, with one study demonstrating a prevalence of 36% in patients hospitalised following a fractured neck of femur.[20]

It is subdivided into three categories:

➤ *Cardio-inhibitory CSS* (CICSS): the primary result of CSM is a pause in HR >3 seconds.
➤ *Vasodepressor CSS* (VDCSS): the primary result is a drop in systolic BP of 50 mmHg or more.
➤ *Mixed CSS*: a simultaneous combination of both of the above.

In a study of 64 elderly patients (mean age 81 years) with CSS, 37% had VDCSS, 29% CICSS and 34% had a mixed picture.[16] The same study found that the most common precipitants of CSS were head movements and prolonged standing, and that 25% of patients with CSS had had a previous associated fracture. Amnesia for witnessed syncope is well recognised in this population.[10,16]

CSS seems to be able to result in a range of presentations, namely syncope, falls, drop attacks and light-headedness.[10] In a study systematically applying CSM to a group of elderly patients with any of these symptoms (mean age 79 years), a positive result was detected in 18% of subjects.[21] The yield being higher in the syncope and falls groups than those with dizziness alone.

Treatment
Pacemakers

A group of 60 patients (mean age 70) with syncope attributed to either CICSS or mixed type CSS were randomly assigned to either pacemaker insertion or a control group.[22] After three years of follow-up there was a 57% recurrence of syncope in the control subjects compared to only 9% in the paced group (p=0.0002).

The role of cardiac pacing in CICSS appears not to be limited to those with syncope. A study compared dual-chamber pacemaker insertion to standard care in a series of 175 patients (mean age 73 years) presenting to the emergency department with an unexplained fall and who were subsequently tested and found to have CICSS.[23] It was found that over the following one-year period there was a significant reduction in the likelihood of falling within the treatment group (OR 0.42, 95% CI 0.23–0.75). The authors speculated that this improvement in falls rather than syncope may be due, in part, to amnesia for actual syncope or may be because older people are more likely to fall with smaller reductions in cerebral perfusion that are insufficient to cause syncope than younger individuals.

Vasodepressor subtype

Treatment for VDCSS is less well established. Education and reassurance about the condition is important. Simple lifestyle adjustments, as outlined on p. 346, should be tried. Any culprit medications (e.g. antihypertensives) should be reduced or discontinued if possible. If these measures fail, a trial of medical therapy as used in orthostatic hypotension may be warranted for frequent events or patients at a high risk of injury.

Orthostatic hypotension

OH is a condition of low BP occurring on postural change that results in reduced cerebral perfusion and associated symptoms. When defined as a drop in BP of >20 mmHg, with or without symptoms, it appears to have a prevalence of 33% in geriatric inpatients.[24]

It is believed that approximately 500–700 mL of blood is pooled in the capacitance blood vessels in the legs, the splanchnic and pulmonary circulations while sitting or lying down.[25] On standing this causes a reduced venous return to the heart and, therefore, a lower cardiac output. In normal individuals, baroreceptors in the walls of the major blood vessels detect this change and initiate a reflex by increasing sympathetic nervous activity. The resultant constriction of peripheral blood vessels and increase in HR prevents a drop in BP. This process can be disturbed in a number of clinical situations (Figure 15.5).

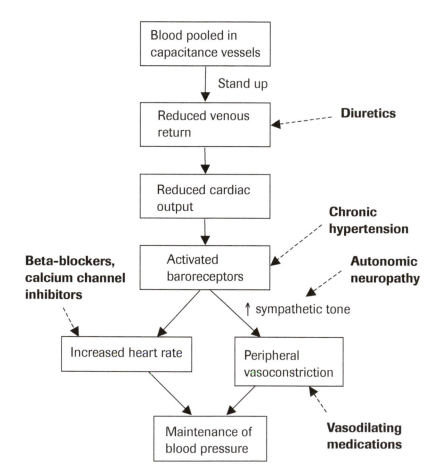

FIGURE 15.5 The causative mechanisms of orthostatic hypotension (OH).

Solid arrows represent the normal physiological steps and dashed arrows represent unhelpful factors.

Autonomic neuropathy impairs the ability to increase sympathetic nervous responses. This deficiency is associated with Parkinson's disease, MSA and diabetes. Also, a number of medications can affect this system, in particular anticholinergic (e.g. TCAs) and dopaminergic (e.g. levodopa) agents.

Chronic hypertension decreases the sensitivity of baroreceptors to change in intra-vascular pressure and also causes reduced vessel wall and vascular compliance.[25] For these reasons OH and hypertension often occur together. Also, cerebral blood flow autoregulation appears to be affected by prolonged hypertension, resulting in small changes in BP dramatically affecting cerebral blood flow.[26] Further, all BP-lowering medications are likely to worsen this problem. Particular culprits are vasodilators and diuretics (by reducing intravascular volume), and agents with pronounced peak and trough levels due to having short half-lives.[27,28] This combination of OH and hypertension is particularly difficult to treat (*see* p. 400).

Post-prandial hypotension

A post-prandial reduction in BP in elderly subjects (mean age 87 years) has been noted.[29] This appears to occur between 30 and 60 minutes after a meal with a mean maximum decrease in systolic BP of 25 mmHg. It was found in symptomatic and asymptomatic subjects but not in a young control group (mean age 27). There was no associated increase in HR, suggesting that this could be related to an impaired autonomic mechanism. In some individuals (i.e. the frail) this reduction is sufficient to cause syncope.

Situational syncope

A range of stimuli can trigger a vasovagal-type reaction resulting in VVS. These are usually attributed to a rise in intra-abdominal pressure secondary to coughing, micturating or defecating. They are sometimes referred to accordingly, for example 'cough syncope'. Treatment should be to reduce the precipitant, for example treating chest disorders, constipation and prostatism. Other treatment as for VVS should then be considered for ongoing symptoms.

Postural orthostatic tachycardia syndrome

Postural orthostatic tachycardia syndrome (POTS) is a condition that has been described in younger individuals (mean age 30, range 14–56 years).[30] It appears to cause symptoms of weakness and light-headedness with associated tachycardia (a rise of 30 beats per minute or more within 10 minutes) but only minor changes in BP on postural change. It is believed to be autonomically mediated and is diagnosed by the HUT. Treatments that may be helpful include fludrocortisone (*see* below) and beta-blockers.

Treatment of OH, VDCSS and VVS

OH, VDCSS and VVS have similar causative mechanisms and so their treatment is similar. The first step is education and reassurance of the patient. A list of things to avoid or to try is given in Table 15.2. The second step is to reduce or discontinue any potentially causative medications (all anticholinergics, dopaminergics and antihypertensive agents, in particular vasodilators, diuretics and drugs with short half-lives). Compression hosiery (preferably full-length stockings) may be tried to reduce the effects of fluid pooling in the legs. In the case of OH, if the above steps do not improve symptoms, a trial of fludrocortisone or midodrine may be warranted. In the past it has been suggested that raising the head of the bed (to provide gravitational exposure during sleep) may be beneficial.[32] But more recent evidence suggests this is not effective.[33]

TABLE 15.2 Lifestyle measures to help with the symptoms of episodic low blood pressure

Things to avoid in order to prevent hypotensive episodes:

    fluid depletion

    prolonged standing

    large meals

    hot rooms

    alcohol

    rapid postural change

    straining

Things to try to improve symptoms:

    small, frequent meals

    increased salt intake (not if history of heart failure)[31]

    lying flat and elevating legs at the onset of symptoms

Fludrocortisone

Fludrocortisone is a synthetic mineralocorticoid, and its main mechanism of action is by promoting renal sodium retention (in exchange for potassium). Its dose is usually started at 50 µg and titrated up to 400 µg if required. Main side-effects are provocation of congestive cardiac failure and hypertension (due to fluid retention), and the development of hypokalaemia. It is contraindicated in people on diuretic medications or with clinical evidence of fluid overload.

Midodrine

Midodrine is an alpha-adrenergic agonist that causes an increase in BP via vasoconstriction of arterioles and venous capacitance vessels. It is absorbed from the gastrointestinal tract and metabolised into its active metabolite (desglymidodrine) in the liver. Its onset of action is about 40 minutes after ingestion and its effects last for four to six hours. Therefore it is taken two to three times a day.[34] The dose is titrated upwards from 2.5 mg tds to 10 mg tds if required and supine BP permits. It does not cross the blood–brain barrier and so has no central side-effects.[35]

In studies, a 10 mg dose of midodrine has caused a mean increase in systolic BP of 28–34 mmHg one hour after ingestion.[35,36] This has been associated with symptomatic improvement in small cohorts with OH.[35-37]

The most problematic side-effect is supine hypertension; others include a scalp-tingling sensation, pruritis, urinary urgency and a goose bumps sensation due to a piloerection. Midodrine does not have a licence for use in the UK, therefore it can only be prescribed by falls specialists on a named-patient basis.

CARDIOGENIC SYNCOPE

A cardiological cause accounts for around 15% of older adults presenting with syncope.[4] It generally carries a worse prognosis than other causes of syncope.[26] There are two broad diagnostic groups of causative conditions. These are structural lesions causing reduced left ventricular outflow and arrhythmias. The most likely structural lesion in the elderly is aortic stenosis. Likely causative dysrhythmias in the elderly include complete heart block, sick sinus syndrome and ventricular tachycardia. In younger people conditions such as long QT syndrome and Brugada syndrome[38] (a cause of sudden death, associated with a characteristic ECG pattern) are more likely to be causative. A number of medications may worsen the situation, for example drugs that prolong the QT interval predispose individuals to torsade de pointes.

Cardiogenic syncope is more likely when there is a history of cardiac disease or a family history of sudden death or in the presence of an abnormal ECG.[39] Symptoms suggestive of a cardiac cause include onset during exertion. Exercise results in peripheral vasodilatation and outflow tract impairment can prevent an appropriate increase in cardiac output resulting in syncope (but a vasovagal causation is more common shortly after finishing exercising).[13] Alternatively ischaemia-related ventricular tachycardia may be triggered. Cardiogenic syncope, unlike most neurocardiovascular syncope, is characteristically unrelated to either postural change or head movements and so should be suspected in individuals with symptom onset while sitting or lying still. A sensation of palpitations may be associated. Preceding shortness of breath is significantly more common with cardiogenic syncope, whereas prodromal autonomic symptoms of sweating, nausea, blurred vision or faintness are more suggestive of non-cardiogenic syncope.[40]

Specific assessments should begin with auscultation of the heart and a standard ECG. When structural disease is suspected, an echocardiogram should be performed. With exercise-induced symptoms an exercise test should be considered. If an arrhythmia is suspected and symptoms are occurring at least every 24 hours, a standard ambulatory ECG should be performed. If symptoms are less frequent a longer period of ambulatory monitoring or an implantable loop recorder can be tried. Some devices are triggered by the patient following a syncopal event and are able to retrospectively record the last 10 or so minutes. An alternative is EPS to try to induce the arrhythmia. If underlying cardiac ischaemia is thought to be triggering an arrhythmia, an angiogram may be indicated.

Treatment should be directed to the underlying cause (Figure 15.6). Potentially worsening medications should be withdrawn if possible. The risk of recurrent episodes of VT, myocardial infarction and sudden death can be reduced with beta-blockers.[41] Alternative anti-arrhythmics are either less effective or have a higher risk of adverse effects. Recurrent VT episodes can also be terminated with an implantable defibrillator, and these are often used in combination with anti-arrhythmic drugs. Ischaemia-related arrhythmias may require revascularisation. Bradyarrhythmias may be appropriate for pacemaker insertion. Surgical options should be explored for structural lesions. For inoperable aortic stenosis, symptoms may be improved by discontinuing any vasodilatory medications.

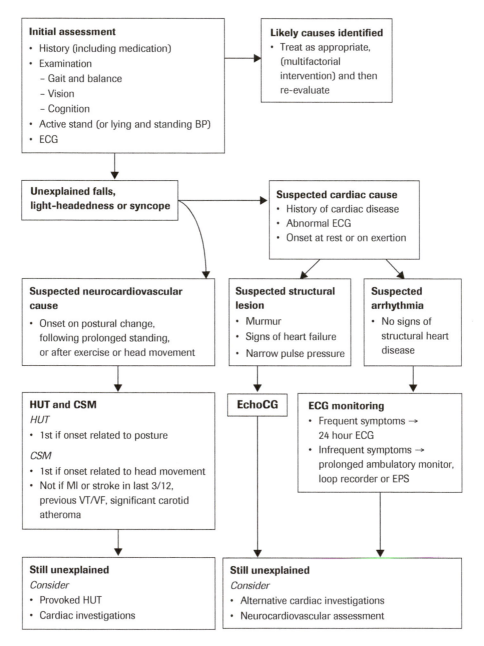

FIGURE 15.6 Suggested procedure for the assessment of elderly patients with falls, light-headedness or syncope.

REFERENCES

1 Lipsitz LA, Wei JY, Rowe JW. Syncope in an elderly, institutionalised population: prevalence, incidence, and associated risk. *Q J Med*, 1985; **55**: 45–54.

2 Zaidi A, Clough P, Cooper P, *et al.* Misdiagnosis of epilepsy: many seizure-like attacks have a cardiovascular cause. *J Am Coll Cardiol*, 2000; **36**(1): 181–4.

3 Brignole M, Alboni P, Benditt D, *et al.* Guidelines on management (diagnosis and treatment) of syncope. *Eur Heart J*, 2001; **22**(15): 1256–1306.

4 Ungar A, Mussi C, Del Rosso A, *et al.* Diagnosis and characteristics of syncope in older patients referred to geriatric departments. *J Am Geriatr Soc*, 2006; **54**(10): 1531–6.

5 Kenny RA, O'Shea D, Parry SW. The Newcastle protocols for head-up tilt table testing in the diagnosis of vasovagal syncope, carotid sinus hypersensitivity, and related disorders. *Heart*, 2000; **83**: 564–9.

6 Fitzpatrick AP, Theodorakis G, Vardas P, *et al.* Methodology of head-up tilt testing in patients with unexplained syncope. *J Am Coll Cardiol*, 1991; **17**(1): 125–30.

7 Del Rosso A, Bartoli P, Bartoletti A, *et al.* Shortened head-up tilt testing potentiated with sublingual nitroglycerin in patients with unexplained syncope. *Am Heart J*, 1998; **135**: 564–70.

8 Parry SW, Gray JC, Newton JL, *et al.* 'Front-loaded' head-up tilt table testing: validation of a rapid first line nitrate-provoked tilt protocol for the diagnosis of vasovagal syncope. *Age Ageing*, 2008; **37**: 411–15.

9 Richardson DA, Bexton R, Shaw FE, *et al.* Complications of carotid sinus massage – a prospective series of older patients. *Age Ageing*, 2000; **29**: 413–17.

10 Kenny RA, Traynor G. Carotid sinus syndrome – clinical characteristics in elderly patients. *Age Ageing*, 1991; **20**: 449–54.

11 Parry SW, Richardson DA, O'Shea D, *et al.* Diagnosis of carotid sinus hypersensitivity in older adults: carotid sinus massage in the upright position is essential. *Heart*, 2000; **83**: 22–3.

12 Kuhne M, Schaer B, Moulay N, *et al.* Holter monitoring for syncope: diagnostic yield in different patient groups and impact on device implantation. *Q J Med*, 2007; **100**: 771–7.

13 National Institute of Health and Care Excellence. *Transient Loss Of Consciousness ('Blackouts') Management in Adults and Young People.* CG109, 2010. Available at: www.nice.org.uk/guidance/cg109 (accessed 3 December 2014).

14 Pierre B, Fauchier L, Breard G, *et al.* Implantable loop recorder for recurrent syncope: influence of cardiac conduction abnormalities showing up on resting electrocardiogram and of underlying cardiac disease on follow-up developments. *Europace*, 2008; **10**: 477–81.

15 Petersen MEV, Williams TR, Sutton R. Psychogenic syncope diagnosed by prolonged head-up tilt testing. *Q J Med*, 1995; **88**: 209–13.

16 McIntosh SJ, Lawson J, Kenny RA. Clinical characteristics of vasodepressor, cardioinhibitory, and mixed carotid sinus syndrome in the elderly. *Am J Med*, 1993; **95**: 203–8.

17 Ballard C, Shaw F, McKeith I, *et al.* High prevalence of neurovascular instability in neurodegenerative dementias. *Neurology*, 1998; **51**: 1760–2.

18 Naschitz JE, Gaitini L, Mazov I, *et al.* The capnography-tilt test for the diagnosis of hyperventilation syncope. *Q J Med*, 1997; **90**: 139–45.

19 Richardson DA, Bexton RS, Shaw FE, *et al.* Prevalence of cardioinhibitory carotid sinus hypersensitivity in patients 50 years or over presenting to the accident and emergency department with 'unexplained' or 'recurrent' falls. *Pace*, 1997; **20**(Part II): 820–3.

20 Ward CR, McIntosh S, Kenny RA. Carotid sinus hypersensitivity – a modifiable risk factor for fractured neck of femur. *Age Ageing*, 1999; **28**: 127–33.

21 Kumar NP, Thomas A, Mudd P, *et al.* The usefulness of carotid sinus massage in different patient groups. *Age Ageing*, 2003; **32**(6): 666–9.

22 Brignole M, Menozzi C, Lolli G, *et al.* Long-term outcome of paced and nonpaced patients with severe carotid sinus syndrome. *Am J Cardiol*, 1992; **69**: 1039–43.

23 Kenny RA, Richardson DA, Steen N, *et al.* Carotid sinus syndrome: a modifiable risk factor for nonaccidental falls in older adults (SAFE PACE). *J Am Coll Cardiol*, 2001; **38**(5): 1491–6.

24 Palmer KT. Studies into postural hypotension in elderly patients. *NZ Med J*, 1983; **96**: 43–5.

25 Lipsitz LA. Orthostatic hypotension in the elderly. *N Engl J Med*, 1989; **321**: 952–7.

26 Kapoor WN. Syncope in older persons. *J Am Geriatr Soc*, 1994; **42**: 426–36.

27 MacFadyen RJ, Lees KR, Reid JL. Differences in first dose response to angiotensin converting enzyme inhibition in congestive heart failure: a placebo controlled study. *Br Heart J*, 1991; **66**: 206–11.

28 Mussi C, Ungar A, Salvioli G, *et al.* Orthostatic hypotension as a cause of syncope in patients older than 65 years admitted to emergency departments for transient loss of consciousness. *J Gerontol*, 2009; **64A**: 801–6.

29 Lipsitz LA, Nyquist RP, Wei JY, *et al.* Postprandial reduction in blood pressure in the elderly. *N Engl J Med*, 1983; **309**(2): 81–3.

30 Grubb BP, Kosinski DJ, Boehm K, *et al.* The postural orthostatic tachycardia syndrome: a neurocardiogenic variant identified during head-up tilt table testing. *Pace*, 1997; **20**(1): 2205–12.

31 El-Sayed H, Hainsworth R. Salt supplementation increases plasma volume and orthostatic tolerance in patients with unexplained syncope. *Heart*, 1996; **75**: 134–40.

32 Ten Harkel ADJ. Van Lieshoult JJ, Weiling W. Treatment of orthostatic hypotension with sleeping in the head-up tilt position, alone and in combination with fludrocortisone. *J Intern Med*, 1992; **232**: 139–45.

33 Fan CW, Walsh C, Cunningham CJ. The effect of sleeping with the head of the bed elevated six inches on elderly patients with orthostatic hypotension: an open randomised controlled trial. *Age Ageing*, 2011; **40**: 187–92.

34 Benditt DG, Fahy GJ, Lurie KG, *et al.* Pharmacotherapy of neurally mediated syncope. *Circulation*, 1999; **100**(11): 1242–8.

35 Wright RA, Kaufmann HC, Perera R, *et al.* A double-blind, dose-response study of midodrine in neurogenic orthostatic hypotension. *Neurology*, 1998; **51**(1): 120–4.

36 Jankovic J, Gilden JL, Hiner BC, *et al.* Neurogenic orthostatic hypotension: a double-blind, placebo controlled study with midodrine. *Am J Med*, 1993; **95**: 38–48.

37 Low PA, Gilden JL, Freeman R, *et al.* Efficacy of midodrine vs placebo in neurogenic orthostatic hypotension: a randomized, double-blind multicenter study. *JAMA*, 1997; **277**(13): 1046–51.

38 Antzelevitch C, Brugada P, Brugada J, *et al.* Brugada syndrome: 1992–2002. *J Am Coll Cardiol*, 2003; **41**(10): 1665–71.

39 Sagrista-Sauleda J, Romero-Ferrer B, Moya A, *et al.* Variations in diagnostic yield of head-up tilt test and electrophysiology in groups of patients with syncope of unknown origin. *Eur Heart J*, 2001; **22**(10): 857–65.

40 Galizia G, Abete P, Mussi C, *et al.* Role of early symptoms in assessment of syncope in elderly people: results from the Italian group for the study of syncope in the elderly. *J Am Geriatr Soc*, 2009; **57**(1): 18–23.

41 Aronow WS. Treatment of ventricular arrhythmias in the elderly. *Cardiol Rev*, 2009; **17**: 136–46.

CHAPTER 16

Osteoporosis

Osteoporosis is a condition of reduced bone density that is associated with micro-architectural changes that reduce bone quality, which leads to an increased risk of fracture. The process of bone loss begins after attaining peak bone mass around the age of 25–30 years. A gradual decline then occurs in all people as they age, mediated by a relative excess of bone resorption compared to bone formation (Figure 16.1). The definition of when this is a pathological condition is based on bone mineral density (BMD) measurements. A BMD of less than 2.5 standard deviations (SD) below the normal value for a person of the same sex aged 25 is defined as osteoporosis, and between 1.0 and 2.5 SD below the norm is termed 'osteopaenia'. Using this definition, around 30% of post-menopausal women are classified as having osteoporosis.[1] This data is derived from studies looking at Caucasian women, and their applicability to other groups is uncertain. People who fulfil this definition may have either failed to reach a normal peak bone mass, have a condition that has accelerated bone loss or have simply lived long enough for their bone density to have declined below this arbitrary level.

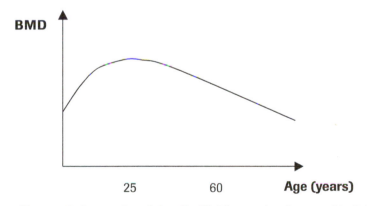

FIGURE 16.1 Changes in bone mineral density (BMD) over time in normal individuals.

Osteoporosis has been subdivided into primary and secondary causes. The primary causes have been further divided into type I (post-menopausal) and type II (related to ageing). Important secondary causes or contributory factors in elderly people with osteoporosis are shown in Table 16.1. There are also genetic factors – a family history of osteoporosis increases an individual's risk.[2] The majority of osteoporosis occurs in women due to the accelerated bone loss that occurs after the menopause.

Fragility fractures are those that occur following minimal trauma, which is conventionally acknowledged as falling from one's own height or less. The occurrence of such a fracture in an elderly person is highly suggestive of osteoporosis. Severe osteoporosis is defined as a BMD <2.5 SD below the normal reference plus one or more fragility fractures.

TABLE 16.1 Important secondary causes of osteoporosis

Causative factor	Comments
Steroids	Usually following exogenous oral steroids for >3 months in a year; occasionally secondary to inhaled formulations; plus the other causes of Cushing syndrome
Osteomalacia	Reduced sunlight exposure, dietary deficiency, malabsorption (e.g. coeliac disease), phenytoin
Hyperparathyroidism	Primary or secondary (e.g. chronic renal disease); paraneoplastic (parathyroid hormone (PTH)-related peptide)
Hyperthyroidism	Over-replacement is also possible
Hypogonadism	For example, pan-hypopituitarism
Multiple myeloma	
Smoking	A meta-analysis has suggested that smokers have an additional 0.2% BMD ↓ per year compared to non-smokers;[3] this may be due to an associated poor diet[4]
Excessive alcohol	Alcohol probably has a direct effect causing the suppression of bone formation when taken in large quantities; alcoholism is also associated with vitamin D deficiency. More than three units per day implies increased risk.[5]
Immobility	
Low body weight	The risk of hip fracture is elevated in thin women[6]
Heparin	
Low calcium intake	Probably less important than vitamin D deficiency

OSTEOPOROSIS IN MEN

Osteoporotic fractures are less common in men than women. The key to this difference is the absence of a post-menopausal acceleration of bone loss in men. Other factors include a higher peak bone mass and a lower incidence of falls.[7] However, the precise incidence of osteoporosis in men is not known. The standard definition of osteoporosis is based on comparing BMD measurements to those of young women. This criterion may result in an underestimation of the incidence as men have a higher peak bone mass. If a comparison is made to the BMD of young men, then an age-adjusted prevalence of 6% is estimated for male osteoporosis.[8] The lifetime fracture risk for men is estimated at 13–25% compared to nearly 50% for women.[8] However, it should be noted that many of these fractures will occur in younger people without osteoporosis and that fractures occurring at a younger age are more common in men than women. The lifetime risk of hip fracture in the UK is 5% in men compared to 12% in women.[7] Given the infrequent use of BMD in older men, it is not surprising to find that asymptomatic osteoporosis is rarely detected and it usually presents with symptoms associated with a fracture.

The secondary causes of osteoporosis are similar to those of women but are more common in men with osteoporosis. Alcohol excess, glucocorticoids and hypogonadism are reported to cause 40–50% of cases.[8]

In relation to hypogonadism, testosterone levels appear to decline from about the fourth decade at a rate that has been estimated to be between 0.5% and 1.6% per year.[9] This is also coupled with a rise in sex hormone binding globulin (SHBG) that has a combined effect in reducing free testosterone levels by 2–3% per year. Plus, there is evidence that testosterone levels transiently reduce at times of intercurrent illness. Other factors, including obesity and diabetes, may also affect levels of free testosterone. The actual number of older men defined as having testosterone deficiency is dependent on the value that is considered as normal. It is estimated that 80-year-old men have a mean testosterone level that is half that of 20-year-olds.[10] Men have been found to suffer progressive BMD reductions after castration.[11] Testosterone replacement has been shown to increase bone mass in deficient males.[10]

It has also been suggested that a relative deficiency in oestrogens is an important factor in osteoporosis in men. Bioavailable oestradiol levels decline in men with advancing age, similar to testosterone.[12] Osteoporosis has been described in young men who have either had inherited oestrogen deficiencies (through lacking the aromatase enzyme) or resistance syndromes.[8] A study comparing the levels of testosterone and oestradiol in younger and older men relative to changes in BMD found that serum oestradiol levels better correlated to bone loss than serum testosterone levels.[13]

The metabolic pathway of testosterone is shown in Figure 16.2. Testosterone is produced by the Leydig cells of the testes under the influence of luteinising hormone (LH). It may then directly interact with androgen receptors or may be converted to

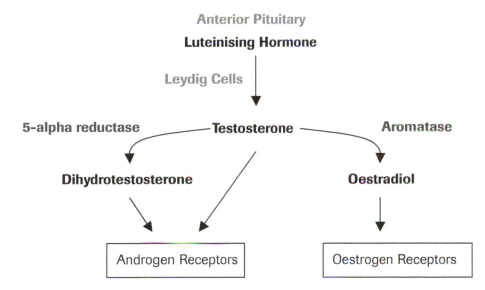

FIGURE 16.2 The metabolic pathway of testosterone.

dihydrotestosterone (DHT) by the enzyme 5-alpha reductase, which acts on a subset of androgen receptors. DHT appears to have actions on the prostate and for this reason 5-alpha reductase inhibitors (e.g. finasteride) are used in the treatment of benign prostatic hyperplasia. Some testosterone is converted to oestradiol by the enzyme aromatase. Testosterone replacement has been shown to produce a rise in oestradiol levels. It may be this increase that mediates the rise in BMD that has been observed.

PHYSIOLOGY

The key components of bone are proteins (especially collagen), cells and calcium salts. Osteoblasts are the cells that form new bone and osteoclasts are the cells that resorb it. They work in balance and in normal bone this produces a constant remodelling process. Their action is coordinated by a number of growth factors, cytokines and hormones. There are two distinct types of bone, termed 'cortical' and 'cancellous' (or 'trabecular'). Long bones are mainly composed of cortical bone and bones of other shapes are mainly composed of cancellous bone (e.g. the pelvis and vertebrae).

The metabolism of bone is influenced by a number of external factors. Bone acts as a reservoir of calcium. Vitamin D and parathyroid hormone (PTH) influence its turnover in order to regulate serum calcium levels. The relationship between vitamin D and PTH is shown in Figure 16.3. They are discussed further, along with calcitonin, below.

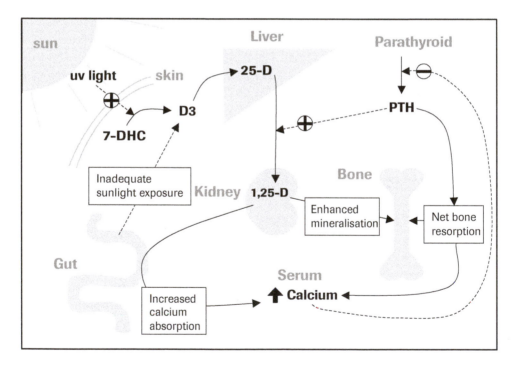

FIGURE 16.3 Simplified schematic of the interactions between vitamin D and parathyroid hormone (PTH) in calcium metabolism.

D3 = cholecalciferol; 25-D = 25-hydroxycholecalciferol; 1,25-D = 1,25-dihydroxycholecalciferol; 7-DHC = 7-dehydroxycholesterol; + = an enhancing effect; − = an inhibitory effect.

Vitamin D

Vitamin D is not a true vitamin as most of it is normally created within the skin by the action of ultraviolet (UV) light from the sun on 7-dehydroxycholesterol to form cholecalciferol (D_3). The remainder comes from dietary intake. If sunlight exposure is inadequate, this intestinal source becomes more important. This precursor is then converted to 25-hydroxycholecalciferol in the liver. This is further hydroxylated in the kidney to form 1,25-hydroxycholecalciferol (also known as 'calcitriol'), which is the active form of vitamin D. The main actions of vitamin D are on the bowel and on bone. In the bowel it causes an increase in both calcium and phosphate absorption by inducing an increase in binding proteins in the intestinal epithelial cells. Its actions on bone are complex but appear to result in enhanced bone mineralisation. Vitamin D receptors have also been found on striated muscle cells. Their role is unclear but vitamin D deficiency is associated with proximal myopathy and an increased risk of falls (*see* p. 331).[14]

Parathyroid hormone

PTH is secreted from the parathyroid glands. It also has complex actions on bone but the net result is increased bone resorption. This causes the release of calcium and phosphate into the circulation. PTH also has a mild inhibitory effect on renal calcium excretion but conversely increases renal phosphate loss. The overall effect is to increase serum calcium and reduce serum phosphate levels. PTH also has a major role in controlling the metabolism of vitamin D as it simulates the conversion of 25-hydroxy to 1,25-hydroxycholecalciferol in the kidney. PTH secretion is controlled by negative feedback on the parathyroid glands by serum calcium. Therefore, its secretion is reduced when serum calcium levels are elevated.

Calcitonin

Calcitonin is a poorly understood hormonal agent that is excreted by the C cells of the thyroid gland. Its effect is essentially the opposite of PTH – it causes a reduction in bone resorption by inhibiting osteoclasts and its release is stimulated by rising serum calcium levels. However, its precise physiological role in humans is, as yet, undefined and people who have undergone a thyroidectomy appear to be able to survive without any.

CLINICAL FEATURES

The three most common osteoporosis-associated fractures in order of frequency are vertebral, hip and distal radius (Colle's fracture), but pelvic and humeral fractures are also frequently seen.

Vertebral fractures

Vertebral fractures most commonly occur in the low thoracic to upper lumbar region. They may be asymptomatic, being detected only on X-rays, or present as progressive spinal curvature with height loss (kyphosis), chronic back pain, or acute back pain following minor trauma. Occasionally spinal cord compression can occur. Patterns of vertebral changes are shown in Figure 16.4. As a consequence of multiple fractures, a spinal kyphosis can cause further complications, for example reduced lung capacity provoking respiratory problems or reduced abdominal wall muscle efficacy leading to constipation. Treatment is usually with analgesia alone. Nasal salmon calcitonin may have a role as an analgesic agent in this situation (*see* p. 365).

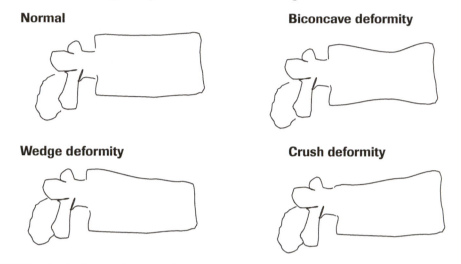

Normal

Biconcave deformity

Wedge deformity

Crush deformity

FIGURE 16.4 Patterns of vertebral deformity seen with osteoporosis.

A technique of percutaneous correction or 'vertebroplasty' has been proposed. This involves the injection of cement into the damaged vertebral body in order to stabilise it and reduce associated pain. Small, non-randomised studies had shown promising results.[15,16] However, a recent randomised trial failed to show an advantage over sham surgery.[17] The technique appears to be well tolerated in the elderly. Potential complications include cement pulmonary emboli and nerve root or spinal cord compression due to cement leakage around the vertebra.

Hip fractures

Hip fractures usually occur after falling from the patient's own height or less (a fragility fracture). The average age of hip fracture is currently around 79–82 years with 80% occurring in women.[18,19]

Assessment

Often there is classical leg shortening and external rotation but an undisplaced or impacted fracture may only cause pain on attempted weight-bearing. Around 1% of initial X-rays do not show a fracture that later becomes apparent (usually by becoming displaced).[20] MRI scanning can increase the fracture detection rate. A 4.4% prevalence of hip or pelvic fracture has been found by MRI scanning patients who attended an emergency department with hip pain but with no fracture seen on initial X-ray.[21] In another study of patients aged 70 and over with negative X-rays but a high clinical suspicion of fracture (persisting pain, unable to weight bear and pain on straight leg raising or hip rotation) MRI scanning detected a proximal femoral fracture in 21 of

25 (84%) people, with a further three having pelvic fractures.[22] CT imaging or isotope bone scans are alternative, but less sensitive detection techniques. Another option is to simply repeat the hip X-ray after 24–48 hours.[23]

Initial evaluation should include assessment for pain, nutrition/hydration, pressure ulcer risk, cognition and functional status.[23] The evaluation of pain should include documentation of its intensity (e.g. on a 0 to 10 scale) with reassessment after giving analgesia. There is evidence of under-treatment of pain in older patients following hip fracture, including infrequent use of opiate drugs.[24] The risk of delirium is not a valid reason to avoid opiates as pain itself could also be a trigger. One study found that 81% of elderly patients (mean age 83 years) with hip fracture complained of pain, but 36% of these people received no analgesia.[25] Of those who did receive analgesia, there was a mean time of 141 minutes from presentation to receipt of medication. Compared to younger people with fractures, patients aged over 70 are less likely to receive analgesia in emergency departments (66% vs 80%) and tend to receive lower doses.[26]

The majority of patients who sustain a fractured neck of femur are frail and are likely to benefit from a comprehensive geriatric assessment (*see* p. 8). Future care should address the reason for the initial fall and treatment of osteoporosis. Yet there is evidence that secondary prevention is suboptimal. In a review of prescriptions between 1995 and 2004 for patients who had a previous hip fracture and now resided in nursing homes (n=4430, mean age 83 years), just 11.5% were prescribed osteoporosis medications.[27]

Management

Guidelines have described the key elements of best care.[23,28] Clinicians should aim to perform a hip X-ray, administer intravenous fluids and analgesia (usually opiates), and move onto a pressure-relieving mattress within two hours of arrival in the emergency department. Admission to orthopaedic care should occur within four hours. Comprehensive assessment by medical, surgical and anaesthetic teams should be rapid, with good communication and collaboration between these specialities.

Treatment is almost always by surgical fixation – either joining the broken bones back together with a dynamic hip screw (for extracapsular fractures) or replacing the broken section of bone with a hemi-arthroplasty (for intracapsular fractures). Surgery should be performed as soon as practically possible, preferably within 48 hours. Those on warfarin with an INR >1.5 should have their warfarin withheld and be given intravenous vitamin K. The use of anti-platelet drugs should not postpone surgery. Osteoporotic bone can be a challenge for the surgeon to repair, and tends to heal more slowly.[28] Regional anaesthesia appears to be associated with lower perioperative mortality rates.[29]

The patient should be able to weight bear directly after surgical repair, and early mobilisation is considered best practice. Various models of postoperative rehabilitation have been proposed. These include rehabilitation on the orthopaedic ward, within a specialised orthogeriatric unit, or at the patient's own home with a supported discharge service.

People with hip fracture are at high risk of underlying malnutrition, which could delay postoperative healing. Screening for malnutrition should be performed and oral supplements should be given when detected. Postoperative delirium is found in around 28–40% of elderly patients with fractured neck of femur.[30,31] Symptomatic deep vein thrombosis develops in around 3% and pulmonary embolus in around 1%.[28] Low molecular weight heparins, factor X inhibitors (e.g. fondaparinux) or mechanical compression devices can reduce the risk of DVT, but can increase the risk of other complications, and there is a lack of widespread consensus on their optimal use.[23,28,29] Early mobilisation is also important. Antibiotic prophylaxis (single dose) reduces the risk of deep wound infections.[32]

Prognosis

Mortality is between 5% and 10% after one month,[33] being higher in the oldest, most frail and those with comorbidities. One study found a 38% one-year mortality rate in patients over the age of 75, and those with extracapsular fractures seemed to have a worse prognosis (probably due to older age and more comorbidities).[18] In those who survive, there is significant associated functional impairment. In a cohort of 536 patients who had sustained a hip fracture (mean age 80 years, mean length of hospital stay 18 days) only 54% were independently mobile at one year, compared to 87% pre-admission.[34] A significant number of patients will require placement within a care home.[18]

Hip protectors

Hip protectors are devices that consist of an underwear-like garment with protective pads overlying the hips on either side. They have been proposed to reduce the likelihood of sustaining a hip fracture following a fall. The evidence here remains inconclusive. When subjected to a Cochrane review, it appeared that a benefit was seen in cluster-randomised trials within institutional care homes with a high background incidence of hip fractures but this was not seen in trials with individual patient randomisation or with community-dwelling individuals.[35] The most recent data is less favourable for their use than earlier studies,[36] even when adherence rates are high.[37] A major problem with this kind of device is patient concordance due to discomfort when wearing them and difficulty getting them on and off. This latter problem may be a particular issue in people with an overactive bladder. It seems hard to justify the costs in terms of personal comfort as well as economics on the basis of available evidence.

Distal radius fractures

Distal radius fractures occur when there is an attempt to lessen the impact of a fall by using an outstretched arm. The treatment of this type of fracture is usually by placing the limb in a cast. Occasionally open or closed reduction is necessary for proper alignment. It does not usually necessitate hospital admission. However, in the elderly living alone, normal functioning may be impaired.

ASSESSMENT
Blood and urine tests

Blood and urine tests should be used to try to exclude secondary causes of osteoporosis. Thyroid stimulating hormone (TSH), calcium, magnesium, phosphate, alkaline phosphatase (ALP), vitamin D, PTH, urea, creatinine, full blood count, serum electrophoresis and urinary Bence–Jones protein are appropriate. Testing for coeliac disease may be indicated (e.g. evidence of iron and vitamin D deficiency).

Dual-energy X-ray absorptiometry scans

Dual-energy X-ray absorptiometry (DEXA) scan measurements taken from the hips of young Caucasian women form the basis of the standard definition of osteoporosis. This technique evaluates the amount of radiation that passes through the tested bone. The calculated density is inversely proportional to the value obtained. Ideally this is done via at least two different sites (e.g. spine and hip). This measurement may give inaccurately high readings in the presence of structural abnormalities, such as vertebral compression fractures. By comparing the data obtained to reference tables, T and Z scores are derived. T scores are based on comparison to the mean value for young people; Z scores are based on age-matched mean values. Readings at particular sites best predict fracture risk at that site; that is, a low femoral neck BMD is a better predictor of hip fracture than a low vertebral BMD.

A 2.6 times increased risk of fractured neck of femur is estimated for each SD drop in femoral neck BMD.[38] A study of 8065 women (median age 72 years) found a baseline prevalence for osteoporosis of 17% based on hip BMD scores.[39] Over a five-year follow-up period, 243 women had hip fractures, but 54% of these women did not have osteoporosis at the start of the assessment. This suggests that a low BMD is a risk factor for fracture, but will fail to detect many people who are at risk. Another study in older women (mean age 69 years), with a 15-year follow-up period, found that prior vertebral fracture was a more accurate predictor of future vertebral fracture than a low BMD score.[40]

Smaller, more portable units are available to scan peripheral sites such as the radius. These are quicker to use and expose the patient to less radiation. The disadvantage is that they may be less accurate and do not allow the comparison of the data to the standard reference tables for hip values.

While DEXA scanning has a role in the diagnosis of osteoporosis, it is less clear what its usefulness is in monitoring response to treatment. Random variations in BMD results obtained may make it a poor guide to the real effects of treatment.[41] Also, there is growing evidence that the relationship between fracture risk and BMD is not a linear one.[42] Treatments may improve bone strength through micro-architectural changes with only small increases in BMD scores.

Women over the age of 75 who have sustained a fragility fracture are very likely to have osteoporosis. Performing a confirmatory DEXA scan in this group is often considered non-mandatory.[5]

FRAX score

A FRAX score can be calculated without the need for performing a DEXA scan and can estimate 10-year fracture risk (available at: www.shef.ac.uk/FRAX (accessed 19 November 2014)). It requires the user to enter data such as the person's age, sex, weight and height, plus information about other risk factors such as pervious fracture, parental hip fracture, smoking, alcohol and steroid use. The tool then stratifies people into high (for treatment), intermediate (do a DEXA and recalculate risk) and low (lifestyle advice only) risk groups.

Quantitative CT

Quantitative computerised tomography (CT) measurements are usually taken at the spine. They allow accurate bone density assessment (expressed as g/cm^3) but are associated with increased costs and radiation exposure.

Quantitative US

Quantitative ultrasound (US) measurements are taken at peripheral sites, such as the calcaneum. The technique is simple, quick and radiation-free but its accuracy has not been fully proven.

Bone biopsy

A bone biopsy may be considered when there is diagnostic uncertainty. This can exclude certain conditions, including malignancy, but is rarely performed.

Biochemical markers of bone turnover

Biochemical markers of bone turnover have been detected in serum and urine samples. They may have the advantage of reflecting responses to treatment faster before BMD changes are detectable on DEXA. They include bone-specific ALP, various breakdown products of collagen, and the non-collagenous bone protein called osteocalcin. They are often utilised in the setting of clinical trials but are infrequently used in routine practice.

TREATMENT OPTIONS

Ideally, osteoporosis or osteopaenia is detected by screening BMD measurements in at-risk groups and treatment is preventative. However, often the first presentation is following a fracture. Non-pharmacological measures include increasing activity levels, stopping smoking and reducing alcohol consumption. If a secondary cause of osteoporosis is identified, this should also be targeted. The pharmacological agents in current use are discussed below. They can be broadly divided into three categories. These are supplementation (calcium and vitamin D), anti-resorptive (e.g. bisphosphonates) and bone-formation stimulating (e.g. PTH).

Calcium and vitamin D

A diet deficient in calcium is associated with bone demineralisation. This is more likely to occur in older adults. Vitamin D is mainly derived from the action of sunlight on the skin. In elderly people who may have reduced mobility and subsequent reduced sunlight exposure, possibly coupled with a diet low in vitamin D, deficiency is a genuine problem. The number of people who are defined as deficient in vitamin D depends on what numerical value is used. For a value of <25 nmol/L in people over the age of 65 years living in the UK, 10–15% who live in private residences and around 30% of those residing in residential care are deficient.[4] However, there is evidence that at levels <50 nmol/L there are increased PTH levels and bone resorption.[43] Using this value, around 55% and 80% of those aged over 65 in private homes or residential care, respectively, are deficient.[4] Trials that have looked at calcium or vitamin D alone have been inconclusive.[43–45] Two of the larger trials using a combination of therapy are discussed below.

The daily supplementation with calcium (1.2 g) and vitamin D (800 IU) of 3270 ambulatory women, with a mean age of 84 years, who lived in nursing homes or apartment houses for the elderly in France has been studied.[46] At baseline, all the subjects had a low calcium intake (less than 800 mg/day) and 44% had low serum 25-hydroxycholecalciferol levels. After 18 months, a 43% lower incidence of hip fractures (p=0.043) and 32% lower total non-vertebral fracture incidence (p=0.015) was seen in the treatment arm. This was associated with a 2.7% increase in femoral BMD compared to a 4.6% reduction in the placebo arm (p<0.001). The PTH levels significantly reduced in the treatment group and increased in the placebo group over this time period. This would be compatible with a rise in PTH being induced by a low intake of calcium with resultant bone resorption to maintain serum calcium levels (i.e. secondary hyperparathyroidism).

A study that recruited 3314 women over the age of 70, with a least one risk factor for hip fracture, gave either daily calcium (1 g) and vitamin D_3 (800 IU) supplementation or placebo.[47] Exclusions were the presence of cognitive impairment or a life expectancy of less than six months. After a median follow-up of 25 months, there were no significant differences in the incidence rates of overall fractures, hip fractures or falls.

Recently, a meta-analysis of trials of vitamin D supplementation with or without calcium found evidence for a benefit with 700–800 IU per day, but not 400 IU per day.[48] The size of the effect was a relative risk reduction of 26% for hip fractures. The variation in doses used within trials may partially explain the mixed results. A component of the Women's Health Initiative study randomised 36 282 healthy women aged between 50 and 79 (mean age 62 years) to receive either calcium (1 g) and vitamin D_3 (400 IU) or placebo over a follow-up period of seven years.[49] It was found that there was a small but statistically significant rise in BMD, but not a significant reduction in fracture rates. There was also a rise in the rates of renal stones in the treatment arm.

So, there have been conflicting results in trials of calcium and vitamin D. Their supplementation may only benefit certain subgroups, such as those with deficiencies at baseline and those who are housebound or in residential care. In addition, there is some evidence that calcium supplementation can increase the risk of myocardial infarction.[50] However, the majority of trials looking at osteoporosis interventions other than calcium or vitamin D also used supplementation with these agents. Therefore, to practise evidence-based medicine, calcium and vitamin D should be added to treatment regimens. The role of vitamin D in the prevention of falls is discussed on p. 331.

Bisphosphonates

Bisphosphonate molecules bind to hydroxyapatite crystals and act by reducing osteo-clast activity (probably by inducing apoptosis) and thereby reduce bone resorption. They have a poor oral absorption and are best taken on an empty stomach without other medication to maximise their bioavailability. Intravenous formulations are also available. The current most commonly used oral agents are alendronate and risedronate. Both of these are available in once-weekly preparations, which appear to have similar efficacy to the daily versions. The main advantage of these preparations is to reduce the inconvenience for the patient.

Erosive oesophagitis and ulceration has been reported with alendronate.[51] Risk factors for this complication appear to be inadequate water intake with the tablet, lying down after ingestion and a history of oesophageal disorders. For this reason patients with gastric or oesophageal problems were excluded from many of the studies and they should not be prescribed alendronate. It is advised that patients consume at least 200 mL of water after ingestion and do not lie down for at least 30 minutes. The medication should be discontinued if oesophageal symptoms develop. This association has not been found with risedronate but similar precautions should be observed while taking this medication.

Risedronate 2.5 mg and 5 mg daily doses were compared to placebo in 2458 ambu-lant post-menopausal women (mean age 69 years), with either two or more vertebral fractures on X-ray or a BMD T score of ≤ 2 plus one vertebral fracture, over a three-year period.[52] All participants also received calcium and vitamin D if baseline levels were low. The 2.5 mg dose arm was discontinued after one year. The 5 mg group had a lower vertebral fracture incidence (11.3%) compared to the placebo group (16.3%), which was significant (RR 0.59, 95% CI 0.42–0.82) and a lower non-vertebral fracture rate (5.2%) compared to placebo (8.4%), which was also significant (RR 0.61, 95% CI 0.39–0.94). BMD was also significantly increased compared to placebo at the lumbar spine (5.4% vs 1.1%) and femoral neck (1.6% vs –1.4%). There did not appear to be any difference in adverse event rates between the treatment and placebo groups.

Risedronate was also compared to placebo in two groups of elderly women at a high risk of hip fracture over a three-year period (the Hip Intervention Program Study Group).[53] Some 5445 women aged between 70 and 79 years (mean age 74) with marked osteoporosis (a T score ≤ 4 or ≤ 3 plus a non-skeletal risk factor for hip fracture) and 3886 women over the age of 80 (mean age 83) with either a non-skeletal risk factor for hip fracture or marked osteoporosis (a T score of at least ≤ 3) were recruited. All participants also received calcium and vitamin D if baseline levels were low. Overall there was a reduction in hip fracture incidence from 3.9% in the placebo arm to 2.8% in the treatment arm (RR 0.7, 95% CI 0.6–0.9). However, there was no benefit in the subgroup of patients without a low BMD score.

Alendronate has been compared to placebo in 2027 women (mean age 71 years, range 55–81 years) with a T score of ≤ 2.1 on BMD and X-ray evidence of previous vertebral fracture over a three-year period (the Fracture Intervention Trial).[54] Women with a history of peptic ulcer disease or dyspepsia were excluded. Participants deemed to have a low calcium intake (82% of the cohort) were given calcium and vitamin D supplements. The incidence of new vertebral fractures was 8.0% in the alendronate group and 15.0% in the placebo group (RR 0.53, 95% CI 0.41–0.68). The incidence of hip fracture was also reduced (RR 0.49, 95% CI 0.23–0.99). There did not appear to be any difference in adverse event rates (including gastrointestinal events) between the treatment and placebo groups.

Another arm of the above study looked at the effect of alendronate compared to placebo in 4432 women with low BMD scores but no evidence of prior vertebral fracture over a four-year period.[55] There was an associated significant increase in BMD scores, but only the subgroup of people with a T score of ≤2.5 had a significant reduction in clinical fracture incidence. This suggests that treating osteopaenic women with bisphosphonates may not be cost-effective – a point upheld by an economic evaluation.[56]

There have been no head-to-head randomised comparison studies between these two agents but meta-analyses have not suggested a significant difference in treatment effects between them.[42] They both appear to significantly reduce vertebral and non-vertebral fracture incidence in osteoporotic women. A more recent retrospective review has found that risedronate, compared to alendronate, appears to be associated with lower rates of nonvertebral (2.0% vs 2.3%) and hip fractures (0.4% vs 0.6%) after one year of therapy.[57] However, 8% of the alendronate patients in this analysis were on a dose lower than currently recommended (35 mg per week), which may have explained some of the observed difference.

Zoledronic acid is available as a once-yearly intravenous infusion. When compared to placebo in a trial randomising 3889 patients (mean age 73 years) with osteoporosis, over a three-year period, it was associated with lower rates of vertebral (3.3% vs 10.9%; RR 0.3, 95% CI 0.24–0.38) and hip (1.4% vs 2.5%; HR 0.59, 95% CI 0.42–0.83) fractures.[58] Also, when compared to placebo in patients who had undergone surgery for hip fracture repair it was associated with lower rates of new fractures.[59] Osteonecrosis of the jaw has been reported following infusion of high doses of intravenous bisphosphonates in patients with malignancy. In the treatment of osteoporosis it is rare, with an estimated incidence of less than one per 100 000 patient years of exposure.[60] Zoledronic acid is recommended for people who are intolerant of oral bisphosphonates.

The optimal duration of treatment with bisphosphonates is unknown but is likely to be around 5–10 years.[2] Antifracture benefits may persist for up to 18 months after discontinuation, which may be of practical importance to the very frail approaching end of life.

Oestrogen

Osteoblasts and osteoclasts have been found to have oestrogen receptors. Oestrogen has been shown to inhibit osteoclast activity and this mechanism is thought to be important in post-menopausal osteoporosis. It is, therefore, not surprising to find that oestrogen replacement therapy has been shown to be beneficial in increasing BMD in older women. In order to reduce the risk of endometrial carcinoma, women who have not had a hysterectomy also take cyclical progestins.

A meta-analysis of trials found a mean increase in BMD compared to control groups of 6.8% at the spine and 4.1% at the femoral neck.[61] There were non-significant trends towards reduced vertebral (RR 0.66, 95% CI 0.41–1.07) and non-vertebral (RR 0.87, 95% CI 0.71–1.08) fracture rates.

The problem with oestrogen therapy is the associated effects on other organ systems. Previously it was thought that oestrogens may increase the risk of breast cancer but were thought to be cardioprotective. A recent large randomised controlled study of women between the ages of 50 and 79 years showed a significant increase in cardiovascular morbidity (coronary heart disease, stroke and pulmonary embolism) as well as breast cancer.[62,63] These were partially offset by significant reductions in hip fractures and colorectal cancer. In those who had not had a hysterectomy, after a mean follow-up of 5.2 years, the hazard ratios were 1.22 (95% CI 1.09–1.36) for total cardiovascular disease, 1.03 (95% CI 0.90–1.17) for total cancer, 0.76 (95% CI 0.69–0.85) for combined fractures and 0.98 (95% CI 0.82–1.18) for mortality.[62] Although overall mortality is not significantly increased, the absolute number of adverse cardiovascular events appears to outweigh the bone protection benefit. They are also associated with an increased risk of urinary incontinence (*see* Box 11.1) and dementia (*see* p. 105). Therefore, it no longer seems reasonable to use these agents routinely in the management of osteoporosis in frail older people.

Selective oestrogen receptor modulators

Selective oestrogen receptor modulators include tamoxifen, which is used in the management of breast cancer, as well as raloxifene, which is used in the management of post-menopausal osteoporosis. Raloxifene is thought to be a useful agent as it has similar actions to oestrogen on bone but an inhibitory effect at the different oestrogen receptor subtype found on breast and endometrial tissue.

The Multiple Outcomes of Raloxifene Evaluation (MORE) trial recruited 7705 women (mean age 67, range 31–80 years) with osteoporosis (defined by BMD scores or radiographic evidence of vertebral fractures) to compare raloxifene (60 mg or 120 mg) to placebo over a three-year period.[64] The participants also received calcium and vitamin D supplements. They found a significant reduction in vertebral fracture incidence (RR for the 60 mg raloxifene group 0.7, 95% CI 0.5–0.8). There was an associated increase in BMD at the femoral neck and spine by around 2.5%. However, there was no significant benefit in terms of non-vertebral fracture reduction (RR 0.9, 95% CI 0.8–1.1). A continuation of the trial to four years did not show a significant change to the above data in either vertebral or non-vertebral fracture incidence.[65]

The most serious side-effect encountered was a significant increased risk of venous thromboembolism (RR 3.1, 95% CI 1.5–6.2). Other side-effects occurring more commonly in the raloxifene group included hot flushes, leg cramps and peripheral oedema. There was a lower incidence of breast cancer in the treatment group (RR 0.3, 95% CI 0.2–0.6). No association with either endometrial hyperplasia or carcinoma was detected.

The role of raloxifene in the management of post-menopausal osteoporosis is unclear. The actual size of the increase in bone density seen appears to be less than that seen with bisphosphonates.[66] This may suggest that is useful only when bisphosphonates are not tolerated. Combination therapy has not been assessed in clinical trials. The increase in venous thromboembolism is certainly a concern, especially in high-risk groups such as hospitalised elderly patients.

Calcitonin

Calcitonin has been proposed as a useful agent in the management of osteoporosis as it has an inhibitory effect on osteoclast activity. It is usually given as salmon calcitonin as this has a 40–50 times greater potency than the human version. It cannot be given by the oral route and is usually taken as a nasal spray or as a subcutaneous injection. It is expensive and long-term use may be associated with the development of antibodies that could negate its efficacy.

The largest study looking at the role of calcitonin in post-menopausal osteoporosis was the PROOF trial.[67] Some 1255 women (mean age 68 years) with osteoporosis were given salmon calcitonin nasal spray at a dose of 100, 200 or 400 IU per day or placebo over a five-year period. All participants also received calcium and vitamin D supplements. Results for the 100 IU and 400 IU doses were not significantly different from the placebo group. The 200 IU daily group had a reduction in vertebral fracture incidence compared with placebo (RR 0.67, 95% CI 0.47–0.97). There was an associated increase in BMD. Rhinitis was the only adverse effect reported. However, it should be noted that there was a 59% drop-out rate in this trial. A meta-analysis of trials found a large heterogeneity in results, raising the concern of publication bias.[68]

There is some evidence for a role in the management of pain associated with acute vertebral crush fractures. A study recruiting 100 men and women (mean age 73 years) who had sustained an osteoporotic vertebral fracture within the last five days gave either nasal salmon calcitonin (200 IU daily) or placebo over a 28-day period.[69] It found a significant reduction in pain and an increase in early mobilisation in the calcitonin group. During the trial the patients were only allowed to take paracetamol as an additional analgesic. No significant adverse effects were reported.

Parathyroid hormone

PTH appears to have both bone creation and bone resorption effects. When bone is exposed to high levels of PTH for long time periods the net effect is bone loss. However, when bone is exposed to intermittent raised levels of PTH it results in osteoblast expression of growth factors and the promotion of new bone formation. It is this finding that underlies the theory for the use of PTH in osteoporosis. It is the only treatment option currently available that acts exclusively by stimulating new bone formation rather than inhibiting resorption. A form of the PTH molecule that includes only the first 34 amino acids (PTH (1-34)) has been developed. It has been produced by recombinant DNA technology and is also known as 'teriparatide'. It is believed that this part of the molecule causes most of its biological effects. It is given parenterally, usually by daily subcutaneous injections. Long-term safety has not yet been established and its administration to rats at supra-physiological values was associated with an increase in osteosarcoma development.

It has previously been shown to have beneficial effects on BMD in younger women treated with gonadotrophin-releasing hormone (GnRH) analogues for endometriosis.[70]

A more recent study (the Fracture Prevention Trial) recruited 1637 post-menopausal women (mean age 69 years) and gave either PTH (1-34) at a dose of 20 or 40 μg/day or placebo.[71] Participants were also given calcium and vitamin D supplements. After a mean duration of 18 months' treatment the subset receiving 20 μg/day of PTH had a significant reduction in vertebral and non-vertebral fracture incidence compared to placebo (RR 0.35, 95% CI 0.22–0.55 and RR 0.47, 95% CI 0.25–0.88, respectively). There was no significant benefit at the higher dose of PTH and it had the cost of increased side-effects. The study was stopped early because of concerns about the elevated osteo-sarcoma incidence in animal models. There were no cases of osteosarcoma within this study. Side-effects occurring more commonly in the treatment group than in the placebo group included nausea, headaches, dizziness and leg cramps. The benefit of this treatment appears to last to some degree up to at least 18 months beyond its discontinuation.[72] When PTH is discontinued, there is evidence that commencing anti-resorptive therapy with a bisphosphonate prevents subsequent reduction in BMD.[73]

So, the role of PTH has not yet been established, in part due to safety concerns. Currently it may be a beneficial treatment for osteoporosis over short periods of administration. Drawbacks to its use include high cost and the need for daily subcutaneous injections.

Strontium

Strontium was first used in the treatment of osteoporosis in the 1950s but fell out of favour due to concerns that it caused bone mineralisation defects and inhibited the synthesis of calcitriol.[74] The development of a new compound, strontium ranelate, has led to the re-emergence of this therapeutic agent. It is believed to promote bone formation while also inhibiting bone resorption. Tissues undergoing osteogenesis actively absorb it. The precise mechanism of action is unknown but may involve, in part, interaction with the calcium-sensing receptor and the suppression of PTH secretion. Due to the heavy atomic weight of strontium, the X-rays utilised in DEXA scanning are more readily absorbed. This leads to artificially elevated BMD estimations. This problem is tackled by using a formula to adjust the readings to more comparative values.

A study involving 1649 post-menopausal women (mean age 69 years) with osteoporosis (defined by BMD) and at least one vertebral fracture gave either 2 g/day of strontium or placebo over a three-year period.[75] Participants were also given calcium and vitamin D supplements. It found a significant reduction in new vertebral fractures (RR 0.59, 95% CI 0.48–0.73) with an associated increase in adjusted BMD of 8.1% at the lumbar spine.

The Treatment of Peripheral Osteoporosis Study (TROPOS) recruited 5091 women (mean age 77) with osteoporosis (defined by BMD) who were given either 2 g/day of strontium ranelate or placebo over a three-year period.[76] Participants were also given calcium and vitamin D supplements. It found an overall 16% RRR in non-vertebral fractures ($p=0.04$), with a RRR for hip fractures of 36% ($p=0.046$). Side-effects observed more frequently in the treatment group included nausea, diarrhoea, headache, dermatitis and eczema. Analysis of available data suggests that strontium is associated with an increased incidence of venous thromboembolism (RR 1.42).[5] Absorption is improved when taken at least two hours after meals – typically patients are advised to take it at bedtime. It is not recommended in those with severe renal impairment.

Therefore, it appears that strontium is a promising therapy for post-menopausal osteoporosis, with benefits in reducing both vertebral and non-vertebral fractures, but data on the long-term safety and efficacy are not yet available.

Denosumab

Denosumab is a monoclonal antibody that binds to the receptor activator of nuclear factor-$\kappa\beta$ ligand (called RANKL) on the surface of osteoclast precursor cells and thus prevents their maturation into osteoclasts.[77] It is given by subcutaneous injection (at intervals of six months).

A trial compared denosumab to placebo in 7808 women (mean age 72; range 60–90 years) with a DEXA T-score between –2.5 and –4.0 over a 36-month period.[78] Participants also received calcium and vitamin D supplements. It found a significant reduction in fractures, including the incidence of hip fracture (0.7% vs 1.2%; HR 0.60, 95% CI 0.37–0.97).

It is currently recommended for the primary or secondary prevention of fractures in postmenopausal women who are at an increased risk of fractures but cannot take bisphosphonates.[79] High risk for primary prevention is defined by a combination of bone densitometry T-score, patient age and other risk factors (parental history of fracture, more than four units of alcohol per day or rheumatoid arthritis).

Statins

Statins (HMG CoA reductase inhibitors) have been linked to increased BMD, possibly by interference with the mevalonate pathway. Two analyses of epidemiological data have suggested that older individuals on current statin therapy have a reduced risk of fractures.[80,81] However, a secondary analysis of the LIPID study did not demonstrate a difference in fracture rate.[82] Randomised controlled trials are required to investigate this association.

Treatment of male osteoporosis

There is very little trial evidence for the treatment of male osteoporosis. Similar to women, the role of calcium and vitamin D alone is unclear, but they have been used in conjunction with other treatments in most trials and so should be considered a standard component of therapy.

Bisphosphonates

A trial has been conducted using alendronate versus placebo in 241 osteoporotic men (mean age 63, range 31–87 years) over a two-year period.[83] All participants were also given calcium and vitamin D supplements. Men with a history of peptic ulcer or oesophageal disease within the last year were excluded. They found mean increases in BMD at the lumbar spine and femoral neck of 7.1% and 2.5% in the alendronate group compared to 1.8% and –0.1% in the placebo group, respectively ($p<0.001$ for both sites). Further, there was a reduction in vertebral fracture incidence from 7.1% in the placebo group to 0.8% in the alendronate group (*p*=0.02). There was no significant difference in side-effect rates between the two groups.

Parathyroid hormone

Although there is no available data to show a benefit in terms of fracture reduction in men, the effects on bone density appear to be more favourable than those seen with alendronate.[84] After 24 months of treatment of osteoporotic men (mean age 58, range 46–85) an increase in BMD at the femoral neck of 9.7% was seen with PTH compared to 3.2% with alendronate (*p*<0.001). The same trial failed to show an additional benefit of combining these two treatments. All participants received vitamin D supplements and additional calcium supplementation if their dietary intake was thought to be inadequate (<1 g per day).

Testosterone

An age-related reduction in testosterone has been described earlier in the chapter (*see* p. 353). A number of problems have been attributed to this reduction, including reduced libido, erectile dysfunction, anaemia, and reduced muscle mass and bone density. It has been proposed that testosterone replacement may benefit all of these. However, the effects of replacement on this decline may be quite different to the replacement of testosterone in other deficiency states, such as pan-hypopituitarism. Testosterone is available in oral, transdermal and injectable preparations.[85]

➤ *Injections*: need to be given regularly and cause fluctuations in serum levels that may increase the risk of some adverse effects, for example erythrocytosis.
➤ *Transdermal*: easy to administer and results in consistent serum levels. May cause skin irritation beneath patches; this is less severe with a gel form of the drug.
➤ *Oral*: associated with hepatotoxicity and neoplasia and for this reason is seldom used.

A study of 108 healthy men over the age of 65 years (mean age 73) looked at the effect of a testosterone patch on BMD.[10] It was found that overall BMD was not increased but there was a positive effect in those individuals who had a low baseline testosterone level. A study using two-weekly intramuscular testosterone injections in hypogonadal men with a mean age of 71 over a three-year period found a significant increase in BMD compared to placebo.[86] There were mean increases of 10.2% and 2.7% at the spine and total hip in the testosterone group compared to 1.3% and –0.2%, respectively, in the placebo group (*p*<0.001 and *p*=0.02). During this study there were significant rises in both haematocrit (mean 42.5% to 48.6%) and PSA levels (mean 1.0 to 1.4) in the testosterone group compared to baseline. Thirty per cent of subjects in the testosterone group required a dose reduction due to a haematocrit level above 52%. There are no studies demonstrating a reduced fracture incidence in osteoporotic men treated with testosterone.

Adverse effects

To date there is no clear evidence that testosterone levels correlate with either cardiovascular disease risk or serum lipid levels. But, given the problems associated with female hormone replacement therapy (*see* p. 363) it would seem prudent to use caution with male replacement until long-term safety data is available. Also, there is little evidence that it induces prostatic hyperplasia and subsequent urinary voiding problems. Some of the problems it does cause are listed below.

➤ *Polycythaemia*: testosterone appears to have an action on bone marrow and higher levels have been found to induce erythropoiesis. The higher peak levels seen with injected doses confer a higher risk. The clinical significance of this is unclear but it is recommended that the haematocrit be monitored during therapy.

➤ *Prostate cancer*: the efficacy of anti-testosterone treatments in the management of prostate cancer has led to concerns that elevating testosterone levels may induce such cancers. To date the available evidence does not support this; however, data from large studies and over long time periods is not yet available. It is recommended that PSA level monitoring be performed during therapy.

➤ *Hepatotoxicity and neoplasia*: appear to be related to oral preparations only.

➤ *Sleep apnoea*: testosterone use has been associated with the development or worsening of sleep apnoea in at-risk individuals. This may be mediated by a central mechanism.

➤ *Fluid retention*: caution may be needed in the presence of cardiac or renal failure.

Monitoring is recommended at three- to six-month intervals. This should include questioning about the above side-effects and measurement of the haematocrit and PSA levels.

B$_{12}$ and folate

A study of Japanese stroke survivors over the age of 65 years has found a reduction in fracture risk with the use of folate and B$_{12}$ supplementation.[87] The theory behind this finding is that low levels of these agents are associated with raised levels of homocysteine, which is associated with osteoporosis. These findings will need to be validated in other cohorts before this becomes standard practice.

Combinations of therapy

The majority of trials investigating therapeutic agents for osteoporosis have used calcium and vitamin D supplements concurrently. Therefore, the combination of any anti-resorptive agent or PTH with calcium and vitamin D is standard practice. There is only limited data to support the combination of agents other than calcium and vitamin D with other osteoporosis treatments. Trials that have looked at a combination of PTH and alendronate have failed to show a benefit of the two agents together.[84,88] This is probably due to alendronate blocking the PTH-induced stimulation of bone formation. A small study has suggested that a combination of teriparatide and denosumab may result in larger gain in BMD than either agent alone, but the impact on fracture rate is so far unknown.[89] The combination of other agents has not been adequately assessed.

TREATMENT RECOMMENDATIONS

If a secondary or contributory cause for osteoporosis is identified, correcting or improving this should also be attempted. A treatment strategy is suggested in Figure 16.5 and on p. 371. In the subgroup of patients with osteopaenia detected on DEXA scanning, optimal treatment is unproven. Given the questionable cost–benefits of anti-resorptive therapy,[56] an alternative strategy may be non-pharmacological measures and the commencement of calcium and vitamin D with repeat BMD measurement in two years' time.

Secondary causes

Identify and, if possible, treat

Lifestyle factors

Stop smoking

Reduce excessive alcohol intake

Increase physical activity

Falls risk

Identify patients at risk of falling and take appropriate action

↓ Plus

Calcium and vitamin D

Plus

Bisphosphonate

Either oral alendronate or risedronate

(if a history of an oesophageal disorder or impaired

swallow, then intravenous zoledronic acid may be more suitable)

↓ Treatment intolerance or failure

Second line agents

• **PTH:** high cost, need injections, maximum duration of 18 months. May be appropriate for severe osteoporosis in people unable to take bisphosphonates

• **Strontium:** promising early trial results but long-term safety and efficacy unknown

• **Denosumab:** 6-monthly subcutaneous injection

• **Raloxifene:** not proven to reduce non-vertebral fractures. Increased risk of thromboembolism. Reduced risk of breast cancer

---

FIGURE 16.5 Suggested strategy to manage osteoporosis in the elderly.

Pharmacological

Currently, the best evidence for efficacy and long-term safety is with the combination of calcium, vitamin D and a bisphosphonate. If a bisphosphonate is not tolerated, the choice of second-line agents includes PTH, strontium and denosumab. Trials studying the efficacy of raloxifene have not demonstrated a clear benefit in reducing non-vertebral fractures. The reason for this may be partly due to the younger age (mean 67 years) of women in the MORE study.[42] However, it must be considered that an older population may also have a significant increase in adverse events, especially venous thromboembolism. Raloxifene may be best suited to people who are at an increased risk of breast cancer and a lower risk of thromboembolism. Oestrogens, testosterone, calcitonin and statins do not have a major role in the management of osteoporosis at the present time.

Non-pharmacological

Helpful lifestyle measures include stopping smoking and reducing excessive alcohol intake. Exercise in earlier life may confer a BMD gain. Increasing activity once osteoporosis has developed is less likely to be beneficial. However, exercise programmes may have a role in the prevention of falls. Those at risk of falls should undergo appropriate risk assessment and intervention (*see* Chapter 14). The role of hip protectors remains controversial.

PROGNOSIS

In the year following a vertebral fracture, osteoporotic women appear to have a 19% risk of sustaining a further vertebral fracture.[90] This risk is increased in women with lower BMD scores and a history of previous fractures. Five-year survival rates are significantly reduced after either hip or vertebral fractures but appear to be unaffected following distal radius fractures.[91]

REFERENCES

1 Cranney A, Tugwell P, Wells G, *et al.* Systematic reviews of randomized trials in osteoporosis: introduction and methodology. *Endocrine Rev*, 2002; **23**(4): 497–507.

2 Sandhu SK, Hampson G. The pathogenesis, diagnosis, investigation and management of osteoporosis. *J Clin Pathol*, 2011; **64**: 1042–50.

3 Law MR, Hackshaw AK. A meta-analysis of cigarette smoking, bone mineral density and risk of hip fracture: recognition of a major effect. *BMJ*, 1997; **315**: 841–6.

4 Hirani V, Primatesta P. Vitamin D concentrations among people aged 65 years and over living in private households and institutions in England: population survey. *Age Ageing*, 2005; **34**: 485–91.

5 National Institute for Health and Care Excellence. *Alendronate, Etidronate, Risedronate, Raloxifene, Strontium Ranelate and Teriparatide for the Secondary Prevention of Osteoporotic Fragility Fractures in Postmenopausal Women.* 2008 (updated 2011). Available at: www.nice. org.uk/TA161 (accessed 18 November 2014).

6 Williams AR, Weiss NS, Ure CL, *et al.* Effect of weight, smoking, and estrogen use on the risk of hip and forearm fractures in postmenopausal women. *Obst Gynae*, 1982; **60**(6): 695–9.

7 Seeman E. Osteoporosis in men: epidemiology, pathophysiology, and treatment possibilities. *Am J Med*, 1993; **95**(Suppl. 5A): S22–8.

8   Bilezikian JP. Osteoporosis in men. *J Clin Endocr Met*, 1999; **84**(10): 3431–4.

9   Allan CA, McLachlan RI. Age-related changes in testosterone and the role of replacement therapy in older men. *Clin Endocr*, 2004; **60**(6): 653–70.

10 Snyder PJ, Peachey H, Hannoush P, *et al.* Effect of testosterone treatment on bone mineral density in men over 65 years of age. *J Clin Endocr Met*, 1999; **84**(6): 1966–72.

11 Stepan JJ, Lachman M, Zverina J, *et al.* Castrated men exhibit bone loss: effect of calcitonin treatment on biochemical indices of bone remodelling. *J Clin Endocr Met*, 1989; **69**(3): 523–7.

12 Ferrini RL, Barrett-Connor E. Sex hormones and age: a cross-sectional study of testosterone and estradiol and their bioavailable fractions in community-dwelling men. *Am J Epidem*, 1998; **147**(8): 750–4.

13 Khosla S, Melton LJ, Atkinson EJ, *et al.* Relationship of serum sex steroid levels to longitudinal changes in bone density in young versus elderly men. *J Clin Endocr Met*, 2001; **86**(8): 3555–61.

14 Venning G. Recent developments in vitamin D deficiency and muscle weakness among elderly people. *BMJ*, 2005; **330**: 524–6.

15 Grados F, Depriester C, Cayrolle G, *et al.* Long-term observations of vertebral osteoporotic fractures treated by percutaneous vertebroplasty. *Rheumatology*, 2000; **38**: 1410–14.

16 Diamond TH, Champion B, Clark WA. Management of acute osteoporotic vertebral fractures: a nonrandomized trial comparing percutaneous vertebroplasty with conservative therapy. *Am J Med*, 2003; **114**: 257–65.

17 Buchbinder R, Osborne RH, Ebeling PR, *et al.* A randomized trial of vertebroplasty for painful osteoporotic vertebral fractures. *N Engl J Med*, 2009; **361**(6): 557–68.

18 Keene GS, Parker MJ, Pryor GA. Mortality and morbidity after hip fractures. *BMJ*, 1993; **307**: 1248–50.

19 Roche JJW, Wenn RT, Sahota O, *et al.* Effect of comorbidities and postoperative complications on mortality after hip fracture in elderly people: prospective observational cohort study. *BMJ*, 2005; doi:10.1136/bmj.38643.663843.55.

20 Pathak G, Parker MJ, Pryor GA. Delayed diagnosis of femoral neck fractures. *Injury*, 1997; **28**: 299–301.

21 Dominguez S, Liu P, Roberts C, *et al.* Prevalence of traumatic hip and pelvic fractures in patients with suspected hip fracture and negative initial standard radiographs – a study of emergency department patients. *Acad Emerg Med*, 2005; **12**: 366–9.

22 Chana R, Noorani A, Ashwood N, *et al.* The role of MRI in the diagnosis of proximal femoral fractures in the elderly. *Injury*, 2006; **37**: 185–9.

23 Scottish Intercollegiate Guidelines Network. *Management of Hip Fracture in Older People*. June 2009. Available at: www.sign.ac.uk/pdf/sign111.pdf (accessed 12 December 2014).

24 Ardery G, Herr K, Hannon BJ, *et al.* Lack of opioid administration in older hip fracture patients. *Geriatr Nurs*, 2003; **24**: 353–60.

25 Hwang U, Richardson LD, Sonuyi TO, *et al.* The effect of emergency department crowding on the management of pain in older adults with hip fracture. *J Am Geriatr Soc*, 2006; **54**: 270–5.

26 Jones JS, Johnson K, McNinch M. Age as a risk factor for inadequate emergency department analgesia. *Am J Emerg Med*, 1996; **14**: 157–60.

27 Parikh S, Mogun H, Avorn J, *et al.* Osteoporosis medication use in nursing home patients with fractures in 1 US state. *Arch Intern Med*, 2008; **168**(10): 1111–5.

28 British Orthopaedic Association. *The Care of Patients with Fragility Fracture*. 2007. Available at: www.fractures.com/pdf/BOA-BGS-Blue-Book.pdf (accessed 12 December 2014).

29 Beaupre LA, Jones CA, Saunders LD, *et al.* Best practices for elderly hip fracture patients: a systematic overview of the evidence. *J Gen Intern Med*, 2005; **20**: 1019–25.

30 Edland A, Lundstrom M, Lundstrom G, *et al.* Clinical profile of delirium in patients treated for femoral neck fractures. *Dement Geriatr Cogn Disord*, 1999; **10**: 325–9.

31 Marcantonio E, Ta T, Duthie E, *et al.* Delirium severity and psychomotor types: their relationship with outcomes after hip fracture repair. *J Am Geriatr Soc*, 2002; **50**: 850–7.

32 Gillespie WJ, Walenkamp GHIM. Antibiotic prophylaxis for surgery for proximal femoral and other closed long bone fractures. *Cochrane Database Syst Rev*, 2010, Issue 3. Art. No.: CD000244. DOI: 10.1002/14651858.CD000244.pub2.

33 Parker M, Johansen A. Hip fracture. *BMJ*, 2006; **333**: 27–30.

34 Magaziner J, Simonsick EM, Kashner TM, *et al.* Predictors of functional recovery one year following hospital discharge for hip fracture: a prospective study. *J Gerontol*, 1990; **45**(3): M101–107.

35 Parker MJ, Gillespie WJ, Gillespie LD. Hip protectors for preventing hip fractures in older people. *Cochrane Database Syst Rev* 2005, Issue 3. Art. No.: CD001255. DOI: 10.1002/14651858. CD001255.pub3.

36 Parker MJ, Gillespie WJ, Gillespie LD. Effectiveness of hip protectors for preventing hip fractures in elderly people: systematic review. *BMJ*, 2006; **332**: 571–3.

37 Kiel DP, Magaziner J, Zimmerman S, *et al.* Efficacy of a hip protector to prevent hip fracture in nursing home residents: the HIP PRO randomized controlled trial. *JAMA*, 2007; **298**(4): 413–22.

38 Cummings SR, Black DM, Nevitt MC. Bone density at various sites for prediction of hip fractures. *Lancet*, 1993; **341**(9): 72–5.

39 Wainwright SA, Marshall LM, Ensrud KE, *et al.* Hip fracture in women without osteoporosis. *J Clin Endocrinol Metab*, 2005; **90**(5): 2787–93.

40 Cauley JA, Hochberg MC, Lui LY, *et al.* Long-term risk of incident vertebral fractures. *JAMA*, 2007; **298**(23): 2761–7.

41 Cummings SR, Palmero L, Browner W, *et al.* Monitoring osteoporosis therapy with bone densitometry: misleading changes and regression to the mean. *JAMA*, 2000; **283**(10): 1318–21.

42 Boonen S, Body J, Boutsen Y, *et al.* Evidence-based guidelines for the treatment of postmenopausal osteoporosis: a consensus document of the Belgian Bone Club. *Osteopor Int*, 2005; **16**: 239–54.

43 Anderson F. Vitamin D for older people: how much, for whom and – above all – why? *Age Ageing*, 2005; **34**: 425–6.

44 Shea B, Wells G, Cranney A, *et al.* Meta-analysis of calcium supplementation for the prevention of postmenopausal osteoporosis. *Endocr Rev*, 2002; **23**(4): 552–9.

45 Papadimitropoulos E, Wells G, Shea B, *et al.* Meta-analysis of the efficacy of vitamin D in preventing osteoporosis in postmenopausal women. *Endocr Rev*, 2002; **23**(4): 560–9.

46 Cahpuy MC, Arlot ME, Duboeuf F, *et al.* Vitamin D3 and calcium to prevent hip fractures in elderly women. *N Engl J Med*, 1992; **327**(23): 1637–42.

47 Porthouse J, Cockayne S, King C, *et al.* Randomised controlled trial of supplementation with calcium and cholecalciferol (vitamin D3) for prevention of fractures in primary care. *BMJ*, 2005; **330**: 1003–6.

48 Bischoff-Ferrari HA, Willet WC, Wong JB, *et al.* Fracture prevention with vitamin D supplementation: a meta-analysis of randomized controlled trials. *JAMA*, 2005; **293**(18): 2257–64.

49 Jackson RD, LaCroix AZ, Gass M, *et al.* Calcium plus vitamin D supplementation and the risk of fractures. *N Engl J Med*, 2006; **354**(7): 669–83.

50 Bolland MJ, Avenell A, Baron JA, *et al.* Effect of calcium supplements on risk of myocardial infarction and cardiovascular events: meta-analysis. *BMJ*, 2010; **341**: c3691.

51 de Groen PC, Lubbe DF, Hirsch LJ, *et al.* Esophagitis associated with the use of alendronate. *N Engl J Med*, 1996; **335**: 1016–21.

52 Harris ST, Watts NB, Genant HK, *et al.* Effects of risedronate treatment on vertebral and non-vertebral fractures in women with non-vertebral osteoporosis: a randomized controlled trial. *JAMA*, 1999; **282**(14): 1344–52.

53 McClung MR, Geusens P, Miller PD, *et al.* Effect of risedronate on the risk of hip fracture in elderly women. *N Engl J Med*, 2001; **344**(5): 333–40.

54 Black DM, Cummings SR, Karpf DB, *et al.* Randomised trial of effect of alendronate on risk of fracture in women with existing vertebral fractures. *Lancet*, 1996; **348**: 1535–41.

55 Cummings SR, Black DM, Thompson DE, *et al.* Effect of alendronate on risk of fracture in women with low bone density but without osteoporosis: results from the fracture intervention trial. *JAMA*, 1998; **280**(24): 2077–82.

56 Schousboe JT, Nyman JA, Kane RL, *et al.* Cost-effectiveness of alendronate therapy for osteopenic postmenopausal women. *Ann Intern Med*, 2005; **142**(9): 734–41.

57 Silverman SL, Watts NB, Delmas PD, *et al.* Effectiveness of bisphosphonates on nonvertebral and hip fractures in the first year of therapy: the risedronate and alendronate (REAL) cohort study. *Osteoporos Int*, 2007; **18**: 25–34.

58 Black DM, Delmas PD, Eastell R, *et al.* Once-yearly zolendronic acid for treatment of postmenopausal osteoporosis. *N Engl J Med*, 2007; **356**(18): 1809–22.

59 Lyles KW, Colon-Emeric CS, Magaziner JS, *et al.* Zolendronic acid and clinical fractures and mortality after hip fracture. *N Engl J Med*, 2007; **357**(18): 1799–809.

60 Khan A. Bisphosphonate-associated osteonecrosis of the jaw. *Can Fam Physician*, 2008; **54**: 1019–21.

61 Wells G, Tugwell P, Shea B, *et al.* Meta-analysis of the efficacy of hormone replacement therapy in treating and preventing osteoporosis in postmenopausal women. *Endocr Rev*, 2002; **23**(4): 529–39.

62 Writing Group for the Women's Health Initiative Investigators. Risks and benefits of estrogen plus progestin in healthy postmenopausal women: principal results from the Women's Health Initiative randomized controlled trial. *JAMA*, 2002; **288**(3): 321–33.

63 Women's Health Initiative Steering Committee. Effects of conjugated equine estrogen in postmenopausal women with hysterectomy: the Women's Health Initiative randomized controlled trial. *JAMA*, 2004; **291**(14): 1701–12.

64 Ettinger B, Black DM, Mitlak BH, *et al.* Reduction of vertebral fracture risk in postmenopausal women with osteoporosis treated with raloxifene: results from a 3-year randomized clinical trial. *JAMA*, 1999; **282**(7): 637–45.

65 Delmas PD, Ensrud KE, Adachi JD, *et al.* Efficacy of raloxifene on vertebral fracture risk reduction in postmenopausal women with osteoporosis: four-year results from a randomized clinical trial. *J Clin Endocr Met*, 2002; **87**(8): 3609–17.

66 Cranney A, Tugwell P, Zytaruk N, *et al.* Meta-analysis of raloxifene for the prevention and treatment of postmenopausal osteoporosis. *Endocr Rev*, 2002; **23**(4): 524–8.

67 Chesnut CH, Silverman S, Andriano K, *et al.* A randomized trial of nasal spray salmon calcitonin in postmenopausal women with established osteoporosis: the prevent recurrence of osteoporotic fractures study. *Am J Med*, 2000; **109**: 267–76.

68 Cranney A, Tugwell P, Zytaruk N, *et al.* Meta-analysis of calcitonin for the treatment of postmenopausal osteoporosis. *Endocr Rev*, 2002; **23**(4): 540–51.

69 Lyritis GP, Paspati I, Karachalios T, *et al.* Pain relief from nasal salmon calcitonin in osteoporotic vertebral crush fractures. *Acta Orthop Scand*, 1997; **68**(Suppl. 275): S112–14.

70 Finkelstein JS, Klibanski A, Arnold AL, *et al.* Prevention of estrogen deficiency-related bone loss with human parathyroid hormone – (1-34): a randomized controlled trial. *JAMA*, 1998; **280**(12): 1067–73.

71 Neer RM, Arnaud CD, Zanchetta JR, *et al.* Effect of parathyroid hormone (1-34) on fractures and bone mineral density in postmenopausal women with osteoporosis. *N Engl J Med*, 2001; **344**(190): 1434–41.

72 Lindsay R, Scheele WH, Neer R, *et al.* Sustained vertebral fracture risk reduction after with-drawal of teriparatide in postmenopausal women with osteoporosis. *Arch Intern Med*, 2004; **164**: 2024–30.

73 Black DM, Bilezikian JP, Ensrud KE, *et al.* One year of alendronate after one year of parathyroid hormone (1-34) for osteoporosis. *N Engl J Med*, 2005; **353**(6): 555–65.

74 Fuleihan GE. Strontium ranelate – a novel therapy for osteoporosis or a permutation of the same? *N Engl J Med*, 2004; **350**(5): 504–6.

75 Meunier PJ, Roux C, Seeman E, *et al.* The effects of strontium ranelate on the risk of vertebral fracture in women with postmenopausal osteoporosis. *N Engl J Med*, 2004; **350**(5): 459–68.

76 Reginster JY, Seeman E, De Vernejoul MC, *et al.* Strontium ranelate reduces the risk of non-vertebral fractures in postmenopausal women with osteoporosis: treatment of peripheral osteoporosis (TROPOS) study. *J Clin Endo Metab*, 2005; **90**(5): 2816–22.

77 Rachner TD, Khosla S, Hofbauer LC. Osteoporosis: now and the future. *Lancet*, 2011; **377**: 1276–7.

78 Cummings SR, San Martin J, McClung MR, *et al.* Denosumab for prevention of fractures in postmenopausal women with osteoporosis. *N Engl J Med*, 2009; **361**: 756–65.

79 National Institute for Health and Care Excellence. *Denosumab for the Prevention of Osteoporotic Fractures in Postmenopausal Women.* TA204, 2010. Available at: www.nice.org.uk/guidance/ta204 (accessed 18 November 2014).

80 Meier CR, Schlienger RC, Kraenzlin ME, *et al.* HMG-CoA reductase inhibitors and the risk of fractures. *JAMA*, 2000; **283**(24): 3205–10.

81 Wang PS, Solomon DH, Mogun H, *et al.* HMG-CoA reductase inhibitors and the risk of hip fractures in elderly patients. *JAMA*, 2000; **283**(24): 3211–16.

82 Reid IR, Hague W, Emberson J, *et al.* Effect of pravastatin on frequency of fracture in the LIPID study: secondary analysis of a RCT. *Lancet*, 2001; **357**: 509–12.

83 Orwoll E, Ettinger M, Weiss S, *et al.* Alendronate for the treatment of osteoporosis in men. *N Engl J Med*, 2000; **343**(9): 604–10.

84 Finkelstein JS, Hayes A, Hunzelman JL, *et al.* The effects of parathyroid hormone, alendronate, or both in men with osteoporosis. *N Engl J Med*, 2003; **349**(13): 1216–26.

85 Rhoden EL, Morgentaler A. Risks of testosterone-replacement therapy and recommendations for monitoring. *N Engl J Med*, 2004; **350**(5): 482–92.

86 Amory JK, Watts NB, Easley KA, *et al.* Exogenous testosterone or testosterone with finasteride increases bone mineral density in older men with low serum testosterone. *J Clin Endocr Met*, 2004; **89**(2): 503–10.

87 Sato Y, Honda Y, Iwamoto J, *et al.* Effect of folate and mecobalamin on hip fractures in patients with stroke: a randomized controlled trial. *JAMA*, 2005; **293**(9): 1082–8.

88 Black DM, Greenspan SL, Ensrud KE, *et al.* The effects of parathyroid hormone and alendronate alone or in combination in postmenopausal osteoporosis. *N Engl J Med*, 2003; **349**(13): 1207–15.

89 Tsai JN, Uihlein UI, Lee H, *et al.* Teriparatide and denosumab, alone or combined, in women with postmenopausal osteoporosis: the DATA study randomised trial. *Lancet*, 2013; **382**: 50–6.

90 Lindsay R, Silverman SL, Cooper C, *et al.* Risk of new vertebral fracture in the year following a fracture. *JAMA*, 2001; **285**(3): 320–3.

91 Cooper C, Atkinson EJ, Jacobsen SJ, *et al.* Population-based study of survival after osteoporotic fractures. *Am J Epidemiol*, 1993; **137**: 1001–5.

QUESTIONS FOR PART D

1 A 78-year-old man complains of a two-month history of an intermittent sensation of the room spinning around. It often occurs when he first lies down in bed at night. There have been no changes in his hearing and he does not have tinnitus. He has a past history of hypertension, and currently takes aspirin, amlodipine and simvastatin. Which of the following diagnoses is most likely?
   A. Benign paroxysmal positional vertigo
   B. Brainstem vascular disease
   C. Orthostatic hypotension
   D. Ménière's disease
   E. Vestibular neuritis

2 Which single intervention is most likely to reduce falls in an old lady on no medication with early cataracts and poor gait and balance?
   A. Hip protectors
   B. Ta'i-chi
   C. Medication review
   D. Occupational therapist home assessment
   E. Cataract surgery

3 A 79-year-old lady is admitted following a fall to the ground that occurred while standing and was associated with preceding light-headedness. A witness reported her unconscious for five minutes. There was associated urinary incontinence and a bite to the tip of the tongue. Which is the most likely cause?
   A. Carotid sinus hypersensitivity
   B. Atrial fibrillation
   C. Epilepsy
   D. Transient ischaemic attack
   E. Vasovagal syncope

4 Which of the following clinical features makes a diagnosis of syncope more likely than epilepsy?
   A. Cyanosis during the attack
   B. Prolonged confusion after the event
   C. Associated urinary incontinence
   D. A history of cerebrovascular disease
   E. Preceding nausea

5 Which of the following clinical features makes a diagnosis of cardiogenic syncope more likely than a neurocardiovascular cause?
   A. Right bundle branch block on the ECG
   B. An onset following prolonged standing
   C. Amnesia for preceding events
   D. Preceding sweating
   E. A history of syncope in childhood

6 Which of the following statements regarding hip fracture in the elderly is most likely to be correct?
   A. Patients with intracapsular fractures generally have worse outcomes than those with extracapsular fractures
   B. Even when surgically corrected within 24 hours, significant lasting functional decline is frequently seen
   C. All patients should receive a bone density scan following hip fracture
   D. Only around 60% of eligible patients currently receive osteoporosis prevention medications following a hip fracture
   E. The 30-day mortality rate is around 30–40%

7 An 87-year-old lady complains of an intermittent feeling of the room spinning round, on each occasion lasting just seconds to a few minutes. Symptoms often occur when she rolls over in bed. There is some associated nausea. She does not report any change in her hearing. Which test would you do next?
   A. MRI scan of the brain
   B. Echocardiogram
   C. Electrocardiogram
   D. Head thrust test
   E. Hallpike's test

8 An elderly lady presents with falls. She usually lives alone and rarely goes outdoors. She is found to have proximal muscle weakness. Her bloods tests are as follows:

Sodium	142	(133–146 mmol/L)
Potassium	4.1	(3.5–5.3 mmol/L)
Urea	3.7	(2.5–7.8 mmol/L)
Creatinine	42	(49–90 umol/L)
ALP	357	(40–117 u/L)
ALT	35	(14–64 u/L)
Albumin	38	(35–50 g/L)
Total calcium	1.69	(2.1–2.6 mmol/L)
Phosphate	0.64	(0.8–1.5 mmol/L)
Haemoglobin	118	(115–165 g/L)
White cell count	6.1	(4–11 $\times 10^9$/L)
Platelets	267	(150–450 $\times 10^9$/L)
Mean cell volume	92	(80–99 fl)

Which of the following factors is most likely to be affecting bone biochemistry?
   A. Reduced conversion of 25-hydroxycholecalciferol to 1,25-dihydroxycholecalciferol
   B. Low levels of cholecalciferol
   C. Low levels of parathyroid hormone
   D. Raised levels of calcitonin
   E. Raised levels of osteocalcin

9 Which of the following statements regarding vitamin D is most likely to be correct?
   A. When given alone to residents of a care facility it has been associated with a reduced rate of falls
   B. Ultraviolet light promotes its formation via the hydroxylation of cholecalciferol
   C. Calcitonin modulates its action on bone calcium uptake
   D. A serum concentration of <25 nmol/L is found in over 50% of people living in residential care in the UK
   E. Long-term supplementation increases the risk of cataract formation

10 Which of the following statements is most accurate regarding investigations used in falls and syncope assessment services?
   A. An active stand test assesses balance
   B. A fall in blood pressure of 50 mmHg or more during head-up tilt testing is diagnostic of vasovagal syncope
   C. Carotid sinus massage has the highest diagnostic yield when performed in the supine position
   D. An implantable loop recorder can be placed in situ for periods of up to two weeks
   E. The use of nitrate provocation increases head-up tilt test sensitivity but reduces its specificity

11 A 73-year-old woman has had a fracture of her hip following a fall. She has been on alendronate and calcium and vitamin D tablets for osteoporosis for the preceding two years. Her bone mineral density T score is −3.2 standard deviations. She is being considered for teriparatide therapy. Which of the following statements is most accurate?
   A. Teriparatide therapy should only be given for six months
   B. Teriparatide is poorly tolerated in those with an impaired swallow
   C. Calcium and vitamin D supplements should be discontinued while on teriparatide
   D. Teriparatide stimulates osteoblast growth factor expression
   E. Teriparatide use is associated with an increased risk of myeloma

12 An 87-year-old woman has been admitted to hospital with urinary sepsis. She develops tinnitus and vertigo. She is on multiple medications. Which of the following is least likely to be causing her current symptoms?
   A. Digoxin
   B. Furosemide
   C. Gentamicin
   D. Ibuprofen
   E. Quinine

13 A woman has two episodes of pre-syncope in six months. On head-up tilt test she has a positive response and a diagnosis of vasovagal syncope is made. She has hypertension and peripheral vascular disease. How would you treat her?
   A. Lifestyle advice only
   B. Fludrocortisone
   C. Midodrine
   D. Selective serotonin reuptake inhibitor
   E. Compression stockings

14 An 84-year-old woman has an episode of loss of consciousness when walking to the shops. Paramedics shock her for ventricular tachycardia. Subsequent ECG, echocardiogram and coronary angiography are all normal. What initial management would you recommend?
A. Beta-blocker
B. Amiodarone
C. Flecainide
D. Implantable cardio-defibrillator insertion
E. 24-hour ECG recording

15 An 81-year-old man presents with vertigo. Which of the following clinical features makes a central cause of his symptoms more likely?
A. A positive head thrust test
B. Nausea and vomiting
C. Nystagmus reduced by optic fixation
D. Unsteady gait
E. Symptoms worsened by head movement

16 A 75-year-old lady has osteoporosis with a bone mineral density T score of −2.7 standard deviations. Her past history is hypertension, reflux oesophagitis, deep vein thrombosis and pulmonary embolus. She takes a calcium and vitamin D preparation, aspirin, bendroflumethiazide and omeprazole (due to a history of severe reflux oesophagitis). What treatment should be added to reduce her future risk of fractures?
A. A weekly oral bisphosphonate
B. Strontium ranelate
C. Denosumab
D. Raloxifene
E. Parathyroid hormone

17 An 87-year-old woman has had five episodes of transient loss of consciousness over a four-week period. The events don't seem to be related to posture or movement. She reports a preceding sweating sensation. Witnesses do not report any seizure activity. She has a past history of hypertension and type 2 diabetes. Clinical examination is unremarkable. An ECG shows sinus rhythm at a rate of 78 beats per minute with left bundle branch block. Which investigation would be most appropriate?
A. Exercise test
B. Tilt test
C. 48 hour ECG (Holter monitor)
D. External event recorder
E. Implantable event recorder

18 Which of the following clinical features is most suggestive of a drop attack?
A. Transient loss of consciousness
B. Absence of warning symptoms
C. Prolonged recovery phase
D. Preceding light-headedness
E. Complete heart block on electrocardiogram

19 What is the approximate percentage of people aged over 80 years who will fall over in a one-year period?
   A. 10%
   B. 20%
   C. 30%
   D. 40%
   E. 50%

20 Which of the following statements regarding the drug midodrine is most likely to be correct?
   A. It is a synthetic mineralocorticoid
   B. It causes constriction of arterioles
   C. Its effects last for 12 hours
   D. Peripheral oedema is a common side-effect
   E. It is contraindicated in people with Parkinson's disease

21 Which of the following lifestyle advice is most suitable for a person with a diagnosis of orthostatic hypotension?
   A. Reduce fluid intake
   B. Avoid prolonged sitting
   C. Eat small and frequent meals
   D. Maintain a high room temperature
   E. Lower legs at onset of symptoms

22 Which of the following statements regarding dizziness in older people is most likely to be correct?
   A. Vertigo is the most common form of dizziness
   B. 25% of people aged over 90 report daily dizziness
   C. The head thrust test has around a 90% sensitivity but only a 60% specificity for detecting peripheral causes of vertigo
   D. Loratadine is similarly effective to betahistine in the management of vertigo of a peripheral causation but has fewer side-effects
   E. Anxiety is a common cause

23 Which of the following statements regarding syncope in older people is most likely to be correct?
   A. A cardiogenic cause is more likely than a neurocardiovascular one
   B. A vasodepressor subtype of carotid sinus hypersensitivity is more common than a cardio-inhibitory one
   C. Syncope has an incidence rate of around 20% per year in people residing in care homes
   D. Neurocardiovascular causes of syncope have the worst prognosis
   E. Vasovagal syncope is a likely cause when the onset occurs shortly after completing physical exertion

24 Which of the following statements regarding denosumab is most likely to be correct?
   A. It is a synthetic form of parathyroid hormone
   B. It promotes bone formation by osteoblasts
   C. It inhibits osteoclast precursor cell maturation
   D. It is given as a weekly subcutaneous injection
   E. It has not been found to reduce rates of hip fracture in osteoporotic women

25 Which of the following statements regarding hip fracture is most likely to be correct?
   A. The average age of people sustaining hip fracture is 90 years
   B. Isotope bone scans have a higher sensitivity than MRI scans to detect fractures not seen on initial X-ray images
   C. Delirium secondary to opiate drug administration is a more significant problem than inadequate pain control
   D. Best practice involves performing a hip X-ray, administering intravenous fluids and analgesia, and moving the patient onto a pressure-relieving mattress within four hours of arrival
   E. A single dose of prophylactic antibiotic reduces the risk of deep wound infection

PART E

Cardiovascular

CHAPTER 17

Heart failure

Heart failure occurs when the heart is no longer able to pump blood at the rate required to meet the body's metabolic requirements. It has been estimated to have a prevalence of around 1% in adults in their fifties, and this rises to around 10% in those aged in their eighties.[1] This failure is attributed to a combination of age-related changes to the cardiovascular system and a higher prevalence of cardiovascular diseases. These changes include increased stiffness of the heart and blood vessels caused by reductions in the amount of elastin with increased collagen deposition. This results in impaired cardiac diastolic relaxation and subsequent inefficient filling. In normal individuals these changes do not affect the resting cardiac output but do reduce the ability to increase the output at times of increased demand (e.g. physical exertion).

Frequent cardiac causes of heart failure are ischaemic, hypertensive and valvular heart diseases. Atrial fibrillation (AF) is also more common in the elderly – usually in association with atrial enlargement secondary to elevated intracardiac pressures. The loss of coordinated atrial contraction may further reduce the efficacy of cardiac filling even if the ventricular rate is normal. Another factor increasing risk in the elderly may be the deterioration seen in renal function with advancing years.

Diastolic heart failure (also called 'heart failure with preserved ejection fraction') is a term used to describe the clinical features of heart failure in individuals with an ejection fraction of 45% or more plus evidence of left ventricular diastolic dysfunction. It appears to account for 30–50% of those with heart failure.[2,3] It occurs more commonly in the elderly probably caused by the increased vascular stiffness. In reality, both systolic and diastolic dysfunction probably coexist to some degree in many older patients with heart failure. Other factors increasing risk include female sex and a history of hypertension, whereas it is less common in people with a history of ischaemic heart disease.[3]

ASSESSMENT

History

Classically, heart failure symptoms are breathlessness on exertion, ankle swelling and orthopnoea. Precipitating medications such as non-steroidal anti-inflammatory drugs (NSAIDs) (which impair renal salt handling and increase fluid overload), calcium channel blockers, dopamine agonists and pioglitazone (which can all cause peripheral oedema) should be identified.

Examination

Signs include a raised jugular venous pressure (JVP), a third heart sound, pitting ankle oedema and basal chest crepitations. Their interpretation can be more difficult in the elderly. For example, leg oedema can be due to calcium channel blockers, a low albumin, or venous congestion, and basal chest crepitations can be a normal variant.

Investigations

An electrocardiograph (ECG) will usually be abnormal with signs of previous ischaemia or chamber enlargement (*see* Figure 17.1). A chest X-ray may show ventricular enlargement, oedema, effusions, Kerley lines or venous congestion. Thyroid disease and anaemia should be excluded by standard blood tests.

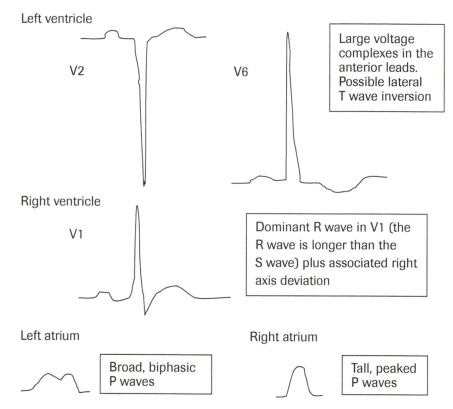

FIGURE 17.1 Electrocardiograph (ECG) signs of heart chamber enlargement.

The natriuretic peptides are a group of naturally occurring, structurally related hormones that include brain natriuretic peptide (BNP), atrial natriuretic peptide (ANP) and C-type natriuretic peptide (CNP) variants. They have a physiological role in the maintenance of fluid homeostasis. Despite its name, BNP comes mainly from the cardiac ventricles – released in response to cardiac wall stretching. It has been proposed as a marker of cardiac failure that can be measured from blood samples.[4] However, it is a non-specific test as levels may rise with other cardiac (e.g. ischaemia and arrhythmias)[5] and non-cardiac conditions (e.g. pulmonary emboli, COPD or, to a lesser degree, with normal ageing),[6] and so it is unclear whether this adds to the information gained from clinical, ECG and chest X-ray evaluation. In a trial that compared the use of BNP levels or clinical symptoms alone to guide treatment, no benefit was found in either vascular outcomes or quality of life.[7] A normal serum level (<100 ng/L) may be helpful in ruling out a diagnosis of heart failure.[6] It also exists in a recombinant form (nesiritide) that has been used as a treatment for acute heart failure. At present this has a high cost and large-sized randomised controlled trials demonstrating a long-term benefit are lacking.

Transthoracic echocardiography should be performed in all patients with a new diagnosis of heart failure. Its functions include the ability to identify any valvular lesions and to distinguish between diastolic and systolic dysfunction. Diastolic heart failure is associated with left ventricular hypertrophy, but not dilatation. There is likely to be left atrial enlargement. Standard techniques for estimating ejection fraction tend to overestimate its value in the presence of left ventricular enlargement (and associated change in shape). Echocardiography is also able to distinguish constrictive pericarditis from diastolic dysfunction.

TREATMENT

A management programme should include patient education, including how to identify the signs of worsening disease and the importance of medication adherence. If any precipitating factors have been identified, attempts should be made to improve them. These may include minor changes such as stopping unhelpful medications or major procedures such as valvular or revascularisation surgery. Secondary prevention of vascular disease with anti-platelets, statins and adequate blood pressure (BP) control may also be appropriate. Smokers should be advised to stop. Left ventricular impairment increases the risk of thromboembolism in the presence of AF. Therefore these patients should be carefully considered for anticoagulation (*see* p. 407).

People with heart failure should be advised to get a one-off pneumococcal and an annual influenza immunisation.[6]

Medications

Most of the evidence for pharmacological management of heart failure is based on trials enrolling patients with systolic dysfunction. There is little direct evidence for the treatment of diastolic problems but it currently appears that similar strategies are probably appropriate.[8] Angiotensin-converting enzyme inhibitors (ACEi) and beta-blockers are considered the usual first-line treatments for heart failure.[6]

Loop diuretics

Loop diuretics (e.g. furosemide or bumetanide) are highly effective at reducing the fluid overload of heart failure. Their site of action is shown in Figure 17.2. They are effective at treating the symptoms of heart failure and improve the quality of patients' lives. They are usually the first medications to be commenced. However, they do not alter the progress or outcome of the condition. Patients with coexistent renal impairment may require large doses for clinical effect.

Patients with bowel oedema due to right heart failure may not absorb furosemide well. In this situation either intravenous furosemide or oral bumetanide may be more effective.

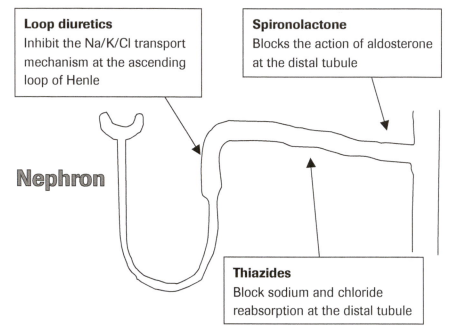

FIGURE 17.2 Sites of action of diuretic drugs.

Thiazide diuretics

Thiazide diuretics are more effective as BP-lowering agents than loop diuretics but are less effective at reducing fluid overload (see Figure 17.2). Therefore, they are not used as first-line therapy. However, in combination with loop diuretics they can be highly effective for patients with oedema that is difficult to control by loop diuretics alone. This is due to their different site of action leading to 'sequential nephron blockade'. Suitable agents include bendroflumethiazide or metolazone at low doses. Their use needs to be closely monitored as fluid loss may be profound and electrolyte disturbances (hyponatraemia and hypokalaemia) are common.

Angiotensin-converting enzyme inhibitors

ACEi have been proven to be effective in the treatment of patients with heart failure. In a study of 2569 patients (mean age 61 years) with ejection fractions below 35% (mean 25%), treatment with enalapril compared to placebo resulted in significantly better mortality rates over a 41-month period (35% vs 40%).[9] A meta-analysis of data from over 12000 patients with heart failure (mean age 61 years, mean ejection fraction 29%) demonstrated lower mortality rates with ACEi compared to placebo over an average follow-up period of 35 months (23% vs 27%).[10] They have also been found to be beneficial in reducing myocardial infarction (MI), stroke or cardiovascular death in patients with vascular risk factors but not known to have left ventricular impairment.[11]

Side-effects include a persistent dry cough due to an increase in bradykinin formation caused by raised levels of angiotensin I (*see* Figure 17.3). This may be severe enough to lead to discontinuation of the medication in up to 10% of patients. They may also cause deteriorating renal function in those with renal artery stenosis. This is due to high renin levels being important for maintaining renal perfusion in these patients. A further potential problem is hyperkalaemia – which may be worse in combination with aldosterone antagonists (e.g. spironolactone). Hypotension is common following initiation of therapy and patients should be warned to avoid rapid postural change. For this reason doses are started low and only gradually increased.

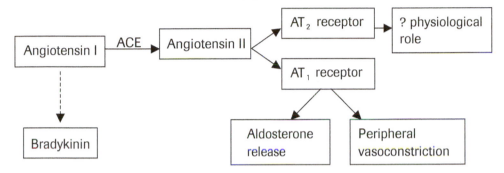

FIGURE 17.3 Normal physiological actions of angiotensin.

ACE = angiotensin converting enzyme; AT1 = angiotensin II type 1; AT2 = angiotensin II type 2.

The commencement of these agents may result in a rise in serum creatinine level. It is generally considered insignificant with a rise of less than 30% from the baseline. Severe renal impairment may be provoked in the presence of bilateral renal artery stenosis. Hyperkalaemia may develop.

Angiotensin type II receptor blockers

Angiotensin type II receptor blockers (ARB) act by directly inhibiting receptor activation (*see* Figure 17.4). As they do not lead to a build-up of bradykinins, they are not associated with a dry cough. They are recommended for use in people intolerant of ACEi.[6]

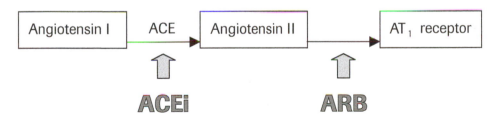

FIGURE 17.4 The sites of action of angiotensin converting enzyme inhibitors (ACEi) and angiotensin receptor blockers (ARB).

AT1 = angiotensin II type 1.

In a trial that compared the addition of valsartan or placebo to standard therapy in 5010 people with advanced heart failure, a significant reduction in the combined endpoint of mortality and morbidity (but not mortality alone) was seen in the treatment arm (RR 0.87, 95% CI 0.77–0.97).[12] A similar study has compared the addition of candesartan or placebo to the treatment of 7599 patients (mean age 66 years) with heart failure.[13] It also demonstrated a benefit with the ARB in cardiovascular death or non-fatal MI compared to placebo (HR 0.87, 95% CI 0.79–0.96).

A trial that recruited 3152 patients (mean age 71 years) with systolic heart failure compared the addition of losartan or captopril to standard medical management.[14] Over an 18-month period they found no difference in mortality rates but fewer patients discontinued therapy because of adverse events in the losartan group (9.7% vs 14.7%) – mainly due to a lower incidence of cough. A trial that randomised 25 577 patients (mean age 66 years) with vascular disease or diabetes to receive an ACEi, an ARB, or both (median follow-up 56 months) did not detect any significant difference in vascular events.[15] More patients developed cough with the ACEi (4.2% vs 1.1%). Side-effects were increased with both drugs in combination. Also, a meta-analysis of trials found that combinations of ARB and ACEi were associated with an increase in adverse events without any survival benefit.[16] Therefore it seems that ARB drugs should not be combined with ACEi.

Beta-blockers

Reduced bodily tissue perfusion results in the activation of the sympathetic nervous system. This process is helpful when the reduction is due to profound blood loss but is counterproductive in the case of heart failure. It may actually reduce cardiac function, and increase the risk of ischaemia and arrhythmias. For these reasons beta-blockers have been tried in heart failure.

Carvedilol has been compared to placebo in 1094 patients with chronic systolic heart failure in addition to standard medical therapy over a follow-up period of 6–12 months.[17] A significantly lower mortality rate was found in the carvedilol group (3.2% vs 7.8%).

The CIBIS-II trial randomised 2647 patients (mean age 61 years) with chronic systolic heart failure to receive either bisoprolol (slowly titrated up to 10 mg per day) or placebo in addition to standard therapy over a period of 1.3 years.[18] It found a lower mortality rate in the bisoprolol group compared to the placebo arm (11.8% vs 17.3%; HR 0.66, 95% CI 0.54–0.81).

The MERIT-HF study randomised 3991 patients (mean age 64 years) with chronic systolic heart failure to receive either metoprolol (slowly titrated up to 200 mg once daily) or placebo in addition to their usual medications over a one-year period.[19] It also found a lower mortality rate with the beta-blocker compared to placebo (7.2% vs 11.0%; RR 0.66, 95% CI 0.53–0.81).

The patients recruited in the above studies were relatively young. However, data derived from a number of randomised controlled trials suggests that these benefits are maintained among older patients.[20] Also, a more recent study has randomised 2128 patients over the age of 70 (mean age 76 years) with heart failure to receive either nebivolol or placebo over a 21-month period.[21] This found a reduction in all-cause mortality and cardiovascular hospital admissions with beta-blocker therapy (HR 0.86, 95% CI 0.74–0.99). Some evidence suggests that all beta-blockers may be equally effective in the elderly.[22]

Doses should be gradually increased at two-weekly intervals. Their use is contraindicated in patients with reversible airway disease, marked bradycardia, or second- or third-degree heart block.

Spironolactone

Spironolactone is a potassium-sparing diuretic that acts by inhibiting the action of aldosterone by blocking the binding with its receptor (*see* Figure 17.2).

A study has compared low-dose spironolactone (25 mg daily) to placebo in 1663 patients with systolic heart failure also on standard medical therapy over a two-year period.[23] The mortality rate was significantly lower in the spironolactone group (35% vs 46%; RR 0.70, 95% CI 0.60–0.82). Spironolactone use was associated with a 10% incidence of gynaecomastia and a 2% incidence of serious hyperkalaemia. The mechanism of the apparent beneficial effects of spironolactone is not fully understood. At the low dose used it has very little diuretic effect. It may have a cardioprotective role. The higher serum potassium levels seen with spironolactone compared to placebo may lead to a lower rate of cardiac arrhythmias induced by hypokalaemia.

Digoxin

Digoxin is proposed to have a mechanism that causes an increased intracellular calcium concentration leading to improved cardiac muscle contraction. Side-effects include nausea and vomiting, diarrhoea and arrhythmias. The risk of toxicity is increased in association with a hypokalaemia. It (at a mean daily dose 250 mcg) has been compared to placebo in 6800 patients with systolic heart failure on standard medical therapy over a three-year period.[24] It did not result in any improvement in mortality rates but was associated with a significantly lower rate of hospitalisation than placebo (RR 0.72, 95% CI 0.66–0.79). However, frail elderly people are more prone to side-effects and unlikely to tolerate such a high dose. It may be considered in people with deterioration despite the use of first and second-line drug treatments.[6]

Hydralazine and nitrates

In patients who are intolerant of ACEi, the combination of hydralazine and nitrates may, occasionally, be a suitable alternative. A study of 642 patients (mean age 58 years) who received either hydralazine (300 mg per day) and isosorbide dinitrate (160 mg per day), prazosin (20 mg per day) or placebo over a mean period of 2.3 years found a reduction in mortality with hydralazine-isosorbide (26%) compared to placebo (34%) or prazosin.[25] However, this combination is significantly less effective than ACEi.[26] The high doses used in the trials are unlikely to be tolerated by many older patients.

Cardiac resynchronisation

The use of biventricular pacemaker devices to restore a more physiological timing of ventricular contraction has been proposed for people with severe heart failure whose ECGs show sinus rhythm plus bundle branch block. This involves pacing the right ventricle in the normal way and also placing a lead through the coronary sinus to be able to pace the left ventricle,[27] the rationale being that improved timing of contractions will improve cardiac output.

In a trial of 813 patients (median age 67 years) in New York Heart Association class III or IV with ejection fractions below 35% and QRS durations of at least 120 ms (median 160 ms), individuals were randomised to receive medical therapy alone or in combination with cardiac resynchronisation over a mean period of 29 months.[28] The primary outcome of death or unplanned hospitalisation for a cardiovascular event occurred in 39% of the resynchronisation group compared to 55% of the controls (HR 0.63, 95% CI 0.51–0.77). This suggests that this treatment is beneficial in such patients, although cost-effectiveness is unclear. They may also be combined with implantable defibrillators to reduce the risk of sudden death due to arrhythmias (*see* below).

Implantable cardioverter-defibrillators

Sudden death caused by cardiac arrhythmias is common in patients with advanced heart failure. In the past some physicians have advocated regular oral amiodarone to prevent this complication. A recent study compared the use of amiodarone to implantable cardioverter-defibrillator (ICD) insertion or placebo in 2521 patients (median age 60 years) with advanced heart failure and ejection fractions at or below 35%.[29] After 46 months of follow-up, the amiodarone group fared no better than those given placebo (28 and 29% mortality, respectively), but the ICD group did significantly better (22% mortality).

Palliative care

It is a requirement that palliative care be incorporated into a patient's heart failure care. Patients who are reaching the palliative stage of their condition typically have had a number of admissions due to uncontrolled heart failure, no clear precipitant for deterioration, worsening renal function, and a poor response to optimal medical management.[30]

Prevention

The adequate control of hypertension has been associated with a reduction in the incidence of heart failure.[31]

Prognosis

The prognosis of heart failure is poor. One-year and five-year survival rates are around 60–80% and 30%, respectively, and older age is associated with a worse outcome.[32,33] The prognoses for systolic and diastolic heart failure are similar.[33]

REFERENCES

1 Kannel WB, Belanger AJ. Epidemiology of heart failure. *Am Heart J*, 1991; **121**(3): 951–7.

2 Aurigemma GP, Gaasch WH. Diastolic heart failure. *N Engl J Med*, 2004; **351**(11): 1097–105.

3 Hogg K, Swedberg K, McMurray J. Heart failure with preserved left ventricular systolic function. *J Am Coll Cardiol*, 2004; **43**(3): 317–27.

4 De Denus S, Pharand C, Williamson DR. Brain natriuretic peptide in the management of heart failure the versatile neurohormone. *Chest*, 2004; **125**(2): 652–68.

5 McKie PM, Burnett JC. B-type natriuretic peptide as a biomarker beyond heart failure: speculations and opportunities. *Mayo Clin Proc*, 2005; **80**(8): 1029–36.

6 National Institute for Health and Care Excellence. *Chronic Heart Failure: management of chronic heart failure in adults in primary and secondary care.* CG 108, 2010. Available at: www.nice.org.uk/guidance/cg108 (accessed 19 November 2014).

7 Pfisterer M, Buser P, Rickli H, *et al.* BNP-guided vs symptom-guided heart failure therapy: the Trial of Intensified vs Standard Medical Therapy in Elderly Patients with Congestive Heart Failure (TIME-CHF) randomized trial. *JAMA*, 2009; **301**(4): 383–92.

8 Crouse M, Flack D, Kerns JW, *et al.* Which medications benefit patients with diastolic heart failure? *J Family Practice*, 2011; **60**: 101–8.

9 The SOLVD Investigators. Effect of enalapril on survival in patients with reduced left ventricular ejection fractions and congestive heart failure. *N Engl J Med*, 1991; **325**(5): 293–302.

10 Flather MD, Yusuf S, Kober L, *et al.* Long-term ACE-inhibitor therapy in patients with heart failure or left-ventricular dysfunction: a systematic overview of data from individual patients. *Lancet*, 2000; **355**: 1575–81.

11 The Heart Outcomes Prevention Evaluation Study Investigators. Effects of an angiotensin-converting-enzyme inhibitor, ramipril, on cardiovascular events in high-risk patients. *N Engl J Med*, 2000; **342**(3): 145–53.

12 Cohn JN, Tognoni G. A randomized trial of the angiotensin-receptor blocker valsartan in chronic heart failure. *N Engl J Med*, 2001; **345**(23): 1667–75.

13 Demers C, McMurray JJV, Swedberg K, *et al.* Impact of candesartan on non-fatal myocardial infarction and cardiovascular death in patients with heart failure. *JAMA*, 2005; **294**(14): 1794–8.

14 Pitt B, Poole-Wilson PA, Segal R, *et al.* Effect of losartan compared with captopril in mortality in patients with symptomatic heart failure: randomised trial – the Losartan Heart Failure Survival Study ELITE II. *Lancet*, 2000; **355**: 1582–7.

15 ONTARGET Investigators. Telmisartan, ramipril, or both in patients at high risk for vascular events. *N Engl J Med*, 2008; **358**(15): 1547–59.

16 Makani H, Bangalore S, Desouza KA, *et al.* Efficacy and safety of dual blockade of the renin-angiotensin system: meta-analysis of randomised trials. *BMJ*, 2013; **346**: f360.

17 Packer M, Bristow MR, Cohn JN, *et al.* The effect of carvedilol on morbidity and mortality in patients with chronic heart failure. *N Engl J Med*, 1996; **334**(21): 1349–55.

18 CIBIS-II Investigators and Committees. The Cardiac Insufficiency Bisoprolol Study II (CIBIS-II): a randomised trial. *Lancet*, 1999; **353**: 9–13.

19 MERIT-HF Study Group. Effect of metoprolol CR/XL in chronic heart failure: Metoprolol CR/XL Randomised Intervention Trial in Congestive Heart Failure (MERIT-FH). *Lancet*, 1999; **353**: 2001–7.

20 Dulin BR, Haas SJ, Abraham WT, *et al.* Do elderly systolic heart failure patients benefit from beta blockers to the same extent as the non-elderly? Meta-analysis of >12,000 patients in large-scale clinical trials. *Am J Cardiol*, 2005; **95**: 896–8.

21 Flather MD, Shibata MC, Coats AJS, *et al.* Randomized trial to determine the effect of nebivolol on mortality and cardiovascular hospital admission in elderly patients with heart failure (SENIORS). *Eur Heart J*, 2005; **26**(3): 215–25.

22 Kramer JM, Curtis LH, Dupree CS, *et al.* Comparative effectiveness of beta-blockers in elderly patients with heart failure. *Arch Intern Med*, 2008; **168**(22): 2422–8.

23 Pitt B, Zannad F, Remme WJ, *et al.* The effect of spironolactone on morbidity and mortality in patients with severe heart failure. *N Engl J Med*, 1999; **341**(10): 709–17.

24 The Digitalis Investigation Group. The effect of digoxin on mortality and morbidity in patients with heart failure. *N Engl J Med*, 1997; **336**(8): 525–33.

25 Cohn JN, Archibald DG, Ziesche S, *et al.* Effect of vasodilator therapy on mortality in chronic congestive heart failure. *N Engl J Med*, 1986; **314**(24): 1547–52.

26 Cohn JN, Johnson G, Ziesche S, *et al.* A comparison of enalapril with hydralazine-isosorbide dinitrate in the treatment of chronic congestive heart failure. *N Engl J Med*, 1991; **325**(5): 303–10.

27 Chow AWC, Lane RE, Cowie MR. New pacing technologies for heart failure. *BMJ*, 2003; **326**: 1073–7.

28 Cleland JGF, Daubert J, Erdmann E, *et al.* The effect of cardiac resynchronization on morbidity and mortality in heart failure. *N Engl J Med*, 2005; **352**(15): 1539–49.

29 Bardy GH, Lee KL, Mark DB, *et al.* Amiodarone or an implantable cardioverter-defibrillator for congestive heart failure. *N Engl J Med*, 2005; **352**(3): 225–7.

30 Ellershaw J, Ward C. Care of the dying patient: the last hours or days of life. *BMJ*, 2003; **326**: 30–4.

31 Moser M, Herbert PR. Prevention of disease progression, left ventricular hypertrophy and congestive heart failure in hypertension treatment trials. *J Am Coll Cardiol*, 1996; **27**: 1214–18.

32 Nieminen MS, Harjola V. Definition and epidemiology of acute heart failure syndromes. *Am J Cardiol*, 2005; **96**(Suppl.): G5–10.

33 Bhatia RS, Tu JV, Lee DS, *et al.* Outcome of heart failure with preserved ejection fraction in a population-based study. *N Engl J Med*, 2006; **355**(3): 260–9.

CHAPTER 18

Hypertension

EPIDEMIOLOGY

Hypertension is a common problem, especially in the elderly, yet it is often under-recognised and under-treated. Data from the Framingham Heart Study found that it had a prevalence of 27% in those below age 60 years, rising to 63% of those aged 60–79, and 74% in those aged over 80.[1] Only 32% of hypertensive subjects were on adequate treatment to control their blood pressure (BP) below 140/90 mmHg. Even normotensive people aged 55–65 years have a 90% chance of developing hypertension at some stage in their lifetime.[2] Isolated systolic hypertension (ISH) is defined as having a systolic BP above 140 mmHg with a diastolic below 90 mmHg. It appears to be particularly common in the elderly, probably due to an increase in stiffness of large arteries.[3] This is mediated by a reduction in elastin and an increase in collagen proteins plus calcification within vessel walls. The result is a widening of the pulse pressure.

ASSESSMENT

It is advised that BP estimates are based on an average of at least two readings while seated, on at least two different occasions.[3] Orthostatic hypotension (OH) is frequently associated with hypertension in the elderly (*see* p. 344). Standing BP readings, especially in those with postural symptoms, may demonstrate it, but an active stand test would provide a more accurate evaluation (*see* p. 328). Twenty-four-hour BP monitoring can provide additional information and is recommended for people with BP readings above 140/90 mmHg.[4] It is discussed below.

TABLE 18.1 The classification of hypertensive retinopathy

Grade	
I	Narrowing of retinal arterioles
II	Arteriovenous 'nipping'
III	Soft exudates or flame haemorrhages
IV	Papilloedema

A physical examination may detect signs of end-organ damage, such as hypertensive retinopathy (*see* Table 18.1), evidence of left ventricular enlargement or proteinuria on urinalysis. Electrocardiograph (ECG) or chest X-ray tests may provide further signs of left ventricular hypertrophy.

24-hour blood pressure monitoring

Several BP recording devices are available for the patient to carry around with them over a period of, usually, 24 hours. They take measurements at regular intervals (usually set to hourly or half-hourly) and this data can be downloaded and analysed when the machine is returned to the healthcare setting. The use of such devices has led to the discovery of different patterns of BP that have differing effects on cardiovascular risk. O'Brien *et al.* have provided a useful review of this topic.[5] The main variants are discussed below.

'Normal' blood pressure

BP usually varies throughout the day with lower values occurring during the night. Normal individuals are currently defined as having an average daytime BP that is at or below 135/85 mmHG and a night-time dip to 120/70 mmHg or less. However, a truly normal BP is hard to define (*see* pp. 399). (*See* Figure 18.1.)

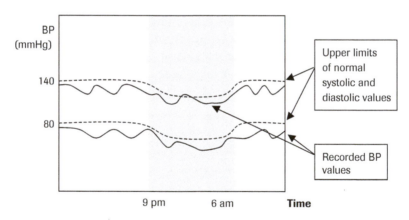

FIGURE 18.1 Representation of a 24-hour pattern of a 'normal' blood pressure.

Hypertension

Hypertension is defined as an average daytime BP of greater than 140/90 mmHg (this value is adjusted for people who have vascular disease (such as a stroke) and those who have diabetes – *see* below). A diurnal variation is usually maintained. A mean nocturnal BP of over 125/75 mmHg is considered abnormal. (*See* Figure 18.2.)

White coat hypertension

This is a term that is used to describe a pattern of hypertension with initial high readings in the presence of a healthcare professional (traditionally a doctor – hence 'white coat'). The BP will then normalise if repeated later. It is estimated to occur in 15–30%

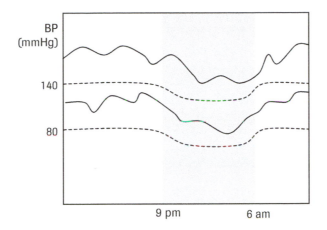

FIGURE 18.2 Representation of hypertension over 24 hours with preserved diurnal variation.

of the population but is more common in elderly people. Its significance is not fully understood but it does not appear to be associated with a major cardiovascular risk. It is represented in Figure 18.3. White coat hypertension should be suspected in people who continue to have high BP readings despite treatment for hypertension but also experience symptoms that suggest over-treatment (e.g. postural light-headedness).

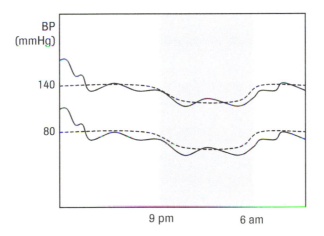

FIGURE 18.3 Representation of a 24-hour blood pressure recording in a person with 'white coat' hypertension.

Loss of diurnal variation
A number of people seem to have lost the normal pattern of BP variation. This pattern appears to be associated with an increased vascular and end organ damage risk,[6] including vascular dementia.[7] The term 'non-dippers' has been used for these people (compared to the normal 'dippers'). (*See* Figure 18.4.)

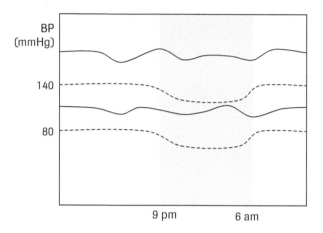

FIGURE 18.4 Representation of a 24-hour blood pressure recording in a person with hypertension associated with a loss of diurnal variation.

Nocturnal hypertension

Some people have higher night-time BP readings than their daytime values. Similar to those with a loss of diurnal variation, they appear to be at an increased risk of vascular events. (*See* Figure 18.5.)

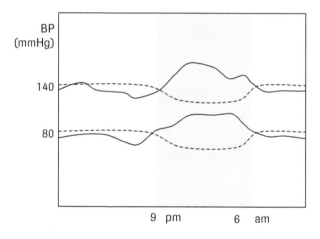

FIGURE 18.5 Representation of a 24-hour blood pressure recording in a person with nocturnal hypertension.

Twenty-four-hour BP monitoring probably has a number of roles in clinical practice. Among those are the enabling of identification of white coat and nocturnal hypertension, guiding the commencement of treatment in patients with borderline BP readings, and assessing the overall control of BP in people with mixed spine hypertension and OH.

The use of ambulatory BP values rather than conventional measurement has been compared.[8] Over a six-month period the ambulatory BP group was prescribed fewer anti-hypertensive medications with similar resultant blood pressures and no evidence of an increase in left ventricular size (assessed by ECG and echocardiography measurements). Another study found that 24-hour recordings offered additional information to predict cardiovascular risk to that derived from conventional measurements alone.[9] The night-time BP reading may be of particular predictive value due to its unfluctuating nature during normal sleep. So, it appears to be an appropriate alternative to conventional methods in selected patients.

TREATMENT

Reducing elevated BP has been shown to reduce the risk of vascular adverse events, in particular stroke (*see* p. 200). Estimates of around a 40% reduction in stroke and 15% reduction in MI with adequate BP treatment have been made.[10] Such benefits appear to be maintained in elderly populations and in those with isolated systolic hypotension (ISH).[11,12] These patients have also been found to have a significantly lower rate of heart failure after BP treatment compared to placebo over a 4.5-year period (RR 0.51, 95% CI 0.37–0.71).[13] Even in those aged over 80 meta-analysis of data from antihypertensive randomised controlled trials suggests a maintained benefit.[14] A more recent trial specifically recruited those aged over 80 (n=3845, mean age 84 years) and reduced BP by 15/6 mmHg on average (from 173/91).[14] After a 1.8-year follow-up period they found a 30% reduction in stroke (95% CI–1 to 51%), 21% reduction in death from any cause (95% CI 4 to 35%), and a 64% reduction in heart failure (95% CI 42 to 78%), with no increase in adverse effects from treatment compared to placebo. Mid-life hypertension is also associated with an increased risk of developing dementia in later life (*see* p. 104). Once hypertension has been identified treatment should be considered immediately, as delays are associated with excess cardiovascular adverse events.[16]

However, the situation may be different in the frail elderly.[11] BP reduction increases the risk of orthostatic hypotension (*see* p. 344) and thus falls and fractures. This may explain why, although a benefit in cardiovascular mortality in maintained in those aged over 80 years (RR 0.75, 95% CI 0.65–0.87), total mortality is uninfluenced by treatment (RR 1.01, 95% CI 0.90–1.13).[17] In addition, available evidence suggests that cardiovascular risk reduction benefits of treatment are not maintained in the very frail. A study found that high BP had no overall mortality effect on those with a walking speed below 0.8 m/s.[18] The relationship between hypertension and frailty is a complex one as high BP increases the risk of cerebral white matter lesions that are associated with the development of functional impairment (*see* p. 15). BP is likely to be lower in the frailest due to a reduction in cardiac output secondary to impairment of diastolic function.[19]

BP targets

There is no apparent 'normal' BP value below which there is no additional treatment benefit, that is, the lower the blood pressure the lower the vascular risk. A meta-analysis of studies suggests that lowering blood pressures down to at least 115/75 mmHg continues to reduce vascular risk.[20] Below this value there is little available data. Between the ages of 40 and 69 years there is a doubling of vascular death rates for every elevation of 20 mmHg systolic, or 10 mmHg diastolic BP.[20] After this age the relative risk reduction is less but the absolute risk is higher and so a significant benefit is still attained. Accepted target blood pressures are better than 140/85 mmHg in non-diabetics and better than 130/80 mmHg in those with diabetes.[10] The lower target of 130/80 mmHg has also been recommended for patients with evidence of secondary organ damage (vascular disease, abnormal renal function, retinopathy, or evidence of left ventricular enlargement on ECG or echocardiogram).[21]

The actual benefit of treatment is proportional to the baseline risk of cardiovascular disease. Indicators of elevated risk include signs of target organ damage (e.g. left ventricular hypertrophy, proteinuria or retinopathy) or associated comorbidities (e.g. diabetes, stroke or renal impairment). More than 50% of people over 65 years in most populations are defined as hypertensive by such targets.[10] Even if these targets cannot be safely achieved (e.g. because of associated OH – *see* Chapter 15), there may still a benefit from smaller BP reductions and so, in some elderly people, less strict goals may be more appropriate. A recent NICE guideline has recommended a BP target of below 150/90 mmHg for people aged over 80 years (or below a daytime average of 145/85 mmHg on 24 hour BP recordings).[4] In some frail elderly patients the risk of adverse effects from any BP-lowering treatment may outweigh beneficial effects.[11] Clinical judgement for each individual is required in this group of people.

Non-pharmacological intervention

Some lifestyle measures can reduce the impact of hypertension. These include weight reduction in the obese, avoiding excess alcohol intake, increasing physical activity, and dietary factors (fresh vegetables, low saturated fat and reduced salt).[10] Additional changes to reduce the chance of vascular disease, such as stopping smoking, are also clearly logical.

Pharmacological intervention

Despite the above measures, pharmacological therapy is usually required. Caution should be used when starting any new drug in a frail older person. An increased risk of falls and subsequent fracture has been demonstrated following the commencement of antihypertensive treatment (incidence rate ratio 1.43, 95% CI 1.19–1.72 in the first 45 days).[22]

The question remains as to which agent or combination of agents is most effective. Analysis of the trials performed suggests that any method of BP reduction will have cardiovascular benefits, and the degree of reduction rather than the drugs used is the key factor.[23] Most patients will require more than one agent to achieve adequate control – especially if the starting BP is above 160/100 mmHg,[3] and 30% will need three or more agents.[10] Other vascular prevention strategies are also of proven benefit in many of these patients (e.g. antiplatelets[24] and statins[25]). This all adds to the burden of polypharmacy seen in elderly people (*see* p. 30). Given the lack of obvious benefit to the individual patient, medication adherence is a particular problem with these drugs, and patient education is especially important. Two recent, large hypertension trials are discussed below.

ALLHAT

The ALLHAT trial randomised 33 357 people over the age of 55 (mean age 67 years) with hypertension and at least one other vascular risk factor to receive either a thiazide (chlorthalidone), angiotensin-converting enzyme (ACE) inhibitor (lisinopril) or a calcium channel blocker (amlodipine) over a mean follow-up of 4.9 years.[26] After this time, there was no significant difference in the primary outcome (combined fatal coronary heart disease and non-fatal myocardial infarction (MI)) with any of the agents. Chlorthalidone resulted in a small but significantly greater reduction in systolic BP than either lisinopril (2 mmHg) or amlodipine (0.8 mmHg). The conclusion of this trial was that, due to their low cost and proven efficacy, thiazides should be considered as first-line agents for BP control.

ASCOT

The ASCOT trial randomised 19 257 people (mean age 63, range 40–79 years) with hypertension plus other vascular risk factors to receive either amlodipine with perindopril if required or atenolol plus bendroflumethiazide if required over a five-year period.[27] The mean initial BP was 164/95 mmHg and this was reduced to 136/77 mmHg in the amlodipine arm and 139/79 mmHg in the atenolol arm. The primary endpoint of non-fatal MI and fatal coronary heart disease failed to reach significance in favour of the amlodipine regimen (8.1 vs 9.2 events per 1000 people-years; $p=0.11$). However, there were significant reductions in total cardiovascular events and procedures (27.4 vs 32.8; $p<0.0001$), stroke (6.2 vs 8.1; $p=0.0003$) and overall mortality (13.9 vs 15.5; $p=0.025$). Only 53% of participants achieved their target BP, which was set at 140/90 mmHg for non-diabetics and 130/80 mmHg for diabetics (of whom only 32% achieved the target). On average 2.2 and 2.3 BP-lowering agents were used in the amlodipine and atenolol groups, respectively. Eight per cent of the subjects were on four or more agents at the end of the study. Twenty-five per cent of each group stopped a treatment because of side-effects. Adverse events occurring more often in the amlodipine arm included cough (19% vs 8%) and oedema (23% vs 6%). Adverse events occurring more often in the atenolol arm included bradycardia (6% vs <1%), dizziness (16% vs 12%), dyspnoea (10% vs 6%), fatigue (16% vs 8%) and cold peripheries (6% vs 1%).

The mean difference in blood pressure of 2.7/1.9 mmHg between the groups would explain at least some of difference in outcomes. Other metabolic features that differed between groups included a higher mean glucose (raised by 0.2 mmol/L), body mass index (by 0.3 kg/m²) and lower HDL cholesterol (by 0.1 mmol/L) in the atenolol group.

PROGRESS

This trial is of particular relevance to BP control post-stroke and is discussed on p. 210.

Individual drugs

The mechanisms of action and main side-effects of the most commonly used agents are discussed on p. 387.

Thiazide diuretics

Thiazide diuretics are considered a first-line agent for the management of hypertension in the elderly[10] – especially in those with ISH. They were used in the ALLHAT, ACSOT and PROGRESS trials as outlined earlier. Newer thiazide-like diuretics, such as chlorthalidone or indapamide, may be preferable to older thiazide diuretics such as bendroflumethiazide or hydrochlorothiazide.[4]

ACE inhibitors

ACE inhibitors were used in the ALLHAT, ACSOT and PROGRESS trials as outlined earlier. Around 5 to 10% of people are intolerant of ACE inhibitors due to cough.

Calcium channel blockers

Dihydropyridines (e.g. amlodipine) are suitable for the management of hypertension, especially in the elderly.[10] Non-dihydropyridines (e.g. diltiazem) are probably less effective in this situation. In the ALLHAT study a calcium channel blocker compared less favourably to a thiazide for the prevention of heart failure (peripheral oedema is a recognised side-effect of calcium channel blockers).

Beta-blockers

A recent meta-analysis of trials into the use of atenolol has brought into question the use of beta-blockers for the treatment of hypertension.[28] In randomised controlled trials comparing atenolol to placebo, despite improvements in BP, no significant reductions in cardiovascular events or mortality were detected. In comparison to alternative antihypertensive agents, there was a significantly higher mortality with atenolol (RR 1.13; 95% CI 1.02–1.25).

Less lipid-soluble agents (e.g. atenolol, bisoprolol and metoprolol) are less likely to cause neuropsychiatric side-effects (sedation, sexual dysfunction and depression) than lipid-soluble alternatives (e.g. propranolol).[3]

Angiotensin receptor blockers (ARBs)

A trial recruiting 15 245 patients compared valsartan to amlodipine (plus other antihypertensive agents as required) in patients aged over 50 years (mean age 67) with hypertension and other vascular risk factors over a mean period of 4.2 years.[29] The amlodipine regimen proved to be more effective at lowering BP (by a mean of 1.5/1.3 mmHg) and was associated with a non-significant lower rate of attaining the combined end-point of cardiac mortality and morbidity (10.4% vs 10.6%).

Losartan has been compared to atenolol in 1326 patients (mean age 70, range 55–80 years) with ISH and evidence of left ventricular hypertrophy in the LIFE study.[30] Other agents (mainly thiazide diuretics) could be added if required for better BP control. Despite similar reductions in blood pressure (28/9 mmHg in both arms), after a mean period of 4.7 years, there was a non-significantly reduced incidence of the combined endpoint of cardiovascular death, stroke or MI in the losartan arm (RR 0.75; 95% CI 0.59–1.01). This suggests that ARBs may be useful BP-lowering agents, but given the emerging evidence that beta-blockers may be less effective than alternatives (*see* above), the more expensive and less well studied ARBs are usually second-line agents. The combination of ARBs with ACE inhibitors appears to increase the risk of side-effects without any benefit.[31,32]

Interpretation of pharmacological data

The benefits seen after BP-lowering are probably mostly due to the degree of pressure reduction rather than any factors related to the class of medications themselves. The above studies suggest that, either alone or (more commonly) in combination, any of thiazide diuretics, ACE inhibitors and dihydropyridine calcium channel blockers (e.g. amlodipine) are suitable first-line agents for the management of hypertension in the elderly. The actual agents chosen may be dictated by the presence of comorbidities, for example ACE inhibitors may be of additional benefit in those with renal impairment, thiazides may be avoided in those with gout. Certain agents (e.g. vasodilators and diuretics) and those in shorter-acting formulations are particularly likely to cause OH (*see* p. 344). This may influence the choice of drug in selected patients. An additional factor influencing prescribing should be cost – as cheaper agents are the more cost-effective.[10]

Beta-blockers should no longer be considered first-line agents unless there is another reason to justify their use – such as the prevention of angina or rate control in AF. ARBs are probably a reasonable choice of second-line agent, or for those intolerant of but with an indication for ACE inhibitors. Alpha-blockers (e.g. doxazosin) may also be appropriate in some patients but the evidence is less clear and an increased association with orthostatic hypotension may limit their use in the elderly. Other drugs, such as central alpha-agonists (e.g. methyldopa and clonidine) or vasodilators (e.g. hydralazine), will occasionally be appropriate but there is less randomised controlled trial evidence of efficacy and side-effects are likely to be significant.

Current guidelines for the British Hypertension Society and NICE recommend either a calcium channel blocker or thiazide diuretic as first-line therapy in the elderly (>55 years).[4] The second step would be to add an ACE inhibitor (or an ARB if ACE inhibitor-intolerant). The third step is to add either a calcium channel blocker or thiazide (whichever has not already been used).

Resistant hypertension (BP >140/90 mmHg despite treatment with three or more antihypertensive drugs) is reported to be present in 10–20% of people with hypertension.[33] Twenty-four-hour BP monitoring is usually required to exclude white coat hypertension plus confirmation of patient therapeutic adherence. Tackling obesity, alcohol excess and high dietary salt intake can all help. Underlying secondary causes of hypertension should be considered (e.g. hyperaldosteronism, renal artery stenosis or phaeochromocytoma). NICE guidance recommends adding in either spironolactone (if serum potassium is 4.5 mmol/L of less) or a higher dose thiazide-like diuretic (if serum potassium >4.5 mmol/L).[4] If this is ineffective then an alpha- or beta-blocker drug should be considered. Expert advice should be obtained if the BP remains uncontrolled. However, more lenient BP targets are suitable for the frail elderly.

REFERENCES

1 Lloyd-Jones DM, Evans JC, Levy D. Hypertension in adults across the age spectrum: current outcomes and control in the community. *JAMA*, 2005; **294**(4): 466–72.

2 Vasan RS, Beiser A, Seshadri S, *et al.* Residual lifetime risk of developing hypertension in middle-aged women and men: the Framingham Heart Study. *JAMA*, 2002; **287**(8): 1003–10.

3 Dickerson LM, Gibson MV. Management of hypertension in older persons. *Am Family Phys*, 2005; **71**(3): 469–76.

4 National Institue of Health and Care Excellence. *Hypertension: clinical management of primary hypertension in adults.* CG127, 2011. Available at: www.nice.org.uk/guidance/cg127 (accessed 8 October 2014).

5 O'Brien E, Coats A, Owens P, *et al.* Use and interpretation of ambulatory blood pressure monitoring: recommendations of the British Hypertension Society. *BMJ*, 2000; **320**: 1128–34.

6 Verdecchia P, Schillaci G, Guerrieri M, *et al.* Circadian blood pressure changes and left ventricular hypertrophy in essential hypertension. *Circulation*, 1990; **81**: 528–36.

7 Yamamoto Y, Akiguchi I, Oiwa K, *et al.* The relationship between 24-hour blood pressure readings, subcortical ischemic lesions and vascular dementia. *Cerebrovasc Dis*, 2005; **19**: 302–8.

8 Staesseu JA, Byttebier G, Buntinx F, *et al.* Antihypertensive treatment based on conventional or ambulatory blood pressure measurement: a randomised controlled trial. *JAMA*, 1997; **278**(13): 1065–72.

9 Staessen JA, Thijs L, Fagard R, *et al.* Predicting cardiovascular risk using conventional vs ambulatory blood pressure in older patients with systolic hypertension. *JAMA*, 1999; **282**(6): 539–46.

10 Williams B, Poulter NR, Brown MJ, *et al.* Guidelines for management of hypertension: report of the fourth working party of the British Hypertension Society, 2004-BHS IV. *J Human Hypertension*, 2004; **18**: 139–85.

11 Muller M, Smulder YM, de Leeuw PW, *et al.* Treatment of hypertension in the oldest old: a critical role for frailty? *Hypertension*, 2014; **63**: 433–41.

12 Perry HM, Davis BR, Price TR, *et al.* Effect of treating isolated systolic hypertension on the risk of developing various types and subtypes of stroke: the Systolic Hypertension in the Elderly Program (SHEP). *JAMA*, 2000; **284**(4): 465–71.

13 Kostis JB, Davis BR, Cutler J, *et al.* Prevention of heart failure by antihypertensive drug treatment in older persons with isolated systolic hypertension. *JAMA*, 1997; **278**(3): 212–16.

14 Gueyffier F, Bulpitt C, Boissel JP, *et al.* Antihypertensive drugs in very old people: a subgroup meta-analysis of randomised controlled trials. *Lancet*, 1999; **353**: 793–6.

15 Beckett NS, Peters R, Fletcher AE, *et al.* Treatment of hypertension in patients 80 years of age or older. *N Engl J Med*, 2008; **358**(18): 1887–98.

16 Staessen JA, Thijs L, Fagard R, *et al.* Effects of immediate versus delayed antihypertensive therapy on outcome in the Systolic Hypertension in Europe Trial. *J Hypertension*, 2004; **22**: 847–57.

17 Musini VM, Tejani AM, Bassett K, *et al.* Pharmacotherapy for hypertension in the elderly. *Cochrane Database Syst Rev*, 2009 Oct 7;(4):CD000028.

18 Odden MC, Peralta CA, Haan MN, *et al.* Rethinking the association of high blood pressure with mortality in elderly adults: the impact of frailty. *Arch Intern Med*, 2012; **172**: 1162–8.

19 van Bemmel T, Holman ER, Gussekloo J, *et al.* Low blood pressure in the very old, a consequence of imminent heart failure: the Leiden 85-plus Study. *J Human Hypertension*, 2009; **23**: 27–32.

20 Prospective Studies Collaboration. Age-specific relevance of usual blood pressure to vascular mortality: a meta-analysis of individual data for one million adults in 61 prospective studies. *Lancet*, 2002; **360**: 1903–13.

21 Joint British Societies' guidelines on prevention of cardiovascular disease in clinical practice. *Heart*, 2005; **91**(Suppl. V): v1–v52.

22 Butt DA, Mamdani M, Austin PC, *et al.* The risk of hip fracture after initiating antihypertensive drugs in the elderly. *Arch Intern Med*, 2012; **172**(22): 1739–44.

23 Blood Pressure Lowering Treatment Trialists' Collaboration. Effects of different blood-pressure-lowering regimens on major cardiovascular events: results of prospectively-designed overviews of randomised trials. *Lancet*, 2003; **362**: 1527–35.

24 Hansson L, Zanchetti A, Carruthers SG, *et al.* Effects of intensive blood-pressure lowering and low-dose aspirin in patients with hypertension: principal results of the Hypertension Optimal Treatment (HOT) randomised trial. *Lancet*, 1998; **351**: 1755–62.

25 Sever PS, Dahlof B, Poulter NR, *et al.* Prevention of coronary and stroke events with atorvastatin in hypertensive patients who have average or lower-than-average cholesterol concentrations, in the Anglo-Scandinavian Cardiac Outcomes Trial – Lipid Lowering Arm (ASCOTT-LLA): a multicentre randomised controlled trial. *Lancet*, 2003; **361**: 1149–58.

26 The ALLHAT Officers and Coordinators for the ALLHAT Collaborative Research Group. Major outcomes in high-risk hypertensive patients randomized to angiotensin-converting enzyme inhibitor or calcium channel blocker vs diuretic: the Antihypertensive and Lipid-Lowering Treatment to Prevent Heart Attack Trial (ALLHAT). *JAMA*, 2002; **288**(23): 2981–97.

27 Dahlof B, Sever PS, Poulter NR, *et al.* Prevention of cardiovascular events with an antihypertensive regimen of amlodipine adding perindopril as required versus atenolol adding bendroflumethiazide as required, in the Anglo-Scandinavian Cardiac Outcomes Trial – Blood Pressure Lowering Arm (ASCOT-BPLA): a multicentre randomised controlled trial. *Lancet*, 2005; **366**: 895–906.

28 Carlberg B, Samuelsson O, Lindholm LH. Atenolol in hypertension: is it a wise choice? *Lancet*, 2004; **364**: 1684–9.

29 Julius S, Kjeldsen SE, Weber M, *et al.* Outcomes in hypertensive patients at high cardiovascular risk treated with regimens based on valsartan or amlodipine: the VALUE randomised trial. *Lancet*, 2004; **363**: 2022–31.

30 Kjeldsen SE, Dahlof B, Devereux RB, *et al.* Effects of losartan on cardiovascular morbidity and mortality in patients with isolated systolic hypertension and left ventricular hypertrophy: a Losartan Intervention For Endpoint Reduction (LIFE) study. *JAMA*, 2002; **288**(12): 1491–8.

31 The ONTARGET Investigators. Telmisartan, ramipril, or both in patients at high risk for vascular events. *N Engl J Med*, 2008; **358**: 1547–59.

32 Makani H, Bangalore S, Desouza KA, *et al.* Efficacy and safety of dual blockade of the renin-angiotensin system: meta-analysis of randomised trials. *BMJ*, 2013; **346**: f360.

33 Myat A, Redwood SR, Qureshi AC, *et al.* Resistant hypertension. *BMJ*, 2012; **345**: 40–5.

CHAPTER 19

Atrial fibrillation

Atrial fibrillation (AF) is more common in older than younger people. It occurs in less than 2% of those below the age of 65 and in 5.9% of those over 65 years.[1] The prevalence rises to between 7% and 14% of the population over the age of 80. However, these figures may underestimate the true prevalence of AF as unsustained episodes (paroxysmal AF (PAF)) are likely to have been missed.

AF can be provoked by almost any cardiac abnormality. Those who have had a previous myocardial infarction (MI), or have left ventricular impairment or atrial enlargement are at an increased risk of its development. Only around 15% occurs in people with structurally normal hearts ('lone' AF).[2] People with a higher pulse pressure (*see* p. 13) are also at a greater risk of developing AF.[3]

The major adverse consequence of AF is the six-fold increased risk of stroke (the rate is even higher in those with AF secondary to mitral valve disease).[2] This is due to the formation and subsequent embolisation of thrombus – most typically from the left atrial appendage. On average the annual risk of stroke in people with AF but no antiplatelet or anticoagulation medication is around 5%, but this varies according to other risk factors. From the Stroke Prevention in AF II trial, the following clinical characteristics were associated with a higher risk of stroke: history of previous stroke or transient ischaemic attack (TIA), systolic blood pressure (BP) above 160 mmHg; left ventricular dysfunction; and age over 75 years.[4] Older age is also a major risk factor for stroke and, given the higher incidence of stroke in old age, the absolute benefit of anticoagulation is greater.[5]

Rating scales to estimate risk have been developed: one of these is the $CHADS_2$ tool.[6] In this scheme one point is given for each of **C**ongestive cardiac failure history, **H**ypertension, **A**ge over 75 years and **D**iabetes, and a history of **S**troke scores **2** points (spelling $CHADS_2$) – giving a score of 0–6. This has since been further extended, to take account of additional risk factors, to form the CHA_2DS_2VASc score.[7] In this scheme two points are scored for age over 75 (A_2), in addition, one point is given for a history of vascular disease (**V** = prior MI, peripheral vascular disease or aortic plaque), age over 65 (**A** – but no additional point if aged over 75) and female sex (**S**) – giving a score of 0–9. The estimated stroke rates for different scores are shown in Table 19.1.[8] The CHA_2DS_2VASc score appears to have better predictive ability than the simpler $CHADS_2$ score.[9]

TABLE 19.1 Estimated stroke rates for $CHADS_2$ and CHA_2DS_2-VASc scores

$CHADS_2$	Rate*	CHA_2DS_2-VASc	Rate*
0	1.9	0	0
1	2.8	1	1.3
2	4.0	2	2.2
3	5.9	3	3.2
4	8.5	4	4.0
5	12.5	5	6.7
6	18.2	6	9.8
		7	9.6
		8	6.7
		9	15.2

* Estimated stroke rate per 100 patient-years (for patients on neither warfarin nor antiplatelet agents)

Overall, around 15% of strokes are associated with AF, but this proportion is elevated in older patients, being around 36% in those over the age of 80.[10] Recurrent episodes of PAF appear to carry a similar thromboembolic risk to sustained AF.[4] However, the relevance of very infrequent, brief episodes, such as a single short run of AF detected on a 24-hour electrocardiograph (ECG), is unclear.

When evaluating a patient with AF it is important to look for reversible secondary causes. These include thyrotoxicosis and excess alcohol intake. Twenty-four-hour ECG recordings may detect previously unknown PAF or may be useful to judge rate control over a prolonged period. Echocardiography may provide information regarding left ventricular function, left atrial size, and valvular lesions but is unlikely to give additional information that would influence the decision regarding the suitability of an elderly patient for anticoagulation.[11]

PREVENTION OF THROMBOEMBOLIC COMPLICATIONS
Warfarin

Warfarin antagonises the effect of vitamin K in the process of production of its dependent clotting factors within the liver (factors VII, IX, X, prothrombin, and proteins C and S) (*see* Figure 10.10). This reduces the risk of forming blood clots within the left atrium due to blood stasis during AF. The overall efficacy of warfarin is in the order of around a 65% reduction in relative risk of stroke.[4,12] When real-life practice has been compared to the results of such trials, similar outcomes have been observed.[13] Of course, the absolute risk reduction depends on the individual's baseline risk of stroke, that is, those at highest risk benefit the most. Patients under the age of 65 years who have no history of vascular disease or diabetes are at a very low risk of thromboembolism and the benefits do not outweigh the risks of warfarinisation.[12]

The main side-effect of warfarin is an elevated bleeding tendency. Traditionally quoted contraindications to anticoagulation include recent bleeding, multiple falls (more than two in the last year), inability to consistently take the prescribed dose, uncontrolled hypertension and excessive alcohol intake.[11] However, risks to older people have probably been overestimated in the past.[14] Falling, in particular, does not seem to be an important factor in deciding whether a patient should receive warfarin.[15]

Despite the evidence of benefit of warfarin in those with AF, only around 30% of such patients who do not have contraindications are receiving this therapy.[16] This is usually due to a perceived low risk of embolus or high risk of haemorrhage within particular patients. Having previously had a patient who sustained a serious bleeding complication appears to reduce the probability of a physician prescribing warfarin.[17]

The anticoagulant response to warfarin is increased with advanced age.[18] This difference is still apparent after correction for confounding variables such as body weight, medication interactions and comorbidity. Part of this difference may be due to dietary change. Vitamin K, which opposes the effect of warfarin, is found in leafy green vegetables. Therefore a diet containing less of these may make the effects of warfarin more pronounced.

Loading

The old regimen of 10 mg on three consecutive days resulted in over a third of patients being over-coagulated on the fourth day.[19] An early loading regimen that commenced with 10 mg but then varied according to international normalised ratio (INR) on day two was described by Fennerty *et al.*[19] This has largely been replaced in the elderly by regimens commencing with a 5 mg dose, which cause lower incidences of over-coagulation.[20] The initial dose may be further reduced in the presence of other factors increasing sensitivity to warfarin, such as liver disease or medication interactions.[21]

Complications

Complications of therapy are mainly due to increased bleeding. Overall, major bleeds occur at a rate of 2–7% per year and fatal ones at a rate of 1% per year.[4,22,23] The risk rises proportionally with increasing INR values.[24] The bleeding risk is also elevated in this first few months of therapy and in those with unstable INRs.[23] Patients who have had one bleed are at a higher risk of additional events within the following year.[23] Age itself, when adjusted for confounding variables, does not appear to be a significant risk factor for overall rates of bleeding complications.[23,25,26] On the other hand, a doubling of risk for subdural haemorrhage with each additional decade has been reported.[25] Other risk factors for bleeding while on warfarin therapy include recent haemorrhage, binge drinking of alcohol, renal impairment, liver disease, NSAID use, and having a diagnosis of cancer.[21]

Intracranial bleeds occur at a rate of 0.3% to 1% per year in patients on warfarin, depending on baseline risk factors (such as hypertension and previous stroke).[27] Around 70% of intracranial bleeding occurring in people on warfarin is due to intra-cerebral haemorrhage (ICH) and most of the rest is due to subdural haematomas.[27] ICH in this population carries a 60% mortality rate. The size of the bleed often increases over a 24-hour period, making urgent reversal of the coagulation impairment imperative. This is best achieved with prothrombin complex concentrate infusion. ICH is further discussed on p. 214.

In a study of 228 very old patients (mean age 81, range 76–94 years) on warfarin over a mean follow-up of 28 months, an annual incidence of 10% for major bleeding and 1% for fatal haemorrhage was detected.[28] Two intracranial bleeds occurred (0.4% per year) and these were both fatal. There was an associated 2.6% ischaemic stroke rate per year. The most common site of major bleeding was gastrointestinal (30%). Forty-two per cent of major bleeds occurred with INRs above the target range (> 3.0), and 60% of fatal bleeds occurred with a very high INR (>5.0). The majority of the adverse bleeding events resulted in complete recovery.

A more recent study randomised 973 patients over the age of 75 (mean age 82 years) who were in AF, but their physician was unsure of the benefits of anticoagulation, to either warfarin or aspirin.[29] Follow-up was for 2.7 years, 72% of patients had a CHADS$_2$ score of 1 or 2. The annual stroke risk was 1.8% with warfarin compared to 3.8% with aspirin (RR 0.48, 95% CI 0.28–0.80). Surprisingly, extracranial bleeding was less common on warfarin (1.4% per year vs 1.6%; RR 0.87, 95% CI 0.43–1.73). This suggests that the benefits of warfarin are still apparent in this age group, and bleeding rates may be lower than previously thought. Good INR control is clearly important. Even elderly patients in a controlled environment may also be at risk of unstable warfarin dosing. There is a high incidence of errors in the management of INRs within nursing homes,[30] with an increased chance of sub-therapeutic INRs or overcoagulation.[31]

A number of scoring tools have been developed to try to estimate the risk of bleeding complications while on oral anticoagulants. One of these is called 'HAS-BLED' – *see* Table 19.2.[32] A score of three or more on the HAS-BLED tool suggests a significantly increased risk of bleeding. However, this is perhaps best used to try to identify potentially reversible factors (e.g. antiplatelet use and alcoholism) or identify those patients who need careful supervision, rather than to justify not prescribing anticoagulation.[9]

TABLE 19.2 The HAS-BLED tool for the evaluation of bleeding risk while on anticoagulation

Clinical feature	Details	Score
Hypertension	Systolic blood pressure > 160 mmHg	1
Abnormal renal or hepatic function	• Renal dialysis/transplant • Cirrhosis or bilirubin more than 2× normal and enzymes more than 3× normal	1 or 2
Stroke		1
Bleeding	History of bleeding or known risk factor	1
Labile INR	Recurrent high INR values or low time in the therapeutic range (<60%)	1
Elderly	Age over 65 years	1
Drugs or alcohol	• Concurrent use of aspirin or NSAIDs • Alcohol abuse	1 or 2
	Maximum possible score	9

Current guidelines recommend anticoagulation with warfarin or a novel anticoagulant (*see* below) is considered for people with AF who have a CHA$_2$DS$_2$VASc score of two or more (or a CHADS$_2$ score of two or more; or age over 75, or two or more of: age over 65, female sex, vascular disease).[8] Those with a CHA_2DS_2VASc score of one should be considered either for anticoagulation or for aspirin (75–325 mg per day). Those with a CHA_2DS_2VASc of zero are recommended to have no treatment.

Novel anticoagulants

The oral drugs dabigatran (a direct thrombin inhibitor), apixaban and rivaroxaban (both factor Xa inhibitors) have recently been developed as alternatives to warfarin. These drugs have the advantage of being a standardised dose that does not need titrating or monitoring. The two potential limitations are the higher cost and the inability to rapidly reverse the anticoagulation effect. Broadly speaking they have a similar efficacy as warfarin in preventing stroke in patients with AF but may have fewer bleeding complication rates.

Dabigatran (at doses of 110 and 150 mg twice daily) has been compared to warfarin in 18 113 patients (mean age 71, mean $CHADS_2$ score = 2.1) in AF plus one or more additional risk factor(s) for stroke (mean follow up 2.0 years).[33] The study found similar rates of ischaemic stroke per year with dabigatran compared to warfarin (110 mg dose: 1.34% vs 1.20% [RR 1.11, 95% CI 0.89–1.40]; 150 mg dose: 0.92% vs 1.20% [RR 0.76, 95% CI 0.60–0.98]), but lower annual rates of haemorrhagic stroke at either dose (110 mg dose: 0.12% vs 0.38% [RR 0.31, 95% CI 0.17–0.56]; 150 mg dose: 0.10% vs 0.38% [RR 0.26, 95% CI 0.14–0.49]) and major bleeding with the 110 mg dose (2.71% vs 3.36% [RR 0.80, 95% CI 0.69–0.93]) but not the 150 mg dose (3.11% vs 3.36% [RR 0.93, 95% CI 0.81–1.07]).

Apixaban (5 mg twice daily) has been compared to warfarin in 18 201 patients (median age 70, mean $CHADS_2$ score = 2.1) in AF plus one or more additional risk factor(s) for stroke (mean follow up 1.8 years).[34] The study found similar rates of ischaemic stroke per year with apixaban compared to warfarin (0.97% vs 1.05% [HR 0.92, 95% CI 0.74–1.13]), but lower annual rates of haemorrhagic stroke (0.24% vs 0.47% [HR 0.51, 95% CI 0.35–0.75]) and major bleeding (2.13% vs 3.09% [HR 0.69, 95% CI 0.60–0.80]).

Rivaroxaban (20 mg once daily) has been compared to warfarin in 14 264 patients (median age 73, mean $CHADS_2$ score = 3.5) in AF at a higher risk of stroke ($CHADS_2$ score 2 or more) with a primary outcome of stroke (ischaemic or haemorrhagic) or systemic embolism (mean follow up 1.9 years).[35] The study found similar rates of the primary outcome per year with rivaroxaban compared to warfarin (1.7% vs 2.2% [HR 0.79, 95% CI 0.66–0.96]) and major bleeding (3.6% vs 3.4% [HR 1.04, 95% CI 0.90–0.120]), but a lower annual rate of haemorrhagic stroke (0.5% vs 0.7% [HR 0.67, 95% CI 0.47–0.93]).

In the above three studies the mean time patients spent in the correct therapeutic window for those on warfarin (INR 2.0 to 3.0) was 55–66%. This figure does not sound very impressive but is likely to reflect real world experience with this drug. A comparison analysis has found that apixaban, dabigatran and rivaroxaban, when used to prevent stroke for patients in AF, appear to have broadly similar outcomes and adverse event rates.[36] If a patient is already established on warfarin and INR values are stable, there may be little to gain from switching to a novel anticoagulant.

Aspirin

Aspirin is less effective than warfarin in reducing the risk of thromboembolism in AF. The size of any benefit is unclear as results of clinical trials have been conflicting. The Stroke Prevention in AF I study found a 42% relative risk reduction with the daily use of 325 mg of aspirin compared to placebo (absolute risks 3.6% vs 6.3% per year).[37] Another study failed to demonstrate a significant benefit in reducing thromboembolic complications with 75 mg of aspirin compared to placebo in 672 people.[38] An analysis of multiple trials concluded that aspirin resulted in approximately a 20% reduction in stroke risk.[4] However, this reduction may simply reflect a reduction in non-thromboembolic strokes. A more recent Japanese study (871 patients, mean age 65, aspirin 150–200 mg daily) has suggested that aspirin may be no more effective than placebo but increase the risk of bleeding complications.[39] Given that a higher proportion of older people have AF, and thus a probable cardioembolic source of stroke, it is perhaps no surprise that aspirin seems to be less beneficial in this age group.[5] As a result of this data, guidelines are tending to move away from aspirin and instead recommend nothing for patients at low risk of stroke (e.g. younger patients with lone AF).[8]

Clopidogrel

The combination of aspirin (75–100 mg) and clopidogrel (75 mg) has been compared to warfarin (INR 2–3) for the prevention of thromboembolic events in patients with AF.[40] In 6706 patients (mean age 70 years) with AF and a least one other risk factor for stroke who were randomised, it was found that both the risk of stroke (RR 1.44, 95% CI 1.18–1.76) and the risk of bleeding complications (RR 1.21, 95% CI 1.08–1.35) were higher in the aspirin and clopidogrel arm (the mean follow-up was 1.28 years). Therefore, warfarin remains the better option.

A further component of this study compared aspirin to aspirin plus clopidogrel in 7554 patients (mean age 71 years) in AF but deemed unsuitable for warfarin.[41] The combined therapy was associated with a lower risk of stroke (2.4% vs 3.3% per year; RR 0.72, 95% CI 0.62–0.83), but this was offset by an increased risk of major haemorrhage (2.0% vs 1.3% per year; RR 1.57, 95% CI 1.29–1.92).

RHYTHM CONTROL

Cardioversion

Reversion of AF back into sinus rhythm is often possible with either DC cardioversion or medications (e.g. flecainide).[2] It is usually not performed in elderly people with reasonable rate control due to the high chance of relapse to AF following the procedure (anticoagulation should be continued). A longer duration of AF and the presence of left atrial enlargement also make the procedure less likely to be effective.[42] When studies have compared outcomes in patients randomly assigned to either a strategy of sinus rhythm restoration or rate control alone, attempts at rhythm control did not appear to offer any long-term benefit.[43,44]

Catheter ablation

Thermal energy (e.g. by radiofrequency) can be used to ablate an area around the pulmonary veins to stop the occurrence of AF. This is achieved by passing a specialised catheter, via a vein, through the intra-atrial septum and into the left atrium.[45] A review of available evidence has suggested that the technique may be more effective at maintaining sinus rhythm than drugs in people who have previously failed medical management.[46] However, the duration of follow-up has typically been 12 months or less, and few studies have recruited older adults. Significant adverse events appear to occur in less than 5% of patients. As the technique is refined it may become more commonly used in practice.

RATE CONTROL

The ideal target for heart rate control is unknown. However, it may not be as low as traditionally thought. A trial compared strict rate control in AF (<80 bpm) to a more lenient regime (<110 bpm).[47] Over a three-year period the average heart rates in the groups were around 75 bpm and 85 bpm respectively. It was easier to achieve target rates in the more lenient group and outcomes were more favourable (serious adverse events in 12.9% compared to 14.9% in the strict group).

Pacemakers

When AF is associated with episodes of very fast and very slow heart rate (the tachycardia–bradycardia syndrome), it is best treated with a combination of pacemaker insertion and the use of rate-slowing drugs. Pacemakers should also be considered in the presence of prolonged and symptomatic pauses (e.g. >3 seconds).

Beta-blockers

Beta-blockers may be used to slow ventricular rate and may prevent episodes of arrhythmia in those with PAF.[48] Sotalol is a beta-blocker that also has some class III anti-arrhythmic activity. In trials it has not proven to be more effective than standard beta-blockers.[48] It is associated with a stronger pro-arrhythmogenic tendency, especially in those with underlying heart disease. It is, therefore, best avoided in the elderly.

Digoxin

Digoxin does not result in an increased rate of reversion to sinus rhythm,[49] nor does it control the rate of AF during exertion,[21] or during episodes of AF in those with PAF.[49] It has a smaller rate-limiting effect than most alternative agents. In a randomised controlled trial that compared intravenous digoxin to placebo, digoxin did not cause cardioversion but did result in a small, significant reduction in heart rate apparent after two hours (heart rate 105 per minute vs 117 per minute with placebo).[50] However, it has been associated with a higher risk of death in people with AF.[51] Older people are also at an increased risk of digoxin toxicity (causing nausea, vomiting, confusion, visual disturbances and cardiac arrhythmias) than younger people due to declines in renal function. Given its limited efficacy and potential toxicity in older adults, it is rarely a suitable drug to use.

Amiodarone

Amiodarone is a highly lipophilic compound and a large loading dose is required to maintain plasma drug levels. It is traditionally described as a Vaughan–Williams class III agent but also has some class I and II activity. It has been demonstrated to have the capacity to convert AF to sinus rhythm (SR), can maintain SR in PAF and can control rate in sustained AF.[52] In comparison to sotalol and various class I drugs it has been found to be superior in maintaining SR.[53] It also appears to be more effective than beta-blockers in preventing the onset of AF in high risk patients.[54]

Along with the potential to induce life-threatening arrhythmias, there are a number of severe adverse reactions associated with amiodarone use – *see* Table 19.3.[55] The most common of these is hypothyroidism, which can be treated simply by hormone replacement. Hyperthyroidism is less common but far harder to treat.[56] Pulmonary infiltrates may occur more commonly after prolonged drug exposure.

TABLE 19.3 Annual incidence of severe adverse reactions to amiodarone

Reaction	Annual incidence (%)
Hypothyroidism	5.9
Pulmonary infiltrates	1.1
Hyperthyroidism	0.9
Hepatic dysfunction	0.6
Peripheral neuropathy	0.3

Calcium channel antagonists

Diltiazem and verapamil may have a role in the slowing of heart rate in some patients who are intolerant to, or inadequately controlled by, alternative agents. They are best avoided in those with heart failure. Verapamil cannot be used in combination with beta-blockers.

REFERENCES

1 Feinberg WM, Blackshear JL, Laupacis A, *et al.* Prevalence, age distribution, and gender of patients with atrial fibrillation: analysis and implications. *Arch Intern Med*, 1995; **155**: 469–73.

2 Peters NS, Schilling RJ, Kanagaratnam P, *et al.* Atrial fibrillation: strategies to control, combat, and cure. *Lancet*, 2002; **359**: 593–603.

3 Mitchell GF, Vasan RS, Keyes MJ, *et al.* Pulse pressure and risk of new-onset atrial fibrillation. *JAMA*, 2007; **297**(7): 709–15.

4 Hart RG, Halperin JL, Pearce LA. Lessons from the *Stroke*, Prevention in Atrial Fibrillation trials. *Ann Intern Med*, 2003; **138**(10): 831–8.

5 van Walraven C, Hart RG, Connolly S, *et al.* Effect of age on stroke prevention therapy in patients with atrial fibrillation: the Atrial Fibrillation Investigators. *Stroke*, 2009; **40**: 1410–16.

6 Gage BF, Waterman AD, Shannon W, *et al.* Validation of clinical classification schemes for predicting stroke: results from the national registry of atrial fibrillation. *JAMA*, 2001; **285**(22): 2864–70.

7 Pamukcu B, Lip GYH, Lane DA. Simplifying stroke risk stratification in atrial fibrillation patients: implications of the CHA_2DS_2–VASc risk stratification scores. *Age Ageing*, 2010; **39**: 533–5.

8 The Task Force for the Management of Atrial Fibrillation of the European Society of Cardiology. Guidelines for the management of atrial fibrillation. *European Heart J*, 2010; **31**: 2369–429.

9 Lane DA, Lip GYH. Use of the CHA2DS2-VASc and HAS-BLED scores to aid decision making for thromboprophylaxis in nonvalvular atrial fibrillation. *Circulation*, 2012; **126**: 860–5.

10 Wolf PA, Abbott RD, Kannel WB. Atrial fibrillation: a major contributor to stroke in the elderly: the Framingham study. *Arch Intern Med*, 1987; **147**: 1561–4.

11 Sudlow M, Thompson R, Thwaites B, *et al.* Prevalence of atrial fibrillation and eligibility for anticoagulants in the community. *Lancet*, 1998; **352**: 1167–71.

12 Atrial Fibrillation Investigators, *et al.* Risk factors for stroke and efficacy of antithrombotic therapy in atrial fibrillation: analysis of pooled data from five randomized controlled trials. *Arch Intern Med*, 1994; **154**: 1449–57.

13 Kalra L, Yu G, Perez I, *et al.* Prospective cohort study to determine if trial efficacy of anticoagulation for stroke prevention in atrial fibrillation translates into clinical effectiveness. *BMJ*, 2000; **320**: 1236–9.

14 Man-Son-Hing M, Laupacis A. Anticoagulant-related bleeding in older persons with atrial fibrillation: physicians' fears often unfounded. *Arch Intern Med*, 2003; **163**: 1580–6.

15 Man-Son-Hing M, Nichol G, Lau A, *et al.* Choosing antithrombotic therapy for elderly patients with atrial fibrillation who are at risk for falls. *Arch Intern Med*, 1999; **159**: 677–85.

16 Bungard TJ, Ghali WA, Teo KK, *et al.* Why do patients with atrial fibrillation not receive warfarin? *Arch Intern Med*, 2000; **160**: 41–6.

17 Choudhry NK, Anderson GM, Laupacis A, *et al.* Impact of adverse events on prescribing warfarin in patients with atrial fibrillation: matched pair analysis. *BMJ*, 2006; **332**: 141–3.

18 Gurwitz JH, Avorn J, Ross-Degnan D, *et al.* Aging and the anticoagulant response to warfarin therapy. *Ann Intern Med*, 1992; **116**: 901–4.

19 Fennerty A, Dolben J, Thomas P, *et al.* Flexible induction dose regimen for warfarin and prediction of maintenance dose. *BMJ*, 1984; **288**: 1268–70.

20 Harrison L, Johnston M, Massicotte MP, *et al.* Comparison of 5-mg and 10-mg loading doses in initiation of warfarin therapy. *Ann Intern Med*, 1997; **126**(2): 133–6.

21 Gage BF, Fihn SD, White RH. Warfarin therapy for an octogenarian who has atrial fibrillation. *Ann Intern Med*, 2001; **134**(6): 465–74.

22 Landefeld CS, Goldman L. Major bleeding in outpatients treated with warfarin: incidence and prediction by factors known at the start of outpatient therapy. *Am J Med*, 1989; **87**: 144–52.

23 Fihn SD, McDonell M, Martin D, *et al.* Risk factors for complications of chronic anticoagulation: a multicenter study. *Ann Intern Med*, 1993; **118**: 511–20.

24 Landefeld CS, Rosenblatt MW, Goldman L. Bleeding in outpatients treated with warfarin: relation to the prothrombin time and important remediable lesions. *Am J Med*, 1989; **87**: 153–9.

25 Hylek EM, Singer DE. Risk factors for intracranial hemorrhage in outpatients taking warfarin. *Ann Intern Med*, 1994; **120**(11): 897–902.

26 Fihn SD, Callahan CM, Martin DC, *et al.* The risk for and severity of bleeding complications in elderly patients treated with warfarin. *Ann Intern Med*, 1996; **124**(11): 970–9.

27 Hart RG, Boop BS, Anderson DC. Oral anticoagulants and intracranial haemorrhage: facts and hypotheses. *Stroke*, 1995; **26**(8): 1471–7.

28 Johnson CE, Lim WK, Workman BS. People aged over 75 in atrial fibrillation on warfarin: the rate of major haemorrhage and stroke in more than 500 patient-years of follow-up. *J Am Geriatr Soc*, 2005; **53**: 655–9.

29 Mant J, Hobbs FD, Fletcher K, *et al.* Warfarin versus aspirin for stroke prevention in an elderly community population with atrial fibrillation (the Birmingham Atrial Fibrillation Treatment of the Aged Study, BAFTA): a randomised controlled trial. *Lancet*, 2007; **370**: 493–503.

30 Gurwitz JH, Field TS, Avorn J, *et al.* Incidence and preventability of adverse drug events in nursing homes. *Am J Med*, 2000; **109**: 87–94.

31 Gurwitz JH, Monette J, Rochon PA, *et al.* Atrial fibrillation and stroke prevention with warfarin in the long-term care setting. *Arch Intern Med*, 1997; **157**: 978–84.

32 Pisters R, Lane DA, Nieuwlaat R, *et al.* A novel user-friendly score (HAS-BLED) to assess 1-year risk of major bleeding in patients with atrial fibrillation: the Euro Heart Survey. *Chest*, 2010; **138**: 1093–100.

33 Connolly SJ, Ezekowitz MD, Yusuf S, *et al.* Dabigatran versus warfarin in patients with atrial fibrillation. *N Engl J Med*, 2009; **361**: 1139–51.

34 Granger CB, Alexander JH, McMurray JJV, *et al.* Apixaban versus warfarin in patients with atrial fibrillation. *N Engl J Med*, 2011; **365**: 981–92.

35 Patel MR, Mahaffey KW, Garg J, *et al.* Rivaroxaban versus warfarin in nonvalvular atrial fibrillation. *N Engl J Med*, 2011; **365**: 883–91.

36 Rasmussen LH, Larsen TB, Graungaard T, *et al.* Primary and secondary prevention with new oral anticoagulant drugs for stroke prevention in atrial fibrillation: indirect comparison analysis. *BMJ*, 2012; **345**: e7097.

37 Stroke Prevention in Atrial Fibrillation Investigators. Stroke Prevention in Atrial Fibrillation Study: final results. *Circulation*, 1991; **84**: 527–39.

38 Petersen P, Boysen G, Godtfredsen J, *et al.* Placebo-controlled, randomised trial of warfarin and aspirin for prevention of thromboembolic complications in chronic atrial fibrillation. *Lancet*, 1989; **1**: 175–9.

39 Sato H, Ishikawa K, Kitabatake A, *et al.* Low-dose aspirin for prevention of stroke in low-risk patients with atrial fibrillation: Japan Atrial Fibrillation Stroke Trial. *Stroke*, 2006; **37**: 447–51.

40 ACTIVE Writing Group. Clopidogrel plus aspirin versus oral anticoagulation for atrial fibrillation in the Atrial fibrillation Clopidogrel Trial with Irbesartan for prevention of Vascular Events (ACTIVE W): a randomised controlled trial. *Lancet*, 2006; **367**(9526): 1903–12.

41 ACTIVE Investigators. Effect of clopidogrel added to aspirin in patients with atrial fibrillation. *N Engl J Med*, 2009; **360**(20): 2066–78.

42 Channer KS. Current management of symptomatic atrial fibrillation. *Drugs*, 2001; **61**(10): 1425–37.

43 Page RL. Newly diagnosed atrial fibrillation. *N Engl J Med*, 2004; **351**(23): 2408–16.

44 Roy R, Talajic M, Nattel S, *et al.* Rhythm control versus rate control for atrial fibrillation and heart failure. *N Engl J Med*, 2008; **358**(25): 2667–77.

45 Lubitz SA, Fischer A, Fuster V. Catheter ablation for atrial fibrillation. *BMJ*, 2008; **336**: 819–26.

46 Terasawa T, Balk EM, Chung M, *et al.* Systematic review: comparative effectiveness of radiofrequency catheter ablation for atrial fibrillation. *Ann Intern Med*, 2009; **151**(3): 191–202.

47 Van Gelder IC, Groenveld HF, Crijns HJGM, *et al.* Lenient versus strict rate control in patients with atrial fibrillation. *N Engl J Med*, 2010; **362**: 1363–73.

48 Steeds RP, Birchall AS, Smith A, *et al.* An open label, randomised, crossover study comparing sotalol and atenolol in the treatment of symptomatic paroxysmal atrial fibrillation. *Heart*, 1999; **82**(2): 170–5.

49 Robles de Medina EO, Algra A. Digoxin in the treatment of paroxysmal atrial fibrillation. *Lancet*, 1999; **354**: 882–3.

50 The Digitalis in Acute Atrial Fibrillation (DAAF) Trial Group. Intravenous digoxin in acute atrial fibrillation: results of a randomized, placebo-controlled multicentre trial of 239 patients. *Eur Heart J*, 1997; **18**: 649–54.

51 Whitbeck MG, Charnigo RJ, Khairy P, *et al.* Increased mortality among patients taking digoxin: analysis from the AFFIRM study. *Eur Heart J*, 2013; **34**: 1481–8.

52 Connolly SJ. Evidence-based analysis of amiodarone efficacy and safety. *Circulation*, 1999; **100**: 2025–34.

53 The AFFIRM First Antiarrhythmic Drug Study Investigators. Maintenance of sinus rhythm in patients with atrial fibrillation: an AFFIRM study of the first antiarrhythmic drug. *J Am Coll Cardiol*, 2003; **42**: 20–9.

54 Solomon AJ, Greenberg MD, Kilborn MJ, *et al*. Amiodarone versus a beta-blocker to prevent atrial fibrillation after cardiovascular surgery. *Am Heart J*, 2001; **142**(5): 811–15.

55 Amiodarone Trials Meta-analysis Investigators. Effect of prophylactic amiodarone on mortality after acute myocardial infarction and in congestive heart failure: meta-analysis of individual data from 6500 patients in randomised trials. *Lancet*, 1997; **350**: 1417–24.

56 Newman CM, Price A, Davies DW, *et al*. Amiodarone and the thyroid: a practical guide to the management of thyroid dysfunction induced by amiodarone therapy. *Heart*, 1998; **79**: 121–7.

QUESTIONS FOR PART E

1 An 84-year-old lady has a history of high blood pressure, for which she takes ben-droflumethiazide 2.5 mg and amlodipine 5 mg once daily. Her BP is recorded as 171/92 mmHg. Examination reveals an ejection systolic murmur and some swelling of her ankles but no other abnormalities. She last had an echocardiogram five months ago. This showed mild aortic stenosis (gradient 24 mmHg) and an ejection fraction of 42%. What would you do?
   A. Repeat the echocardiogram
   B. Refer for valve surgery
   C. Increase the dose of bendroflumethiazide and amlodipine
   D. Add a loop diuretic
   E. Stop amlodipine and start an ACE inhibitor

2 Which of the following statements regarding atrial fibrillation (AF) in older adults is most likely to be correct?
   A. It has a prevalence of approximately 10% in people aged over 80
   B. AF is associated with approximately 10% of strokes in people over the age of 80
   C. Older patients treated with warfarin are more likely to have a haemorrhagic, rather than ischaemic, stroke
   D. Only two-thirds of people without contraindications currently receive warfarin
   E. A combination of aspirin and clopidogrel is less effective at reducing stroke risk, but is associated with less bleeding complications

3 An independent 81-year-old man is found to have a systolic blood pressure in the range of 150–160 mmHg, and a diastolic blood pressure of 65–75 mmHg on three separate occasions. He has no past history of disease and takes no regular medications. His ECG shows evidence of left ventricular hypertrophy. Which of the following statements is most correct?
   A. Blood pressure-lowering treatment would significantly reduce his risk of future heart failure
   B. The side-effects of blood pressure-lowering medications are likely to outweigh their benefits
   C. His pulse wave velocity is likely to be reduced
   D. He is likely to have white coat hypertension
   E. His blood pressure should simply be repeated in three months' time

4 Regarding diastolic heart failure in the elderly, which statement is most likely to be correct?
   A. It is present in a third of people over the age of 65 with heart failure
   B. It has a better prognosis than systolic heart failure
   C. ACE inhibitors are contraindicated
   D. It rarely causes pulmonary oedema
   E. Beta-blockers are typically recommended

5 The risk of intracerebral bleeding while on warfarin is most likely to be increased by which of the following factors?
  A. History of falls
  B. Unstable INR readings
  C. Advanced age
  D. After a long duration of warfarin therapy
  E. History of previous gastric ulcer

6 Which of the following medications is *least* associated with an increased survival rate in older adults with congestive cardiac failure?
  A. Digoxin
  B. ACE inhibitors
  C. Beta-blockers
  D. Spironolactone
  E. Angiotensin type II receptor blockers

7 Which of the following statements regarding blood pressure in the elderly is most likely to be correct?
  A. In normal individuals blood pressure does not alter significantly between day and night
  B. White coat hypertension is less common in older than younger people
  C. Treatment of hypertension is less beneficial in older than younger people
  D. Thiazide diuretics are less likely to cause orthostatic hypotension than ACE inhibitors
  E. Calcium channel blockers are more effective at controlling blood pressure than beta-blockers

8 A 73-year-old woman presents with a new onset of atrial fibrillation. She has no significant past medical history and takes no regular medications. She lives alone and is fully independent. Her pulse rate is 116 beats per minute and her blood pressure 138/76 mmHg. She has mild ankle oedema and some fine bibasal chest crackles. Which of the following treatment options is most likely to provide long-term benefit?
  A. DC cardioversion
  B. Digoxin
  C. A beta-blocker
  D. Flecainide
  E. Amiodarone

9 A 67-year-old woman presents with atrial fibrillation. Her blood pressure is recorded as 124/73 mmHg. She has no significant past medical history and examination is otherwise normal. She is concerned about potential side-effects of any medications. Which treatment option should you recommend to prevent future stroke and minimise bleeding risks?
  A. Aspirin
  B. Aspirin + clopidogrel
  C. Aspirin + dipyridamole
  D. Warfarin
  E. Dabigatran

10 A 78-year-old woman was referred with hypertension. She also had gout and osteoarthritis. Her current medications were candesartan, atenolol, paracetamol, and calcium
and vitamin D. She was intolerant of many medications, such as amlodipine, perindopril
and allopurinol. On examination, her blood pressure was 179/95 mmHg. Her investigation results were as below.

Haemoglobin	146 g/L	(normal range 115–165)
Serum sodium	137 mmol/L	(137–144)
Serum potassium	4.8 mmol/L	(3.5–4.9)
Serum creatinine	71 µmol/L	(60–110)
Urinalysis	normal	
Electrocardiogram	sinus rhythm	
Chest X-ray	normal	

What is the most appropriate next investigation?
A. Ambulatory blood pressure monitoring
B. Echocardiogram
C. Renal tract ultrasound
D. 24-hour urinary catecholamines
E. 24-hour urinary cortisol

11 A 76-year-old woman has a past history of hypertension and sustained a stroke three
years ago. Despite this she is independent in her daily activities. Her current medications
are clopidogrel 75 mg od, bendroflumethiazide 2.5 mg od and atorvastatin 80 mg nocte.
Her last three blood pressure readings have been 136/75, 138/79 and 135/78 mmHg.
Her blood tests are as below.

Haemoglobin	123 g/L	(normal range 115–165)
Serum sodium	139 mmol/L	(137–144)
Serum potassium	4.1 mmol/L	(3.5–4.9)
Serum urea	8.4 mmol/L	(2.5–7.8)
Serum creatinine	109 µmol/L	(60–110)
Serum glucose	5.6 mmol/L	

According to current UK guidelines, what is the most appropriate course of
action?
A. Continue current medication
B. Change thiazide to an ACE inhibitor
C. Add a calcium channel blocker
D. Add an ACE inhibitor
E. Add a beta-blocker

12 A 74-year-old man is found to be in atrial fibrillation. He has a past medical history of hypertension, type 2 diabetes and a stroke five years ago. What is his CHA_2DS_2-VASc score?
   A. 1
   B. 2
   C. 3
   D. 4
   E. 5

13 Which of the following statements is most likely to be correct regarding frail elderly patients with atrial fibrillation?
   A. Successful cardioversion removes the need to anticoagulate
   B. Controlling heart rate to an average below 80 beats per minute improves symptom control
   C. Digoxin reduces hospitalisation rates
   D. Novel anticoagulants are contraindicated
   E. Aspirin is less effective at reducing stroke risk compared to younger people

14 Current NICE guidelines recommend a target blood pressure of below which value for people aged over 80 years?
   A. 130/80 mmHg
   B. 130/85 mmHg
   C. 140/85 mmHg
   D. 150/90 mmHg
   E. 160/90 mmHg

15 Which of the following medications is *least* likely to precipitate peripheral oedema in an elderly person?
   A. Amlodipine
   B. Ibuprofen
   C. Pioglitazone
   D. Ropinirole
   E. Quetiapine

16 Which of the following echocardiographic features is most likely to be detected in people with a diagnosis of diastolic heart failure (or 'heart failure with preserved ejection fraction')?
   A. Ejection fraction more than 80%
   B. Left ventricular dilatation
   C. Right atrial enlargement
   D. Left ventricular hypertrophy
   E. Constrictive pericarditis

17 A 73-year-old-man is seen in a stroke review clinic. He had a left lacunar stroke six months earlier but has made a good functional recovery and is independent in his daily activities. He has been found to have an average daily blood pressure of 142/85 mmHg on 24-hour blood pressure monitoring. He currently takes chlorthalidone 25 mg od, amlodipine 10 mg od and lisinopril 20 mg od for his blood pressure. His blood tests are as below.

Sodium	139 mmol/L	(137–144)
Potassium	4.3 mmol/L	(3.5–4.9)
Urea	5.1 mmol/L	(2.5–7.8)
Creatinine	78 µmol/L	(60–110)

Which of the following medication changes would be most appropriate?
A. Add spironolactone 25 mg daily
B. Increase chlorthalidone dose to 50 mg daily
C. Add irbesartan 75 mg daily
D. Add doxazosin modified release 4 mg daily
E. No change

18 A 71-year-old woman is found to have atrial fibrillation. She has a past history of hypertension and type 2 diabetes but has no other known health problems. According to her CHA_2DS_2-VASc score, which of the following is the best estimate of her risk of stroke over the following year while not taking anticoagulant or anti-platelet medications?
A. 2%
B. 4%
C. 7%
D. 10%
E. 15%

PART F

Selected topics

This section includes a mix of clinical topics that are of particular importance to older adults. Key aspects are briefly reviewed. The topics covered are as listed below:

➤ Anaemia
➤ Arthritis
➤ Chronic obstructive pulmonary disease
➤ Epilepsy
➤ Influenza
➤ Leg ulcers
➤ Methicillin resistant *Staphylococcus aureus*
➤ Motor neuron disease
➤ Myopathy
➤ Pneumonia
➤ Pressure ulcers
➤ Type 2 diabetes

ANAEMIA

The development of anaemia is not a normal component of healthy ageing. Anaemia is traditionally defined according to World Health Organization (WHO) criteria of a haemoglobin (Hb) level <130 g/L in men and <120 g/L in women. Using these criteria it has been estimated to have an overall prevalence of 11–17% in people over the age of 65, possibly rising to 40% of this age group who are admitted to hospital.[1–3] Its prevalence rises with age from 8% of those aged 65 to 74, 13% of those aged 75 to 84, and 23% of those aged 85 and over.[1] However, most of this anaemia is mild. Less than 1% of older adults have an Hb <100 g/L.[1] The association of anaemia with ageing may be partly due to declining renal function or testosterone levels. It may be another marker of frailty. However, anaemia is associated with worse outcomes, which include functional decline, falls and cognitive impairment.[4–7] It is unknown whether anaemia plays a causative role or is simply a bystander in these processes. Even a mild anaemia may indicate a serious underlying disorder. It is important to look for treatable causes.

Iron deficiency anaemia

Iron deficiency anaemia (IDA) constitutes around 17–20% of anaemia in community-dwelling over sixty-fives.[1] It is associated with red blood cell microcytosis (mean cell volume (MCV) <80 fL), which may also be seen in anaemia of chronic disease, sideroblastic anaemia and haemoglobin disorders (e.g. thalassaemia). It may present with normocytosis when coupled with deficiency in folate or B_{12}. In addition to microcytosis, a low ferritin, serum iron, and transferrin saturation ratio, and a raised total iron binding capacity all suggest IDA. Of these additional tests, a serum ferritin level is most often helpful. A ferritin level <12 mcg/dL always indicates iron deficiency, but a level of 12–45 mcg/dL is also suggestive.[8] Ferritin levels may be in the normal range if an inflammatory process is also present. Bone marrow examination would reveal decreased bodily iron stores.

Unless an alternative source of blood loss is present, IDA usually indicates bleeding into the gastrointestinal (GI) tract. A study that performed upper and lower GI endoscopy on 100 patients (mean age 60 years, range 20 to 85) with IDA found causative lesions in 62, with 36 being in the upper GI tract (peptic ulceration being most frequent in 19 (51%)) and 25 being in the lower GI tract (colonic cancer being most frequent in 11 (42%)).[9] A study in older people with IDA found that upper GI endoscopy revealed a potentially causative lesion in 49%, and lower GI endoscopy a potentially causative lesion in 32%.[10] Colonoscopy is usually well tolerated in older adults and more likely to reveal significant pathology compared to when performed in younger people.[11]

Iron supplementation is the usual treatment and should be continued for three months to ensure adequate replacement of body iron stores. Blood transfusion is rarely necessary in asymptomatic patients with a haemoglobin concentration above 8 g/dL.

B_{12} and folate deficiency

B_{12} and folate deficiency each contribute to 8–10% of anaemias in the over sixty-fives.[1] They are associated with macrocytosis (MCV >100 fL). There may also be associated leucopaenia and thrombocytopaenia. Severe deficiency may lead to neuropsychiatric symptoms. Blood levels for these vitamins should be established. Alcoholism and hypothyroidism should be excluded.

B_{12} deficiency may be caused by reduced gastric intrinsic factor secretion (e.g. partial gastrectomy or atrophic gastritis), depletion due to bacterial overgrowth (*see* p. 305), or malabsorption (e.g. pancreatic insufficiency or ileal resection). Atrophic gastritis can be secondary to chronic *Helicobacter pylori* infection or autoimmune in aetiology. Autoimmune causation (i.e. pernicious anaemia) is associated with antiparietal cell or anti-intrinsic factor antibodies in the serum. Dietary insufficiency of B_{12} is very uncommon (occasionally in vegans). Absorption of B_{12} may be reduced by metformin. In a series of 172 older adults (mean age 76 years) with B_{12} deficiency who underwent extensive testing, just 33% was due to pernicious anaemia.[12]

Folate deficiency may be due to dietary insufficiency, coeliac disease (*see* p. 304), high cell turnover states (e.g. malignancy) or drugs (e.g. phenytoin and methotrexate).

Renal impairment

Chronic renal impairment is associated with lower secretion of erythropoietin, this may lead to a normocytic or mildly microcytic anaemia. Studies have suggested an increased risk of anaemia once glomerular filtration rate (GFR) falls below 60 mL/min per 1.73 m^2, especially once below 30 mL/min per 1.73 m^2.[2,13] Using a definition of GFR <30 mL/min per 1.73 m^2 it has been deemed to be responsible for around 8–12% of anaemia in the over sixty-fives.[1]

Anaemia of chronic disease

Anaemia of chronic disease (ACD) is also referred to as anaemia of chronic inflammation. Typically it occurs in people with chronic infectious, inflammatory or neoplastic conditions. It accounts for around 20–24% of anaemia in the over sixty-fives.[1] It is associated with elevated levels of ferritin and ESR. The serum iron concentration is low, but body iron stores are normal (detected by bone marrow examination). A cytokine-induced impairment of iron mobilisation is believe to play a causal role.[14] MCV values may be normal or mildly microcytic (i.e. 70–80 fL).

Other causes of anaemia

One series found that 'unexplained' anaemia accounted for around 34% of anaemia in the over sixty-fives.[1] Most of these people had an Hb >110 g/L (88%), and few were below 100 g/L (1%). Features consistent with myelodysplasia (i.e. raised MCV, low white cell or platelet count) were present in 17% of these people. It is caused by ineffective haematopoiesis. Appearances of the peripheral blood film or bone marrow specimen may aid diagnosis. Additional possible contributors could include moderate renal impairment (e.g. GFR between 30 and 60 mL/min per 1.73 m^2) or an age-related decline in bone marrow function. Other causes of anaemia are rare in old age. Haemolytic anaemia can occasionally be caused by adverse drug reactions (e.g. penicillins, cephalosporins, NSAIDs, methyldopa, levodopa or quinine). It is associated with a positive direct Coombs' test, raised reticulocyte count and low haptoglobin levels (which binds free haemoglobin). It may only present after several months of drug exposure.

ARTHRITIS

Osteoarthritis

Osteoarthritis (OA) accounts for around two-thirds of joint diseases.[15] Age is the most important risk factor, but congenital abnormalities, obesity and previous trauma all increase the probability of its development. In people aged over 60 years the prevalence of hip OA is around 7%, and knee OA around 12%.[16] Pathologic changes include loss of cartilage, osteophyte formation plus bone sclerosis and cyst formation around joint margins. Its key clinical manifestation is pain. Typically ESR levels are not elevated. X-rays demonstrate the classic pathological changes.

Non-pharmacological interventions include physiotherapy, weight reduction and increased exercise.[17] NSAIDs are often used in younger patients, but carry a high risk of toxicity in older adults (including gastric bleeding, renal impairment, hypertension and heart failure). Cyclooxygenase 2 (COX-2) inhibitors may be less prone to causing gastric bleeding, but have all the other risks of harm plus a possible increase in cardiac ischaemic events. For these reasons all NSAIDs should be avoided in older adults unless absolutely necessary. Paracetamol (acetaminophen) and weak opioids are safer options for analgesia.

Joint replacement surgery may be considered in those who have significant disability despite other therapeutic measures. In a cohort of older adults (mean age 75 years) with severe OA who underwent hip or knee replacement, postoperative complications occurred in 17% (none fatal), median time to independent walking was 12 days, and surgery was associated with significant symptomatic benefits at 12 months.[18]

Rheumatoid arthritis

Rheumatoid arthritis (RA) is the commonest inflammatory arthropathy affecting older adults, and has a prevalence of around 2% in this age group.[19] The majority of these patients will have had an onset of their disease in earlier life. However, 10 to 20% of RA presents in patients over the age of 60 years. This later group is referred to as elderly onset rheumatoid arthritis (EORA). When compared to those with a younger onset, this group is less likely to develop rheumatoid nodules, and large proximal joints are more often affected (e.g. shoulder and knee). Whereas younger onset disease affects women two to three times more frequently than men, in EORA the gender distribution is approximately 1:1. Morning stiffness lasting over one hour is characteristic. Presentation may be with non-specific symptoms (e.g. weight loss and fatigue). It may be associated with sicca syndrome (dry eyes and mouth). The condition is autoimmune in aetiology and has some genetic linkage, being more concordant in monozygotic twins.

Rheumatoid factor (RF) is positive in around 66% of those with EORA, compared to 80–90% of those with younger onset disease.[20] It may also be weakly positive in a number of healthy older people. Anti-cyclic citrullinated peptide (anti-CCP) antibodies are an alternative diagnostic test. They are also present in around two-thirds of those with RA, but less common outside this condition.[20] ESR is characteristically elevated. The differential diagnosis includes polymyalgia rheumatica (*see* p. 437). Synovitis may be seen in the hands, usually affecting the wrists, proximal interphalangeal and metacarpal phalangeal joints. X-rays may show erosive changes (typically juxta-articular) and joint space narrowing.

Options for analgesia are as discussed for OA. The balance or risks and benefits of treatment with low dose steroids (e.g. prednisolone 5 mg per day or less) may make this a suitable option for disease control in some older adults. Alternatively, disease modifying anti-rheumatic drugs (DMARDs) that are used frequently in older adults include methotrexate, sulphasalazine and hydroxychloroquine. The role of tumour necrosis factor (TNF) antagonists in the elderly is not yet well defined. These drugs may carry an unacceptably high risk of side-effects including infections and tumours.

Gout and pseudogout

Gout is caused by the formation of monosodium urate crystals within joints – typically distally in the hands and feet. Pseudogout is caused by the deposition of calcium pyrophosphate crystals and tends to affect larger, more proximal joints such as the shoulder, wrist and knee. They typically present as an acute mono- or oligo- (affecting less than five joints) arthritis. The conditions can be distinguished by the appearance of the crystals under microscopic examination of aspirated synovial fluid.

Gout is more common in younger men than women, but affects women more frequently in older age.[21] In older age it is frequently associated with diuretic use. It can also be precipitated by declining renal function or myeloproliferative disorders, and is associated with obesity and hypertension. A diet high in red meat, seafood and alcohol (especially beer) make gout more likely. After a first attack of gout the majority of people will have a further attack within one year if untreated. Chronic gout is associated with the formation of tophi (collections of monosodium urate crystals usually on the fingers, toes or elbows). Serum urate levels are often, but not always, elevated. Pseudogout may occur secondary to a number of disorders. These include hypothyroidism, hyperparathyroidism, haemochromatosis and hypomagnesaemia. X-rays may reveal chondrocalcinosis, but this may also be seen in other conditions (e.g. OA). A definitive diagnosis of gout or pseudogout is made by finding the relevant crystals by synovial joint fluid aspiration.

Acute attacks of either condition can be treated with steroids (oral or intra-articular), colchicine or NSAIDs. All of these are potentially harmful to older patients. In the longer term, the prevention of recurrence of gout is achieved by using urate-lowering therapy (e.g. allopurinol) and dietary modification.

CHRONIC OBSTRUCTIVE PULMONARY DISEASE

Chronic obstructive pulmonary disease (COPD) is a progressive disorder of irreversible, or only partially reversible, airflow limitation. It is defined on spirometry as having a forced expiratory volume in one second/forced vital capacity (FEV_1/FVC) ratio of <70% of the predicted value. Stage two COPD is said to occur when the FEV_1 is <80% of the predicted value. Pathological processes include chronic bronchitis and emphysematous changes. In the developed world it is almost always associated with smoking (rare causes include coal dust inhalation). There is some overlap with asthma in clinical features, and in some individuals the two conditions may coexist.

FEV_1 declines with age. FVC also declines, but to a lesser extent. This has led to concern that older patients with FEV_1/FVC ratios of just below 70% may be over-diagnosed with COPD. But evidence suggests that such patients are at a higher risk of COPD-related adverse events.[22] However, in those who have never smoked, 35% of healthy people over the age of 70 years, and 50% of those aged over 80, have been found to have an FEV_1/FVC of <70%.[23] Additionally, 18% of those over 80 years would be classified as having stage two COPD.

The disease typically has a pattern of slowly progressive decline in respiratory function, with superimposed acute exacerbations. These are often caused by infections with either bacteria (e.g. *H. influenzae*, *Ps. aeruginosa*, *Strep. pneumoniae*, *Moraxella catarrhalis*, *Mycoplasma*, or *Chlamydia pneumoniae*) or viruses (e.g. rhinoviruses, RSV, coronavirus, influenza, and parainfluenza).

Treatment

Smoking is also likely to increase the risk of exacerbations of COPD by causing increased mucous viscosity and bacterial adhesions. Patients who manage to stop smoking have a rate of lung function decline that is half that of continued smokers.[24] Therefore, discontinuing smoking is very important, even in older patients. Yet smoking cessation advice is rarely given to the elderly.[25]

Inhaled beta-agonists (e.g. salbutamol) lead to relaxation of the smooth muscles in the airway walls. Long-acting agents (e.g. salmeterol) may reduce the frequency of exacerbations. Inhaled anticholinergic drugs can also relax airway smooth muscle. They are poorly absorbed and so cause few systemic side-effects. However, a recent meta-analysis of studies comparing inhaled anticholinergics to placebo or other active drug found an increased rate of cardiovascular death, MI, or stroke in the anticholinergic treated group (1.8% vs 1.2%; RR 1.58, 95% CI 1.21–2.06).[26] This increased risk may only be justifiable if significant symptomatic benefits are found with this therapy alone. Oral theophylline has been used as a bronchodilator in COPD. It has a number of side-effects, including precipitating seizures and cardiac arrhythmias. Toxicity is increased in older adults, even at similar blood levels compared to younger individuals.

Steroids are generally less effective in COPD compared to asthma. However, their use in exacerbations is associated with a reduction in length of stay in hospital. Short-term response does not predict future response, and so trials of steroids to look for airway reversibility are unhelpful. Inhaled steroids have fewer side-effects than oral preparations. However, there will be some oropharyngeal deposition, which may result in local irritation, candidiasis, and some systemic absorption. A systematic review of trials of inhaled steroids in stable COPD did not show a benefit in reduced mortality.[27] Also, there was an increased risk of pneumonia in those on inhaled steroids (RR 1.34, 95% CI 1.03–1.75). A trial that compared inhaled fluticasone and salmeterol, alone or in combination, to placebo in 6112 patients (mean age 65 years) over a three-year period did not demonstrate a significant survival benefit.[28] However, the combined treatment did reduce the number of exacerbations and improved health status and spirometry values.

Older adults may have less benefit from inhaled medications due to poor inhaler technique. The commonest reason for this is poor timing of actuation and inhalation. Reduced mental function and weakness of the hands may also be factors. Dry powder devices may be helpful, as their use is not dependent on timing or muscle strength. In a study of older adults (mean age 74 years) with COPD, 46% reported finding their metered dose inhaler device difficult to use, and 17% found a dry powder device difficult to use.[29] Yet older people often do not have their inhaler technique checked. The use of spacer devices can result in increased intrapulmonary drug delivery, with reduced oropharyngeal deposition, leading to increased efficacy. However, older adults provided with spacer devices often do not use them.[29] A randomised trial found that older adults were more likely to use either breath-actuated aerosol devices or dry powder inhalers correctly than metered dose inhalers with spacers.[30]

Mucolytic agents (e.g. carbocisteine) may be of benefit if the production of large amounts of viscous sputum is a problem, but there is no randomised controlled trial evidence of a benefit in acute exacerbations. During severe exacerbations the use of non-invasive ventilation may be appropriate. Suitable patients typically have a rising pCO_2 and acidosis despite usual therapy. It can remove the need for intubation and reduce both mortality and length of stay. When used in older adults it appears to be similarly tolerated and similarly beneficial as to when used in younger adults.[31]

Long-term oxygen is associated with increased survival and quality of life in advanced COPD plus hypoxia (probably by reducing pulmonary artery pressure and increasing cardiac output). Pulmonary rehabilitation is beneficial in moderate to advanced disease; especially if there is evidence of deconditioning, weight loss, depression and social isolation. It can result in increased muscle mass and exercise tolerance, with reduced breathlessness. Effects in older people seem to be similar to those in younger age groups.[32]

EPILEPSY

The prevalence of epilepsy is highest in the elderly, having been diagnosed in around 0.8% of those over age 85 years.[33] Epilepsy can be idiopathic or secondary to underlying structural brain changes. In the elderly idiopathic epilepsy is rare. Seizures secondary to stroke account for 30–40% of cases.[34] Seizures occur in 10–20% of people with advanced dementia, and this represents 10–20% of epilepsies in older adults.[34,35] Tumours, subdural haematomas, drugs (e.g. antipsychotics, theophylline, baclofen or benzodiazepine withdrawal), alcohol or metabolic disturbances (e.g. hypoglycaemia or hyponatraemia) can also provoke seizures. Seizures can be partial (localised symptoms) or generalised (affecting most of the brain). Examples of generalised seizures include tonic-clonic episodes and absences. Partial seizures can be simple (no change in consciousness) or complex (altered consciousness). Partial seizures can also become secondarily generalised, e.g. focal symptoms followed by a tonic-clonic seizure. In older adults around 70% of seizures are of focal onset, with or without secondary generalisation.[36]

A major differential diagnosis is syncope (*see* p. 337). Features suggesting epilepsy include: onset not related to posture, onset while in bed at night, confusion following the event (>1 hour duration), and bites to the lateral tongue. A witness history is extremely valuable for assessment. Relevant blood tests, brain imaging (preferably

MRI) and an ECG should be performed.[37] Electroencephalography (EEG) is neither a sensitive nor specific test for diagnosing epilepsy in the elderly. It is only appropriate for use by specialists. Following a diagnosis, driving advice should be given to those who still drive.

Whether treatment should be started after a first seizure is unclear. It probably makes sense when an underlying pathology is present that makes recurrence more likely. Otherwise the decision may be guided by patient preference. They are likely to be on lifelong treatment.

Comparative treatment data in the elderly is limited. All medications are probably similarly effective.[36] The choice of drug is often mainly guided by potential side-effects. Drugs are usually started at low doses and gradually titrated upwards until seizures are controlled or unacceptable toxicity occurs. A study has compared carbamazepine to lamotrigine and gabapentin in 593 older patients (mean age 72 years) with a new diagnosis of epilepsy (most commonly secondary to stroke) over a 12-month period.[38] Seizure control was similar with all three drugs. Discontinuation due to side-effects was most common with carbamazepine (31%) compared to lamotrigine (12%) or gabapentin (22%).

Due to toxicity, especially sedation and cognitive impairment, phenobarbital is best avoided in the elderly. Phenytoin has zero order kinetics, which increases its risk of toxicity with small dose changes, which may lead to ataxia. It can also cause bone loss (anti-vitamin D effects) and megaloblastic anaemia (anti-folate effects). For these reasons it is no longer a drug of first choice. Lamotrigine's potential side-effects include rash, insomnia and tremor. Doses have to be slowly titrated upwards at two-week intervals. Sodium valproate may cause tremor, Parkinsonism and weight gain. Carbamazepine can cause a rash and hyponatraemia (secondary to SIADH). It is recommended that controlled release formulations of carbamazepine are used.[37] Gabapentin is associated with weight gain, tremor and ataxia.

Sodium valproate and lamotrigine are recommended as first-line drugs in the UK for the management of both partial and generalised epilepsy.[37,39] Despite evidence that some medications may be less appropriate for older adults, many remain on suboptimal therapeutic agents. In an American study it was found that 54% of elderly patients were taking phenytoin and 17% phenobarbital.[40]

Non-convulsive status epilepticus

Non-convulsive status epilepticus (NCSE) is a form of status epilepticus where there is minimal obvious seizure activity clinically, but evidence of its presence on EEG testing. It can result in a range of clinical presentations from mild confusion to coma.[41] It may have a fluctuating pattern and be difficult to distinguish from other causes of delirium. There may be a past history of epilepsy, but this is less commonly found in older people.[42] Women appear to be more commonly affected than men. Clues to the diagnosis include subtle rhythmical twitching or myoclonus of the eyelids, periorally or in the extremities. Automatisms can also be present. These are repetitive, unconscious, purposeless movement patterns. Examples include orofacial movements (e.g. lip smacking, chewing, yawning, grimacing or rapid blinking) and hand/arm movements (e.g. picking at clothes, rubbing or tapping).[43] A diagnosis should be supported by characteristic EEG appearances (ideally with resolution following treatment). However, there may be practical issues with obtaining timely EEG testing in all patients. Anti-epileptic drug administration (typically intravenous benzodiazepines) should result in an improvement in clinical condition in cases of NCSE.

INFLUENZA

Influenza is caused by an RNA virus of the orthomyxoviridae family. It is more likely to cause serious illness in older adults due to immune senescence and the high prevalence of comorbidities. It may spread rapidly in nursing home environments. Outbreaks are increased in the winter (typically between November and April in the northern hemisphere). It typically presents with a cough and fever, following a two-day incubation period. Death may result from secondary bacterial pneumonia (thought to be responsible for >90% of influenza-related deaths in the over sixty-fives). It affects around 5–20% of the population each year. The virus has two glycoproteins on its surface. These are haemagglutinin, which allows adhesion of the virus to respiratory epithelial cells and subsequent viral entry, and neuraminidase, which is an enzyme involved in the release of newly formed virions from the host cell (*see* Figure 20.1).

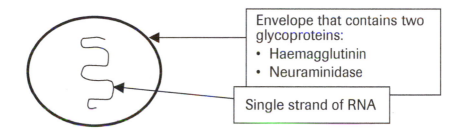

FIGURE 20.1 The structure of the influenza virus.

It has been identified in three types, called A, B and C, but only A and B are clinically important. They exist in numerous subtypes due to variations in haemagglutinin (H) and neuraminidase (N) proteins. The three subtypes that commonly affect humans are H1N1, H2N2 and H3N2. Seasonal variation in virus strains also occurs. 'Antigenic drift' causes minor change that results in annual epidemics, as the virus is able to avoid memory T cells and circulating antibodies. 'Antigenic shift' occurs following major change of the virus (i.e. recombination of RNA), which leads to pandemics. The virus rarely spreads beyond the respiratory tract. Bacterial infection typically occurs at five to seven days following initial symptoms – especially *Strep. pneumoniae*.

Viral culture takes three to five days. More rapid serological tests have been developed for diagnosis. Antiviral medications need to be commenced within 48 hours of symptoms to be effective. Barrier nursing may reduce spread of infection around hospitals or nursing homes.

Treatment

Neuraminidase inhibitors reduce the duration of symptoms by one to two days. No resistance has yet been reported. Oseltamivir is taken orally. Side-effects include nausea and vomiting. Zanamivir is an inhaled medication. It may cause bronchospasm and it is advised that it be avoided in people with COPD or asthma. Amantadine is an M2 channel inhibitor (also used in Parkinson's disease; *see* p. 165). A Cochrane review was unable to indentify any evidence of efficacy in the elderly.[44] It may cause confusion, hallucinations, and seizures (possibly by an anticholinergic action). It is not currently recommended in the treatment of influenza.

Influenza vaccine

Vaccination is potentially the most cost-effective approach. The vaccine is made of non-infectious particles. It may take four to six weeks for sufficient antibody response following administration. The effects last a few months and so it is typically given around October–November in the northern hemisphere. Age-related changes in immune function make vaccines less effective in older adults. Unfortunately most studies have possible bias due to their population design. Efficacy estimations are difficult. Influenza varies in both severity of outbreak and strain of virus between seasons. A Cochrane review of the efficacy of vaccinations for elderly people suggested only modest benefits for those in care homes and no benefit for those living in the community.[45] Another Cochrane review did not find convincing evidence that vaccinating healthcare workers would reduce influenza among nursing home residents.[46]

Influenza vaccination may reduce the risk of developing secondary bacterial pneumonia, but available data is inconclusive. A retrospective study looking at data from a large elderly (mean age 74 years) cohort over a 10-year period (over 700 000 person seasons of data) found that influenza vaccination was associated with a 27% reduction in the risk of hospitalisation for influenza or pneumonia (adjusted OR 0.73, 95% CI 0.68–0.77) and a 48% reduction in the risk of death (adjusted OR 0.52, 95% CI 0.50–0.55).[47] This latter figure appears to defy logic as other causes of death (e.g. cardiovascular disease) would be expected to be more prevalent. It is estimated that less than 10% of deaths each year are attributable to influenza.[48] A problem may be the lack of adjustment for confounding variables such as comorbidities that lead to bias (i.e. healthier people may be more likely get vaccinated).[49] In a study that did attempt to adjust for such factors in a cohort of people aged over 65, influenza vaccination was not associated with a significant reduction in risk of community-acquired pneumonia (OR 0.92, 95% CI 0.77–1.10).[50] So, the actual benefits of influenza vaccination in reducing pneumonia in the elderly remain unclear.

Current UK recommendations are for all people aged over 65 years to have an annual influenza immunisation.

LEG ULCERS

Leg ulcers are estimated to have a prevalence of 1–2% in the over sixty-fives.[51] The vast majority are caused by venous insufficiency, arterial, diabetic and mixed aetiologies.

Venous insufficiency

In around 70% of people with leg ulcers the mechanism includes increased venous blood pressure caused by incompetent venous valves, inadequate blood pumping due to reduced mobility, or occluded veins following venous thrombosis.[52] Venous incompetence may affect up to 10% of the population.[53] Venous ulcers are most commonly found around the ankle malleoli. Clinical examination may reveal signs of venous insufficiency: oedema and trophic skin changes (e.g. lipodermatosclerosis and hyperpigmentation). Lipodermatosclerosis is caused by fibrotic changes in the dermis and subcutaneous tissues and results in toughening of the skin that can lead to an 'inverted champagne bottle' appearance.[53] The hyperpigmentation is due to the leakage and subsequent breakdown of blood cells. This may stimulate melanin deposition, causing a brown colouration.[53] Treatment usually involves compression bandaging. As there is a risk of an arterial component, an ankle–brachial pressure index (ABPI) should be performed prior to bandaging. This test compares the standard blood pressure (BP) measured at the arm to the pressure at the ankle. The lower the figure, the more likely that arterial insufficiency is a factor. A value of 0.8 or above should be obtained if compression bandaging is to be applied.

Pressure bandaging has been shown to increase healing rates compared to no compression in clinical trials.[54] The amount of pressure that should be exerted by the treating bandages has been an area of uncertainty. In a trial comparing elasticated (higher pressure) with unelasticated (lower pressure) bandages in 112 people with venous leg ulcers failed to demonstrate any significant difference in efficacy or adverse events.[52] Approximately 60% of ulcers had healed at six months in both groups. Large ulcers heal more slowly than small ones.

Simple measures to treat ulceration and prevent recurrence include leg elevation, improved mobility and nutrition, and reductions in obesity.[55] Antibiotics are necessary only when the lesions become infected. Likely organisms are *Staphylococcus aureus*, *Pseudomonas aeruginosa* and beta-haemolytic streptococci.[53] Surgical debridement may be appropriate in certain circumstances. This is most often undertaken when there are signs of infection.[56] The removal of the dead tissue is thought to increase the chance of wound granulation and reduce infection risk. Removed tissues can be sent for culture. For large ulcers that fail to heal, skin grafting has been tried. There is some evidence that, in combination with compression bandaging, this can improve healing rates.[57]

Larval therapy is an old technique of debridement that has been reintroduced recently. Sterile fly maggots are now commercially available. The larvae are placed onto the wound and covered in a dressing. Their use has been evaluated in both leg and pressure ulcers (*see* later) with high rates (88%) of complete debridement.[58] However, more recent data from a randomised trial that recruited 269 patients did not find a benefit in leg ulcer healing time.[59] Pain was significantly more common with larval therapy. Potential barriers include psychological and aesthetic aspects.

Arterial ulcers

Large vessel ischaemia is associated with signs of arterial insufficiency, i.e. pallor, reduced temperature, prolonged capillary refill time and absent pulses. These signs may be absent if small vessel disease is the cause of the ulceration. Assessment should include identifying vascular risk factors. An ABPI should be performed; it is usually below 0.5 in cases of arterial insufficiency. Vascular surgery may be indicated to restore adequate blood flow. Secondary vascular prevention medication should be commenced (e.g. antiplatelets and statins). Smoking-cessation and diabetic control may also be appropriate.

Diabetic ulcers

Peripheral neuropathy and arterial insufficiency may be present alone or in combination in diabetic foot ulcers. Prevention is aided by careful footwear selection, tight glucose control and revascularisation where appropriate. Surgical debridement and eradication of infection, including osteomyelitis, is necessary once an ulcer has developed.

Other aetiologies

Pressure ulcers may develop on the leg, especially over the heel. Less common causes of ulceration include vasculitis and malignancy. Vasculitis may initially present as an area of cutaneous purpura. It is associated with unexplained raised inflammatory markers, black necrosis and irregular borders to the ulcers. Malignancies causing ulceration are most likely to be squamous cell or basal cell carcinomas. They usually occur on sun-exposed skin areas. Rarely, other skin conditions can present as ulcers in the elderly, for example pyoderma gangrenosum associated with inflammatory bowel disease.

METHICILLIN RESISTANT *STAPHYLOCOCCUS AUREUS*

Methicillin resistant *Staphylococcus aureus* (MRSA) produces a protein that confers resistance to beta-lactam antibiotics (e.g. penicillins and cephalosporins). It is readily spread by direct person-to-person contact or via contaminated environments. The organism can survive for months on fomites (inanimate objects that harbour organisms – e.g. dead skin cells, cleaning cloths and stethoscopes).[60] The organism is strongly associated with healthcare facilities and is currently much less common in community settings.[61] It is associated with increased length of stay and healthcare costs. Older adults appear to be at increased risk of colonisation. This may be partly due to higher rates of hospital admission and high rates of prevalence within care home populations. Carriers are typically asymptomatic. One study isolated MRSA from nasal swabs in 159 of 715 (22%) asymptomatic care home residents in the UK.[62]

It was estimated that there were around 94 000 cases of invasive MRSA infections in the USA in 2005 (75% being bacteraemia), and the incidence was highest in the over sixty-fives.[63] Invasive infection is most likely in patients with indwelling lines or following surgical procedures. Compared to non-MRSA *Staphylococcus aureus* infections, mortality appears to be higher with MRSA bacteraemia.[64,65] Infection rates have been increasing over the past decade, but there is now some evidence that rates may be declining.[60,64]

Detection is usually from culturing swabs of the nose and throat, which takes several days. More rapid tests (e.g. polymerase chain reaction) to detect MRSA have been developed but are currently less reliable.

Treatment

Hand washing and patient isolation are highly important. There is some evidence that isolation may be effective even in endemic settings.[66] Appropriate use of antibiotics may also reduce spread. There is some evidence that fluoroquinolone use is particularly implicated.[67,68] Topical colonisation is usually treated with nasal mupirocin and antiseptic body washes.

For invasive infection the choice of effective antibiotics is limited. Vancomycin is the most commonly used antibiotic at present. Sodium fusidate or rifampicin may be used in combination with vancomycin or used together for soft tissue infections that fail to respond. Tetracycline or clindamycin may be appropriate for some soft tissue infections and bronchiectasis. Urinary tract infections may respond to tetracycline, trimethoprim or nitrofurantoin. Newer agents include teicoplanin, linezolid, daptomycin and tigecycline. All have potentially significant side-effects and high financial costs. Alarmingly there have been cases of vancomycin resistant *Staphylococcus aureus* (VRSA) detected in the USA.[69]

MOTOR NEURON DISEASE

Motor neuron disease (MND) consists of a spectrum of presentations, all affecting anterior horn cell functioning. It can affect both upper (UMN) and lower motor neurons (LMN). Amyotrophic lateral sclerosis (ALS) is the commonest form (65%). It is due to loss of neurons from the corticospinal tract and anterior horn cells, causing a mixed picture of UMN and LMN signs. Pseudobulbar palsy is caused by bilateral UMN loss, leading to dysarthria, dysphagia and emotional lability. It can also affect cranial nerve nuclei to give a clinical picture of progressive bulbar palsy. These patients usually present with dysarthria and dysphagia. In this situation wasting and fasciculations may be seen in the facial muscles and tongue. Additionally it can cause a pure LMN deficit in the limbs (progressive muscular atrophy) – presenting as atrophy and fasciculations, or pure UMN signs in the limbs (primary lateral sclerosis). Symptoms gradually progress over time. It does not cause any sensory, cerebellar or oculomotor deficits. The bladder is not affected.

The underlying cause is mostly unknown.[70] Its incidence is around two per 100 000 per year, and its prevalence approximately six per 100 000 people.[71] It affects men more commonly than women. The condition is usually sporadic, but 5–10% have a family history (possibly linked to a superoxide dismutase gene variation).[71] Most cases present within the age range 40–70 years, with a mean age of onset around 60 years. Half of patients die within three years,[71] but 25% are alive at five years, and 10% live beyond 10 years. A worse prognosis is suggested by an older age and presentation with bulbar features. Patients presenting after the age of 70 years are more likely to have initial bulbar signs (perhaps 50% of cases). A small proportion of cases are associated with a form of frontotemporal dementia (termed MND-FTD), which may be autosomal dominantly inherited.[72]

Electromyogram (EMG) is likely to show muscle denervation with preserved velocities. The significance of antibodies in the serum is unclear. Brain or spine imaging is likely to appear normal.

There is no curative treatment. Riluzole has been associated with decreased death at 12 months, but no benefit on muscle strength. It probably works by reducing glutamate-induced excitotoxicity. The median survival increase is around two to three months.[73] Tube feeding may be appropriate for selected patients with dysphagia. Non-invasive ventilation can prolong survival in appropriate patients. Analgesia may be necessary for joint pains. Spasticity may be present and require treatment (*see* p. 39). Advanced planning and palliative care are important aspects of management.

MYOPATHY

The symptoms of myopathy tend to present as proximal weakness, which in the arms may affect combing the hair, and in the legs the climbing of stairs. Reflexes are present but may be diminished (whereas they may be lost in polyneuropathies), sensation is intact. There are many potential causes. These include Cushing's syndrome, thyroid disorders, vitamin D deficiency, and drug-induced. Discussion here is limited to polymyositis, giant cell arteritis and statin-induced myopathy.

Polymyositis

Polymyositis causes a slowly progressive, symmetrical, proximal weakness. It is usually painless. It may be associated with dysphagia, and polyarthritis or arthralgia. There can also be cardiopulmonary involvement causing pneumonitis, conduction defects, pericarditis, or myocarditis. A number of people will have another underlying disease. Around 20% have a connective tissue disease (e.g. systemic lupus erythematosus or rheumatoid arthritis). It is more common in women than men. Dermatomyositis causes a rash in addition to muscular symptoms and has a more frequent association with malignancy. Gottron's papules are areas of macular erythematous scaling over the knuckles and extensor surfaces of the knees and elbows. It can also cause a heliotrope periorbital rash, or less commonly macular erythema over the anterior chest or shoulders. It may be associated with malignancy, especially in the elderly, and most commonly with ovarian, gastrointestinal, lung, or breast cancer.[74]

Blood tests may show an elevated creatine kinase (CK). The electromyogram shows characteristic changes. Autoantibodies are more common in people with a younger onset (e.g. antinuclear antibody and anti-Jo-1 antibody). Muscle biopsy may help diagnosis. An underlying cause should be sought. Treatment is with immunosuppressant drugs.

Giant cell arteritis

Giant cell arteritis (GCA) is a term for a form of vasculitis that may present either as polymyalgia rheumatica (PMR) or temporal arteritis (TA). These later two conditions are similar in that they occur after age 50, respond rapidly to steroids, and have a poorly understood aetiology (*see* Table 20.1).[75] Additionally there is some overlap, around 20% of patients with PMR also have TA, and around 40% of patients with TA also have PMR. PMR is commoner than TA.

Polymyalgia rheumatica

PMR occurs in patients over the age of 50, and 90% of cases present in those over 60 years. It is twice as common in women as men. It causes a slowly progressive pain and stiffness of the proximal muscles. Fever, malaise, night sweats, and weight loss are present in around a third of people. Morning stiffness lasting over 30 minutes is characteristic. A mild polyarthritis similar to rheumatoid arthritis may be seen. Diagnosis relies on the exclusion of other diseases. Inflammatory markers are elevated. The ESR is typically over 40 mm/hour, the serum C-reactive protein is also likely to be elevated. Autoantibodies and CK are usually normal. There may be anaemia of chronic disease (two-thirds of people) and abnormal liver enzymes (a third of people). Treatment is with steroids, typically prednisolone at a dose of 10–20 mg per day. The steroids can usually be slowly reduced and withdrawn over a period of several months. Bone protection should be considered for people on steroids (*see* Chapter 16).

Temporal arteritis

TA is an inflammatory process of the medium to large-sized vessels, particularly vessels arising from the proximal aorta. It rarely affects the intracranial vessels. The condition often presents with fever, malaise and weight loss. Headache occurs in most patients (>2/3). There may be TA tenderness or reduced palpable pulsation. Other symptoms include jaw claudication (50% of cases), scalp tenderness (50%), and visual loss (20%). This latter problem is due to involvement of the retinal vessels. It is painless. Examination may reveal papilloedema and retinal haemorrhages. It is an emergency as visual loss is typically irreversible. The condition may present as pyrexia of unknown origin in around 15% of people. The formation of a thoracic aortic aneurysm (possibly with dissection) is a rare late feature.

An ESR is usually over 50 mm/hour. A temporal artery biopsy (ideally before steroids, but may be positive up to two weeks after their commencement) may reveal a characteristic pattern of vasculitis (e.g. monocyte infiltration and granuloma formation). The artery may only show segmental involvement, so a 2 cm length sample is required.

Treatment is with steroids (typically prednisolone at a dose of 40 to 60 mg per day). This can gradually be reduced over several months.

TABLE 20.1 A comparison of polymyalgia rheumatica (PMR) and temporal arteritis (TA).

	PMR	TA
Age	>50	>50
ESR (mm/hour)	>40	>50
Symptoms/signs	Pain in proximal muscles or morning stiffness	1. Headache 2. Artery tenderness or reduced pulsation
Other criteria	1. Rapid response to steroids 2. Exclusion of other disease	Vasculitic changes on temporal artery biopsy
For diagnosis	All of the above	3 or more of the above

Statin-induced myopathy

Myopathy has a known association with statin drugs. They may cause a range of presentations, from being asymptomatic to developing rhabdomyolysis. The incidence of rhabdomyolysis is around four per 100 000 per year on atorvastatin, simvastatin or pravastatin.[76] Myopathy, defined as weakness and a raised CK, occurs in 12 per 100 000 per year. Typical symptoms include myalgia, muscle tenderness, weakness, nocturnal cramps, and tendon pain. Muscle symptoms may be worse following exercise. The duration of therapy prior to developing symptoms has a mean of six months (range one week to four years). The symptoms persist for a mean two months (one week to four months) following discontinuation of the drug. Statins are unlikely to be causative if the patient has been on them for several years. Known risk factors include old age, female sex, low BMI, reduced hepatic or renal function, and alcohol excess. Other drugs that may increase the risk include those that are inhibitors or substrates of cytochrome P450 pathway (e.g. calcium channel blockers, amiodarone, macrolide antibiotics, and warfarin). It may be more likely to occur with lipophilic drugs: i.e. simvastatin and atorvastatin.

PNEUMONIA

The risks of developing pneumonia rise with increasing age. Those aged over 90 years are five times more likely to develop pneumonia and twice as likely to die from it compared to people aged 65 to 69 years (mortality 7.8% vs 15.4%).[77] Those with comorbidities are at particular risk. The mortality for those over the age of 65 years admitted to hospital with community-acquired pneumonia (CAP) is around 11%, and a further 34% die within one year of discharge.[78] In those aged over 85 the annual risk of hospitalisation with pneumonia is around 5%.[79] These increases may be partly explained by an increased risk of aspiration pneumonia (*see* below). Smoking is an additional factor.[80]

Older people may present atypically. They are less likely to report cough, shortness of breath or pleuritic chest pain, but are more likely to have an elevated respiratory rate compared to younger people.[81] They are also more likely to be afebrile and lack a raised white blood cell count than younger people.[82,83] Patients who develop pneumonia in nursing homes are more likely to present with confusion.[84,85]

Similar to younger people, *S. pneumoniae* is the most common pathogen-causing CAP in the elderly.[86] However, infections with, *Staph. aureus* and gram-negative bacteria (e.g. *H. influenzae*, *E. coli* and *Klebsiella pneumoniae*) make up a larger proportion of cases. *Pseudomonas aeruginosa* may be a more likely cause in those undergoing tube feeding.[87] A proportion of cases are caused by viruses. In many patients the underlying organism is never identified as frail elderly patients are often unable to provide suitable sputum samples for testing.

Simple scales have been developed to help rate severity of CAP. The CURB-65 score gives one point for each of **C**onfusion, a raised serum **U**rea (>7 mmol/L), a respiratory **R**ate of 30 breaths per minute or over, a low **B**lood pressure (systolic <90 mmHg or diastolic <60 mmHg), and aged **65** or above. A modified version, the CRB-65, omits blood urea so that it can be more useful for initial assessment in the community. A study of older people (mean age 77 years) with CAP found that 30-day mortality rates with this latter score were <1% for a score of zero or one, 8% for a score of two, and 17% for a score of three (no patients had a score of four).[88] Hospitalisation should be considered for those with a score of two or above.

Pneumococcal polysaccharide vaccine (available as 7-valent and 23-valent versions) has been developed for the prevention of pneumonia caused by *S. pneumoniae*. A meta-analysis that excluded trials judged to be of low methodological quality did not find a reduction in overall pneumonia rates in the elderly (RR 0.89, 95% CI 0.69–1.14) or invasive pneumococcal disease (RR 0.90, 95% CI 0.46–1.77).[89] However, more recent studies have found a benefit. A Japanese study found a 23-valent vaccine, compared to placebo, reduced rates of pneumococcal pneumonia (2.8% vs 7.3%, $p<0.001$) and related death rates (0% vs 35%, $p<0.01$) in nursing home residents.[90] Also a study conducted in the US has associated a fall in hospital admission rates due to pneumonia with the introduction of a vaccination programme, and the greatest benefits were seen in those aged over 85 years.[91] In the UK people over the age of 65 without relevant comorbidities are advised to have a one-off pneumococcal immunisation. Repeat injections are recommended five-yearly for those with splenectomy or chronic kidney disease. Influenza vaccination may reduce the risk of secondary bacterial pneumonia (*see* p. 432).

Aspiration pneumonia

Aspiration pneumonia or pneumonitis occurs following either oropharyngeal or gastric contents entering the lower respiratory tract. These two entities may be hard to distinguish clinically as they may both cause similar clinical symptoms and signs, blood test results and chest X-ray appearances.

Aspiration pneumonitis is an inflammation of the lungs in response to the inhalation of acidic gastric contents. The event is often witnessed. It is most likely to occur in people with reduced consciousness (e.g. postoperative, drug overdose or major stroke). These contents cause a chemical injury but are typically sterile. It is believed that 20 mL or more of liquid with a pH <2.5 is required to trigger a significant reaction.[92] This is unlikely to occur in people on acid-suppressing medications. Presenting symptoms may range from acute respiratory distress syndrome and shock to mild cough with low oxygen saturation. The symptoms usually commence soon after the aspiration event but some are asymptomatic. A late complication of pneumonitis may be secondary infection. Following witnessed aspiration upper airway suction is recommended. In this situation a sterile pneumonitis is likely and antibiotics are probably unnecessary unless symptoms last beyond 24 hours.[93]

Aspiration pneumonia is an infectious process following the inhalation of the contents of the oropharynx, which contains bacteria. Silent aspiration occurs even in healthy older adults more commonly than in younger individuals.[94] Up to half of normal healthy individuals may aspirate small amounts of matter during sleep.[92] Pneumonia is more likely to occur when larger volumes are aspirated and more pathogenic organisms have colonised the oropharynx. This is more common in people with an impaired swallow, or cough reflex, or those on medications that are either sedating or reduce saliva production (e.g. anticholinergics).[86] Individuals with poor dentition and the elderly in general (probably due to comorbidities) are at an increased risk. Aspiration events are often unwitnessed. Presenting features are similar to those of other pneumonias. Chest X-ray will show infiltrates in a characteristic distribution. If it occurred when lying down these will be the posterior segments of the upper lobes or apical segments of the lower lobes, if sitting up then the basal segments of the lower lobes are most likely to be affected.[92] Untreated they have an increased risk of abscess formation compared to non-aspiration pneumonia. Accurate data on incidence is lacking. It is estimated that possibly 5–15% of community-acquired pneumonias are secondary to aspiration.[92] It is a more common cause of pneumonia in people with neurological disorders (e.g. stroke or neurodegenerative diseases) or those who reside in nursing homes. Dysphagia is common immediately following stroke, and aspiration may be silent. It still occurs in those fed by nasogastric or PEG tubes (*see* p. 115).[86]

Antibiotics are indicated in aspiration pneumonia. Bacteria isolated from early studies suggested a major role for anaerobic organisms. However, more recent studies have not detected anaerobes as frequently. Bacteria implicated in community-acquired aspiration pneumonia include *Strep. pneumoniae*, *H. influenzae* and *Staph. aureus*, and in hospital-acquired cases gram-negative organisms, including *Ps. aeruginosa*, are more likely.[92] A study of elderly patients (mean age 80 years) presenting from nursing home with severe aspiration pneumonia found gram-negative organisms in 49%, anaerobes in 16% and *Staph. aureus* in 12%.[95] Anaerobes were more commonly found in those with poor dentition. However, anaerobes were often found in combination with gram-negative organisms, and most infections responded well to initial non-anaerobic antibiotic coverage. So the impact of anaerobic organisms in these cases is unclear. Therefore, the choice of antibiotic will partly depend on the location of its onset. Broad-spectrum agents such as piperacillin-tazobactam are typically recommended.[92] Agents to cover anaerobic organisms (e.g. metronidazole) may be most helpful in those with poor dentition. One study of 100 older patients (median age 82 years), mainly residing in nursing homes, found that clindamycin was as effective as combinations of a penicillin and a beta-lactamase inhibitor for treating aspiration pneumonia.[96] However, this antibiotic may cause unacceptably high rates of *C. difficile* diarrhoea in older populations.

Ideally steps would be taken to prevent aspiration pneumonia. Simple bedside tests have been developed to detect those at risk of aspiration. Observing the patient's response to small volumes of oral water has been found to be a good indicator of aspiration risk.[97] More formal videofluoroscopy (a radiographic examination using radio-opaque barium mixed with food of varying consistency, performed by a radiologist and a speech and language therapist – *see* p. 40), may be useful in selected cases. However, abnormal results may be obtained in healthy older people. A trial that compared the use of either thickened liquids or chin-down posturing on swallowing for 515 older adults (mean age 81 years) at risk of aspiration (suffering from dementia or Parkinson's disease) to try to prevent pneumonia did not detect a significant difference between methods.[98] However, no control group was included. A neurotransmitter named 'substance P' is involved in the cough and swallow reflexes. ACE inhibitors (but not angiotensin receptor blockers) prevent the breakdown of this agent. A meta-analysis of studies has suggested a lower risk of pneumonia in people on ACE inhibitors.[99] The use of antipsychotic drugs is associated with an increased risk of pneumonia (probably through aspiration) (odds ratio 1.6, 95% CI 1.3–2.1).[100] So this is another reason why their use should be limited (*see* pp. 28 and 110). Improving dental hygiene in susceptible individuals may also have a beneficial effect. In general there is little robust data in this field.[101]

PRESSURE ULCERS

Pressure ulcers (PU) are also known as 'pressure sores', 'bedsores' or 'decubitus ulcers'. They develop in areas where pressure on the skin overlying a bony prominence restricts capillary blood flow, resulting in tissue hypoxia then necrosis and breakdown. Classic sites are over the sacrum, ischial tuberosities and heels (*see* Figure 20.2). This process is worsened by a reduction in the natural padding provided by subcutaneous fat associated with poor nutrition and other factors such as moisture levels (including incontinence), shear and friction forces (e.g. sliding down the bed or when being transferred), and superimposed infections. Elderly patients are at an increased risk, especially following hip fracture or spinal injury. The prevalence of PU in hospitalised people is around 3–14%.[102]

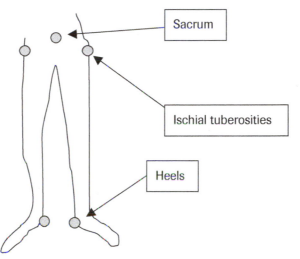

FIGURE 20.2 Common sites of pressure ulcers.

The pathogenesis has been subdivided into four stages but progression of the lesions does not always follow this linear pattern.[103] This grading system is outlined below.
➤ Stage 1: Superficial skin changes (e.g. erythema, bogginess, increased temperature).
➤ Stage 2: Shallow ulcer due to loss of epidermis and/or dermis.
➤ Stage 3: Full thickness skin loss with necrosis of subcutaneous fat.
➤ Stage 4: Involvement of bone, tendon or muscle.

Assessment

The site and stage of pressure damage should be recorded for all patients entering a geriatric unit. Assessment and monitoring of progression may be aided by the use of photographs. Swabs taken from wounds will always identify bacterial growth – often multiple organisms. This is probably only clinically significant when there is evidence of infection such as surrounding erythema, the characteristic odour of anaerobic organisms (usually *Bacteroides* species) or suspected osteomyelitis. Bone beneath deep ulcers is at risk of osteomyelitis (*see* below). An elevated serum white cell count (WCC) and inflammatory markers (e.g. ESR or CRP) may accompany infection.

Prevention

Various screening tools have been developed to try to identify those patients most at risk and therefore try to target intervention strategies. Among those commonly used are the Waterlow and Braden scores.[104,105] In the Waterlow scale a score of 15 or more indicates high risk of PU development, in the Braden scale a score of 18 or less signifies increased risk. However, their actual predictive value is questionable.[106] It seems that, to date, an ideal tool has not been developed and, in addition, clinical judgement is still required to identify those at risk. People at high risk often have reduced mobility, nutritional deficiency, inability to reposition themselves and cognitive impairment.[107]

The more frequently the patient is repositioned the better. Ulcer formation has been known to occur after time intervals as short as two hours. The aim is at least four-hourly repositioning for those at high risk, and at least every six hours for those judged at risk.[107] This should begin from the time of admission.

Mattresses are subdivided into static and dynamic designs. Static devices are simply air-filled or made of foam. Dynamic devices are filled with air at alternating pressures. Specialised foam mattresses have been found to be superior to standard hospital mattresses in the prevention of PU.[108] In a study comparing the use of a foam mattress and four-hourly turning regimen to an alternating pressure air mattress without turning in patients at high risk of PU, no difference in the incidence of ulceration was noted (15.6% vs 15.3%; n=447; median age 82 years).[109] In an intensive therapy unit (ITU) setting, air-filled beds have been shown to be superior to standard ITU beds in reducing PU incidence.[110] A trial has compared dynamic mattresses with dynamic overlays (a thinner device placed on top of a standard mattress) and did not find any difference in PU incidence.[111]

Barrier creams should also be considered for application to areas of intact, but at-risk, skin as these can reduce the risk of skin damage.[107]

Treatment

PU can be associated with significant pain. When it occurs, analgesia is an important part of therapy. Logic suggests that measures to correct malnutrition should aid PU healing. To date, there is no evidence from clinical trials of a benefit for replacing vitamins or minerals to treat PU in the absence of a known deficiency.[112] Recently a study failed to find a benefit of using an anabolic steroid (oxandrolone) to try to aid PU healing compared to placebo.[113]

Non-gauze dressings are usually preferred, as they require less frequent changes (typically every three to four days) and are associated with mildly improved healing rates.[114] A wide range of dressings is available with differing clinical indications. The usual aim is to keep the ulcer bed moist and clean. The frequency of dressing changes can vary according to the product used; at each change the ongoing suitability of that type of dressing should be reassessed. Commonly used types of dressings are outlined in Table 20.2.[115]

TABLE 20.2 Types of dressings frequently used in the management of pressure ulcers

Dressing type	Comments
Hydrocolloid	Used for stage 2 ulcers or non-infected shallow grade 3 ulcers. Can also be used to protect body areas at risk of damage
Transparent film	Can be used to protect at-risk skin from friction injury. Can act as a second dressing to help retain a wound filler (e.g. alginate) within the ulcer bed. Not suitable when there is moderate to heavy exudate
Hydrogel	For shallow and minimally exuding ulcers. Can be used to moisten dry ulcer beds. May be useful for painful ulcers.
Alginate	Used when there is moderate to heavy exudate. Can be useful for infected ulcers (while receiving concurrent treatment for infection)
Foam	For exudative stage 2 or shallow stage 3 ulcers. Can be used on painful ulcers or to protect at-risk skin from shear injury
Silver-impregnated	For ulcers that are infected or at high risk of infection
Cadexomer iodine	Used when there is moderate to heavy exudate. Not for people with iodine sensitivity. Iodine acts as an antiseptic

Vacuum-assisted dressings have also been developed. These create a negative pressure gradient across a suitably sized piece of polyurethane foam fitted into the wound cavity. It is felt that this may reduce wound healing times by the more effective reduction of wound exudates, surrounding oedema and bacterial colonisation.[116] Current guidance suggests their use for wounds with a large amount of exude in order to reduce the number of dressing changes required.[107]

Larval therapy has been used to debride pressure ulcers. In an unrandomised, retrospective study, the use of larvae for chronic pressure ulcers was associated with more rapid healing than conventional therapy.[117] The main side-effect noted was pain (in 4–24% of patients). Randomised controlled trials are required to confirm these findings. Larval therapy may be most useful when sharp debridement is contraindicated or if there is associated vascular insufficiency.[107]

Surgical intervention is usually only recommended for grade 3 or 4 ulcers in patients suitable to undergo an operation. Debridement is believed to improve wound healing by removing the necrotic tissue that has harmful effects on the wound. It has the added benefits of potentially unmasking underlying abscesses and allowing samples to be taken for culture, for example bone to diagnose osteomyelitis. Skin repair techniques include direct closure, skin grafts and the use of skin flaps.[118] They are associated with high recurrence and adverse event rates in elderly, immobile patients and, therefore, appropriate patient selection is important.

Antibiotics should only be used if there is evidence of systemic sepsis, spreading cellulitis or underlying osteomyelitis.[107] Osteomyelitis is most commonly caused by

Staphylococcus aureus (in some cases MRSA).[119] It should be suspected when there is a raised serum WCC, ESR and/or CRP without an alternative explanation. Imaging with plain X-ray, isotope bone scanning or MRI can be useful. X-rays only become abnormal beyond two weeks when significant bone mineral content has been lost. MRI and isotope bone scanning are more able to detect early changes, with MRI usually being the preferred method. A positive culture from bone biopsy provides a definitive diagnosis, but a positive blood culture with supportive imaging studies may make this unnecessary. Treatment may require surgical debridement and a prolonged course of antibiotics (e.g. four to eight weeks) with the choice of agent dependent on culture sensitivities.

TYPE 2 DIABETES

More than half of diabetes in the Western world occurs in people over the age of 65 years. Around 10% of those aged over 75 and 14% those over 85 in the UK have diabetes.[120] Approximately 25% of nursing home residents have diabetes.[121] Over 90% of older diabetics have type 2 diabetes. Type 1 diabetes is due to destruction of pancreatic beta cells. It is linked with autoimmune disease. Its onset is rare in the old, but some people may survive with it into old age.

In type 2 diabetes the pancreatic beta cells are preserved, but their insulin secretion is reduced. Risk factors for type 2 diabetes include a family history, obesity and a past history of gestational diabetes. Over 80% of those with type 2 diabetes are overweight or obese.[122] Advanced age is another strong risk factor. Ageing leads to reduced insulin secretion, peripheral insulin resistance, and an increased proportion of body fat (*see* p. 10). Insulin resistance may be mediated through reduced intracellular signalling processes. Increased central adiposity and reduced physical exercise are common in older age and may increase insulin resistance. Homeostasis of serum glucose concentration is impaired. A slowing of the return to normal levels is seen following a meal. Raised levels of glucose may lead to enhanced protein glycation, which may further accelerate the ageing process. In the elderly, diabetes is associated with physical function impairment.[123] The 'metabolic syndrome' is defined as a combination of hypertension, raised lipids, central obesity and glucose intolerance. Some commonly used drugs may increase serum glucose levels. These include beta-blockers, nifedipine, thiazide diuretics, atypical antipsychotics and steroids.

Diabetes leads to long-term complications. These are usually distinguished as microvascular (small vessel) – nephropathy, retinopathy and neuropathy; and macrovascular (large vessel) – ischaemic heart disease (IHD), stroke and peripheral vascular disease (PVD). Diabetic people are also at a risk of hypoglycaemia (usually secondary to treatment), which may also cause lasting harm. A history of one or more episodes of severe hypoglycaemia is associated with an increased risk of developing dementia.[124] The risk of serious hypoglycaemia is increased if on beta-blockers or in the presence of autonomic neuropathy (via reduced counter-regulatory responses). Cognitive impairment, taking irregular meals, and a high alcohol intake all make it more likely.

Hyperosmolar hyperglycaemic state (HHS) may develop in people with inadequately controlled type 2 diabetes. This condition incorporates hyperglycaemia (blood glucose >33 mmol/L), hyperosmolarity (serum osmolarity >320 osmol/L), volume depletion and renal insufficiency. Patients don't have ketoacidosis but may develop lactic acidosis. It may evolve over several days. Infection is a common precipitant and delirium often develops. Mortality rates increase with age, being <10% in those <75 years, 19% in those aged 75 to 84, and 35% in those >85 years.[125] Treatment includes correcting the, typically large, fluid deficit and an intravenous infusion of insulin.[126]

Diabetic ketoacidosis is more common in type 1 diabetes, but can still occur in type 2. It has the three features of hyperglycaemia, ketonaemia and acidosis. It can be precipitated by acute illness (e.g. sepsis) or inadequate insulin administration. Management guidelines are available elsewhere.[127]

Diagnosis

Typical symptoms may occur less commonly in the elderly. Atypical symptoms or a presentation with complications are more likely. Standard diagnostic definitions of diabetes are listed below (just one of the three is required).

1. Typical symptoms (polyuria, polydipsia and weight loss) plus a random glucose of 11.1 mmol/L or above.
2. A fasting glucose at or above 7.0 mmol/L.
3. A glucose level of 11.1 mmol/L or higher two hours after an oral glucose tolerance test (OGTT).

Impaired glucose tolerance (IGT) is defined as a serum glucose level between 7.8 and 11.1 mmol/L two hours after an OGTT. Impaired fasting glucose is defined as a fasting glucose level between 5.6 and 7.0 mmol/L. These two categories are likely to include similar patients, but the latter removing the need for performing an OGTT.

Glucose attaches to red blood cells to form glycosolated haemoglobin (termed 'HbA$_{1C}$'). As red blood cells survive in the circulation for two to three months, its value reflects blood sugar levels over this preceding period. It is used to measure glucose control and has recently also been used in diagnosis. Traditionally it has been reported as a percentage, but laboratories are now moving towards using mmol/mol units. A value above 48 mmol/mol (6.5%) suggests a diagnosis of diabetes (HbA$_{1C}$ may be inaccurate in some situations, e.g. acute illness or anaemia).[128]

Once the diagnosis is established it is appropriate to look for the associated complications. Serum creatinine should be measured and urinary protein (dipsticks or 24-hour urine) evaluated to look for evidence of nephropathy. Retinal examination should be performed (annual ophthalmology checks are recommended). Examination should look for evidence of neuropathy.

Treatment

Education should be given, including how to recognise and treat hypoglycaemia, titrate medication, and monitor blood sugar. A reduction in weight and an increase in exercise may prevent the onset of diabetes in those with IGT.[129,130] This benefit is probably still present in older adults.[131] Dietary advice and calorie restriction may be appropriate (especially in those with a BMI >30 kg/m²). A small proportion of patients will achieve HbA$_{1C}$ targets with diet alone.[132] As part of a vascular risk reduction, those who smoke should be helped to stop. Aspirin and statin medications may be indicated. Blood pressure control is recommended to 130/80 mmHg or below. Reducing blood pressure leads to a reduction in both micro and macrovascular complications. The size of the effect is equivalent to a 12% reduction in complication risk and a 15% reduction in risk of death related to diabetes for every 10 mmHg fall in BP.[133] ACE inhibitors or angiotensin receptor blockers (ARBs) are usually used first as they have been believed to reduce the risk of progressive deterioration in renal function. However, recent trials have questioned this belief.[134,135] A more intense therapeutic regime using aspirin, ACE inhibitors, statins and better blood pressure control has been found to reduce death in patients with type 2 diabetes.[136]

Glucose control

It is necessary to establish a treatment target HbA_{1C} level for each patient. Factors involved in this decision include life expectancy, comorbidities, social set-up, hypoglycaemia risk, and the presence of cognitive impairment.[137] Over-treatment can lead to harm to older people. For example, admissions for hypoglycaemia are associated with a higher risk of developing dementia.[138] It is typically recommended to aim for an HbA_{1C} of 53 mmol/mol (7.0%) or less in younger adults. This may still be appropriate for healthy independent elders. Some authors recommend a target of 53–64 mmol/mol (7.0 to 8.0%) in the healthy elderly and a target of 64–75 mmol/mol (8.0 to 9.0%) in the frail.[139] Metabolic decompensation with cachexia is unlikely below the 75 mmol/mol (9.0%) level. Sadly, despite the high prevalence in older people, there is very little trial data for patients aged over 75 years.

Studies have found that tighter glucose control reduces the risk of microvascular complications. The UKPDS study found that intensive control of glucose resulted in a 25% reduction in microvascular complications (HbA_{1C} values of 7.0% vs 7.9%) after a 10-year study period.[140] However, similar results have not been demonstrated regarding a reduction in macrovascular complications. A different trial randomised 11 140 patients (mean age 66 years) to intensive (mean HbA_{1C} 6.5%) or standard control (7.3%) over a five-year period.[141] No significant reduction in macrovascular events or death was detected. However, microvascular events (mainly nephropathy) were reduced (9.4% vs 10.9%; HR 0.86, 95% CI 0.77–0.97). Another trial randomised 10 251 patients (mean age 62 years) to intensive glucose lowering (mean HbA_{1C} 6.4%) or standard control (7.5%).[142] The trial was discontinued after 3.5 years due to excess mortality in the intensive control arm, without a reduction in cardiovascular events. Hypoglycaemia requiring assistance was more common (16.2% vs 5.1%) as was weight gain in excess of 10 kg (27.8% vs 14.1%).

However, a meta-analysis of trials (n=33 040; mean age 62 years) did find that a 0.9% average reduction in HbA_{1C} (6.6% vs 7.5%), after a five-year follow-up period, was associated with a 17% reduction in non-fatal MI (OR 0.83, 95% CI 0.75–0.93).[143] But no reduction in stroke or all-cause mortality was detected.

Various treatment options are discussed below, followed by a recommendation for their practical implementation in the elderly (*see* Figure 20.3).

Biguanides (metformin)

Metformin is the only currently available biguanide. It causes reduced hepatic gluconeogenesis, increased peripheral glucose uptake, and increased insulin sensitivity. Typically HbA_{1C} values reduce by 1–2%.[122] Hypoglycaemia is rare. It may be associated with reduced appetite and weight loss, making it a particularly useful therapy in those who are obese. Self blood sugar monitoring is usually unnecessary.[122] Lactic acidosis is a rare but reported serious complication of metformin therapy. However, a Cochrane review was unable to confirm this association.[144] It is usually not recommended in those with marked hepatic failure, hypoxia or renal failure (caution with eGFR below 45 mL/min/1.73 m^2, avoid if below 30). Treatment with metformin is associated with a lower risk of cardiovascular mortality compared to any other oral hypoglycaemic agent or placebo (OR 0.74, 95% CI 0.62–0.89).[145] For this reason it is usually considered a first-line therapy.

Sulphonylureas

Sulphonylureas stimulate insulin release from pancreatic beta cells. Hypoglycaemia is an associated risk; 10–20% of patients have been found to have one or more hypoglycaemic events per year while on this type of medication. Longer-acting drugs (e.g. glibenclamide and chlorpropramide) have a higher risk of hypoglycaemia and are best avoided in the elderly (chlorpropramide may also cause SIADH). Risks are lower with shorter-acting agents (e.g. gliclazide and tolbutamide). Weight gain is another potential problem (approx. 2 kg). They reduce HbA_{1C} values by around 1–2%.[122]

Alpha-glucosidase inhibitors

Alpha-glucosidase inhibitors (e.g. acarbose) reduce HbA_{1C} by around 0.5%.[122] They delay carbohydrate digestion and lower peak glucose levels. Weight gain and hypoglycaemia are less likely than with sulphonylureas in the elderly.[146] Flatulence, abdominal pain and diarrhoea are the most common adverse events. In trials these symptoms led 25–45% of patients to discontinue treatment.[122]

Thiazolidinediones

Thiazolidinediones (e.g. rosiglitazone and pioglitazone) stimulate peroxisome proliferator-activated receptor-gamma (PPAR-gamma) causing increased transcription of insulin sensitive genes 'insulin sensitizers', i.e. reduced insulin resistance. They typically reduce HbA_{1C} levels by around 1%.[122] It is recommended to monitor liver blood tests at the start of therapy and every few months. They may cause oedema and are not recommended in patients with heart failure. They may increase weight, affect bone metabolism and cause anaemia. They have been associated with an increased risk of fractures.[147] A meta-analysis of trials comparing rosiglitazone to placebo (mean age of patients 56 years) found a significant increase in risk of myocardial infarction in patients receiving rosiglitazone (OR 1.43, 95% CI 1.03 to 1.98).[148] The mechanism of this may be by alteration in serum lipids or fluid retention. The risk may be even higher in older adults who have a greater risk of IHD. Rosiglitazone is not recommended if there is a history of heart failure, IHD or PVD. A trial comparing pioglitazone to placebo in

5238 patients (mean age 62 years) found that it reduced HbA_{1C} (7.0% vs 7.6%) but this did not lead to a significant benefit in the primary outcome of combined mortality and vascular events (HR 0.90, 95% CI 0.08–1.02).[149] It did, however, lead to an increased incidence of heart failure (11% vs 8%) and weight gain (average 3.6 kg vs –0.4 kg). For all of these reasons, this class of medications will rarely be indicated in older adults.

Insulin

Insulin is usually considered when glucose control is inadequate on two or three treatments. In this instance there is probably no benefit in continuing oral agents other than metformin. There is no maximum dose, and doses exceeding one unit per kilogram may be required in patients with type 2 diabetes due to insulin resistance.[122] Insulin therapy is associated with weight gain (typically 2 to 4 kg) and a risk of hypoglycaemia.

Several different formulations of insulin are available. They include short- and long-acting types, and as a mix of both (biphasic insulin). Once-daily basal insulins are also available (e.g. glargine and detemir). This latter group has a low incidence of nocturnal hypoglycaemia, and are recommended by NICE for those with type 2 diabetes where assistance is needed for injecting the insulin or there is a high risk of recurrent hypoglycaemia.

A trial randomised 708 people (mean age 62 years) with suboptimal diabetic control (HbA_{1C} 7.0 to 10.0%, mean 8.5%) who were already taking metformin and a sulphonylurea to receive biphasic insulin twice a day, prandial insulin three times a day (before meals), or basal insulin once daily (at bedtime).[150] After one year the basal insulin was less effective at lowering HbA_{1C} than either biphasic or prandial regimens (mean values 7.6, 7.3 and 7.2% respectively), but was associated with less weight gain (1.9 vs 4.7 and 5.7 kg) and lower rates of hypoglycaemic events (2.3 vs 5.7 and 12.0 per patient per year). A more recent study found similar results and patient satisfaction was higher with basal insulin,[151] perhaps partly due to less blood sugar testing being required.

Other glucose-lowering options

Several newer agents for glycaemic control are now available. These include glucagon-like peptide-1 agonists, glinides, amylin agonists and dipeptidylpeptidase-4 inhibitors. However, data on their use in older adults and long-term safety is limited. Currently they are rarely used in the elderly and so are not discussed further here.

Usually it is recommended to start on metformin (unless contraindicated), and make a change once the HbA_{1C} is above the target value. Second-line options include adding a sulphonylurea, insulin or acarbose (see Figure 20.3). After three years around 50% of patients will require more than one agent to control their blood sugar.[132] This may be due to progressive beta cell failure. Guidelines typically recommend adding insulin to metformin; however, this may have no benefit over using insulin alone.[152]

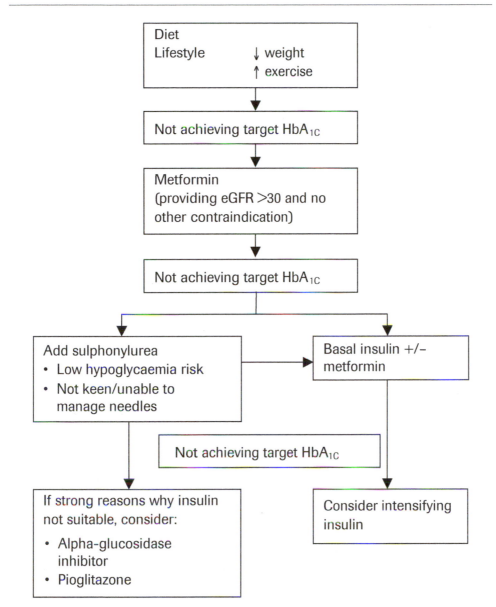

FIGURE 20.3 Suggested algorithm for glycaemic control in the frail elderly.

REFERENCES

1 Guralnik JM, Eisenstaedt RS, Ferrucci L, *et al.* Prevalence of anemia in persons 65 years and older in the United States: evidence for a high rate of unexplained anemia. *Blood*, 2004; **104**(8): 2263–8.

2 Ble A, Fink JC, Woodman RC, *et al.* Renal function, erythropoietin, and anaemia of older persons. *Arch Intern Med*, 2005; **165**: 2222–7.

3 Gaskell H, Derry S, Moore RA, *et al.* Prevalence of anaemia in older persons: systematic review. *BMC Geriatrics*, 2008; **8**(1): 1–8.

4 Penninx BWJH, Pahor M, Cesari M, *et al.* Anemia is associated with disability and decreased physical performance and muscle strength in the elderly. *J Am Geriatr Soc*, 2004; **52**(5): 719–24.

5 Chaves PHM, Carlson MC, Ferrucci L, *et al.* Association between mild anaemia and executive function in community-dwelling older women: the Women's Health and Aging Study II. *J Am Geriatr Soc*, 2006; **54**(9): 1429–35.

6 Duh MS, Mody SH, Lefebvre P, *et al.* Anaemia and the risk of injurious falls in a community-dwelling elderly population. *Drugs Aging*, 2008; **25**(4): 325–34.

7 Andro M, Le Squere P, Estivin S, *et al.* Anaemia and cognitive performances in the elderly: a systematic review. *Eur J Neurol*, 2013; **20**: 1234–40.

8 Guyatt GH, Patterson C, Ali M, *et al.* Diagnosis of iron-deficiency anemia in the elderly. *Am J Med*, 1990; **88**(3): 205–9.

9 Rockey DC, Cello JP. Evaluation of the gastrointestinal tract in patients with iron-deficiency anemia. *N Engl J Med*, 1993; **329**: 1691–5.

10 Joosten E, Ghesquiere B, Linthoudt H, *et al.* Upper and lower gastrointestinal evaluation of elderly inpatients who are iron deficient. *Am J Med*, 1999; **107**(1): 24–9.

11 Ure T, Dehghan K, Vernava AM, *et al.* Colonoscopy in the elderly. Low risk, high yield. *Surg Endosc*, 1995; **9**(5): 505–8.

12 Andres E, Affenberger S, Vinzio S, *et al.* Food-cobalamin malabsorption in elderly patients: clinical manifestations and treatment. *Am J Med*, 2005; **118**(10): 1154–9.

13 Astor BC, Munter P, Levin A, *et al.* Association of kidney function with anaemia: the third National Health and Nutrition Examination Survey (1988–1994). *Arch Intern Med*, 2002; **162**: 1401–8.

14 Joosten E. Strategies for the laboratory diagnosis of some common causes of anaemia in elderly patients. *Gerontology*, 2004; **50**: 49–56.

15 Gorevic PD. Osteoarthritis: a review of musculoskeletal aging and treatment issues in geriatric patients. *Geriatrics*, 2004; **59**(8): 28–32.

16 Quintana JM, Arostegui I, Escobar A, *et al.* Prevalence of knee and hip osteoarthritis and the appropriateness of joint replacement in an older population. *Arch Intern Med*, 2008; **168**(14): 1576–84.

17 Penninx BWJH, Messier SP, Rejeski J, *et al.* Physical exercise and the prevention of disability in activities of daily living in older persons with osteoarthritis. *Arch Intern Med*, 2001; **161**: 2309–16.

18 Hamel MB, Toth M, Legedza A, *et al.* Joint replacement surgery in elderly patients with severe osteoarthritis of the hip or knee: decision making, postoperative recovery, and clinical out-comes. *Arch Intern Med*, 2008; **168**(13): 1430–40.

19 Kerr LD. Inflammatory arthropathy: a review of rheumatoid arthritis in older patients. *Geriatrics*, 2004; **59**(10): 32–5.

20 Lopez-Hoyos M, Ruiz de Algeria C, Blanco R, *et al.* Clinical utility of anti-CCP antibodies in the differential diagnosis of elderly-onset rheumatoid arthritis and polymyalgia rheumatica. *Rheumatol*, 2004; **43**: 655–7.

21 Cassetta M, Gorevic PD. Crystal arthritis: gout and pseudogout in the geriatric patient. *Geriatrics*, 2004; **59**(9): 25–31.

22 Mannino DM, Buist AS, Vollmer WM. Chronic obstructive pulmonary disease in the older adult: what defines abnormal lung function? *Thorax*, 2007; **62**: 237–41.

23 Hardie JA, Buist AS, Vollmer WM, *et al.* Risk of over-diagnosis of COPD in asymptomatic elderly never-smokers. *Eur Respir J*, 2002; **20**: 1117–22.

24 Scanlon PD, Waller LA, Altose MD, *et al.* Smoking cessation and lung function in mild-to-moderate chronic obstructive pulmonary disease. The Lung Health Study. *Am J Respir Crit Care Med*, 2000; **161**: 381–90.

25 Ruse CE, Molyneux AWP. A study of the management of COPD according to established guidelines and the implications for older patients. *Age Ageing*, 2006; **35**: 299–301.

26 Singh S, Loke YK, Furberg CD. Inhaled anticholinergics and risk of major adverse cardiovascular events in patients with chronic obstructive pulmonary disease: a systematic review and meta-analysis. *JAMA*, 2008; **300**(12): 1439–50.

27 Drummond MB, Dasenbrook EC, Pitz MW, *et al.* Inhaled corticosteroids in patients with stable chronic obstructive pulmonary disease: a systematic review and meta-analysis. *JAMA*, 2008; **300**(20): 2407–16.

28 Calverley PMA, Anderson JA, Celli B, *et al.* Salmeterol and fluticasone propionate and survival in chronic obstructive pulmonary disease. *N Engl J Med*, 2007; **356**(8): 775–89.

29 Jervis S, Ind PW, Shiner RJ. Inhaled therapy in elderly COPD patients; time for re-evaluation? *Age Ageing*, 2007; **36**: 213–18.

30 Jones V, Fernandez C, Diggory P. A comparison of large volume spacer, breath-activated and dry powder inhalers in older people. *Age Ageing*, 1999; **28**: 481–4.

31 Balami JS, Packham SM, Gosney MA. Non-invasive ventilation for respiratory failure due to acute exacerbations of chronic obstructive pulmonary disease in older patients. *Age Ageing*, 2006; **35**: 75–9.

32 Katsura H, Kanemaru A, Yamada K, *et al.* Long-term effectiveness of an inpatient pulmonary rehabilitation program for elderly COPD patients: comparison between young-elderly and old-elderly groups. *Respirology*, 2004; **9**(2): 230–6.

33 Wallace H, Shorvon S, Tallis R. Age-specific incidence and prevalence rates of treated epilepsy in an unselected population of 2,052,922 and age-specific fertility rates of women with epilepsy. *Lancet*, 1998; **352**: 1970–3.

34 Mendez MF, Lim GTH. Seizures in elderly patients with dementia: epidemiology and management. *Drugs Aging*, 2003; **20**: 791–803.

35 Brodie MJ, Elder AT, Kwan P. Epilepsy in later life. *Lancet Neurol*, 2009; **8**: 1019–30.

36 Brodie MJ, Kwan P. Epilepsy in elderly people. *BMJ*, 2005; **331**: 1317–22.

37 National Institute for Health and Care Excellence. The epilepsies: the diagnosis and management of the epilepsies in adults and children in primary and secondary care. CG 137, 2012. Available at: www.nice.org.uk/guidance/cg137 (accessed 12 November 2014).

38 Rowan AJ, Ramsay RE, Collins JF, *et al.* New onset geriatric epilepsy: a randomized study of gabapentin, lamotrigine, and carbamazepine. *Neurology*, 2005; **64**: 1868–73.

39 Scottish Intercollegiate Guidelines Network. Clinical guideline 70. *Diagnosis and Management of Epilepsy in Adults*, 2003. Available at: www.sign.ac.uk/pdf/sign70.pdf (accessed 12 November 2014).

40 Pugh MJV, Cramer J, Knoefel J, *et al.* Potentially inappropriate antiepileptic drugs for elderly patients with epilepsy. *J Am Geriatr Soc*, 2004; **52**(3): 417–22.

41 Haffey S, McKernan A, Pang K. Non-convulsive status epilepticus: a profile of patients diagnosed within a tertiary referral centre. *J Neurol Neurosurg Psychiatry*, 2004; **75**: 1043–4.

42 Tu TM, Loh NK, Tan NCK. Clinical risk factors for non-convulsive status epilepticus during emergent electroencephalogram. *Seizure*, 2013; **22**: 794–7.

43 Kaplan PW. Nonconvulsive status epilepticus in the emergency room. *Epilepsia*, 1996; **37**: 643–50.

44 Galvao MGA, Santos MARC, Alves da Cunha AJL, *et al.* Amantadine and rimantadine for influenza A in children and the elderly. *Cochrane Database Syst Rev* 2008, Issue 1. Art. No.: CD002745. DOI: 10.1002/14651858.CD002745.pub2.

45 Rivetti D, Jefferson T, Thomas RE, *et al.* Vaccines for preventing influenza in the elderly. *Cochrane Database Syst Rev* 2006, Issue 3. Art. No.: CD004876. DOI: 10.1002/14651858. CD004876.pub2.

46 Thomas RE, Jefferson T, Demicheli V, *et al.* Influenza vaccination for healthcare workers who work with the elderly. *Cochrane Database Syst Rev* 2006, Issue 3. Art. No.: CD005187. DOI: 10.1002/14651858.CD005187.pub2.

47 Nichol KL, Nordin JD, Nelson DB, *et al.* Effectiveness of influenza vaccine in the community-dwelling elderly. *N Engl J Med*, 2007; **357**(14): 1373–81.

48 Simonsen L, Reichert TA, Viboud C, *et al.* Impact of influenza vaccination on seasonal mortality in the US elderly population. *Arch Intern Med*, 2005; **165**: 265–72.

49 Simonsen L, Taylor RJ, Viboud C, *et al.* Mortality benefits of influenza vaccination in elderly people: an ongoing controversy. *Lancet Infect Dis*, 2007; **7**: 658–66.

50 Jackson ML, Nelson JC, Weiss NS, *et al.* Influenza vaccination and risk of community-acquired pneumonia in immunocompetent elderly people: a population-based, nested case-control study. *Lancet*, 2008; **372**: 398–405.

51 Callam MJ, Ruckley CV, Harper DR, *et al.* Chronic ulceration of the leg: extent of the problem and provision of care. *BMJ*, 1985; **290**: 1855–6.

52 Meyer FJ, Burnand KG, Lagattolla NRF, *et al.* Randomized clinical trial comparing the efficacy of two bandaging regimens in the treatment of venous leg ulcers. *Br J Surg*, 2002; **89**: 40–4.

53 Grey JE, Enoch S, Harding KG. Venous and arterial leg ulcers. *BMJ*, 2006; **332**: 347–50.

54 Cullum N, Nelson EA, Fletcher AW, *et al.* Compression for venous leg ulcers. *Cochrane Database Syst Rev* 2001, Issue 2. Art. No.: CD000265. DOI: 10.1002/14651858.CD000265.

55 Simon DA, Dix FP, McCollum CN. Management of venous leg ulcers. *BMJ*, 2004; **328**: 1358–62.

56 Brem H, Kirsner RS, Falanga V. Protocol for the successful treatment of venous ulcers. *Am J Surg*, 2004; **188**(Suppl.): S1–8.

57 Jones JE, Nelson EA. Skin grafting for venous leg ulcers. *Cochrane Database Syst Rev* 2000, Issue 2. Art. No.: CD001737. DOI: 10.1002/14651858.CD001737.pub2.

58 Mumcuoglu KY, Ingber A, Gilead L, *et al.* Maggot therapy for the treatment of intractable wounds. *Int J Derm*, 1999; **38**(8): 623–7.

59 Dumville JC, Bland JM, Cullum N, *et al.* Larval therapy for leg ulcers (VenUS II): randomised controlled trial. *BMJ*, 2009; **338**: 1047–50.

60 Kluytmans J, Stuelens M. Methicillin resistant *Staphylococcus aureus* in the hospital. *BMJ*, 2009; **338**: 532–7.

61 Grundmann H, Tami A, Hori S, *et al.* Nottingham *Staphylococcus aureus* population study: prevalence of MRSA among elderly people in the community. *BMJ*, 2002; **324**: 1365–6.

62 Barr B, Wilcox MH, Brady A, *et al.* Prevalence of methicillin-resistant *Staphylococcus aureus* colonization among older residents of care homes in the United Kingdom. *Infect Control Hosp Epidemiol*, 2007; **28**(7): 853–9.

63 Klevens MR, Morrison MA, Nadle J, *et al.* Invasive methicillin-resistant *Staphylococcus aureus* infections in the United States. *JAMA*, 2007; **298**(15): 1763–71.

64 Wyllie DH, Crook DW, Peto TEA. Mortality after *Staphylococcus aureus* bacteraemia in two hospitals in Oxfordshire, 1997–2003: cohort study. *BMJ*, 2006; **333**: 281–6.

65 Laupland KB, Ross T, Gregson DB. *Staphylococcus aureus* bloodstream infections: risk factors, outcomes, and the influence of methicillin resistance in Calgary, Canada, 2000–2006. *J Infect Dis*, 2008; **198**(3): 336–43.

66 Cooper BS, Stone SP, Kibbler CC, *et al.* Isolation measures in the hospital management of methicillin resistant *Staphylococcus aureus* (MRSA): systematic review of the literature. *BMJ*, 2004; **329**: 533–40.

67 Weber SG, Gold HS, Hooper DC, *et al.* Fluoroquinolones and the risk for methicillin-resistant *Staphylococcus aureus* in hospitalized patients. *Emerg Infect Dis*, 2003; **9**(11): 1415–22.

68 Charbonneau P, Parienti JJ, Thibon P, *et al.* Fluoroquinolone use and methicillin-resistant *Staphylococcus aureus* isolation rates in hospitalized patients: a quasi experimental study. *Clin Infect Dis*, 2006; **42**(6): 778–84.

69 Sievert DM, Rudrik JT, Patel JB, *et al.* Vancomycin-resistant *Staphylococcus aureus* in the United States, 2002–2006. *Clin Infect Dis*, 2008; **46**(5): 668–74.

70 Orrell RW. Understanding the causes of amyotrophic lateral sclerosis. *N Engl J Med*, 2007; **357**(8): 822–3.

71 Mitchell JD, Borasio GD. Amyotrophic lateral sclerosis. *Lancet*, 2007; **369**: 2031–41.

72 Le Ber I, Camuzat A, Berger E, *et al.* Chromosome 9p-linked families with frontotemporal dementia associated with motor neuron disease. *Neurology*, 2009; **72**: 1669–76.

73 Miller RG, Mitchell JD, Lyon M, *et al.* Riluzole for amyotrophic lateral sclerosis (ALS)/motor neuron disease (MND). *Cochrane Database Syst Rev* 2007, Issue 1. Art. No.: CD001447. DOI: 10.1002/14651858.CD001447.pub2.

74 Dalakas MC, Hohlfeld R. Polymyositis and dermatomyositis. *Lancet*, 2003; **362**: 971–82.

75 Salvarani C, Cantini F, Hunder GG. Polymyalgia rheumatica and giant-cell arteritis. *Lancet*, 2008; **372**: 234–5.

76 Sathasivam S, Lecky B. Statin induced myopathy. *BMJ*, 2008; **337**: 1159–62.

77 Kaplan V, Angus DC, Griffin MF, *et al.* Hospitalized community-acquired pneumonia in the elderly: age- and sex-related patterns of care and outcome in the United States. *Am J Respir Crit Care Med*, 2002; **165**: 766–72.

78 Kaplan V, Clermont G, Griffin MF, *et al.* Pneumonia: still the old man's friend? *Arch Intern Med*, 2003; **163**: 317–23.

79 Fry AM, Shay DK, Holman RC, *et al.* Trends in hospitalizations for pneumonia among persons aged 65 years or older in the United States, 1988–2002. *JAMA*, 2005; **294**(21): 2712–19.

80 Nuorti JP, Butler JC, Farley MM, *et al.* Cigarette smoking and invasive pneumococcal disease. Active Bacterial Core Surveillance Team. *N Engl J Med*, 2000; **342**(10): 681–9.

81 Metlay JP, Schulz R, Li Y, *et al.* Influence of age on symptoms at presentation in patients with community-acquired pneumonia. *Arch Intern Med*, 1997; **157**: 1453–9.

82 Marrie TJ, Haldane EV, Faulkner RS, *et al.* Community-acquired pneumonia requiring hospitalisation: is it different in the elderly? *J Am Geriatr Soc*, 1985; **33**: 671–80.

83 Harper C, Newton P. Clinical aspects of pneumonia in the elderly veteran. *J Am Geriatr Soc*, 1989; **37**: 867–72.

84 Marrie TJ, Blanchard W. A comparison of nursing home-acquired pneumonia patients with patients with community-acquired pneumonia and nursing home patients without pneumonia. *J Am Geriatr Soc*, 1997; **45**: 50–5.

85 Lim WS, Macfarlane JT. A prospective comparison of nursing home acquired pneumonia with community acquired pneumonia. *Eur Respir J*, 2001; **18**: 362–8.

86 Marik PE, Kaplan D. Aspiration pneumonia and dysphagia in the elderly. *Chest*, 2003; **124**: 328–36.

87 Furman CD, Rayner AV, Tobin EP. Pneumonia in older residents of long-term care facilities. *Am Fam Physician*, 2004; **70**(8): 1495–500.

88 Bont J, Hak E, Hoes AW, *et al.* Predicting death in elderly patients with community-acquired pneumonia: a prospective validation study reevaluating the CRB-65 severity assessment tool. *Arch Intern Med*, 2008; **168**(13): 1465–8.

89 Huss A, Scott P, Stuck AE, *et al.* Efficacy of pneumococcal vaccination in adults: a meta-analysis. *CMAJ*, 2009; **180**(1): 48–58.

90 Maruyama T, Taguchi O, Niederman MS, *et al.* Efficacy of 23-valent pneumococcal vaccine in preventing pneumonia and improving survival in nursing home residents: double blind, randomised and placebo controlled trial. *BMJ*, 2010; **340**: c1004.

91 Griffin MR, Zhu Y, Moore MR, *et al.* U.S. Hospitalizations for pneumonia after a decade of pneumococcal vaccination. *N Engl J Med*, 2013; **369**: 155–63.

92 Marik PE. Aspiration pneumonitis and aspiration pneumonia. *N Engl J Med*, 2001; **344**(9): 665–71.

93 Mylotte JM, Goodnough S, Gould M. Pneumonia versus aspiration pneumonitis in nursing home residents: prospective application of a clinical algorithm. *J Am Geriatr Soc*, 2005; **53**(5): 755–61.

94 Butler SG, Stuart A, Kemp S. Flexible endoscopic evaluation of swallowing in healthy young and older adults. *Ann Otol Rhinol Laryngol*, 2009; **118**(2): 99–106.

95 El-Solh AA, Pietrantoni C, Bhat A, *et al.* Microbiology of severe aspiration pneumonia in institutionalized elderly. *Am J Respir Crit Care Med*, 2003; **167**: 1650–4.

96 Kodowaki M, Demura Y, Mizuno S, *et al.* Reappraisal of clindamycin iv monotherapy for treatment of mild-to-moderate aspiration pneumonia in elderly patients. *Chest*, 2005; **127**(4): 1276–82.

97 Teramoto S, Matsuse T, Fukuchi Y, *et al.* Simple two-step swallowing provocation test for elderly patients with aspiration pneumonia. *Lancet*, 1999; **353**: 1243.

98 Robbins A, Gensler G, Hind J, *et al.* Comparison of 2 interventions for liquid aspiration on pneumonia incidence: a randomized trial. *Ann Intern Med*, 2008; **148**(7): 509–18.

99 Caldeira D, Alarcao J, Vaz-Carneiro A, *et al.* Risk of pneumonia associated with use of angiotensin converting enzyme inhibitors and angiotensin receptor blockers: systematic review and meta-analysis. *BMJ*, 2012; **345**: 15.

100 Knol W, van Marum RJ, Jansen PAF, *et al.* Antipsychotic drug use and risk of pneumonia in elderly people. *J Am Geriatr Soc*, 2008; **56**: 661–6.

101 Loeb MB, Becker M, Eady A, *et al.* Interventions to prevent aspiration pneumonia in older adults: a systematic review. *J Am Geriatr Soc*, 2003; **51**(7): 1018–22.

102 Grey JE, Enoch S, Harding KG. ABC of wound healing: pressure ulcers. *BMJ*, 2006; **332**: 472–5.

103 Parish LC, Witkowski JA. Controversies about the decubitus ulcer. *Dermatol Clin*, 2004; **22**: 87–91.

104 Waterlow J. A risk assessment card. *Nurs Times*, 1985; **81**(48): 49–55.

105 Braden BJ, Bergstrom N. Predictive validity of the Braden scale for pressure sore risk in a nursing home population. *Res Nurs Health*, 1994; **17**: 459–70.

106 Schoonhoven L, Haalboom JRE, Bousema MT, *et al.* Prospective cohort study of routine use of risk assessment scales for prediction of pressure ulcers. *BMJ*, 2002; **325**: 797–800.

107 National Institute for Health and Care Excellence. *Pressure Ulcers: prevention and management of pressure ulcers.* CG 179, 2014. Available at: www.nice.org.uk/guidance/cg179 (accessed 21 November 2014).

108 Cullum N, McInnes E, Bell-Syer SEM, *et al.* Support surfaces for pressure ulcer prevention. *Cochrane Database Syst Rev* 2004, Issue 3. Art. No.: CD001735. DOI: 10.1002/14651858.CD001735.pub2.

109 Vanderwee K, Grypdonck MHF, Defloor T. Effectiveness of an alternating pressure air mattress for the prevention of pressure ulcers. *Age Ageing*, 2005; **34**: 261–7.

110 Inman KJ, Sibbald WJ, Rutledge FS, *et al.* Clinical utility and cost-effectiveness of an air suspension bed in the prevent of pressure ulcers. *JAMA*, 1993; **269**(9): 1139–43.

111 Nixon J, Cranny G, Iglesias C, *et al.* Randomised, controlled trial of alternating pressure mattresses compared with alternating pressure overlays for the prevention of pressure ulcers: PRESSURE (pressure relieving support surfaces) trial. *BMJ*, 2006; **332**: 1413–15.

112 Langer G, Schloemer G, Knerr A, *et al.* Nutritional interventions for preventing and treating pressure ulcers. *Cochrane Database Syst Rev* 2003, Issue 4. Art. No.: CD003216. DOI: 10.1002/14651858.CD003216.

113 Bauman WA, Spungen AM, Collins JF, *et al.* The effect of oxandrolone on the healing of chronic pressure ulcers in persons with spinal cord injury: a randomized trial. *Ann Intern Med*, 2013; **158**: 718–26.

114 Xakellis GC, Chrischilles EA. Hydrocolloid versus saline-gauze dressings in treating pressure ulcers: a cost-effectiveness analysis. *Arch Phys Med Rehabil*, 1992; **73**: 463–9.

115 European Pressure Ulcer Advisory Panel and National Pressure Ulcer Advisory Panel. *Treatment of Pressure Ulcers: quick reference guide.* Washington DC: National Pressure Ulcer Advisory Panel; 2009. Available at: www.epuap.org/guidelines/Final_Quick_Treatment.pdf (accessed 27 November 2014).

116 Baxter H, Ballard K. Vacuum-assisted closure. *Nursing Times*, 2001; **97**(35): 51–2.

117 Sherman RA. Maggot versus conservative therapy for the treatment of pressure ulcers. *Wound Rep Regen*, 2002; **10**(4): 208–14.

118 Sorensen JL, Jorgensen B, Gottrup F. Surgical treatment of pressure ulcers. *Am J Surg*, 2004; **188**(Suppl.1A): S42–51.

119 Hatzenbuehler J, Pulling TJ. Diagnosis and management of osteomyelitis. *Am Fam Physician*, 2011; **84**: 1027–33.

120 Croxson SC, Burden AC, Bodington M, *et al.* The prevalence of diabetes in elderly people. *Diabet Med*, 1991; **8**(1): 28–31.

121 Resnick HE, Stone R, Heineman J, *et al.* Diabetes in U.S. nursing homes, 2004. *Diabetes Care*, 2008; **31**(2): 287–8.

122 Nathan DM, Holman RR, Buse JB, *et al.* Medical management of hyperglycaemia in type 2 diabetes: a consensus algorithm for the initiation and adjustment of therapy. *Diabetes Care*, 2009; **32**(1): 193–203.

123 Sinclair AJ, Conroy SP, Bayer AJ. Impact of diabetes on physical function in older people. *Diabetes Care*, 2008; **31**: 233–5.

124 Whitmer RA, Karter AJ, Yaffe K, *et al.* Hypoglycemic episodes and risk of dementia in older patients with type 2 diabetes mellitus. *JAMA*, 2009; **301**(15): 1565–72.

125 Gaglia JL, Wyckoff J, Abrahamson MJ. Acute hyperglycemic crisis in the elderly. *Med Clin N Am*, 2004; **88**(4): 1063–84.

126 Kitabchi AE, Umpierrez GE, Miles JM, *et al.* Hyperglycaemic crisis in adult patients with diabetes: a consensus statement from the American Diabetes Association. *Diabetes Care*, 2009; **32**: 1335–43.

127 Savage MW, Dhatariya KK, Kilvet A, *et al.* Joint British Diabetes Society guideline for management of diabetic ketoacidosis. *Diabetic Med*, 2011; **28**: 508–15.

128 Kilpatrick ES, Atkin SL. Using haemoglobin A1c to diagnose type 2 diabetes or to identify people at high risk of diabetes. *BMJ*, 2014; **348**: 37–9.

129 Lindstrom J, Ilanne-Parikka P, Peltonen M, *et al.* Sustained reduction in the incidence of type 2 diabetes by lifestyle intervention: follow-up of the Finnish Diabetes Prevention Study. *Lancet*, 2006; **368**: 1673–9.

130 Lindstrom J, Uusitupa M. Lifestyle intervention, diabetes, and cardiovascular disease. *Lancet*, 2008; **371**: 1731–3.

131 Mozaffarian D, Kamineni A, Carnethon M, *et al.* Lifestyle risk factors and new-onset diabetes mellitus in older adults: the Cardiovascular Health Study. *Arch Intern Med*, 2009; **169**(8): 798–807.

132 Turner RC, Cull CA, Frighi V, *et al.* Glycemic control with diet, sulfonylurea, metformin, or insulin in patients with type 2 diabetes mellitus: progressive requirement for multiple therapies (UKPDS 49). *JAMA*, 1999; **281**(21): 2005–12.

133 Adler AI, Stratton IM, Neil AW, *et al.* Association of systolic blood pressure with macrovascular and microvascular complications of type 2 diabetes (UKPDS 36): prospective observational study. *BMJ*, 2000; **321**: 412–19.

134 Mauer M, Zinman B, Gardiner R, *et al.* Renal and retinal effects of enalapril and losartan in type 1 diabetes. *N Engl J Med*, 2009; **361**(1): 40–51.

135 Bilous R, Chaturvedi N, Sjolie, AK, *et al.* Effect of candesartan on microalbuminuria and albumin excretion rate in diabetes. *Ann Intern Med*, 2009; **151**(1): 11–20.

136 Gaede P, Lund-Andersen H, Parving H, *et al.* Effect of a multifactorial intervention on mortality in type 2 diabetes. *N Engl J Med*, 2008; **358**(6): 580–91.

137 Lee SJ, Eng C. Goals of glycaemic control in frail older patients with diabetes. *JAMA*, 2011; **305**: 1350–1.

138 Whitmer RA, Karter AJ, Yaffe K, *et al.* Hypoglycaemic episodes and risk of dementia in older patients with type 2 diabetes mellitus. *JAMA*, 2009; **301**: 1565–72.

139 Sherman FT. Tight blood glucose control and cardiovascular disease in the elderly diabetic? *Geriatrics*, 2008; **63**(8): 8–10.

140 UK Prospective Diabetes Study Group. Intensive blood glucose control with sulphonylureas or insulin compared with conventional treatment and risk of complications in patients with type 2 diabetes (UKPDS 33). *Lancet*, 1998; **352**: 837–53.

141 ADVANCE Collaborative Group. Intensive blood glucose control and vascular outcomes in patients with type 2 diabetes. *N Engl J Med*, 2008; **358**: 2560–72.

142 Action to Control Cardiovascular Risk in Diabetes Study Group. Effects of intensive glucose lowering in type 2 diabetes. *N Engl J Med*, 2008; **358**: 2545–59.

143 Ray KK, Seshasai SRK, Wijesuriya S, *et al.* Effect of intensive control of glucose on cardiovascular outcomes and death in patients with diabetes mellitus: a meta-analysis of randomised controlled trials. *Lancet*, 2009; **373**: 1765–72.

144 Salpeter SR, Greyber E, Pasternak GA, *et al.* Risk of fatal and nonfatal lactic acidosis with metformin use in type 2 diabetes mellitus. *Cochrane Database Syst Rev* 2006, Issue 1. Art. No. CD002967. DOI: 10.1002/14651858.CD002967.pub2.

145 Selvin E, Bolen S, Yeh H, *et al.* Cardiovascular outcomes in trials of oral diabetes medications. *Arch Intern Med*, 2008; **168**(19): 2070–80.

146 Johnston PS, Lebovitz HE, Coniff RF, *et al.* Advantages of alpha-glucosidase inhibition as monotherapy in elderly type 2 diabetic patients. *J Clin Endocrinol Metab*, 1998; **83**(5): 1515–22.

147 Hampton, T. Diabetes drugs tied to fractures in women. *JAMA*, 2007; **297**(15): 1645.

148 Nissen SE, Wolski K. Effect of rosiglitazone on the risk of myocardial infarction and death from cardiovascular causes. *N Engl J Med*, 2007; **356**(24): 2457–71.

149 Dormandy JA, Charbonnel B, Eckland DJ, *et al.* Secondary prevention of macrovascular events in patients with type 2 diabetes in the PROactive Study (PROspective pioglitAzone Clinical Trial In macroVascular Events): a randomised controlled trial. *Lancet*, 2005; **366**: 1279–89.

150 Holman RR, Thorne KI, Farmer AJ, *et al.* Addition of biphasic, prandial, or basal insulin to oral therapy in type 2 diabetes. *N Engl J Med*, 2007; **357**(17): 1716–30.

151 Bretzel RG, Nuber U, Landgraf W, *et al.* Once-daily basal insulin glargine versus thrice-daily insulin lispro in people with type 2 diabetes on oral hypoglycaemic agents (APOLLO): an open randomised controlled trial. *Lancet*, 2008; **371**: 1073–84.

152 Hemmingsen B, Christensen LL, Wetterslev J, *et al.* Comparison of metformin and insulin versus insulin alone for type 2 diabetes: systematic review of randomised clinical trials with meta-analyses and trial sequential analyses. *BMJ*, 2012; **344**: 16.

QUESTIONS FOR PART F

1 An 84-year-old woman resides in a nursing home. There has been a confirmed outbreak of influenza A within the home over the last 24 hours. She has not been vaccinated for influenza this year. Her past medical history is of osteoarthritis and COPD. Which strategy, if started immediately, is most appropriate to reduce the risk of her developing influenza during this outbreak?
   A. Amantadine capsules
   B. Oseltamivir capsules
   C. Zanamivir inhaled powder
   D. Vaccination against influenza
   E. Vitamin C supplements

2 A 79-year-old man presents with pain in his thighs and shoulders that has been gradually increasing for two weeks. Examination reveals tenderness over the muscles of his upper arms and thighs, but no other abnormalities are detected. He sustained a stroke 10 months ago and was found to be in atrial fibrillation. Since that time he has been on warfarin, amiodarone and simvastatin. His blood tests show:

Sodium	136	(133–146 mmol/L)
Potassium	4.2	(3.5–5.3 mmol/L)
Urea	6.7	(2.5–7.8 mmol/L)
Creatinine	103	(64–104 umol/L)
ALP	104	(40–117 u/L)
ALT	126	(14–64 u/L)
TSH	6.7	(0.3–4.5 mu/L)
Creatine kinase	1437	(20–192 u/L)
Haemoglobin	132	(130–180 g/L)
White cell count	5.9	(4–11 $\times 10^9$/L)
Platelets	265	(150–450 $\times 10^9$/L)
INR	3.1	
ESR	63	(0–20 mm/hour)

What is the most likely cause of his symptoms?
   A. Statin-induced myopathy
   B. Polymyositis
   C. Hypothyroidism
   D. Polymyalgia rheumatica
   E. Neuroleptic malignant syndrome

3 Which of the following statements is most likely to be correct regarding the management of COPD in older adults?
   A. Stopping smoking has less effect on delaying lung function decline in older adults than that seen in younger people
   B. A failure to show improvement in spirometry in response to a two-week course of oral steroids suggests that future steroid treatment will be ineffective
   C. Theophylline has a higher risk of toxicity in older adults even at similar blood concentrations than in younger people
   D. Long-acting inhaled beta-agonists do not reduce the frequency of acute exacerbations
   E. Inhaled anticholinergic medications have been shown to reduce long-term morbidity

4 A 90-year-old man with a history of type 2 diabetes is found to have an HbA_{1C} of 88 mmol/mol (10.2%) at his annual review. His estimated GFR is 58 mL/min/1.73 m^2. He is currently taking metformin 500 mg tds. He lives alone. His past history includes a myocardial infarction a year ago and a venous leg ulcer (which the district nurse attends daily to dress). He was admitted to hospital last year following a severe episode of hypoglycaemia. He scores 23/30 on the MMSE. Which change to his medication would be most appropriate?
   A. Change metformin to a short-acting sulphonylurea twice daily
   B. Add a long-acting sulphonylurea
   C. Add rosiglitazone
   D. Add a basal insulin once daily
   E. Add a twice daily biphasic insulin

5 A 67-year-old man presents with a three-month history of progressive difficulty with swallowing. His wife reports that he has had variable emotions recently. On examination he is dysarthric, he has normal eye movements and limb tone, power and coordination are normal. He scores 29/30 on the MMSE. What is the most likely diagnosis?
   A. Progressive supranuclear palsy
   B. Brain stem ischaemia
   C. Myasthenia gravis
   D. Motor neuron disease
   E. Miller-Fisher variant of Guillain-Barré syndrome

6 Regarding macrocytic anaemia in older adults, which of the following statements is most likely to be correct?
   A. The majority of cases of B_{12} deficiency are caused by autoimmune pernicious anaemia
   B. Folate deficiency is commonly due to small bowel bacterial overgrowth
   C. Dietary deficiency of vitamin B_{12} is an important cause
   D. An associated raised white cell count suggests myelodysplasia
   E. It can be caused by chronic *Helicobacter pylori* infection

7 Which of the following statements regarding aspiration on to the lungs in older adults is most likely to be correct?
   A. Aspiration pneumonia and aspiration pneumonitis cause similar chest X-ray appearances
   B. Aspiration of oropharynx contents during sleep is rare in healthy older adults
   C. Rapid commencement of antibiotics improves outcome in people with aspiration pneumonitis
   D. The majority of pneumonias are caused by anaerobic organisms
   E. Angiotensin receptor blocking drugs are associated with a lower risk of aspiration pneumonia

8 Which of the following statements regarding arthritis in older adults is most likely to be correct?
   A. The prevalence of hip osteoarthritis is around 25% in people aged over 60 years
   B. Elective joint replacement surgery is associated with a 5% 30-day mortality rate in people aged over 70 years
   C. Around 30% of patients with rheumatoid arthritis present after the age of 60
   D. Late onset rheumatoid arthritis characteristically affects small distal joints more than larger proximal ones
   E. Rheumatoid nodules are less likely to occur in people with later onset rheumatoid arthritis

9 Which of the following statements regarding epileptic seizures in the elderly is most likely to be correct?
   A. The prevalence of epilepsy declines after the age of 80 years
   B. Around 35% of seizures are thought to be secondary to stroke
   C. Carbamazepine is more effective at preventing seizures than lamotrigine
   D. Sodium valproate use is associated with weight loss
   E. Around 30% of seizures are of focal onset

10 An 84-year-old man has a cutaneous ulcer on his left lateral malleolus. It has been present for over a month. Which statement is most likely to be correct?
   A. It is most likely to be of diabetic aetiology
   B. Fibrosis and hyperpigmentation of the surrounding skin suggests cellulitis
   C. An ankle–brachial pressure index of 0.8 or above suggests that compression bandaging can safely be tried
   D. The presence of normal foot pulses excludes significant peripheral vascular disease
   E. Surgical debridement should not be undertaken if there is a suspicion of infected tissue surrounding the ulcer

11 Which of the following statements regarding pressure ulcers is most likely to be correct?
   A. Patients should be turned twice a day to prevent pressure ulcer formation
   B. Foam-filled and dynamic mattresses are similarly effective at preventing pressure ulcer formation
   C. Supplementation with vitamin C improves ulcer healing time
   D. Larval therapy is associated with pain in around 10–20% of cases
   E. Non-gauze dressing need to be changed daily

12 Regarding methicillin resistant *Staphylococcus aureus* (MRSA), which statement is most likely to be correct?

A. It produces a protein that confers resistance to beta-lactam antibiotics
B. It cannot survive more than 24 hours outside a living organism
C. Over 50% of care home residents are colonised with MRSA
D. Infection rates are rising exponentially
E. The organism is only sensitive to vancomycin

13 Which of the following statements regarding type 2 diabetes in the over 75s is most likely to be correct?

A. Acarbose is well tolerated but only mildly effective at reducing blood glucose
B. Sulphonylureas reduce insulin resistance
C. Pioglitazone is associated with an increased risk of myocardial infarction, but not heart failure
D. Sulphonylureas can be expected to reduce HbA_{1C} values by around 1 to 2%
E. Lactic acidosis occurs in around 1 in 1000 patients treated with metformin per year

14 A 93-year-old man is admitted from his nursing home. He is found to have a grade 4 pressure ulcer on his sacrum with surrounding erythema. A pelvic X-ray suggests underlying osteomyelitis. Which organism is most likely to be responsible?

A. *Streptococcus pyogenes*
B. *Staphylococcus aureus*
C. *Haemophilus influenzae*
D. *Escherichia coli*
E. *Mycobacterium tuberculosis*

15 A 68-year-old man who is fully healthy enquires if he needs to receive the influenza vaccination. What would you advise him?

A. Immunisation not required
B. Immunise and repeat yearly
C. Immunise and repeat five-yearly
D. Immunise and repeat 10-yearly
E. One-off immunisation

16 A 68-year-old man who is fully healthy enquires if he needs to receive the pneumococcal vaccination. What would you advise him?

A. Immunisation not required
B. Immunise and repeat yearly
C. Immunise and repeat five-yearly
D. Immunise and repeat 10-yearly
E. One-off immunisation

17 An 86-year-old woman is admitted with increased dyspnoea, productive cough and delirium. Her temperature is 38.2°C, respiratory rate 24 breaths per minute and blood pressure 108/66 mmHg. Chest radiography shows right middle lobe consolidation. Her blood tests are as below.

Serum white blood cell count	27.1 ×10^9/L
C-reactive protein	124 mg/L
Urea	9.4 mmol/L
Creatinine	158 umol/L

What is her CURB-65 score?
A. 1
B. 2
C. 3
D. 4
E. 5

18 Compared to younger people presenting with pneumonia, older adults are more likely to be found to have which of the following clinical features?
A. Cough
B. Shortness of breath
C. Elevated respiratory rate
D. Pleuritic chest pain
E. Consolidation on chest X-ray

19 Which of the following clinical features is associated with a *lower* risk of developing aspiration pneumonia?
A. Residing in a nursing home
B. Antipsychotic drug use
C. History of Parkinson's disease
D. Poor dentition
E. Angiotensin converting enzyme inhibitor use

20 Regarding pneumonia in people aged over 75 years, which is the commonest causative organism?
A. *Pseudomonas aeruginosa*
B. *Streptococcus pneumoniae*
C. *Klebsiella pneumoniae*
D. *Staphylococcus aureus*
E. *Haemophilus influenzae*

21 A 91-year-old woman has a sacral pressure ulcer. There is full thickness skin loss with exposure of some underlying subcutaneous fat. There is some slough at the base of the ulcer. Which classification would you attach to this ulcer?
A. Category I
B. Category II
C. Category III
D. Category IV
E. Unclassifiable

22 A nurse new to your unit asks what type of dressing should be applied to a sacral pressure ulcer of one of your patients. The ulcer has been classified as stage 3. There is a moderate to heavy exudate associated with the wound. Which dressing type would be most appropriate?
A. Hydrocolloid
B. Hydrogel
C. Gauze
D. Alginate
E. Transparent film

23 An 80-year-old woman presents with shortness of breath and fatigue. Her past history is of Parkinson's disease that is well controlled on co-careldopa 62.5 mg tds, which was started five months ago. Examination reveals mild jaundice only. Her blood tests results are as below.

Haemoglobin	57 g/L	Ferritin	294
MCV	92.8	Reticulocytes	16%
White cell count	7.8	Urea	6.3
Platelets	186	Creatinine	91
Haematocrit	18%	Bilirubin	51
Haptoglobin not detected			

What would the most appropriate initial action?
A. Refer for bone marrow biopsy
B. Start oral prednisolone
C. Serum and urine electrophoresis
D. Stop co-careldopa
E. Blood transfusion

24 The proportion of anaemia caused by iron deficiency in community-dwelling people over the age of 65 years is closest to which of the following estimates?
A. 10%
B. 20%
C. 30%
D. 40%
E. 50%

25 Which of the following statements regarding non-convulsive status epilepticus in older people is most likely to be correct?
   A. During seizures the EEG appearance is likely to be normal
   B. Consciousness is preserved
   C. By definition there are no abnormal motor signs
   D. Automatisms are present in most cases
   E. Women are more commonly affected than men

26 Which of the following medications is most likely to be associated with reduced vitamin B_{12} absorption?
   A. Atenolol
   B. Simvastatin
   C. Metformin
   D. Ibuprofen
   E. Amitriptyline

Rating scales

ABBEY PAIN SCALE

The Abbey Pain Scale is useful in assessing pain in people who cannot vocalise their symptoms effectively (e.g. those with delirium and dementia). It has six domains (*see* below) all scored with the scheme: absent = 0, mild = 1, moderate = 2, severe = 3. This gives a total score of 0 to 18. Moderate pain is suggested by a score of 8 to 13, and severe pain by a score of 14 or more.

Clinical feature	Example
Vocalisation	Groaning or crying
Facial expression	Grimacing or looking frightened
Change in body language	Fidgeting, guarding or appearing withdrawn
Behavioural change	Increased confusion or reduced oral intake
Physiological change	Tachycardia, hypertension or sweating
Physical changes	Physical injuries including skin breaks/ulcers

ABBREVIATED MENTAL TEST

The Abbreviated Mental Test (AMT) is a quick to use 10-point scale for screening for cognitive impairment. It predominantly assesses short- and long-term memory, attention and orientation. A score of less than 8 is usually taken to imply a significant cognitive deficit,[1] such as delirium or dementia, the cause of which can only be determined by more detailed evaluation. A four-question version (AMT4) has also been devised (age, date of birth, place and year).[2]

ALZHEIMER'S DISEASE ASSESSMENT SCALE – COGNITIVE SUBSCALE

The Alzheimer's Disease Assessment Scale – cognitive subscale (ADAS-cog)[3] is a score to assess severity of cognitive dysfunction in Alzheimer's disease (AD). It gives values for a variety of clinical features, including language, recall, praxis and orientation, which are then added up. The total score is between 0 and 70. A higher score suggests a more severely impaired patient.

BARTHEL INDEX

The Barthel index is a rating scale used to assess recovery with rehabilitation.[4] Scores are given for various daily activities, including continence, self-care, mobility and transfers. The value ranges from 0 to 20 (or sometimes 0 to 100 when 5 marks is awarded per item), with a higher score suggesting greater functionality and independence. Scores achieved by the time of discharge appear to reflect eventual destination. Those scoring less than 10 commonly requiring nursing home placement.[5]

CONFUSION ASSESSMENT METHOD

The Confusion Assessment Method is a screening test for the detection of delirium.[6] For a positive result the patient must have evidence of both items 1 and 2, plus either 3 or 4 as listed below:
1. Acute confusion with a fluctuating pattern
2. Inattention
3. Disorganised speech
4. Altered level of consciousness

GERIATRIC DEPRESSION SCALE

The Geriatric Depression Scale (GDS) was initially developed as a 30-question form[7] but more recently in a 15-question version of yes/no answers. It can be self- or carer-administered. A cut-off score of 5 or more is suggestive of depression. Depending on cut-off used, sensitivities and specificities of 82–100% and 72–82%, respectively, have been demonstrated.[8]

The five-item GDS – an abbreviated version of the GDS that appears to be as effective as the standard GDS, yet administered in less time.[9] The five questions are as follows:
➤ Are you basically satisfied with your life?
➤ Do you often get bored?
➤ Do you often feel helpless?
➤ Do you prefer to stay at home rather than going out and doing new things?
➤ Do you feel pretty worthless the way you are now?

A score of 2 or more is suggestive of depression.

HOSPITAL ANXIETY AND DEPRESSION SCALE

The Hospital Anxiety and Depression Scale (HAD) is a screening tool for anxiety and depression. The patients fill in the questionnaire themselves. There are 14 questions, seven of which look for signs of anxiety and seven for depression. Each is given a score between 0 and 3, leading to maximum scores of 21 for each aspect. A higher score suggests more significant impairment. A score of 11 or above is usually taken to indicate a significant disorder.[10]

HOEHN AND YAHR

The Hoehn and Yahr[11] is a rating scale used to assess the severity of Parkinson's disease (PD). There are five stages as outlined below:

I   Unilateral disease.
II   Bilateral disease.
III   Postural instability.
IV   Advanced disease with severe disability but still able to walk.
V   Confined to wheelchair or bed.

More recently, a modified version of this has been developed.[12]
Stage 0.0   No signs of PD.
Stage 1.0   Unilateral disease.
Stage 1.5   Unilateral and axial disease.
Stage 2.0   Bilateral disease.
Stage 2.5   Mild bilateral disease and recovery on the pull test.
Stage 3.0   Postural instability.
Stage 4.0   Advanced disease with severe disability but still able to walk.
Stage 5.0   Confined to wheelchair or bed.

MINI MENTAL STATE EXAMINATION

The Mini Mental State Examination (MMSE)[13] is a 30-point assessment scale used in the diagnosis and monitoring of cognitive impairment. The higher the score, the better the cerebral function. A score of 25 or below is usually used to indicate significant impairment. It covers only limited cognitive domains (mainly orientation, memory and language), with no assessment of executive function and only one question regarding visuospatial ability. Therefore, its clinical utility is limited and it may well not detect impairment due to frontal lobe dysfunction in the early stages of frontotemporal dementia (FTD). A score of 30 does not automatically mean no impairment (ceiling effect) and a score of 0 does not mean no brain function (floor effect). Its value may be hard to interpret in the presence of illiteracy, dysphasia or visual loss, or in people who do not speak English. Scores achieved also reflect baseline intelligence. When used to monitor dementia, a rate of decline around three points per year is commonly seen. It also appears to have a role in the diagnosis and monitoring of patients with delirium.[14] It takes an average of around eight minutes to peform in the elderly.[15]

MODIFIED RANKIN SCALE

The modified Rankin scale (mRS) is used to assess degree of disability following a stroke.[16] Scores range from 0 (asymptomatic) to 6 (dead). A score of 1 or 2 means some residual symptoms or disability but maintaining independence. Scores of 3, 4 and 5 relate to increasing levels of dependence on others for daily tasks.

NATIONAL INSTITUTES OF HEALTH STROKE SCALE

The National Institutes of Health Stroke Scale (NIHSS) is a rating scale for severity of stroke.[17] The range of scores is from 0 to 42, with higher scores indicating worse severity of stroke. Typically values of 25 or above are considered very severe, and values below 5 are considered mild. Its chief clinical use is in the assessment of patients for suitability for thrombolysis and in monitoring their subsequent progress.

NEUROPSYCHIATRIC INVENTORY

The Neuropsychiatric Inventory (NPI)[18] is a score to assess behavioural problems in dementia. It assesses 10 domains (delusions, hallucinations, agitation/aggression, depression/dysphoria, anxiety, elation/euphoria, apathy/indifference, disinhibition, irritability/lability and aberrant motor behaviour). Each domain is scored out of 12 (by multiplying a severity (0–3) and frequency (0–4) value together). The total score is the sum of these domain scores, which will be between 0 and 120. A higher score suggests a worse behavioural disturbance.

NOTTINGHAM EXTENDED ACTIVITIES OF DAILY LIVING

The Nottingham Extended Activities of Daily Living scale (NEADL) has 22 items that are scored from 0 to 3 (0 = unable to do, 1 = can do with help, 2 = can do alone with difficulty, 3 = can do alone easily) giving a total score of 0 to 66 (i.e. higher scores = more independent).[19] The items are mainly to do with instrumental activities of daily living and cover areas such as use of transport, preparation of meals, using the telephone, managing money and doing the shopping.

SIX-ITEM SCREENER

The Six-Item Screener (SIS) is a brief screening tool for cognitive impairment. The patient is given three items to repeat (e.g. apple, table and penny). They are then asked the day of the week, month and year (each scores one point). Following this they are asked to recall the three items repeated earlier (each scores one point). A score of 0 to 6 is obtained, with 4 or less suggesting significant cognitive impairment.[20]

UNIFIED PARKINSON'S DISEASE RATING SCALE

The Unified Parkinson's Disease Rating Scale (UPDRS)[21] is an assessment tool for use with patients with PD. The total score is between 0 and 199. A higher score suggests a more severe impairment. It has four main parts (the maximum scores for the individual sections are shown in brackets):

I   Mentation, behaviour and mood (16)
II   Activities of daily living (52)
III   Motor (108)
IV   Complications of therapy (23).

REFERENCES

1 Jitapunkul S, Pillay I and Ebrahim S. The abbreviated mental test: its use and validity. *Age Ageing*, 1991; **20**: 332–6.
2 Swain DG, Nightingale PG. Evaluation of a shortened version of the Abbreviated Mental Test in a series of elderly patients. *Clin Rehabil* 1997; **11**: 243–8.
3 Doraiswamy PM, Bieber F, Kaiser L, *et al*. The Alzheimer's disease assessment scale: patterns and predictors of baseline cognitive performance in multicenter Alzheimer's disease trials. *Neurology*, 1997; **48**: 1511–17.
4 Mahoney F, Barthel D. Functional evaluation: Barthel index. *Md State Med J*, 1965; **14**: 61–5.
5 Stone SP, Ali B, Auberleek I, *et al*. The Barthel index in clinical practice: use on a rehabilitation ward for elderly people. *J Royal Coll Phys*, 1994; **28**(5): 419–23.

6 Inouye SK, van Dyck CH, Alessi CA, *et al.* Clarifying confusion: the confusion assessment method. A new method for detection of delirium. *Ann Intern Med*, 1990; **113**(12): 941–8.

7 Brink TL, Yesavage JA, Lum O, *et al.* Screening tests for geriatric depression. *Clin Gerontol*, 1982; **1**: 37–43.

8 Watson LC, Pignone MP. Screening accuracy for late-life depression in primary care: a systematic review. *J Fam Prac*, 2003; **52**(12): 956–64.

9 Hoyl TM, Alessi CA, Harker JO, *et al.* Development and testing of a five-item version of the Geriatric Depression Scale. *JAGS*, 1999; **47**: 873–8.

10 Zigmond AS, Snaith RP. The Hospital Anxiety and Depression Scale. *Acta Psychiatr Scand*, 1983; **67**: 361–70.

11 Hoehn MM, Yahr MD. Parkinsonism: onset, progression and mortality. *Neurology*, 1967; **17**: 427–42.

12 Lang AE, Fahn S. Assessment of Parkinson's disease. In: Munsat TL, *Quantification of Neurologic Deficit*. Stoneham: Butterworth-Heineman, 1989.

13 Folstein MF, Folstein SE, McHugh PR. 'Mini-mental state'. A practical method for grading the cognitive state of patients for the physician. *J Psychiatr Res*, 1975; **12**: 189–98.

14 O'Keeffe ST, Mulkerrin EC, Nayeem K, *et al.* Use of serial mini-mental state examinations to diagnose and monitor delirium in elderly hospital patients. *JAGS*, 2005; **53**: 867–70.

15 Swain DG, O'Brien AG, Nightingale PG. Cognitive assessment in elderly patients admitted to hospital: the relationship between the Abbreviated Mental Test and the Mini-Mental State Examination. *Clin Rehabil*, 1999; **13**: 503–8.

16 Available at: www.strokecenter.org/trials/scales/rankin.html

17 Available at: www.ninds.nih.gov/doctors/NIH_Stroke_Scale_Booklet.pdf

18 Cummings JL, Mega M, Gray K, *et al.* The Neuropsychiatric Inventory: comprehensive assessment of psychopathology in dementia. *Neurology*, 1994; **44**: 2308–14.

19 Available at: www.nottingham.ac.uk/shared/shared_iwho/documents/NEADL.pdf

20 Wilber ST, Lofgren SD, Mager TG, *et al.* An evaluation of two screening tools for cognitive impairment in older Emergency Department patients. *Acad Emerg Med* 2005; **12**(7): 612–16.

21 Fahn S, Elton RL, UPDRS Development Committee. Unified Parkinson's Disease Rating Scale. In: Fahn S, Marsden CD, Calne DB, *et al.*, *Recent Developments in Parkinson's Disease*, Vol. 2. Florham Park, NJ: MacMillan Healthcare Information, 1987. pp. 153–63.

Abbreviations

ABC	antecedents, behaviour and consequences
ABG	arterial blood gas
ABPI	ankle–brachial pressure index
ACA	anterior cerebral artery
ACD	anaemia of chronic disease
ACE	angiotensin-converting enzyme
ACEi	angiotensin-converting enzyme inhibitor
ACE-III	Addenbrooke's Cognitive Examination (third version)
ACh	acetylcholine
ACLS	advanced cardiac life support
AD	Alzheimer's disease
ADLs	activities of daily living
ADAS	Alzheimer's Disease Assessment Scale
ADAS-cog	Alzheimer's Disease Assessment Scale – cognitive sub-scale
ADP	adenosine diphosphate
AF	atrial fibrillation
AFO	ankle–foot orthosis
ALP	alkaline phosphatase
ALS	amyotrophic lateral sclerosis
ALT	alanine aminotransferase
AMD	age-related macular degeneration
AMP	adenosine monophosphate
AMT	Abbreviated Mental Test
ANP	atrial natriuretic peptide
ARB	angiotensin type II receptor blockers
ARD	alcohol-related dementia
ARR	absolute risk reduction
ASA	American Society of Anesthesiologists
ASB	asymptomatic bacteriuria
AVM	arteriovenous malformation
BADLS	Bristol Activities of Daily Living Scale
bd	twice daily

BMD	bone mineral density
BMI	body mass index
BMR	basal metabolic rate
BMT	behavioural management techniques
BNP	brain natriuretic peptide
BP	blood pressure
BPH	benign prostatic hyperplasia
BPPV	benign paroxysmal positional vertigo
BPSD	behavioural and psychological symptoms of dementia
BT	behavioural treatment
CAA	cerebral amyloid angiopathy
CADASIL	cerebral autosomal dominant arteriopathy with subcortical infarcts and leukoencephalopathy
CAM	Confusion Assessment Method
CAP	community-acquired pneumonia
CAUTI	catheter-associated UTI
CBD	corticobasal degeneration
CBT	cognitive behavioural therapy
CCF	congestive cardiac failure
CE	carotid endarterectomy
CGA	comprehensive geriatric assessment
CI	confidence interval
CICSS	cardio-inhibitory carotid sinus syndrome
CJD	Creutzfeld–Jakob disease
CK	creatine kinase
CNP	C-type natriuretic peptide
CNS	central nervous system
COMT	catechol-o-methyltransferase
COMTi	catechol-o-methytransferase inhibitor
COPD	chronic obstructive pulmonary disease
COX-2	cycloxygenase 2
CPR	cardiopulmomary resuscitation
CR	controlled-release
CRP	C-reactive protein
CSF	cerebrospinal fluid
CSH	carotid sinus hypersensitivity
CSM	carotid sinus massage
CSS	carotid sinus syndrome
CT	computerised tomography
DAT	dopamine transporter
DBS	deep brain stimulation
DDS	dopamine dysregulation syndrome
DEXA	dual-energy X-ray absorptometry
DHEA	dehydroepiandrosterone

DHT	dihydrotestosterone
DI	dual incontinence
DIC	disseminated intravascular coagulation
DLB	dementia with Lewy bodies
DMARD	disease modifying anti-rheumatic drug
DVLA	Driver and Vehicle Licensing Agency
DVT	deep vein thrombosis
ECG	electrocardiograph/electrocardiogram
ECT	electroconvulsive therapy
ED	emergency department
EEG	electroencephalography
eGFR	estimated glomerular filtration rate
ELD	external lumbar drainage
EMG	electromyogram
EMI	elderly mentally infirm
ENT	ear, nose and throat
EORA	elderly onset rheumatoid arthritis
EPS	electrophysiological studies
ER	extended release
ERAS	Enhanced Recovery After Surgery
ESR	erythrocyte sedimentation rate
ET	essential tremor
FBC	full blood count
FEV_1	forced expiratory volume in one second
FFP	fresh frozen plasma
FI	faecal incontinence
FTD	frontotemporal dementia
FVC	forced vital capacity
GABA	gamma-aminobutyric acid
GAD	generalised anxiety disorder
GBM	glioblastoma multiforme
GCA	giant cell arteritis
GCS	Glasgow Coma Scale
GDNF	glial cell derived neurotrophic factor
GDS	Geriatric Depression Scale
GFR	glomerular filtration rate
GGT	gamma-glutamyltransferase
GI	gastrointestinal
GnRH	gonadotrophin-releasing hormone
GPi	globus pallidus interna
GTN	glyceryl trinitrate
HAD	Hospital Anxiety and Depression Scale
Hb	haemoglobin
HHS	hyperosmolar hyperglycaemic state

HIV	human immunodeficiency virus
HR	hazard ratio
HRT	hormone replacement therapy
HUT	head-up tilt
IADLs	instrumental activities of daily living
IBS	irritable bowel syndrome
ICA	internal carotid artery
ICD	implantable cardioverter-defibrillator
ICD	impulse control disorder
ICH	intracerebral haemorrhage
IDA	iron deficiency anaemia
IGT	impaired glucose tolerance
IHD	ischaemic heart disease
IM	intramuscular
INR	international normalised ratio
IPC	intermittent pneumatic compression
ISH	isolated systolic hypertension
ITU	intensive therapy unit
IV	intravenous
JVP	jugular venous pressure
LACI	lacunar circulation infarct
LACS	lacunar circulation stroke
LDL	low-density lipoprotein
LE	leukocyte esterase
LH	luteinsing hormone
LMN	lower motor neuron
LP	lumbar puncture
MAOi	monoamine oxidase inhibitor
MCA	middle cerebral artery
MCI	mild cognitive impairment
MCV	mean cell volume
MDMA	methylenedioxymethamphetamine
MDRD	Modification of Diet in Renal Disease
MELAS	mitochondrial encephalomyopathy, lactic acidosis and stroke-like episodes
MI	myocardial infarction
MMSE	Mini Mental State Examination
MND	motor neuron disease
MOCA	Montreal Cognitive Assessment
MRI	magnetic resonance imaging
mRS	Modified Rankin scale
MRSA	methicillin resistant *Staphylococcus aureus*
MSA	multiple system atrophy
MSU	mid-stream urine

MUST	Malnutrition Universal Screening Tool
n	sample size
NCSE	non-convulsive status epilepticus
NEADL	Nottingham Extended Activities of Daily Living scale
NG	nasogastric
NH	nursing home
NHISS	National Institute of Health Stroke Scale
NHS	National Health Service
NICE	National Institute for Health and Care Excellence
NMDA	N-methyl-D-aspartate
NMS	neuroleptic malignant syndrome
NNT	number needed to treat
NPH	normal pressure hydrocephalus
NPI	Neuropsychiatric Inventory
NPV	negative predictive value
NSAID	non-steroidal anti-inflammatory drug
nvCJD	new variant Creutzfeld-Jakob disease
OA	osteoarthritis
OGTT	oral glucose tolerance test
OH	orthostatic hypotension
OR	odds ratio
OSA	obstructive sleep apnoea
PACI	partial anterior circulation infarct
PACS	partial anterior circulation stroke/syndrome
PAF	paroxysmal atrial fibrillation
PCA	posterior cerebral artery
PCC	prothrombin complex concentrate
PD	Parkinson's disease
PDD	Parkinson's disease dementia
PE	pulmonary embolism
PEA	pulseless electrical activity
PEG	percutaneous endoscopic gastrostomy
PET	positron emission tomography
PFO	patent foramen ovale
PG	polyethylene glycol
PMC	pseudomembranous colitis
PMR	polymyalgia rheumatica
PPI	proton pump inhibitor
POCD	postoperative cognitive decline
POCI	posterior circulation infarct
POCS	posterior circulation stroke/syndrome
POPS	Proactive care of Older People undergoing Surgery
POTS	paroxysmal orthostatic tachycardia syndrome
PR	per rectum

PSA	prostate specific antigen
PSP	progressive supranuclear palsy
PTH	parathyroid hormone
PU	pressure ulcers
PVD	peripheral vascular disease
PWV	pulse wave velocity
qds	four times a day
RA	rheumatoid arthritis
RCT	randomised controlled trial
REM	rapid eye movement
RF	rheumatoid factor
RH	residential home
RLS	restless legs syndrome
RR	relative risk
RRR	relative risk reduction
rt-PA	recombinant tissue plasminogen activator
RV	residual volume
SAH	subarachnoid haemorrhage
SC	subcutaneous
SD	standard deviation
SE	standard error
SHBG	sex hormone binding globulin
SIADH	syndrome of inappropriate anti-diuretic hormone
SICH	symptomatic intracerebral/intracranial haemorrhage
SIS	Six-Item Screener
SLE	systemic lupus erythematosus
SPECT	single-photon emission computed tomography
SSRI	serotonin specific reuptake inhibitor
SR	sinus rhythm
STN	subthalamic nucleus
TA	temporal arteritis
TACI	total anterior circulation infarct
TACS	total anterior circulation stroke/syndrome
TCA	tricyclic antidepressant
TD	tardive dyskinesia
tds	three times daily
TENS	transcutaneous electrical nerve stimulation
TGA	transient global amnesia
TIA	transient ischaemic attack
TLC	total lung capacity
TNF	tumour necrosis factor
TOE	transoesophageal echocardiography
TPHA	*Treponema pallidum* haemagglutin antibody
TSH	thyroid stimulating hormone

TURP	trans-urethral resection of prostate
UI	urinary incontinence
UMN	upper motor neuron
UPDRS	Unified Parkinson's Disease Rating Scale
UTI	urinary tract infection
UV	ultraviolet
VaD	vascular dementia
VC	vital capacity
Vd	volume of distribution
VDCSS	vasodepressor carotid sinus syndrome
VDRL	venereal disease research laboratory test
VF	ventricular fibrillation
VP	vascular Parkinsonism
VRSA	vancomycin resistant *Staphylococcus aureus*
VT	ventricular tachycardia
VVS	vasovagal syndrome (or syncope)
WCC	white cell count
WHO	World Health Organization

Answers to questions

PART A

1. B	2. B	3. D	4. C	5. C	6. E
7. D	8. B	9. B	10. E	11. A	12. C
13. C	14. D	15. C	16. D	17. C	18. D
19. B	20. C	21. A	22. B	23. A	24. D
25. D	26. E	27. C	28. B	29. B	30. E
31. A	32. E	33. E	34. B	35. D	36. A
37. B	38. C	39. E	40. E	41. A	42. B
43. D	44. D	45. D	46. B	47. E[1]	48. D
49. B	50. D	51. A	52. D	53. A	54. B[2]
55. C	56. C				

PART B

1. D	2. C	3. A	4. D	5. B	6. D
7. E	8. C[3]	9. B	10. D	11. C[4]	12. B
13. E	14. C	15. E	16. D	17. B	18. B
19. A	20. D[5]	21. C	22. A	23. C	24. E
25. C	26. C	27. D[6]	28. E	29. C	30. D
31. D	32. C	33. A	34. C	35. E	36. D
37. B	38. A	39. E	40. B	41. E	42. C
43. E	44. C	45. A	46. C	47. A	48. D
49. D	50. A	51. A	52. C	53. D	54. E
55. A	56. E	57. C			

PART C

1. A[7]	2. D	3. E[8]	4. C	5. D	6. A[9]
7. A	8. E	9. B[10]	10. E	11. B	12. D
13. D	14. B	15. A	16. A	17. A	18. B

PART D

1. A	2. D	3. E	4. E	5. A	6. B
7. B	8. B[11]	9. A	10. E	11. D	12. A

13. A   14. A   15. D   16. C   17. D   18. B
19. D   20. B   21. C   22. B   23. E   24. C
25. E

PART E

1. E[12]   2. A   3. A   4. E   5. B   6. A
7. E   8. C[13]   9. E   10. A   11. D   12. E
13. E   14. D   15. E   16. D   17. A   18. B

PART F

1. B[14]   2. A[15]   3. C   4. D   5. D   6. E
7. A   8. E   9. B   10. C   11. D   12. A
13. D   14. B   15. B   16. E   17. C   18. C
19. E   20. B   21. C   22. D   23. D   24. B
25. E   26. C

NOTES

1 Ibuprofen is the only medication that will provide symptomatic benefit.
2 ARR for one year = (8.6–4.6)/2. NNT = 100/ARR
3 Intrinsic factor production may be reduced following gastric surgery.
4 Normal pressure hydrocephalus.
5 Quinine may cause confusion. Dopamine antagonists are potentially dangerous in DLB. Ropinirole may worsen confusion.
6 The other answers are suggestive of a frontal or subcortical dementia, which would make VaD more likely.
7 Sounds like stress incontinence. A catheter may be appropriate in this situation.
8 High bladder pressure + low flow = obstruction. It is normal to have a desire to pass urine after >300 mL instilled. Leakage when intra-abdominal pressure is high = stress UI. High flow + high bladder pressure is normal in uroflowmetry. Rising bladder pressure alone suggests detrusor overactivity.
9 Low folate and ferritin best explained by coeliac disease.
10 Donepezil is most likely to cause diarrhoea.
11 Osteocalcin is a bone protien used as a biomarker of bone turnover. Low vitamin D leads to low calcium and high phosphate levels.
12 Amlodipine may cause ankle oedema. Her aortic stenosis is only mild and unlikely to have changed significantly in five months.
13 Beta-blockers are helpful in heart failure. Other options are less likely to be effective, or more likely to have significant side-effects.
14 Zanamivir is not recommended in people with COPD. Vaccination may take weeks to be effective.
15 Amiodarone can increase serum levels of statins. A raised CK does not suggest PMR.

Index

Entries in **bold** denote tables; entries in *italics* denote figures.

CPD with Radcliffe

You can now use a selection of our books to achieve CPD (Continuing Professional Development) points through directed reading.

We provide a free online form and downloadable certificate for your appraisal portfolio. Look for the CPD logo and register with us at: www.radcliffehealth.com/cpd

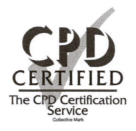